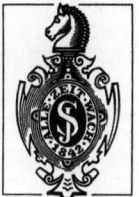

B.G. Weber
F. Magerl

# THE EXTERNAL FIXATOR

AO/ASIF-Threaded Rod System
Spine-Fixator

With a Chapter by Ch. Brunner
Foreword by A. Sarmiento

With 362 Partly Colored Figures

Springer-Verlag
Berlin Heidelberg NewYork Tokyo 1985

Prof. Dr. Bernhard G. Weber
Dr. Friedrich Magerl
Dr. Christian Brunner

Klinik für Orthopädische Chirurgie,
Kantonsspital,
CH-9007 St. Gallen

Translated from the German by
Terry C. Telger

Title of the German Edition
B.G. Weber · F. Magerl: Fixateur externe
© Springer-Verlag Berlin Heidelberg 1985
ISBN-13: 978-3-642-70017-0


ISBN-13: 978-3-642-70017-0          e-ISBN-13: 978-3-642-70015-6
DOI: 10.1007/978-3-642-70015-6

Library of Congress Cataloging in Publication Data. Weber, B.G. (Bernhard Georg), 1927–    . The external fixator. Translated from the German with title: Fixateur externe. Includes bibliographies and index. 1. External skeletal fixation (Surgery) I. Magerl, F. (Friedrich), 1931–    . II. Brunner, Christian Ferdinand, 1937–    . III. Title. IV. Title: Spine-fixator. [DNLM: 1. Fracture Fixation — methods. WE 185 W373e] RD103.E88W43  1985  617′.15  84-24045

Reproduction of the figures: Gustav Dreher GmbH, Stuttgart

2124/3130-543210

# Foreword

Professor B.G. WEBER has once again and in a very timely fashion produced a superb book on an orthopaedic subject of great importance. "The External Fixator" is the most comprehensive text on the subject in orthopaedic literature to date. Professor WEBER thoroughly discusses external fixation with clarity, organization, profuse illustrations and roentgenograms.

Professor WEBER acknowledges that the use of external fixation in orthopaedic surgery is not new and traces its history over the years. He points out clearly the fact that though at various times the "method" has experienced periods of disrepute, modern sophistication, improved technology and a better understanding of its philosophy have given the system a new and perhaps permanent place in the armamentarium of the orthopaedic surgeon.

All methods of treatment have critics as well as supporters, and not infrequently the strongest criticisms are the result of poor understanding of the philosophy proposed and its proper implementation. Professor WEBER, in his carefully detailed and well illustrated book, has made it abundantly clear that the use of external fixators in the treatment of fractures must be clearly understood by the orthopaedic surgeon in order to obtain satisfactory clinical results. His discussion of its philosophy, pathomechanics and technology are most comprehensive and leave "no stone unturned" and because of this the book represents a most comprehensive text on the subject.

I have long held the belief that immobilization in the treatment of long bone fractures is unphysiological and that fracture care should avoid, as much as possible, rigid fixation of fracture fragments. I recognize, however, there are situations where the creation of a healthy environment in which controlled motion is present cannot be attained. Severely open fractures and certain nonunions are representative examples of that situation. It is primarily in these circumstances where rigid fixation may be the treatment of choice. External fixation, as Professor WEBER has so well documented, is an excellent method to obtain osseous repair while maintaining function and cosmesis.

AUGUSTO SARMIENTO, M.D.
Professor and Chairman
Department of Orthopaedics
University of Southern California
School of Medicine

# Preface

The use of an external fixation device for the stabilization of bone fragments probably dates back to LAMBOTTE in 1902. But despite its long history, the external fixator has not gained the same degree of acceptance in fracture management as the "closed" methods of BÖHLER, WATSON-JONES and SARMIENTO, or true internal fixation.

Operative fracture treatment itself was not widely practiced until it was popularized in 1958 by the Swiss Association for the Study of Internal Fixation (ASIF). It is important to note that the principal authors of the ASIF technique, Drs. MÜLLER, ALLGÖWER and WILLENEGGER, have never represented their technique as the only "correct" one, and in the preface to their book *Technique of Operative Fracture Management* (Springer-Verlag, 1963) they state, "We caution very strongly against internal fixations performed without proper training, instrumentation and surgical asepsis ..." The potential risks of internal fixation have sparked renewed interest in conservative treatment strategies, with the result that SARMIENTO's "functional bracing" technique is now practiced as widely as the ASIF method.

But neither internal fixation nor functional bracing is adequate for the management of the highly complex extremity injuries that are being seen with increasing frequency as a result of motorcycle and other high-speed vehicular accidents ("Honda disease"). This accounts in large part for the many recent articles and books devoted to the subject of external skeletal fixation (BROOKER, EDWARDS 1979; UHTHOFF 1982; MEARS 1983; ACKROYD, O'CONNOR, DE BRUYN 1983). The shear volume of these publications suggests that the external fixator is being "rediscovered" in the English-speaking world after ANDERSON put the external fixation concept into practice in the United States in 1934.

When the first ASIF book was published in 1963, Dr. MÜLLER and other Swiss orthopedic surgeons had already been practicing external fixation for some years — first in reconstructive orthopedics and later fracture management. The threaded-rod external fixator, for example, is described in the first ASIF book.

At the Department of Orthopedic Surgery of Kantonsspital St. Gallen, Switzerland, external fixations with the threaded-rod device have become as routine as internal fixations by the ASIF method. This "routineness" may explain why no major publications on external fixation have yet appeared in Switzerland, and we feel that a text on the subject is overdue. In the present book we shall examine the use of the external fixator not only in fracture treatment, but also in other areas of orthopedic surgery.

The following colleagues had a hand in the preparation of the book: Mrs. URSULA OETLIKER and Mrs. MYRTHA ZWEIFEL, who undertook repeated typescript revisions with thireless diligence and technical expertise; KATRIN and HORST SCHUMACHER, who prepared the excellent drawings; and Mrs. MARIANNE SCHAFFNER, Mrs. DORIS CLERICI and Mrs. ANNELISE SPITZ, who prepared the photographic illustrations.

I express special thanks to my closest medical colleagues: Dr. FRITZ MAGERL, assistant department head, who described the spinal external fixation device; and Dr. CHRISTIAN BRUNNER, chief of pediatric orthopedics, who wrote a chapter on external fixations in children and adolescents.

I am also grateful to my present and former straff colleagues who "tended to business" on the clinical level.

In his capacity as engineer and manufacturer, Dr. h.c. ROBERT MATHYS has worked closely with the Technical Committee of the ASIF and with us to improve the quality of the surgical armamentarium. His work is gratefully acknowledged.

Finally, I express thanks to the staff at Springer-Verlag, who once again did outstanding work in the publication of this text.

St. Gallen, Summer, 1984                                                                 B.G. WEBER

# Contents

**External Spinal Skeletal Fixation.** F. Magerl

# Preamble

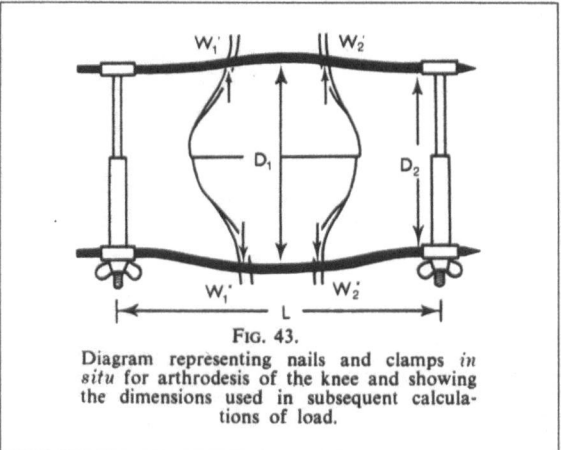

FIG. 43.
Diagram representing nails and clamps *in situ* for arthrodesis of the knee and showing the dimensions used in subsequent calculations of load.

In the book *Compression Arthrodesis,* published in 1953, J. CHARNLEY and his coauthor J.A.L. MATHESON, an engineer, describe the different forces that are required to deform a transfixing pin whose free ends are clamped rigidly or loosely to external rods. The original drawings, Figs. 40 and 42, show the experimental result: When the ends of the pin are "loose," four times less force is needed to produce a given deflection than when the ends are "fixed." This is equivalent to saying that the "fixed" pin exerts a four-times-greater compressive force than the "loose" pin.

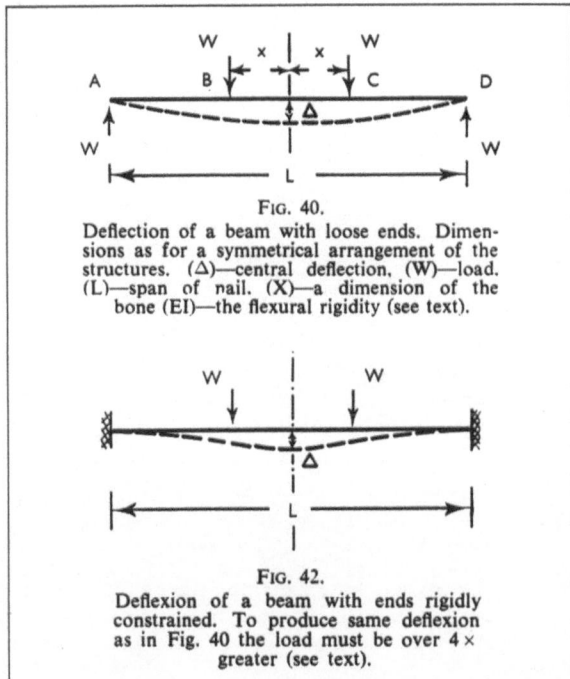

FIG. 40.
Deflection of a beam with loose ends. Dimensions as for a symmetrical arrangement of the structures. (△)—central deflection, (W)—load. (L)—span of nail. (X)—a dimension of the bone (EI)—the flexural rigidity (see text).

FIG. 42.
Deflexion of a beam with ends rigidly constrained. To produce same deflexion as in Fig. 40 the load must be over 4 × greater (see text).

Fig. 43 from CHARNLEY and MATHESON shows the CHARNLEY compression device with its rigidly clamped pins and the manner in which the transfixing pins are deformed by compression, with each pin showing both 1 main deflection and 2 counterflections. The adjacent drawing shows a mounting in which the transfixing pins are held in swiveling clamps. The pins are showing here not the complex triple deformation, but 1 single deflection only. MATHESON's and CHARNLEY's conclusion: The stabilizing pressure of the ridigdly clamped pins was approximately triple that of the pins held in swivel clamps.

A survey of the pertinent literature reveals no references at all to this observation by CHARNLEY, although the stability of the external fixator is a central concern for all authors. Indeed, other systems are praised because they avoid the "rigidity" of the CHARNLEY device, and because the pins can be mounted in any desired orientation relative to the external elements. Overlooked is the fact that with a rigid pin placement, several times more stabilizing compression can be transmitted to the bone, and so fewer pins are needed to achieve the desired stability.

Accordingly, "loose-end" fixators tend to have a more complicated design than "fixed-end" devices. This superiority of rigid pin clamping is why we favor the threaded external fixation device.

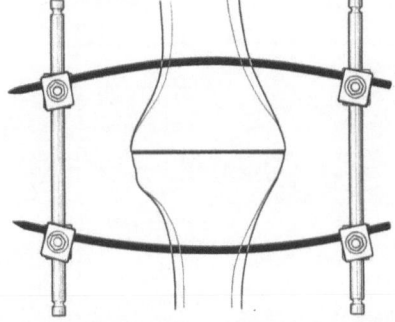

We have devoted a special preamble to the CHARNLEY principle because we feel that it deserves wider recognition among the orthopedic community.

B.G. WEBER

Figs. 40, 42 and 43 from *Compression Arthrodesis* by JOHN CHARNLEY and J.A.L. MATHESON. Livingstone, Edinburgh and London, 1953.

# The ASIF Threaded External Fixator in General Orthopedic and Trauma Surgery of the Extremities

# A General Part

B.G. Weber

## 1 Introduction

Recently several large works, mostly the collected reports from symposia, have been published on the subject of external skeletal fixation. The external fixator merits the particularly close attention of trauma surgeons. With its help, it appears possible to obtain better results in complex open fractures than have previously been achieved with Sarmiento's functional bracing or with the classic nonoperative methods of Böhler or Watson-Jones.

It is fitting that this book is being published during the 25th anniversary of the founding of the Swiss Association for the Study of Internal Fixation. It is interesting to·note that, as early as 1961, the main founder of the ASIF, Dr. Maurice Edmond Müller, described the use of a threaded external fixator for upper tibial and supramalleolar osteotomies and for knee- and ankle-joint arthrodeses in *Operative Fracture Treatment – Papers of the Association for the Study of Internal Fixation.* The first ASIF text, *Technique of Operative Fracture Treatment* (1963) by Müller, Allgöwer and Willenegger, makes no reference at all to external fixation, but it is mentioned again in the first edition of the *Manual of Internal Fixation* (1969). Again, the threaded fixator is discussed with reference to the management of osteotomies, arthrodeses and nonunions. It was not until the second edition of the *Manual,* published in 1977, that external fixation was recommended for the treatment of acute fractures. This time, however, the fixator was not the "old" threaded device, but a new tubular system developed by R. Mathys[1]. Through a worldwide program of instruction, the tubular system of the ASIF has gained wide acceptance very rapidly, just as the Hoffmann apparatus did in its own fashion.

Many different variants of the external frame are on the market today. Even the threaded fixator of the ASIF is currently being used at many centers. In the Department of Orthopedic Surgery at the Kantonsspital St. Gallen, Switzerland, we

have come to prefer the threaded external fixator absolutely over the ASIF tubular system and other devices. This has been true since 1960–1967, when M.E. Müller was department head and the author was a staff physician, and in the years since then. But even at the Balgrist Clinic in Zurich, from 1956 to 1960, I had the opportunity of working with the threaded fixator as a resident under M.E. Müller, who then was a staff physician.

In *Pseudarthrosis* (Weber and Čech, 1973), the threaded fixator is discussed with reference to the management of infected nonunions.

Nearly 30 years' experience with the threaded external fixator in orthopedic and trauma surgery, as well as experience with the tubular system, provide the basis for the present book. The threaded device surpasses all other systems in its versatility and has demonstrated a variety of applications in fractures, nonunions, osteotomies, arthrodeses, and the correction of soft-tissue contractures. While most previous publications on the external fixator have been limited to its use in fractures, the present book deals with the entire range of applications practiced at our center.

At the outset it should be emphasized that numerous methods are available for the management of fractures, nonunions, osteotomies and arthrodeses, as the list below illustrates:

*Methods of Fracture Management*

1. Simple supervision
2. Functional treatment by the Steinmann method
3. Conservative treatment by the Böhler or Watson-Jones method
4. Functional bracing by the Sarmiento method
5. ASIF internal fixation with screws, plates, and intramedullary nails
6. External fixation, e.g. with the ASIF threaded fixator, tubular design, or other systems.

While the first four methods represent closed techniques, methods 5 and 6 are quite complex by comparision. With method 5, for example, an exacting operative technique must be mastered. The same may be said of external fixation, of course, but in the case of open and infected frac-

---

1 Engineer for the Swiss ASIF

tures or infected nonunions, "technique" alone is
a far less critical factor than with other methods.

But what specifically is involved in the use of
an external fixator?

- Debridement
- Sequestrectomy
- Drainage
- Cancellous bone grafting
- Soft-tissue coverage
- Decisions relating to further management, i.e.,
  - Secondary internal fixation
  - An orthosis
  - Tertiary corrective procedures, i.e. arthrode-
    sis, osteotomy, soft-tissue flaps, amputa-
    tion
- Problems relating to infection, local and system-
  ic antibiotics, and local antisepsis.

Because external fixation generally is reserved
for the most challenging clinical problems, the patient and surgeon often are confronted with a difficult situation from the outset. Open and infected
fractures and septic nonunions have a certain
"chronic" character, and rarely is one operation
sufficient to achieve a satisfactory outcome.

The surgeon can find the best solution for a
given problem only if certain personal and technical criteria are met. Specifically:

- The surgeon must be well versed in the various
  treatment methods that are available;
- he must know and be able to treat all complications that may arise;
- a given method must be feasible (e.g., internal
  fixation requires proper asepsis, anesthesia and
  instrumentation);
- the patient must understand the nature of his
  treatment well enough that he can cooperate ac-
  tively with the surgeon during the course of
  treatment.

There is no question that every method has
its ideal and poor indications. It would be absurd
to attempt to solve all or even most problems opti-
mally with only one or two methods.

The principle of choosing the right method for
the right indication is illustrated in Table 1, which
gives a list of the methods practiced at our clinic,
together with sample indications.

It is not possible to discuss the many indications for the various methods, because after all,
external fixation is the subject of the present book.
For the ASIF, external fixation is just one of several possible forms of operative fixation; here our
scope must be more limited. In order to read the
book in the proper light, it is important first to

**Table 1.** Methods for the treatment of fractures, osteotomies
and arthrodeses, and their optimum indications

| Method | Examples of optimum indications | |
|---|---|---|
| | Trauma | Orthopedics |
| No immobili-zation | Impacted abduction fracture of the femoral neck | HELAL-type sub-capital metatarsal osteotomy |
| Traction | Pediatric femoral fracture with shortening | Congenital disloca-tion of the hip |
| Primary plaster | Transverse tibial fracture | Pediatric tibial osteotomy (NICHOL-SON's reed osteo-tomy in continuity) |
| Kirschner wire fixation | Lisfranc fracture-dislocation | Certain types of corrective foot surgery |
| Internal fixa-tion by ASIF technique | Intra-articular fractures | Aseptic nonunions |
| External fixation | Grade III open fracture of the tibial shaft | Certain pediatric osteotomies |

understand the following points, which are based
on clinical experience:

a) External fixation has a definite place in the
management of many orthopedic and trauma
cases, despite the considerable difficulties involved
in the handling of the device and associated treatment.

b) Most new indications for external fixation
are in patients who previously were not selected
for surgical treatment. Thus, external fixation does
not compete with internal fixation, but comple-
ments it.

c) The design of the external frame should be
kept as simple as possible, and the device should
not hinder the patient by its presence or size. A
"humanization" of many external fixation systems is desirable in this regard.

d) The external fixator need not be as rigid
as compression plates and screws. This has to do
with the goals of the fixation. With internal plates
and screws, primary bone healing is the intent,
and so the implants must remain in place for a
year or more. This protective function is beyond
the capabilities of the external fixator, which
should be removed after 3–4 months. Generally,
secondary bone healing with the formation of a
"fixation callus" is the only repair mechanism
which can ensure adequate stability after so short

a time, and some degree of instability, like that seen in conservative treatment or intramedullary nailing, is necessary for this type of healing to occur. In this respect external fixation is more akin to conservative fracture management than to internal fixation. Like internal fixation, however, the external frame offers the opportunity for early postoperative mobilization.

# 2 The History of External Fixation

The history of external fixation can be briefly outlined as follows:

1902 Lambotte: First unilateral frame
1936 Cuendet: First bilateral frame
1938 Hoffmann: First frame allowing pin placement in multiple planes.
1953 Charnley: Bilateral compression frame for the fixation of arthrodeses.
1956 Judet R., Judet J., Lagrange L.: Unilateral compression frame for the fixation of nonunions.
1956 Müller, Allgöwer: Compression frame for diaphyseal nonunions.
1970 Vidal, Rabischong, Bonnel, Adrey: Double frame for compression, distraction or neutralization.
1970 Connes: Describes all indications for the Hoffmann bilateral frame.
1973 Weber, Cech: Combine the ASIF unilateral and bilateral frames for nonunions.
1975 Hierholzer: Describes a triangular fixation frame.
1976 Boltze: Describes the tubular frame of Müller.
1976 Burny: Advocates elastic external fixation.
1979 Magerl: Special external fixator for the spine.
1980 Mears and Fu: Enthusiastic advocates of external fixation in the United States.
1981 Brunner, Weber: Describe prestressing of transfixing pins, adjunctive internal minifixation, transverse compression, and the correction of soft-tissue contractures.
1981 Green: Monograph on the complications of external fixation.
1983 Mears: Most comprehensive publication on external fixation up to now.

# 3 Bone Healing in the Presence of an External Fixator

*Secondary fracture healing* with the formation of a "fixation callus" (PAUWELS) is characteristic of fractures that are treated nonoperatively (Fig. 1).

Fractures that are operatively stabilized tend to undergo *primary healing,* in which the fragments are united by direct, angiogenic bone formation (SCHENK, WILLENEGGER) (Fig. 2).

In the presence of an external fixator, no new type of bone healing occurs. One may observe primary healing, secondary healing or a failure of healing (nonunion), depending on the stability of the device, motion at the fracture site, and fragment viability. Thus, typical patterns of bone healing are observed in fractures and osteotomies of the diaphysis (cortex), epiphysis (cancellous bone), and in nonunions.

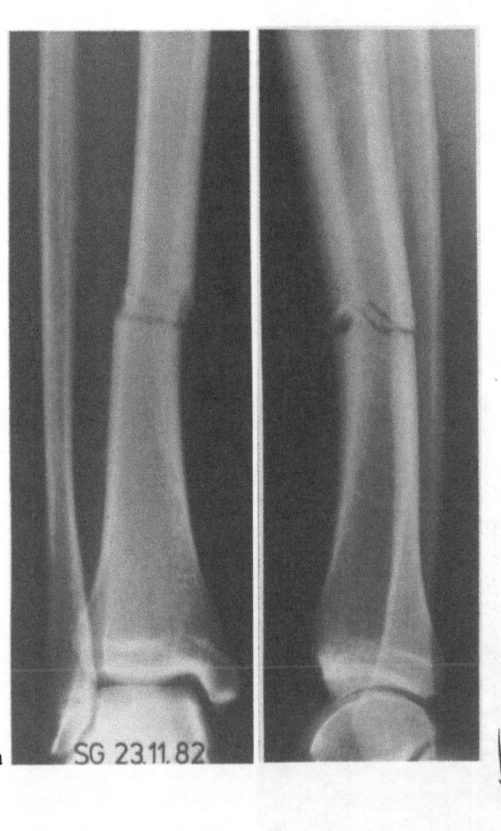

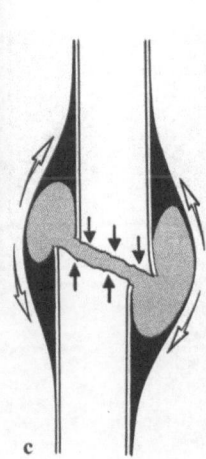

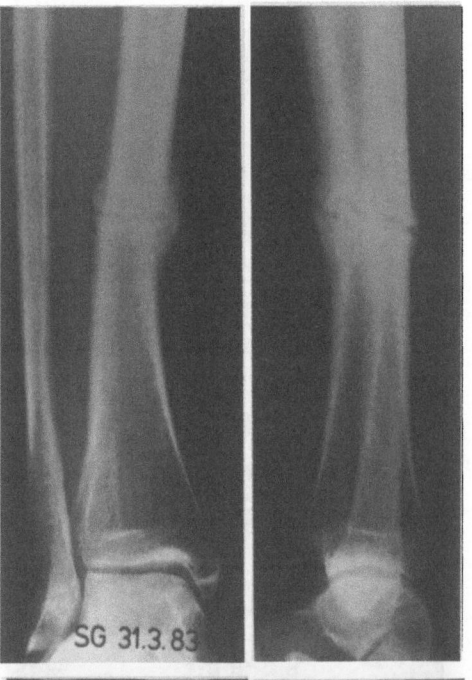

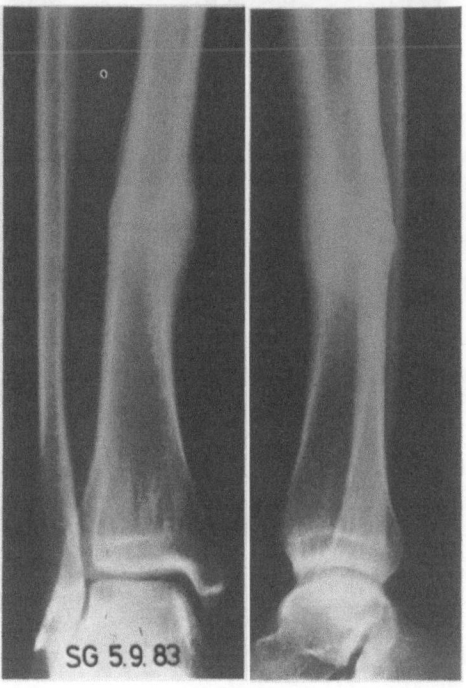

**Fig. 1 a–d.** Secondary fracture healing. V.A.A., 1955, 27 years, ♂, 265761.

**a** Transverse fracture of the tibia.
**b** Unstructured callus at 4 months postinjury.
**c** Features of secondary fracture healing (PAUWELS): The fracture hematoma is enclosed by a tension-resistant envelope. Connective-tissue cells and then cartilage cells develop in its interior. The intercellular substance calcifies to form stable masses that are invaded by blood vessels, along which osteons (Haversian systems) are formed. This pathway from connective tissue to cartilage to calcification characterizes the process of secondary fracture repair.
**d** By 9 months postinjury the initially unstructured "motion" callus has been transformed into a structured fixation callus

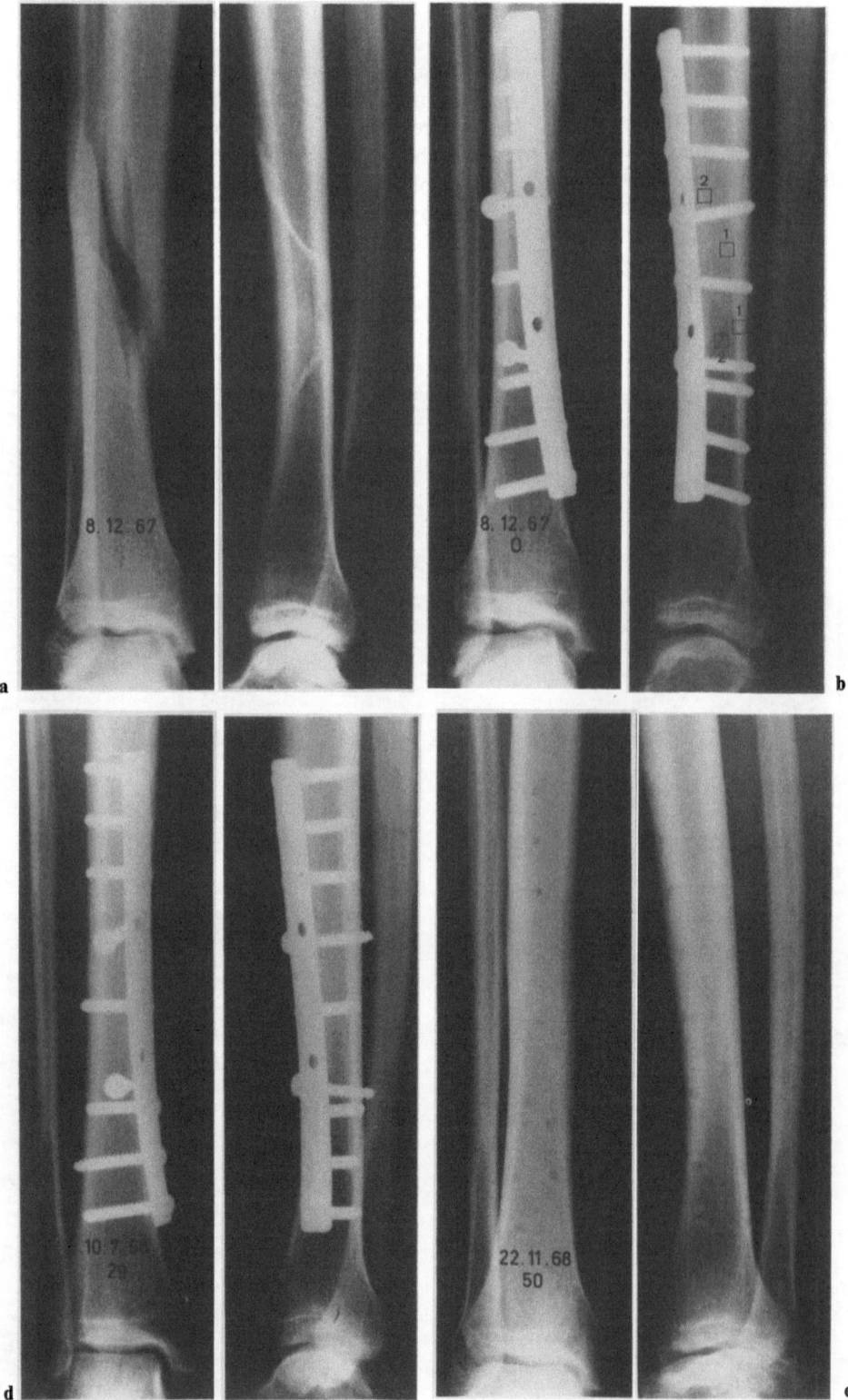

Fig. 2a, b, d, e

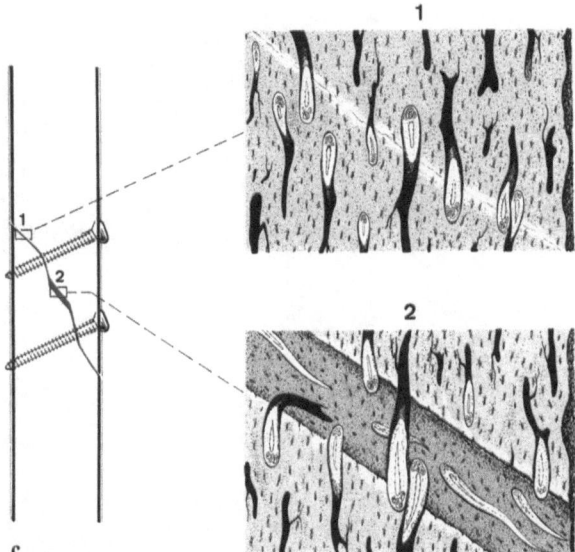

**Fig. 2 a–e.** Primary fracture healing. S.R., 1946, 37 years, ♂, 118379.

**a** Spiral fracture of the tibia.

**b** Internal fixation with lag screws and neutralization plate: *1* Sites of anatomic interfragmental contact; *2* sites where the fragments are separated by a gap.

**c** Histology of primary fracture healing (Schenk and Willenegger): *1* Sites of contact healing. Vessels bridge the fracture site directly, and osteons form along the new vessels. Haversian canals traverse the fracture line from one fragment to the next, creating a directional, osseous union of the bone ends. *2* Sites of gap healing. The gap is invaded by blood vessels, along which lamellar bone is formed. Only after this stage do we see an axial uniting of the fragments by the proliferation of Haversian canals, as in contact healing.

**d** At 29 weeks postinjury neither a fracture gap nor callus is apparent.

**e** At 50 weeks postinjury and 1 week after removal of the implants, the bone (except for screw holes) is completely healed

## 3.1 Healing of a Diaphyseal Fracture

With a *diaphyseal fracture,* the following *types of healing* may occur:

a) Primary healing
b) Secondary healing
c) Nonunion

The different types of healing are illustrated by case examples:

### 3.1.1 Primary Healing of the Cortex (Fig. 3)

By its very nature as an indirect method, external fixation cannot stabilize a fracture, osteotomy, arthrodesis or nonunion as rigidly as direct, internal fixation with plates and screws. Hence, we rarely see pure primary bone healing in the radiographs of our patients.

### 3.1.2 Secondary Healing of the Cortex (Fig. 4)

The imperfect immobilization produced by external fixation gives rise to the formation of an irritation callus, which is gradually converted to a hard fixation callus. This is followed by a remodeling process in which the size of the callus is decreased and a bony cicatrix is formed. This is the typical pattern of secondary fracture healing and is, in fact, the essential advantage of external fixation: after only a few weeks, the irritation and fixation callus stabilize the fracture sufficiently for the frame to be removed.

Internal plates and screws could not be removed at such an early date, because in 8–12 weeks primary angiogenic ossification cannot unite the bone ends as solidly as the callus cuff produced by secondary bone healing.

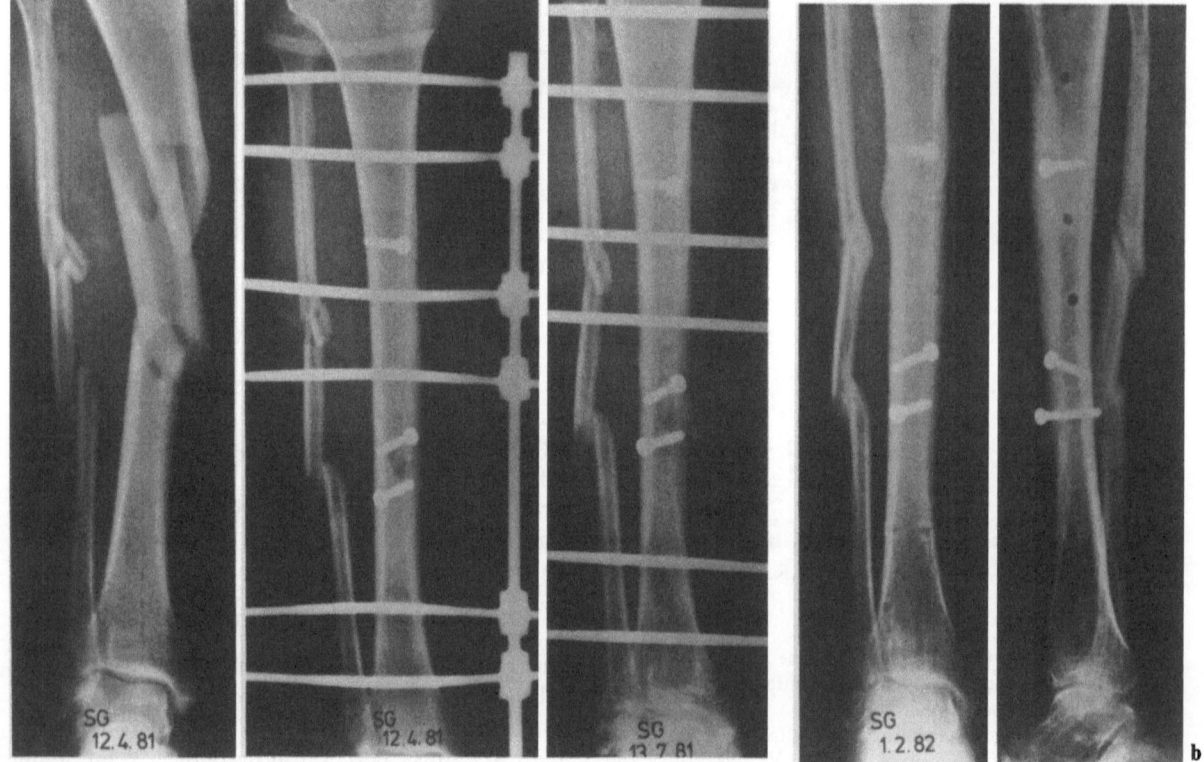

**Fig. 3a, b**

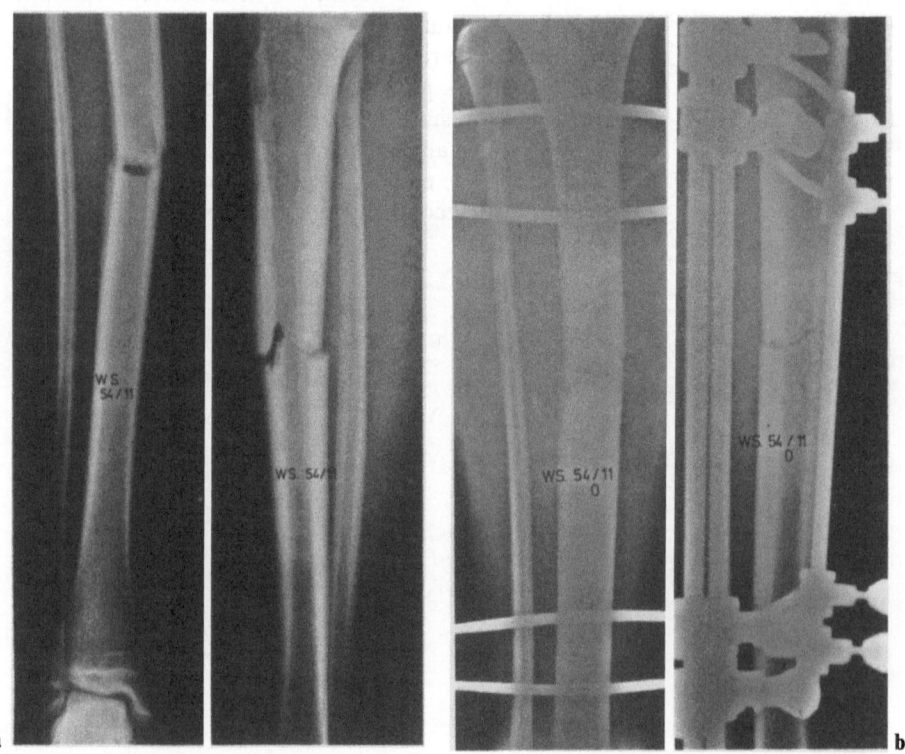

**Fig. 4a, b**

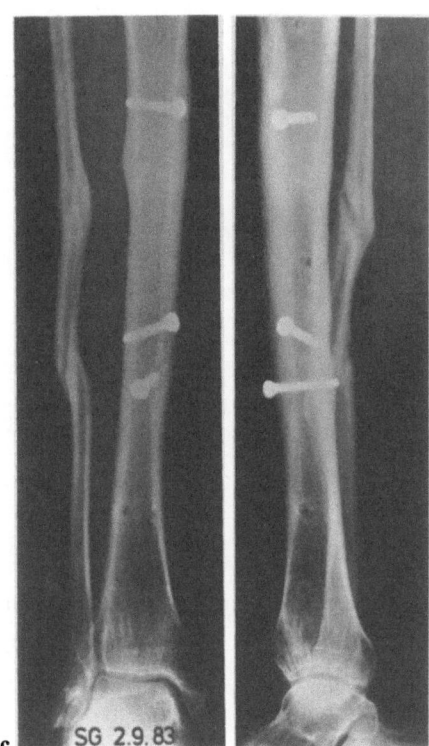

**Fig. 3 a–c.** Primary healing of cortical bone. E.A., 1928, 53 years, ♂, 248755.

**a** Grade II open tibial fracture treated by minimal internal fixation plus external fixation. At 3 months postinjury there is primary healing with no visible callus.

**b** At 10 months postinjury the fracture is clinically solid, and the limb bears weight normally. The proximal fracture line is still faintly visible, and a trace of callus can be seen posterolaterally. No fracture line is apparent distally; the gap is filled, and no callus is seen.

**c** At $2^1/_2$ years postinjury the tibia is normal. A small callus cuff is visible proximally (=secondary fracture healing), and there is virtually no callus distally (=primary fracture healing)

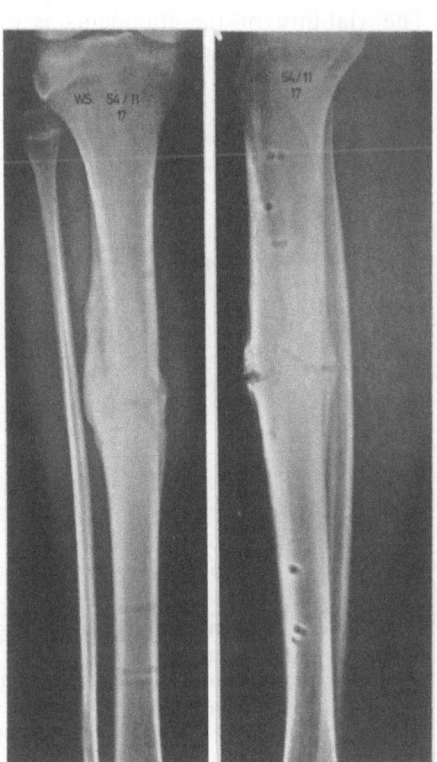
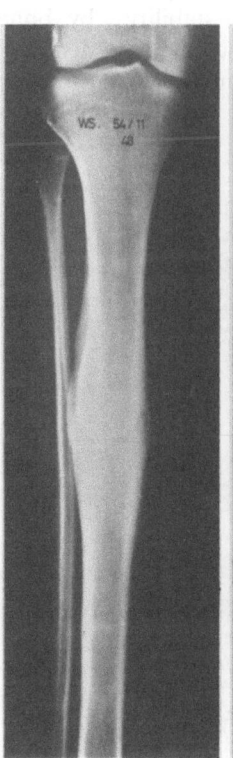
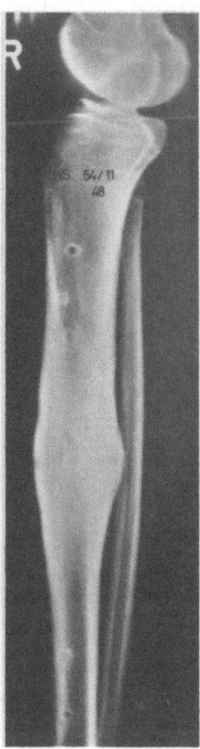

**Fig. 4 a–d.** Secondary healing of cortical bone. W.M., 1963, 17 years, ♂, 198964.

**a** Grade I open tibial fracture.

**b** External fixation was applied for 6 weeks, followed by a walking cast for 4 weeks.

**c** At 17 weeks postinjury there is evidence of typical secondary fracture healing with marked callus formation.

**d** By 11 months the callus has undergone functional remodeling

### 3.1.3 Nonunion

The pathogenesis of a nonunion may be mechanical or biological.

If the bone fragments have a good blood supply, creating conditions favorable for osteogenesis, a mechanical pathogenesis is predominant. This is called a *vascular nonunion* (Fig. 5).

If the bone fragments have little or no blood supply and thus lack osteogenic potential, or if a significant osseous defect is present, then a biological pathogenesis is predominant. This is an *avascular nonunion* (Fig. 6).

Radiographically, fragments with a good blood supply are characterized by hypertrophy, osteoporosis without hypertrophy, or osteoporosis with atrophy.

Poorly perfused fragments also have a characteristic radiographic appearance: relative sclerosis of the bone ends compared with bone remote from the fracture site, or an obvious bone defect.

Vascular nonunions will ossify completely when adequately stabilized. For avascular nonunions, it is necessary to combine stabilization with a biological stimulation of osteogenesis.

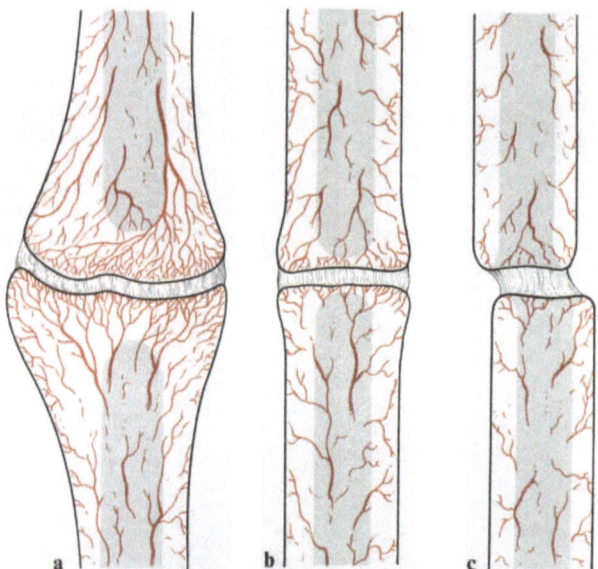

**Fig. 5 a–c.** Classification of nonunions: Vascular nonunions.

**a** Hypertrophic nonunion.
**b** Normotrophic nonunion + osteoporosis.
**c** Atrophic nonunion + osteoporosis

### 3.1.3.1 Pathogenesis of Vascular Nonunion
(Fig. 7)

A vascular nonunion can develop under the protection of an external fixator if the total stability provided by the fixator and callus is inadequate to immobilize the fracture site. True immobility would be required in order for the fibrocartilage to become mineralized, vascularized and replaced by bone. The viability of the fragments is evidenced radiographically by an increasing amount of callus, or in some cases by osteoporosis.

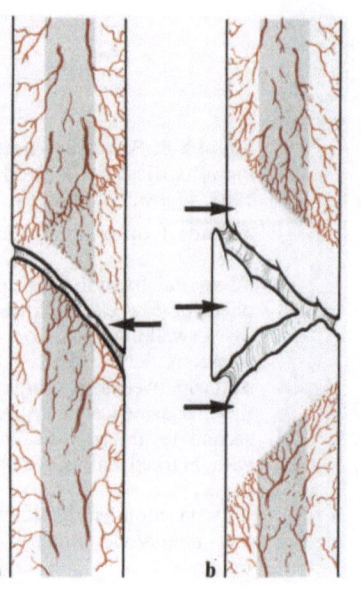

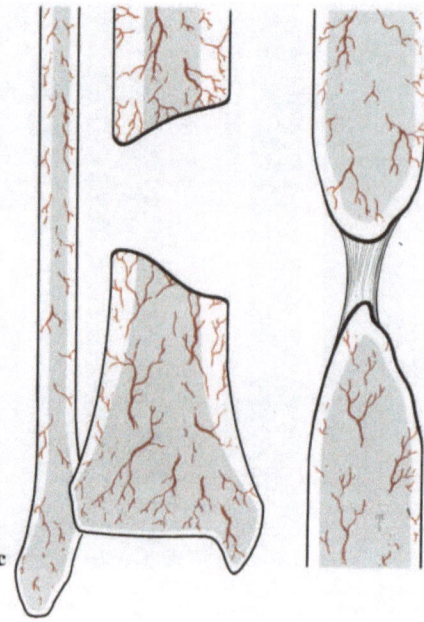

**Fig. 6 a–c.** Classification of nonunions: Avascular nonunions.

**a** Sclerosis or necrosis of one bone end.
**b** Sclerosis or necrosis of multiple fragments.
**c** Osseous defect (= nonunion with bone loss)

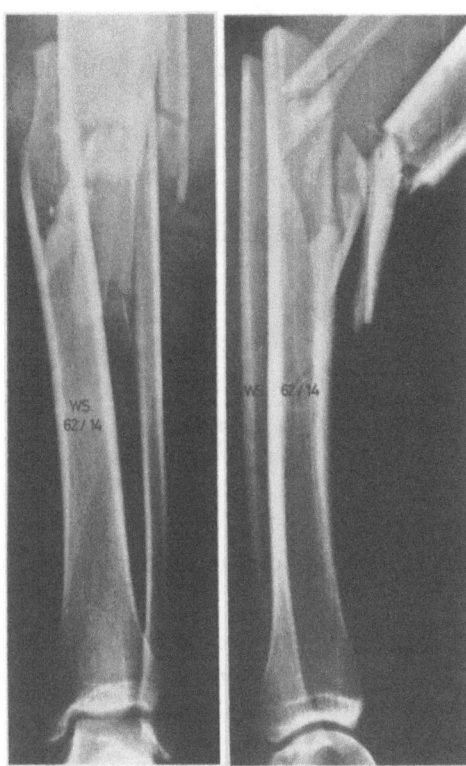

**Fig. 7 a–c.** Development of a vascular nonunion. P.S., 1960, 21 years, ♂, 248908.

**a** Grade III open fracture.
**b** Primary stabilization by lag screw + external fixation. Fifteen weeks later all fragments are osteoporotic, and there is no visible callus.
**c** At 5 months postinjury there is a normotrophic nonunion with osteoporosis of all fragments and minimal callus

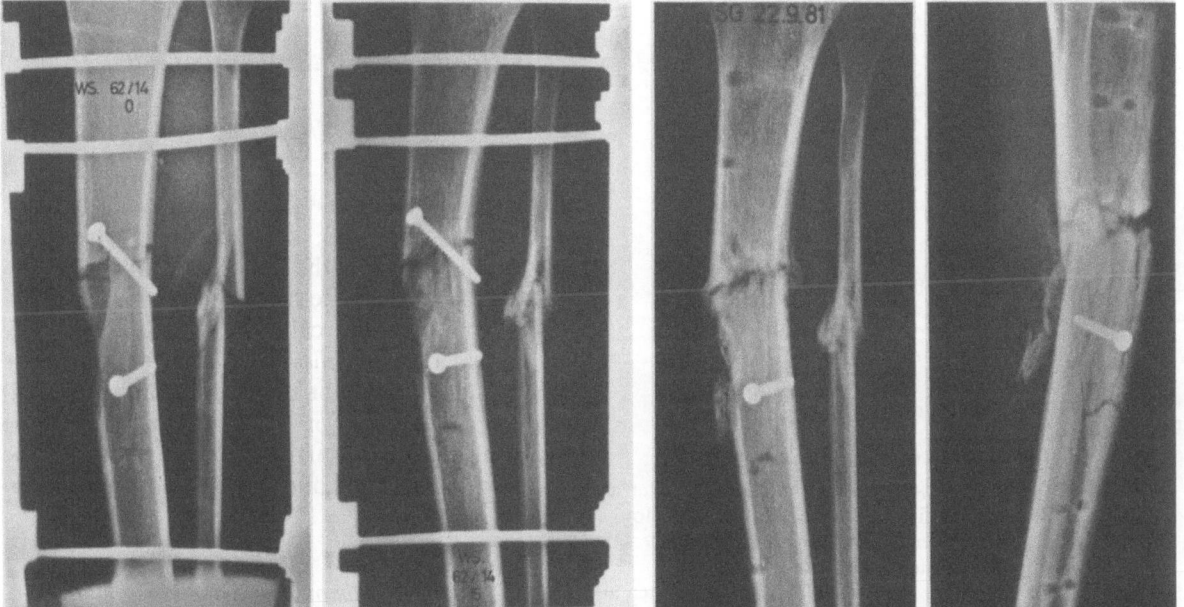

### 3.1.3.2 Pathogenesis of Avascular Nonunion
(Fig. 8)

An avascular nonunion is one in which the fragments lack an adequate blood supply. Even the most stable external fixation is of no benefit in cases of this type. The fragments may lose their blood supply due to stripping of the periosteum by a traumatizing event or by surgery (iatrogenic), or as a result of infection. Radiographically, no irritation or fixation callus is apparent. The bone ends show a relative sclerosis and lack the osteoporotic features of adjacent perfused bone. In other cases a bone defect may be evident, also precluding the possibility of osteogenesis.

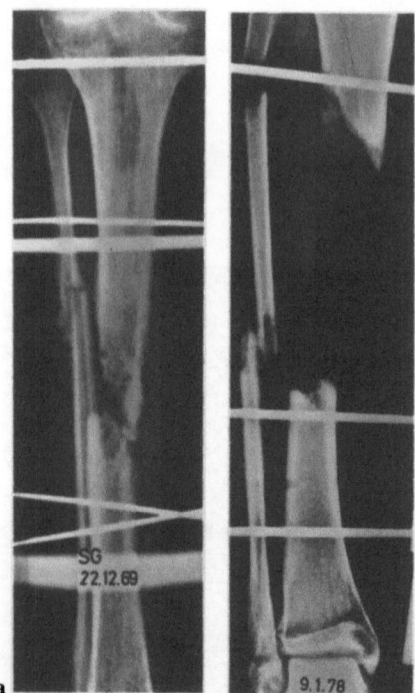

**Fig. 8 a, b.** Development of an avascular nonunion.
**a** S.W., 1927, 42 years, ♂, 146678. Eight months after an open fracture, external fixation, infection, sequestrectomy, and drilling of the bone ends, the bone margins are sclerotic compared to adjacent osteoporotic bone.
**b** H.W., 1950, 28 years, ♂, 210749. $4^1/_2$ months after an open segmental fracture, external fixation, infection, sequestrectomy and Thiersch grafting, the central fragment is osteoporotic, and there is relative sclerosis of the peripheral fragment with a major loss of bony substance

## 3.2 Healing of Cancellous Bone

Three *types of healing* are observed in cancellous bone:
a) Primary healing
b) Secondary healing
c) Nonunion

The different types of healing are illustrated by case examples:

### 3.2.1 Primary Healing of Cancellous Bone
(Fig. 9)

Well perfused, well stabilized cancellous bone surfaces will unite without the formation of a visible callus.

### 3.2.2 Secondary Healing of Cancellous Bone
(Fig. 10)

Well perfused cancellous bone surfaces that are maintained in reasonably stable contact can still unite once the irritation callus has converted to a fixation callus. However, this process takes about twice as long as primary healing.

### 3.2.3 Nonunion of Cancellous Bone

### 3.2.3.1 Pathogenesis of Vascular Nonunion
(Figs. 11, 12)

If the cancellous bone surfaces are well perfused but poorly stabilized, healing may not progress beyond the stage of the irritation callus. This occurs when fracture site motion outstrips the stabilizing ability of the callus. The bone ends may be separated by an interposed layer of connective tissue and cartilage, or by a double layer of cartilage enclosed by a joint capsule containing true synovial fluid (pseudarthrosis). In both forms the fragments are viable and have a good blood supply.

### 3.2.3.2 Pathogenesis of Avascular Nonunion
(Fig. 13)

If one or especially both of the fragments have lost their blood supply, or if an osseous defect is present, a "nonreactive" nonunion will develop. Radiographs show no evidence of callus formation that could compensate for the lack of interfragmental stability.

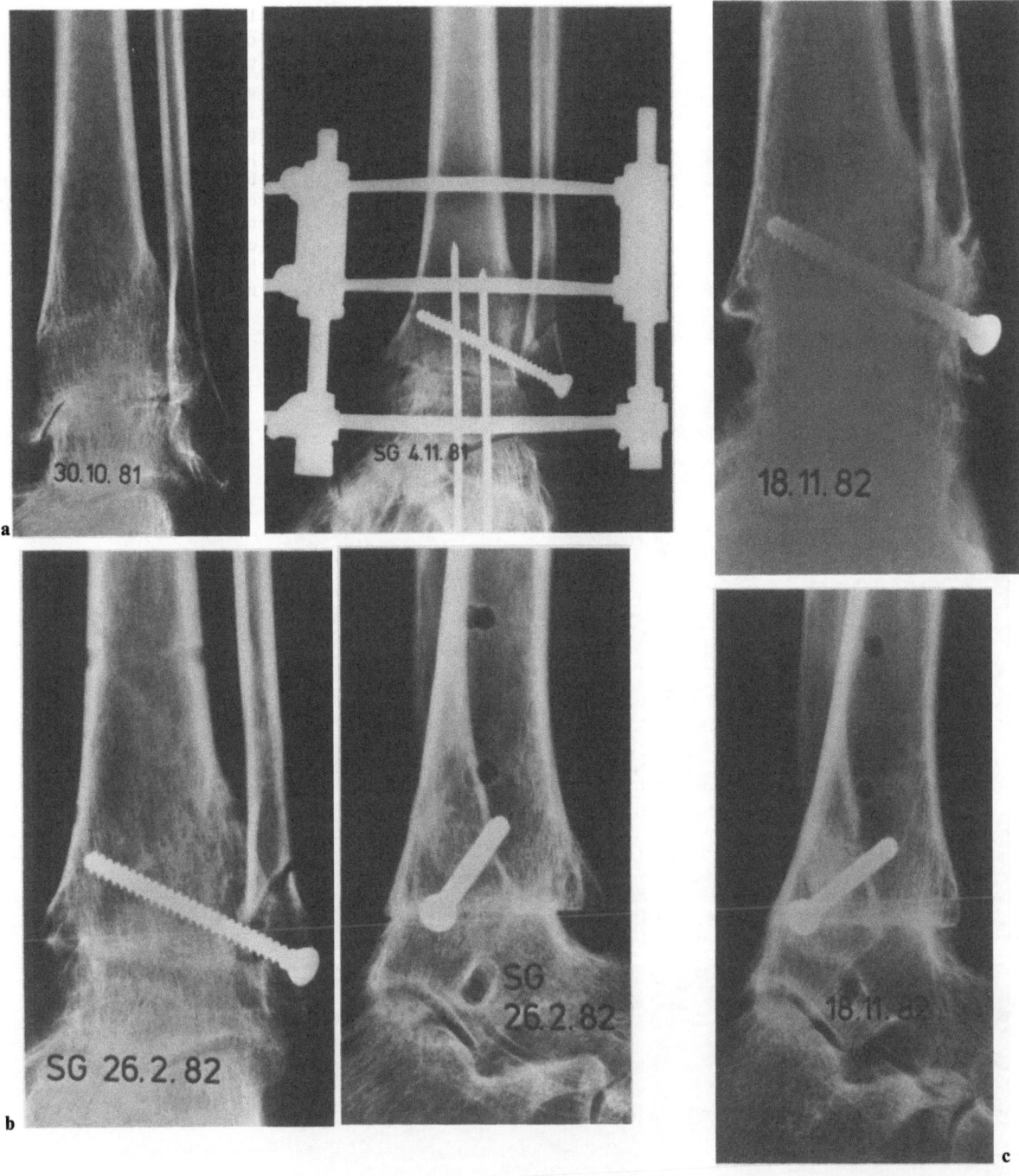

**Fig. 9 a–c.** Primary healing of cancellous bone. P.H., 1945, 36 years, ♂, 134512.

**a** Osteoarthritis of the ankle joint treated by compression arthrodesis.
**b** At 15 weeks postoperatively the bone has consolidated without a callus.
**c** At 1 year postoperatively the bone is still undergoing functional remodeling of its trabecular structure

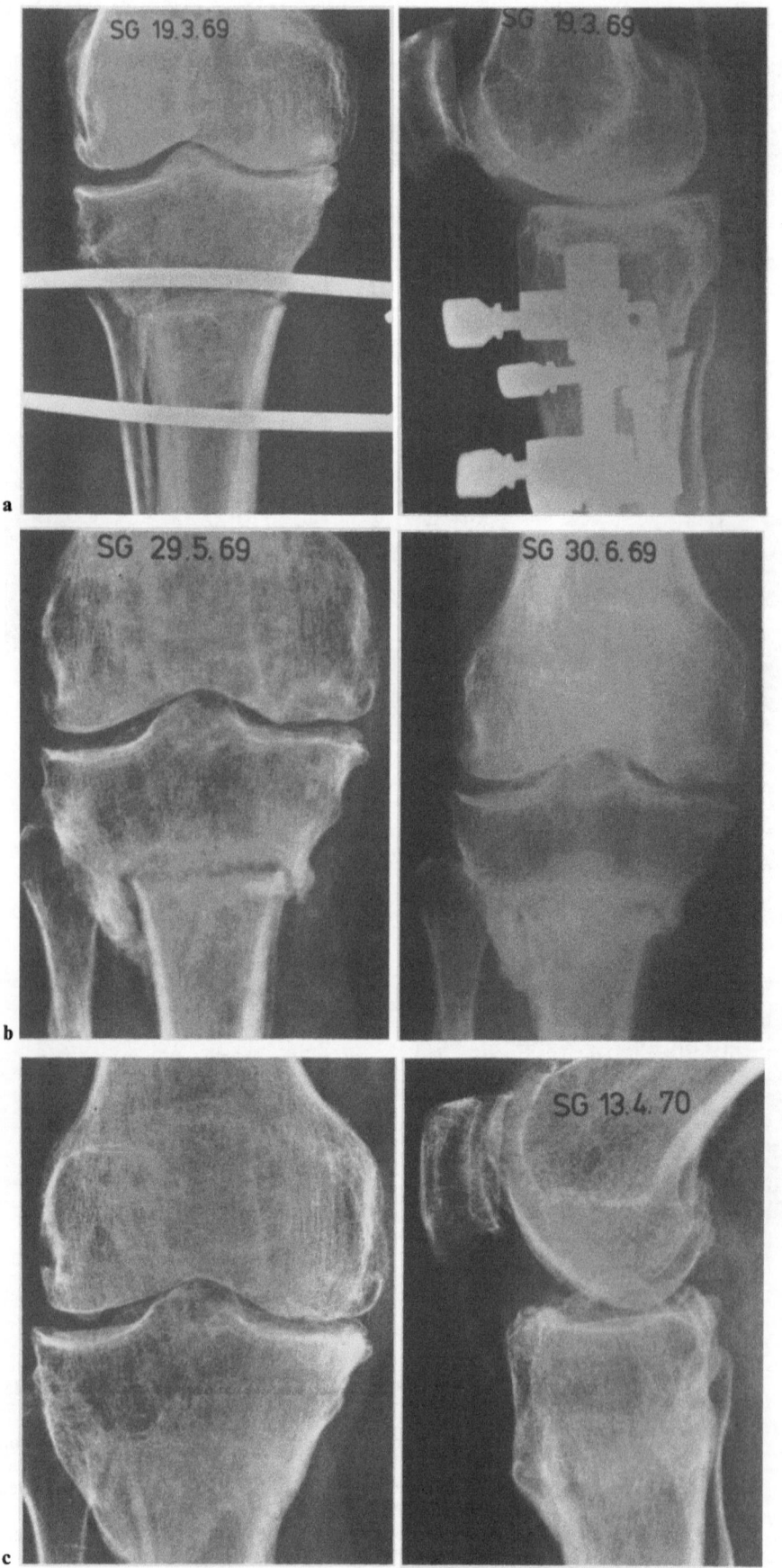

**Fig. 10 a–c.** Secondary healing of cancellous bone. T.A., 1902, 67 years, ♀, 56990.

**a** Osteoarthritis of the knee with varus deformity managed by valgus osteotomy of the proximal tibia.
**b** A motion callus and fixation callus are seen at 2 and 3 months postoperatively.
**c** At 1 year the fixation callus has undergone functional remodeling

**Fig. 11 a–c.** Development of a vascular nonunion. K.H., 1927, 43 years, ♀, 139242.

**a** A proximal tibial osteotomy was performed for osteoarthritis of the knee with varus deformity. Four months later the osteotomy is not solid, and the fragments are osteoporotic.

**b** By 7 months postoperatively a nonunion had developed. Two compression plates were applied without freshening the bone or applying cancellous grafts. Ten weeks later the nonunion is ossified.

**c** By $12^1/_2$ years postoperatively the site of the old osteotomy and nonunion shows a long-established functional remodeling

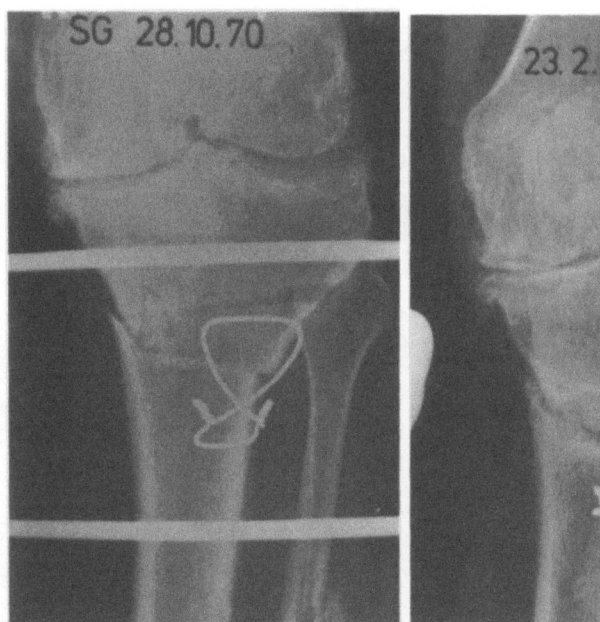

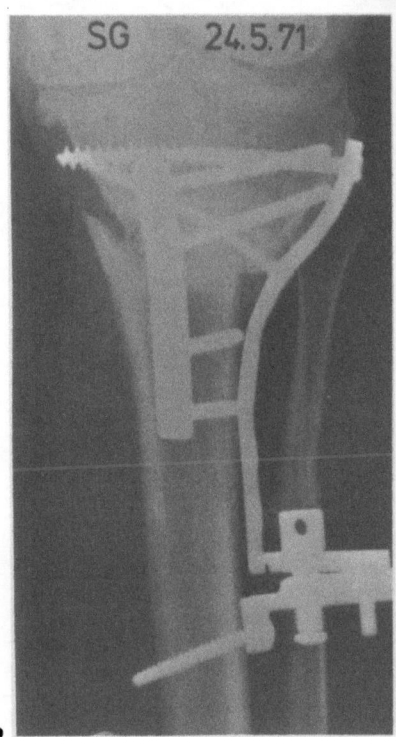

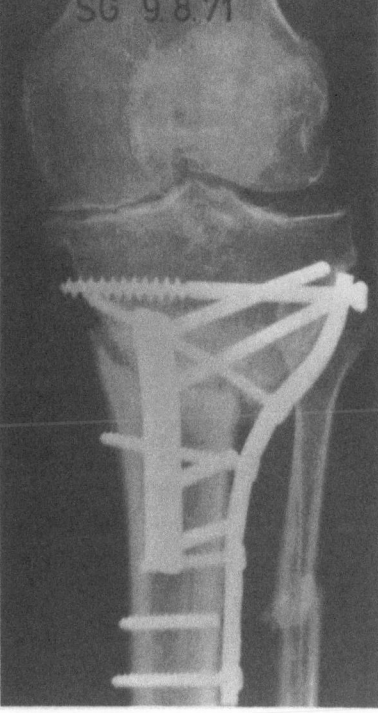

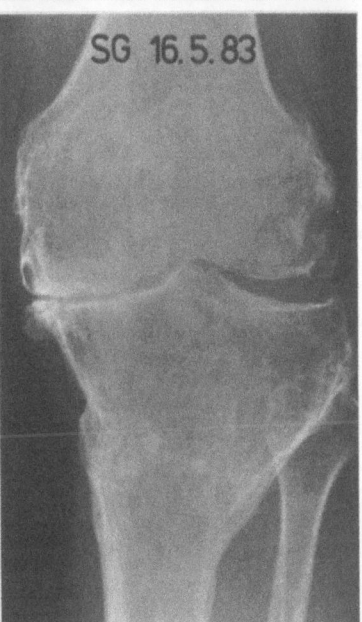

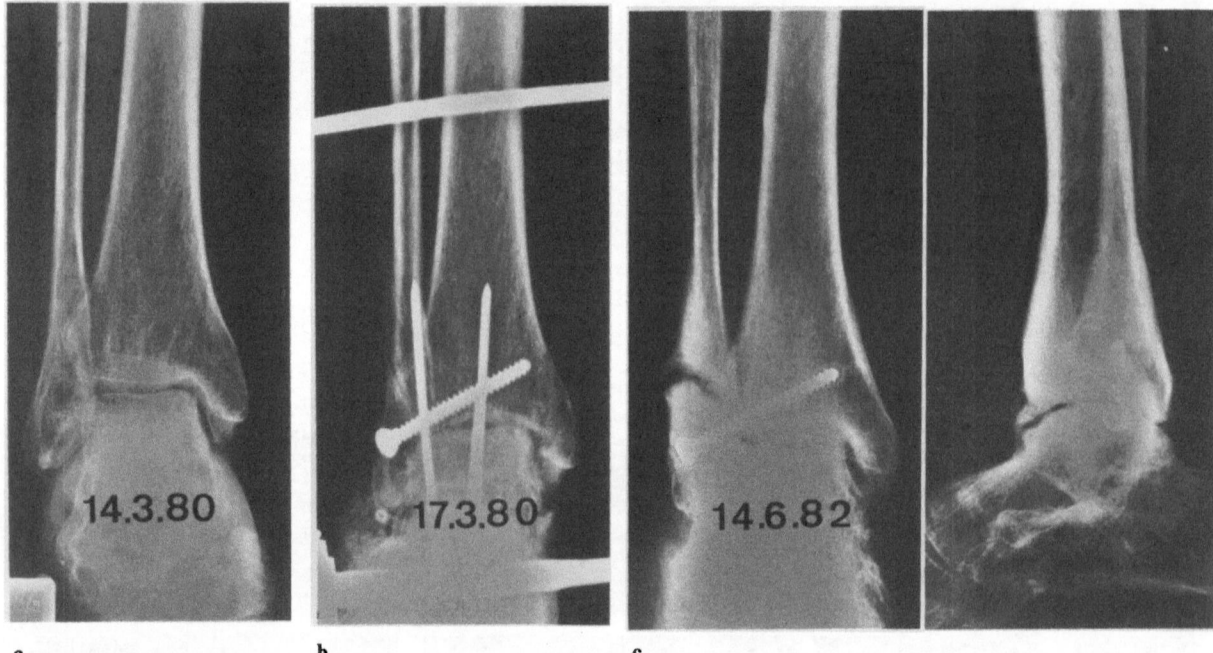

a          b          c

**Fig. 12 a–c.** Development of a vascular nonunion. T.G., 1921, 59 years, ♀, 222558.

**a** Post-traumatic osteoarthritis of the ankle joint.
**b** Compression arthrodesis of the ankle joint with minimal resection of bone.
**c** At 2 years, 3 months postoperatively: hypertrophic nonunion

**Fig.13 a–c.** Development of an avascular nonunion. M.G., 1917, 59 years, ♂, 161164.

**a** Osteoarthritis of the ankle joint secondary to congenital clubfoot. There is partial necrosis of the talar dome.
**b** Status 5 weeks after compression arthrodesis with inadequate bone resection.
**c** At 7 months postoperatively the fragments are nonreactive, there is a relative sclerosis of the bone ends, and a nonunion is apparent

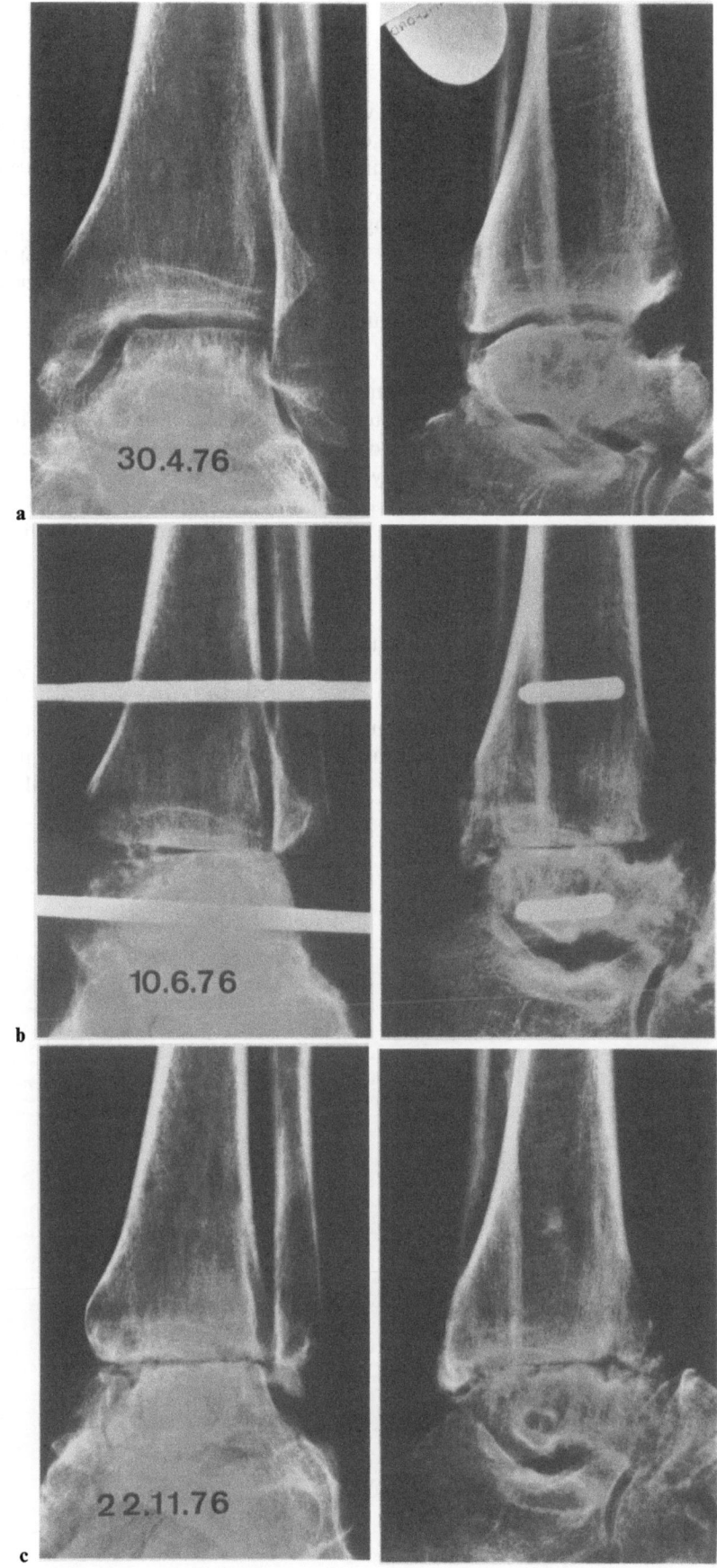

## 3.3 Healing of Nonunions

In nonunions that are stabilized with an external fixator, the type of healing that occurs will vary depending on whether the nonunion is vascular, avascular, or is associated with bone loss.

The different types of healing are illustrated by case examples:

### 3.3.1 Healing of a Vascular Nonunion (Figs. 14, 15)

Radiographically, a vascular nonunion shows either a hypertrophic callus or osteoporosis of the bone ends. Both hypertrophy and atrophy are indicative of a good blood supply. The nonunion should ossify under stable external fixation.

### 3.3.2 Healing of an Avascular Nonunion (Fig. 16)

An avascular nonunion with devitalized fragments requires for its consolidation, in addition to stable fixation, a stimulation of osteogenesis and in most cases an augmentation of live bone. By decorticating the bone ends and applying autogenous cancellous bone, the surgeon creates an artificial "irrita-

**Fig. 14 a–d.** Healing of a vascular nonunion (cortex). P.S., 1960, 21 years, ♂, 248908 (see also Fig. 7).

**a** At 5 months postfracture, following external fixation, there is a normotrophic nonunion with osteoporosis of all fragments and little visible callus.
**b** An tension-band fixation by external fixation was carried out.
**c** Three months later the callus is structured, and the nonunion is clinically solid.
**d** By 1 year, 10 months after external fixation, remodeling is complete ⟶

tion callus" which is gradually transformed into a fixation callus. Care is taken to place the bone grafts in a bed of well perfused tissue; poorly perfused cicatrices generally should be resected before grafts are applied.

### 3.3.3 Healing of a Nonunion with Bone Loss (Figs. 17, 18)

In nonunions with bone loss, autogenous cancellous bone grafting is necessary to replace the deficient bone stock. Again, the graft must be transplanted into a mechanically stable bed with a good blood supply if it is to survive.

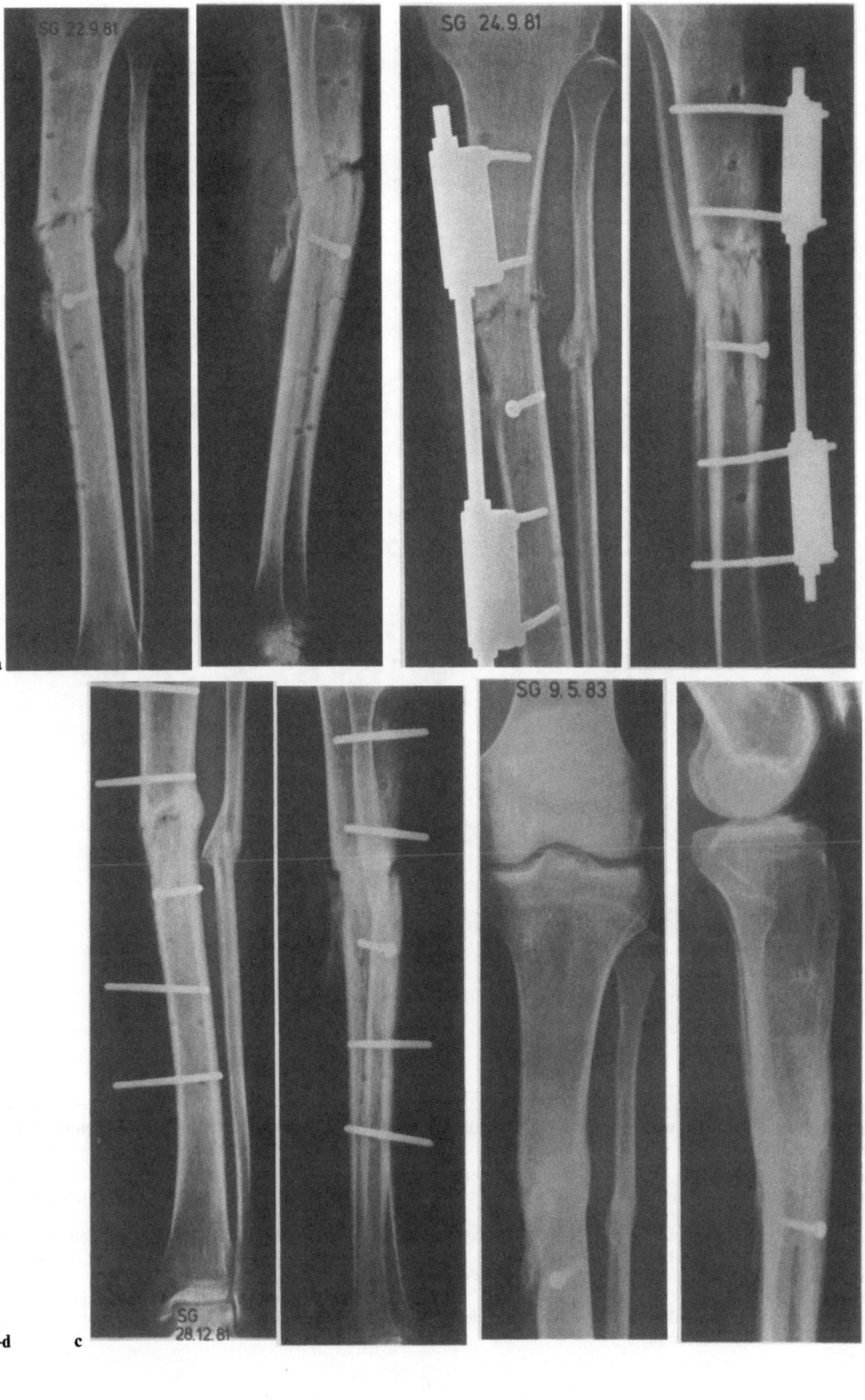

Fig. 14a–d

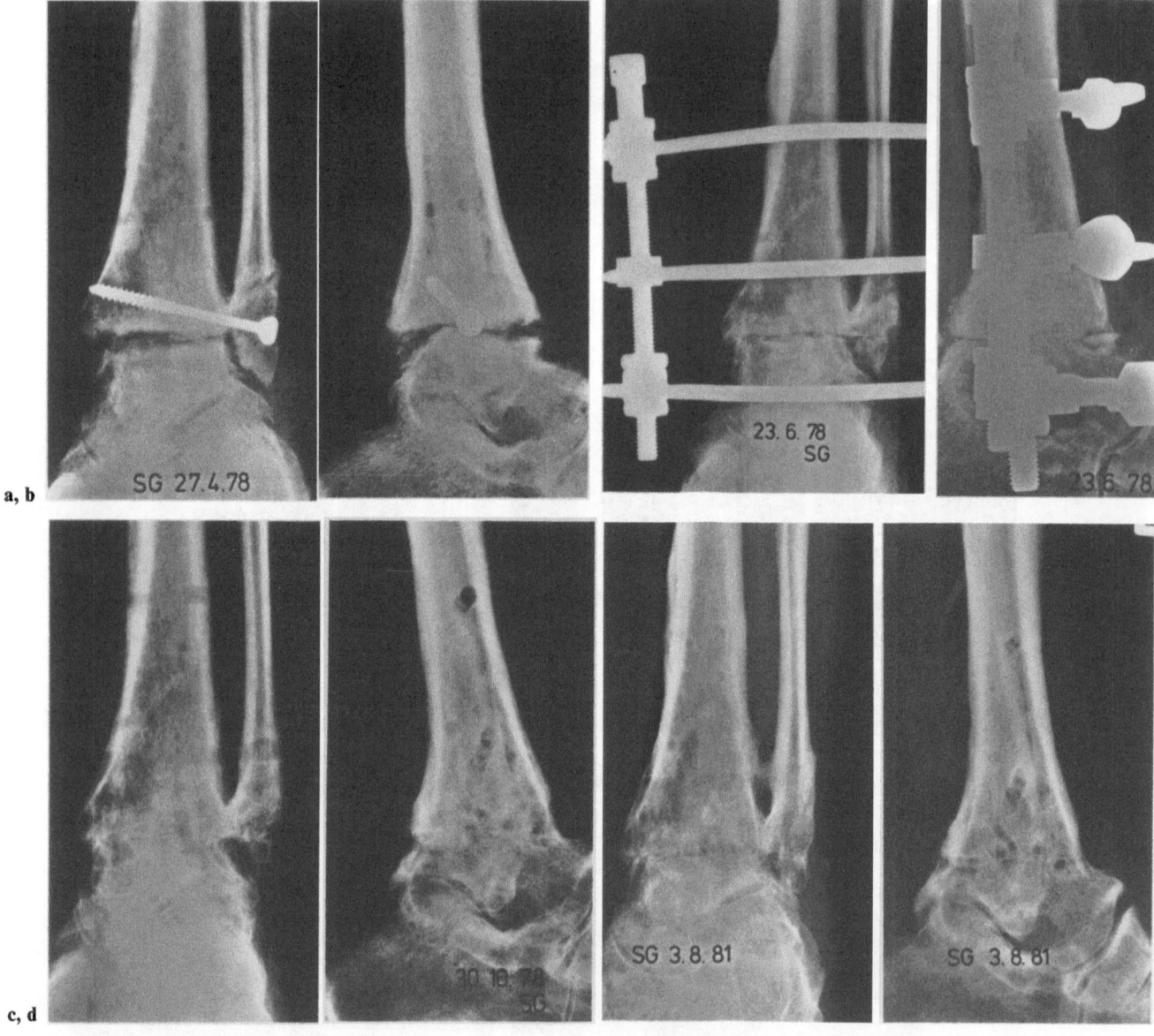

a, b

c, d

**Fig. 15 a–d.** Healing of a vascular nonunion (cancellous bone). F.K., 1928, 50 years, ♂, 113600.

**a** Vascular nonunion of the ankle joint 6 months after an attempted arthrodesis. There is osteoporosis and some atrophic resorption of the bone ends.

**b** Status 2 weeks after a repeat arthrodesis with sparing resection of the well perfused bone ends.

**c** At 5 months after repeat arthrodesis the nonunion is consolidated.

**d** By 3 years after repeat arthrodesis, functional remodeling of the trabecular bone is complete

**Fig. 16 a–d.** Healing of an avascular nonunion (cortex). ▶ C.F., 1940, 29 years, ♂, 127884.

**a** Six months following a corrective osteotomy, infection and plate removal, an inactive nonunion has developed. Note the sclerosis of the bone ends.

**b** At 2 and 16 weeks after external fixation, decortication and autogenous cancellous bone grafting, bridging of the nonunion is apparent.

**c** At 9 months postoperatively the nonunion is solid.

**d** At 22 months the bone has healed completely and is fully remodeled

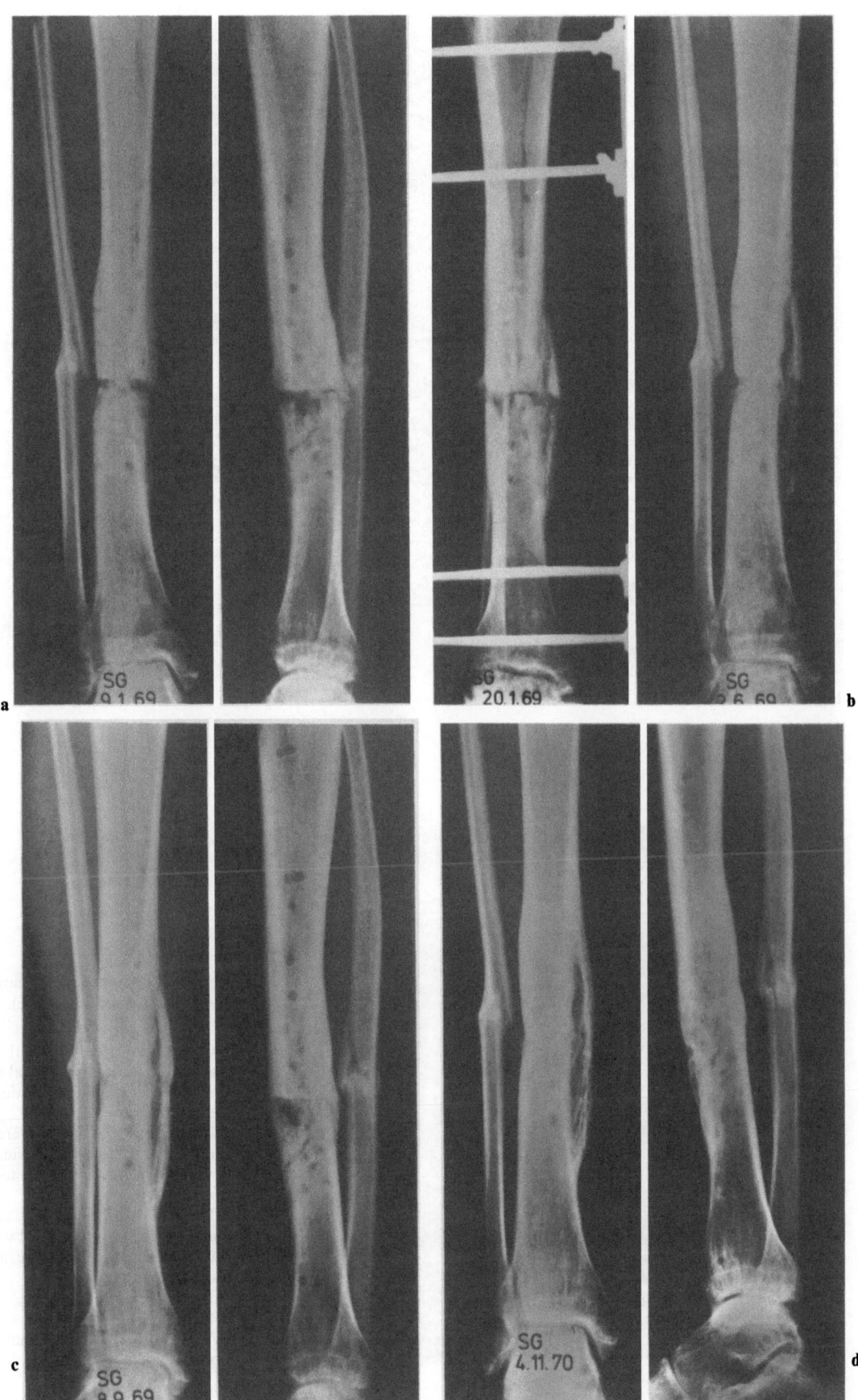

Fig. 16a–d

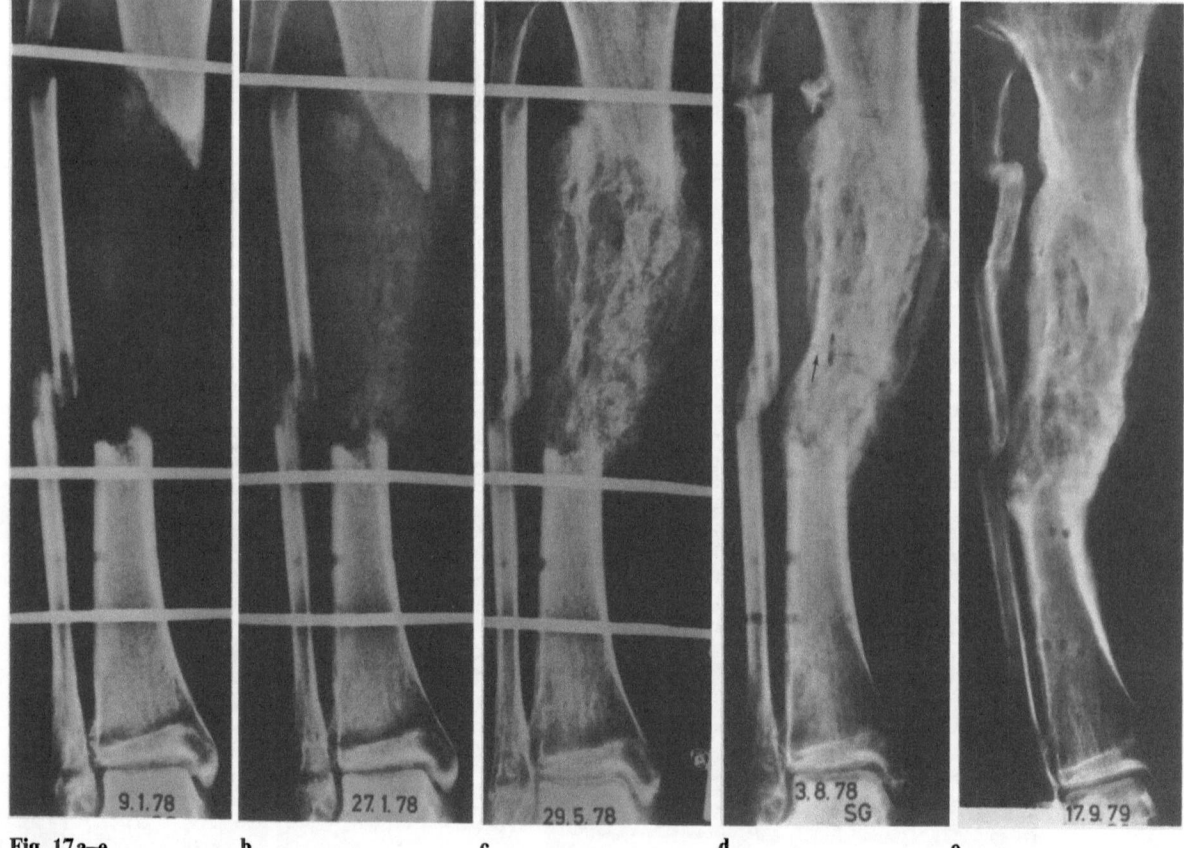

**Fig. 17a–e**

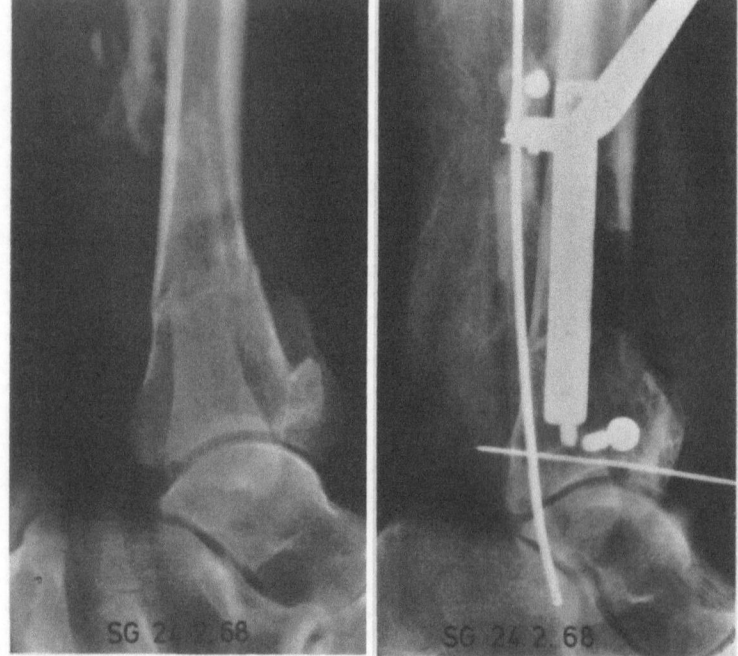

**Fig. 18 a–e.** Healing of a nonunion with bone loss (cancellous bone). K.R., 1942, 26 years, ♀, 120204.

**a** Compression fracture of the ankle joint managed by primary internal fixation with inadequate cancellous grafting of the osseous defect.

**b** At 6 months postinjury there is a nonunion with bone loss associated with both a varus deformity and posterior angulation.

**c** The axial deformities were corrected, the enlarged defect was packed with pieces of autogenous cancellous bone, and an external frame was applied.

**d** Three months later the nonunion is solid.

**e** At 5 months after external fixation the nonunion is healed

**Fig. 17 a–e.** Healing of a nonunion with bone loss (cortex). H.W., 1950, 28 years, ♂, 210749.

**a** Osseous defect in the midshaft of the tibia $4^1/_2$ months after an open segmental fracture, infection, sequestrectomy and Thiersch skin grafting.
**b** First cancellous bone graft.

**c** One month after 2nd cancellous bone graft.
**d** At 8 months after bone grafting there is a stress fracture of the cancellous bone. Further ambulation was done in a leg brace.
**e** At 1 year, 8 months after the 1st bone graft and functional postoperative therapy there is full consolidation of the nonunion

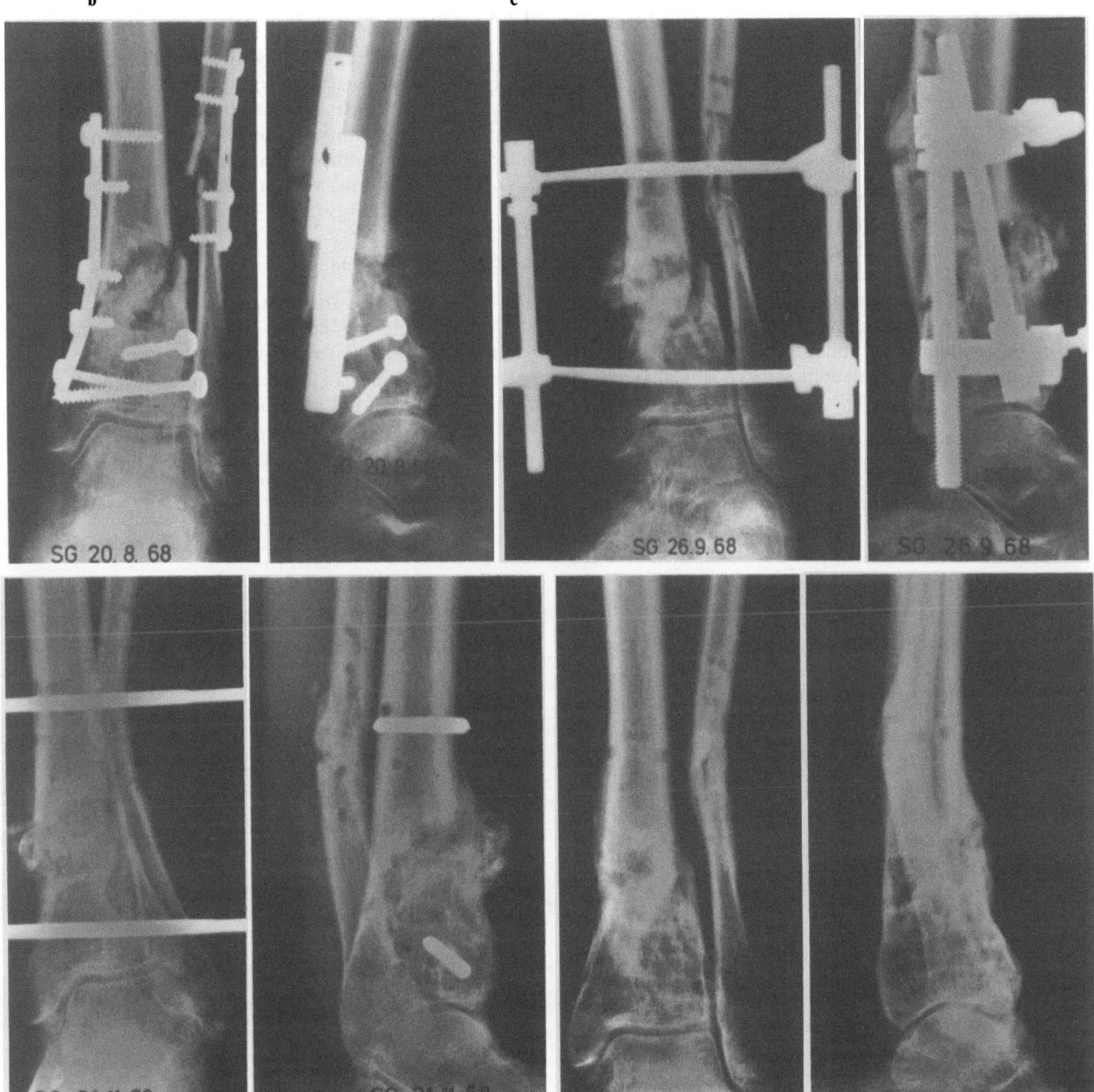

b

c

SG 20. 8. 68

SG 26.9. 68

SG 26 9 68

SG 21. 11. 68

SG 21. 11. 68

SG 1. 3. 69

SG 1. 3. 69

d

e

# 4 Goals of Treatment with the External Fixator

The goals of treatment with an external fixator depend on the function the device is intended to perform: lengthening (distraction), compression, neutralization, or soft-tissue extension.

## 4.1 Lengthening Frame

The lengthening frame effects a gradual distraction of the diaphyseal fragments formed by an osteotomy. In most cases a bone defect is formed as the lengthening progresses. ANDERSON has developed a bilateral threaded frame for limb lengthening, while WAGNER prefers a unilateral frame. Once the desired amount of lengthening has been achieved, it generally is necessary to perform a second operation in which the defect is packed with cancellous bone and plated. ILIZAROV uses his device to create an artificial epiphyseal plate fracture in his pediatric patients. The physiologic repair of the resulting defect obviates the need for a secondary operation. ILIZAROV's corticotomy in the metaphysis in adults serves a similar function.

## 4.2 Neutralization Frame

The purpose of the neutralization frame is to maintain reduction of the fragments with a mini-mum of implant material (transfixing and half pins) in order to facilitate the surveillance and healing of soft-tissue lesions. As a rule, secondary procedures are necessary to achieve consolidation.

Typical indications for the neutralization frame are open shaft fractures and infected nonunions with bone loss involving the tibia, femur or humerus.

## 4.3 Compression Frame

The compression frame is used in arthrodeses, osteotomies, nonunions and fractures to stabilize the fragments by interfragmental pressure, thereby shortening healing time. In this respect it is comparable to internal compression plates and screws. Secondary procedures are not required.

## 4.4 Soft-Tissue Frame

The purpose of the soft-tissue frame is to exert a gradual stretching action on soft tissues. An equinus deformity, for example, can be gradually corrected by means of a bilateral frame applied across the ankle joint. A bilateral frame applied to the distal femur can exert up to 30 kg of traction for short periods of time, e.g. to relieve contractures secondary to an untreated posterior dislocation of the hip.

# B On the Biomechanics of External Fixation

B.G. WEBER

The external fixator is used to move bone fragments relative to each other (lengthening, staged
angulation), maintain the alignment of bone fragments (open comminuted fractures), or apply compression across a bony interface (fractures, osteotomies, arthrodeses).

If we examine the total stability of a skeletal
region that is treated by external fixation, we find
marked variations from one case to the next. The
total stability depends on the type of fixator that
is used, and on whether or not the bone contrib-
utes to the stability.

## 1 Intrinsic Stability of the External Fixator

The bilateral frame is intrinsically more stable than
the unilateral frame. Axial loading (tension or
compression) of the bilateral frame causes a
marked bowing of the Steinmann pins, but deformation of the external rods is negligible (Fig. 19).
Tension and compression are distributed symmet-
rically to both rods.

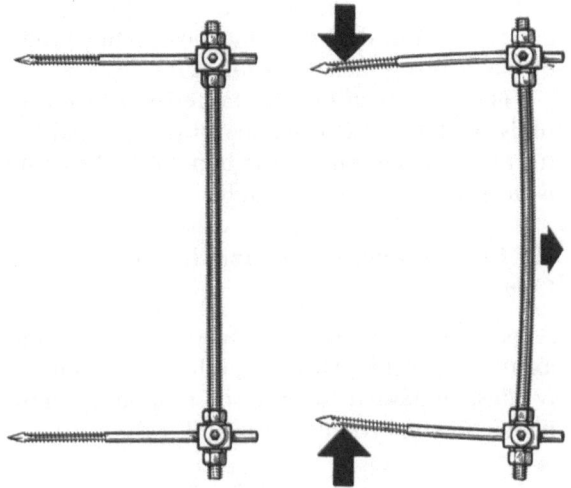

**Fig. 20 a, b.** Intrinsic stability of the unilateral frame.

**a** Simplest configuration of the unilateral frame.
**b** Weight bearing causes a marked bowing of the Schanz
screws and the rod

Due to the asymmetry of the unilateral frame,
the same load will not only produce a greater bowing of the Schanz screws, but also will cause a
marked deformation of the rod (Fig. 20).

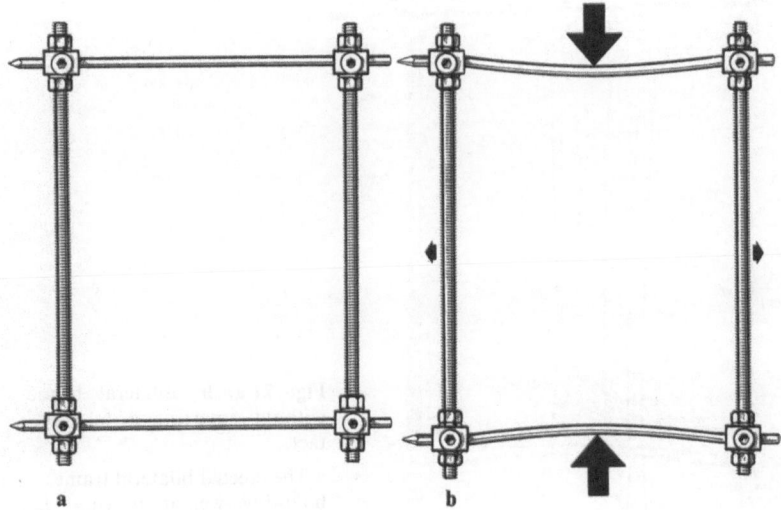

a        b

**Fig. 19a, b.** Intrinsic stability of the bilateral frame.

**a** Simplest configuration of the bilateral frame.
**b** Weight bearing causes a marked
bowing of the transfixing pins but negligible deformation of the rods

# 2 The External Fixator and Bone as a Composite System

## 2.1 External Fixation without Interfragmental Contact

When the external fixator is used for lenghtening or neutralization, the bone ends are not apposed, and so the bone does not contribute to the stability of the involved skeletal region (Figs. 21, 22).

The stability of the skeletal region depends entirely on the inherent stability of the external fixator and its anchorage in the bone; i.e., the fixator is the sole load-bearing member.

## 2.2 External Fixation with Interfragmental Contact

Apposed bone fragments are capable of absorbing axial compression. However, other forces can easily cause undesired fracture site motion, including distraction and rotation (Figs. 23, 24).

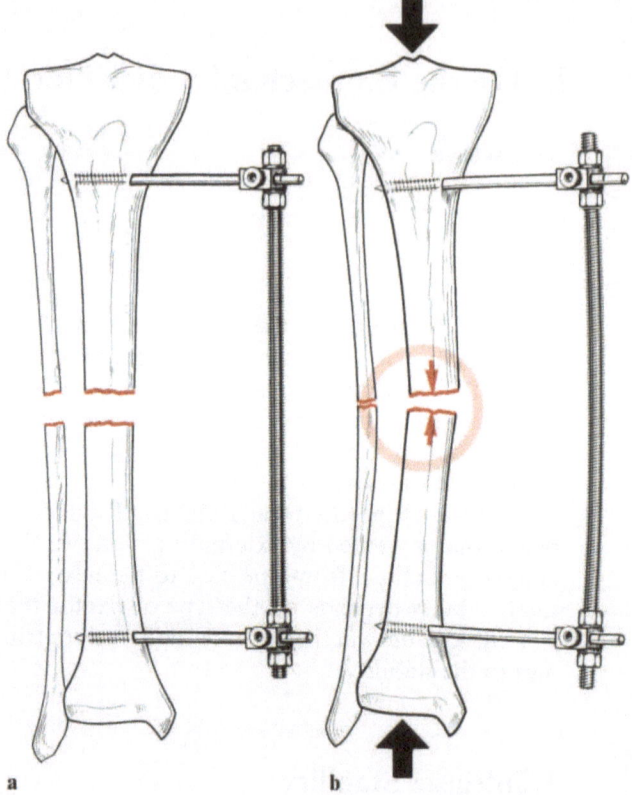

a   b

**Fig. 22 a, b.** Unilateral frame without interfragmental contact.

**a** The erected unilateral frame. **b** During weight bearing the frame is the only load-bearing member and shows a greater deformation than the bilateral frame

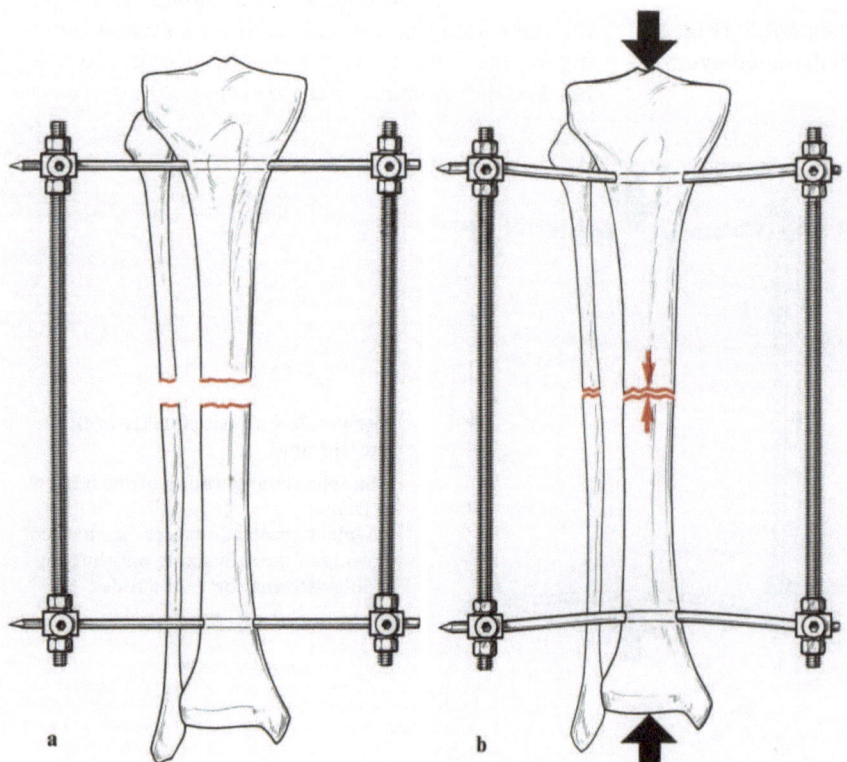

a   b

**Fig. 21 a, b.** Bilateral frame without interfragmental contact.

**a** The erected bilateral frame.
**b** During weight bearing the frame is the only load-bearing member and is markedly deformed

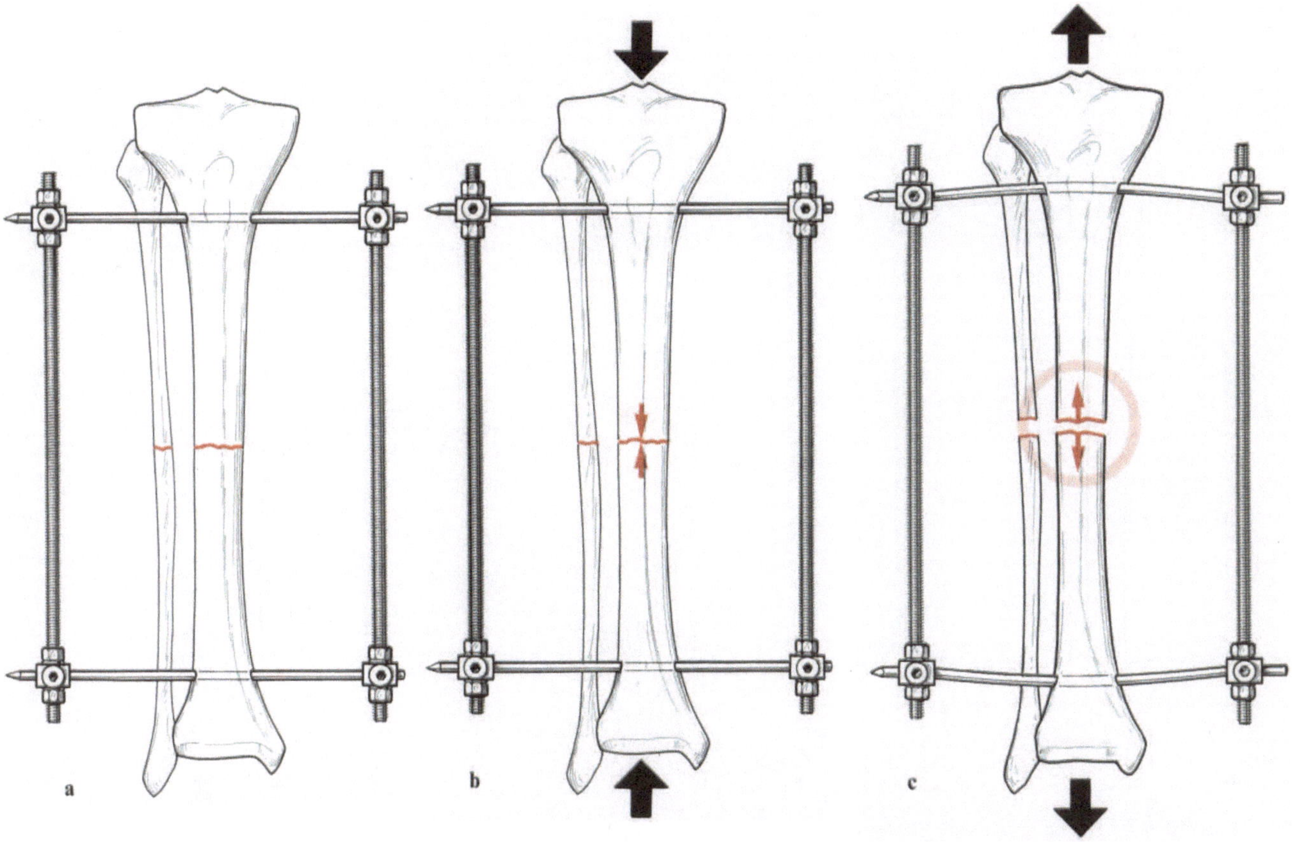

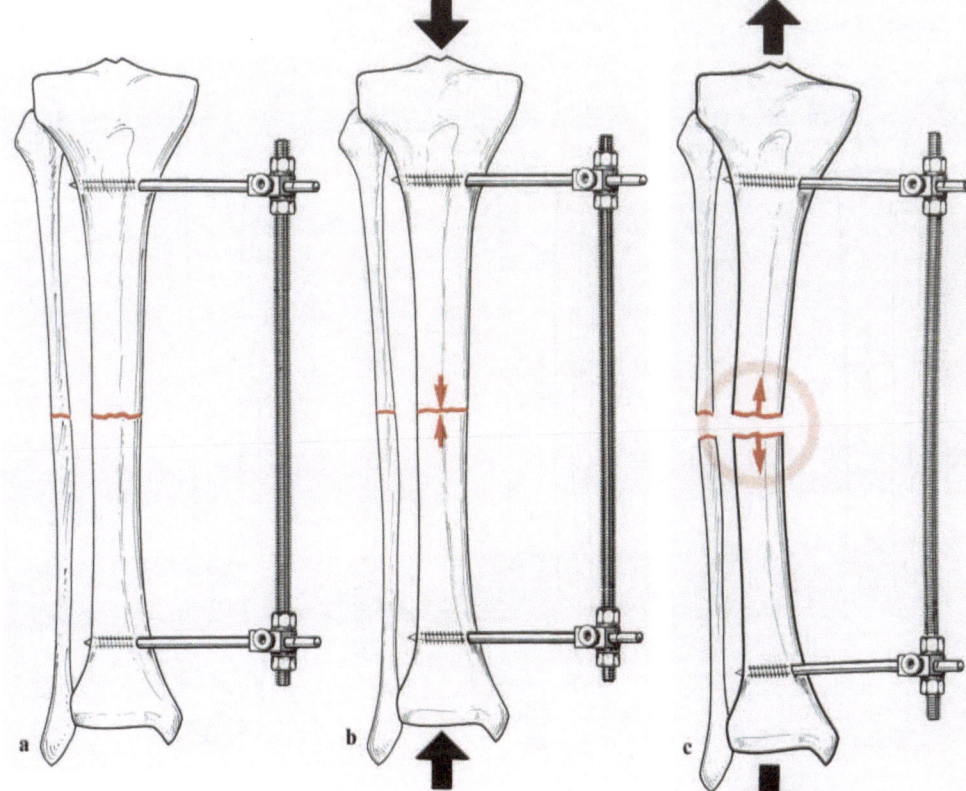

**Fig. 23 a–c.** Bilateral frame with interfragmental contact.

**a** The erected bilateral frame. **b** During weight bearing the bone absorbs all compression; the frame is free of stresses and is not deformed. **c** A distracting force deforms the frame and separates the fragments; axial alignment is not disturbed

**Fig. 24 a–c.** Unilateral frame with interfragmental contact.

**a** The erected unilateral frame. **b** During weight bearing the frame is not stressed, and the bone absorbs all compression. **c** A distracting force causes greater deformation than with a bilateral frame; interfragmental contact is lost, and axial alignment is disturbed

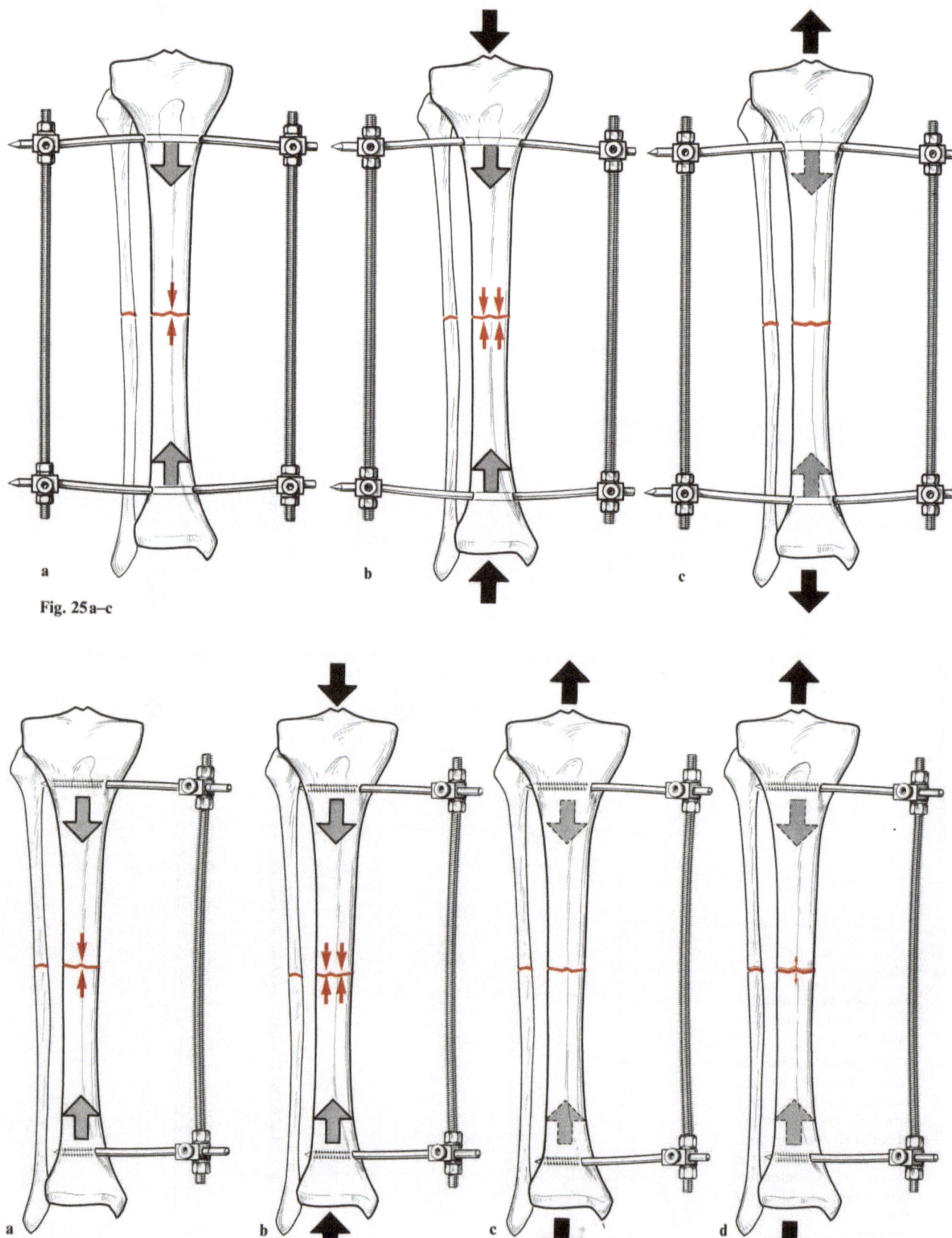

Fig. 25a–c

Fig. 26a–d

**Fig. 25 a–c.** The bilateral compression frame.

**a** The erected bilateral compression frame. The pins are prestressed in compression, and a uniform axial pressure is applied across the fracture. **b** During weight bearing the amount of compression across the fracture increases with the amount of weight borne. **c** A distracting force will nullify the interfragmental compression only if its magnitude equals that of the compressive force produced by prestressing of the frame

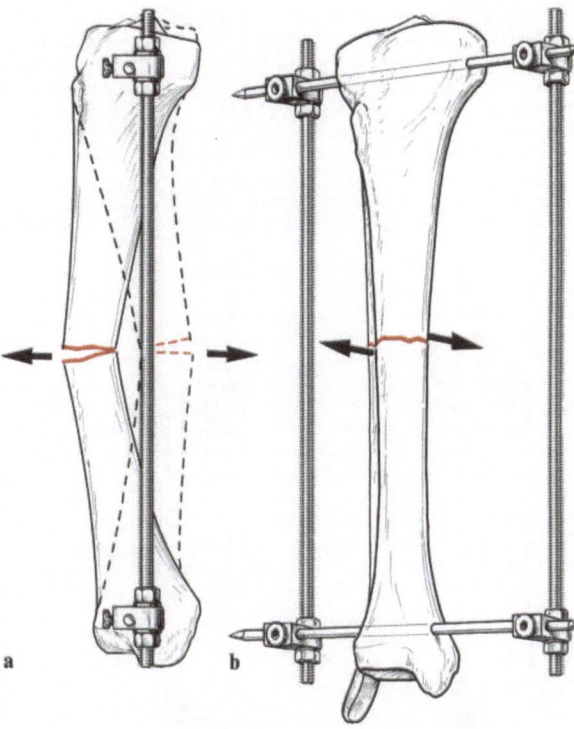

**Fig. 27 a, b.** The limited stability of the simplest external fixator. **a** Unilateral and bilateral frames with only 2 pins or screws offer scant protection against AP angulation. **b** Stability against rotation and shear is also slight

## 2.3 External Fixation with Interfragmental Compression

When a compression frame is used, the fixator and bone form a prestressed composite system of compression-resistant bone and tension-resistant metal.

Under axial loading, all compressive stresses are absorbed by the bony column; the pins, screws and rods are not deformed as when bone contact is absent. The frame prevents varus or valgus angulation of the fragments. The stabilizing action of the bilateral frame is equally good in both directions. The unilateral frame stabilizes better on one side than the other, because the rod provides tension resistance on one side only (Figs. 25, 26).

The compression frame also protects the fixation against distraction, which is not the case in other biomechanical situations. Even at rest, the two pins or screws are elastically deformed, exerting a sustained compression in the order of 20–30 kg. Under loading, the load pressure is added to the pressure from the prestressed pins or screws, and so the interfragmental pressure is always positive (no cycling between tension and compression). In biomechanical terms this means excellent stability of the bone-frame system, with little danger of loosening or fatigue fracture of the implants (SCHNEIDER).

While conventional unilateral and bilateral frames employing two pins or screws stabilize very well against varus and valgus angulation, they are less effective in preventing anteroposterior (AP) angulation, and they offer little protection against torsion. As a result, "minimal" fixators are rarely satisfactory in practice (Fig. 27).

Before discussing means of augmenting the stability of the external fixator, let us first see how biomechanics influences the selection of a suitable type of frame.

**Fig. 26 a–d.** The unilateral compression frame.

**a** The erected unilateral compression frame. The screws are prestressed in compression, and a uniform axial pressure is applied across the fracture. **b** During weight bearing the compression across the fracture increases with the amount of weight borne. **c** A distracting force will nullify the compression only if its magnitude equals that of the compressive force produced by prestressing of the frame. **d** If the distracting force exceeds the prestressing force, the fracture will gape, and axial alignment will deteriorate

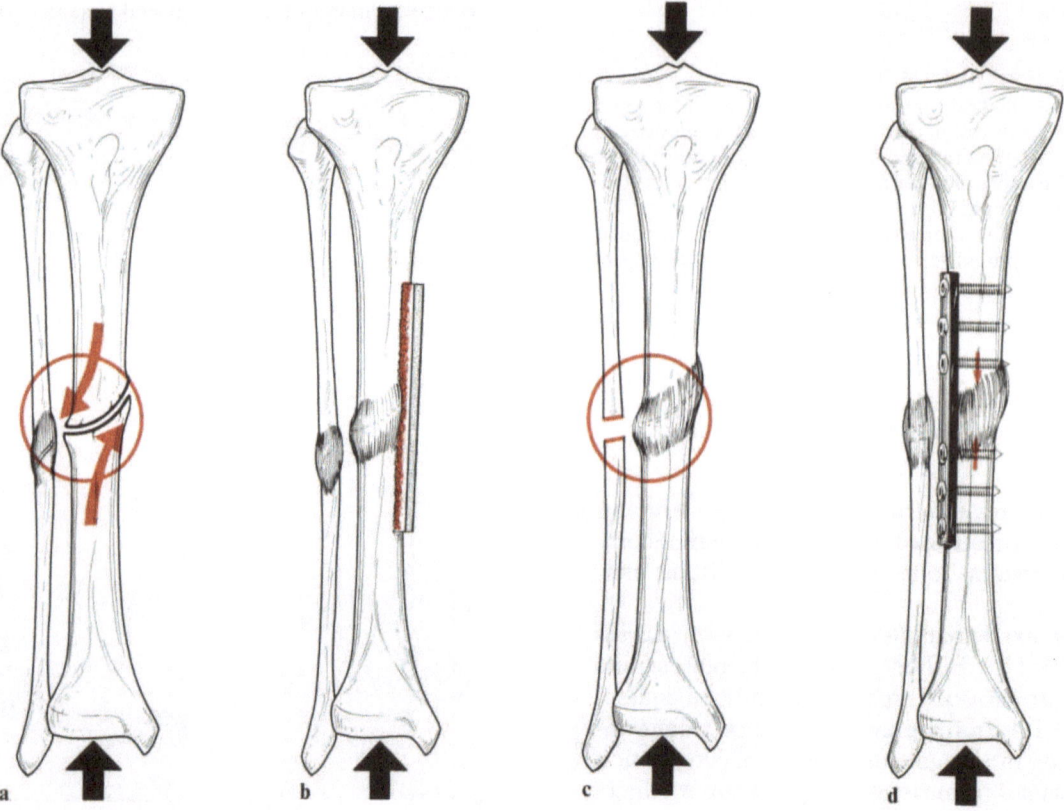

## 2.4 Biomechanics and Selection of the Frame

PAUWELS has pointed to the causative role of "pivotal bending" in failures of osseous union, citing the tibial nonunion as an example.

Three methods are available for correcting the "pivotal bending" effect and thus promoting consolidation of the nonunion (Fig. 28):

- *Bridge grafting* (SCHLÖSSMANN, PAUWELS, MCFARLAND)
- *Fibular osteotomy* (BÖHLER)
- *Tension band fixation* (MÜLLER, WEBER and CECH).

In each case shear motion at the bone ends is eliminated so that the nonunion comes under pure axial compression. The *absence of disruptive forces* (shear, bending, torsion) is the *mechanical prerequisite* for the healing of nonunions as well as fractures, osteotomies and arthrodeses, regardless of the nature of the treatment (plaster, internal fixation, external fixation).

Given the fact that axial compression is desirable while shear and other disruptive forces are not, we can draw the following conclusions with regard to frame selection:

- When the *fragments are not in contact,* a bilateral frame is required.

**Fig. 28 a–d.** Pivotal bending. **a** In a tibial fracture with an intact fibula or a fibular fracture that has healed quickly, the fibula may act as a "pivot" for the tibial fragments, which move relative to each other (bending, shear, overriding) when weight is borne. **b** Bridge graft. **c** Fibular osteotomy (to remove the eccentric pivot). **d** Tension-band plate

- When the *fragments are in contact,* a unilateral frame is sufficient.

In both situations the compressive stresses associated with loading are absorbed by two pillars:
- When the fragments are not in contact, the two pillars consist of *metal only* (Fig. 29).
- When the fragments are in contact, the *bone* forms one of the pillars (Fig. 30).

If a *unilateral frame* is used *in the absence of bone contact,* the resulting mechanical configuration is like that which PAUWELS holds responsible for tibial nonunion. Pivotal bending and shear at the fracture site hamper bone healing (Fig. 31).

When a bilateral frame is used *in the presence of bone contact,* the resulting stability is more than adequate, and a unilateral frame would suffice (Fig. 32).

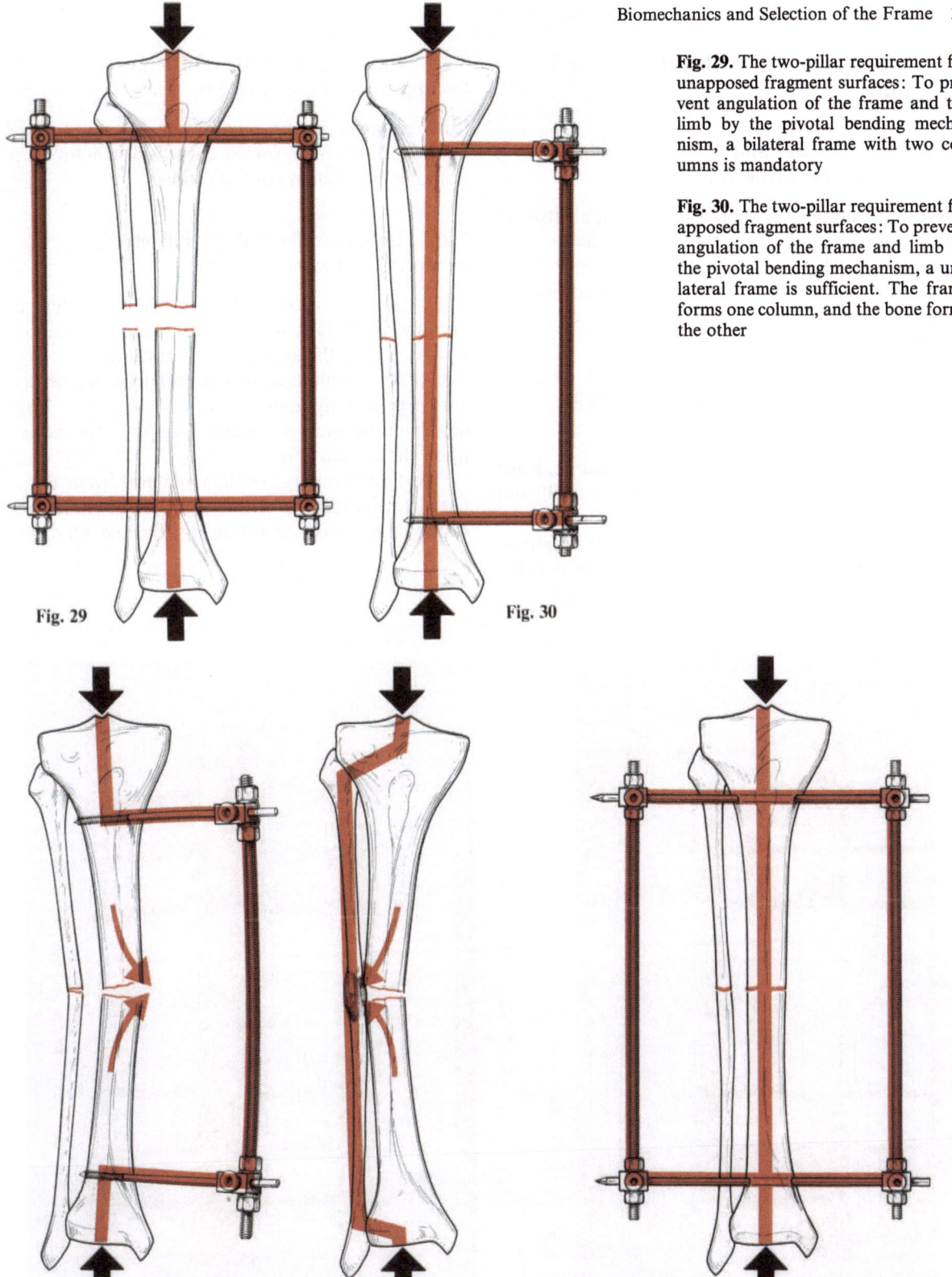

**Fig. 29.** The two-pillar requirement for unapposed fragment surfaces: To prevent angulation of the frame and the limb by the pivotal bending mechanism, a bilateral frame with two columns is mandatory

**Fig. 30.** The two-pillar requirement for apposed fragment surfaces: To prevent angulation of the frame and limb by the pivotal bending mechanism, a unilateral frame is sufficient. The frame forms one column, and the bone forms the other

**Fig. 31 a, b.** The unilateral frame without interfragmental contact. **a** Weight bearing causes pivotal motion at the fracture, with the fixation device as the pivot. **b** The situation is analogous to that in which the fibula acts as a pivot for tibial fracture motion

**Fig. 32.** The "extravagance" of a bilateral frame with interfragmental contact. In this configuration the two-column principle is more than satisfied, with the bone (tibia) providing one load-bearing column, and the frame providing two

# 3 Stress Transfer with the External Fixator

## 3.1 Stress Transfer with the Neutralization and Lengthening Frame (Fig. 33)

When the bone ends are not in contact, all stresses are transferred through the external fixator, regardless of whether a unilateral or bilateral frame is used. The frame is the sole load-bearing member, for it bridges a zone that is not stress-competent.

## 3.2 Stress Transfer in the Presence of Bone Contact

With both the unilateral and bilateral frame, some stress is transferred through the device itself, but most is transmitted through the bone. Because the frame neutralizes disruptive forces (bending, shear, torsion, distraction), stabilizing compression is the only force acting on the bone ends.

### 3.2.1 Stress Transfer with a Bilateral Compression Frame (Fig. 34)

Stress transfer in the bone-frame system is symmetrical. Disruptive forces, such as distraction, do not alter the system configuration.

### 3.2.2 Stress Transfer with a Unilateral Compression Frame (Fig. 35)

Stress transfer through the bone-frame system is asymmetrical. Disruptive forces, such as distraction, can alter the system configuration.

Some deformation of the unilateral frame occurs when compression is initially applied. This deformation increases when disruptive forces act upon the system (Fig. 36).

This disadvantage of the unilateral frame compared to the bilateral frame can be eliminated by employing one of the following *three countermeasures:*

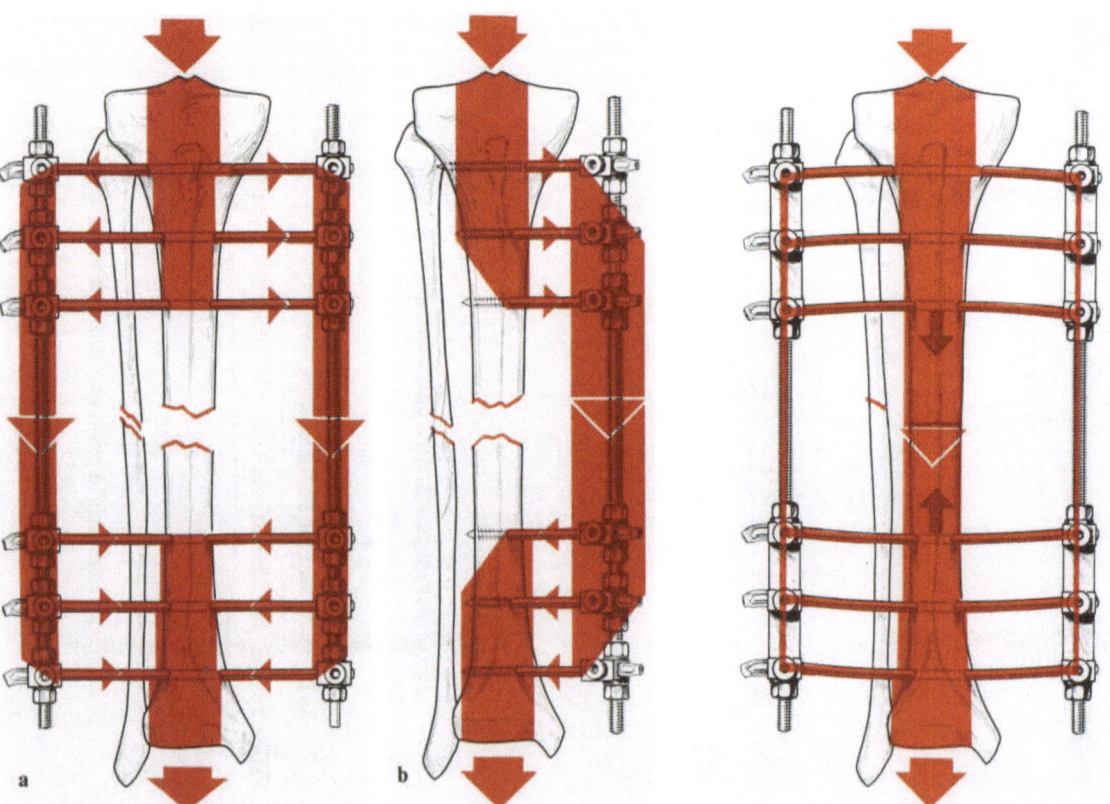

**Fig. 33 a, b.** Stress transfer with the neutralizing frame. Interfragmental contact is absent, and so all stresses are transmitted through the external frame

**Fig. 34.** Stress transfer with the bilateral compression frame. The bony column is the principal conduit for stress transfer. The frame stabilizes the fracture and neutralizes disruptive forces

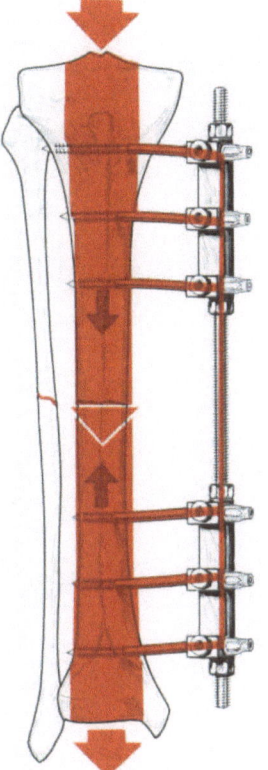

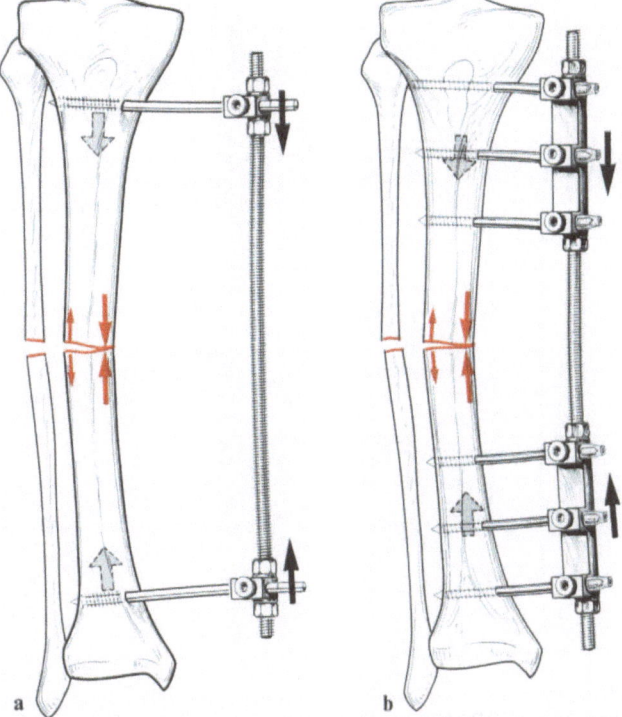

**Fig. 35.** Stress transfer with the unilateral compression frame. Most stresses are transferred through the bony column. The frame stabilizes the fracture and neutralizes disruptive forces, though less effectively than the bilateral frame

**Fig. 36 a, b.** Prestressing of the unilateral frame. **a** When primary stress (i.e., interfragmental compression) is applied, the frame is deformed, axial limb alignment is disturbed, and the fracture gapes on the side opposite the frame. Only the cortices adjacent to the frame are under compression. **b** Increasing the number of Schanz screws has no effect on this phenomenon

### 3.2.2.1 "Prebending" of the Rod

In internal fixation by compression plating, the stability of the fixation is increased by "prebending" the plate so that interfragmental pressure is distributed evenly over the cross-section of the bone. Without this prebending, only the cortex directly adjacent to the plate would come under compression, while the fracture or osteotomy line on the opposite side would gape, and the plate would tend to bend away from the bone axis (PERREN) (Fig. 37).

The "prebending" principle is also applicable to the unilateral frame (Fig. 38):

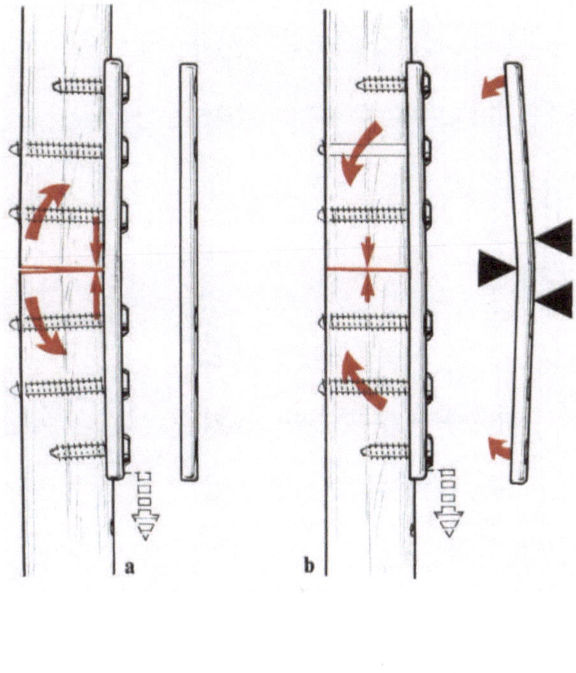

**Fig. 37 a, b.** "Prebending" of a compression plate. **a** The application of a flat compression plate, such as a DCP, causes the fracture line to gape opposite the plate. **b** The same compression plate, when "prebent" before application, prevents this gaping and provides uniform axial compression across the fracture surfaces

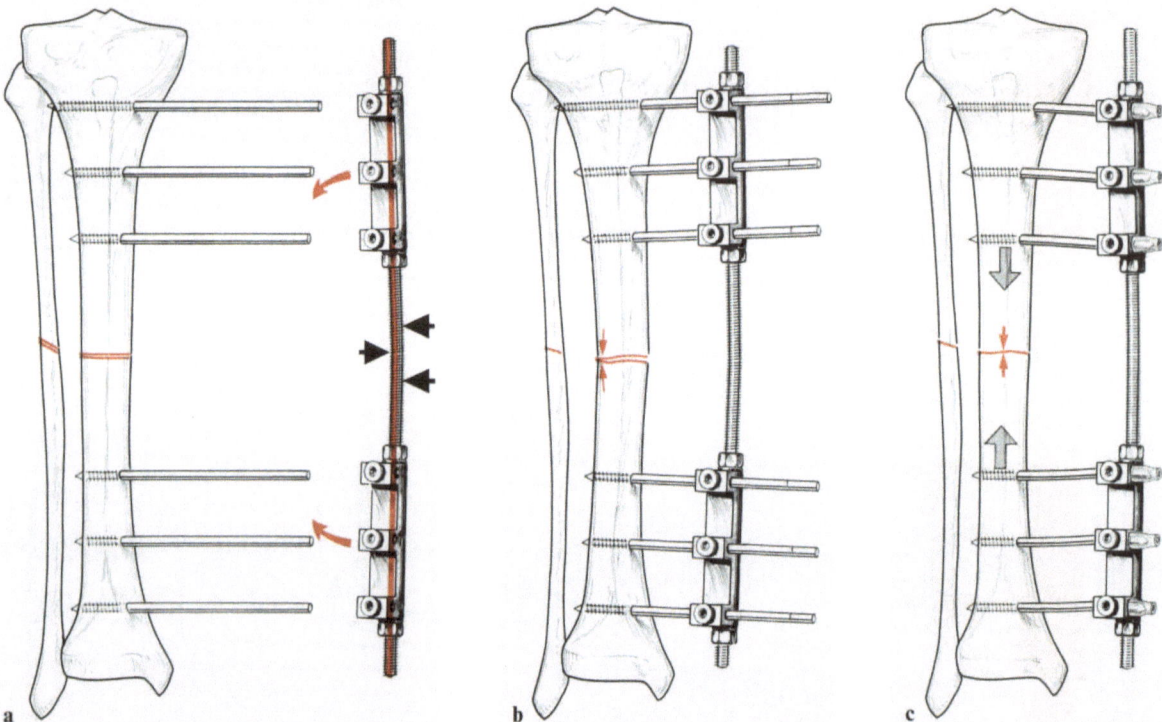

**Fig. 38 a–c.** "Prebending" the rod of a unilateral frame. **a** Like the compression plate, the rod is "prebent" before it is applied. **b** Before compression is initiated, the fracture gapes adjacent to the rod. **c** As compression is applied, the fracture line closes, and the angulation of the rod is reduced by elastic deformation. Interfragmental pressure is distributed evenly over the cross-section of the fracture

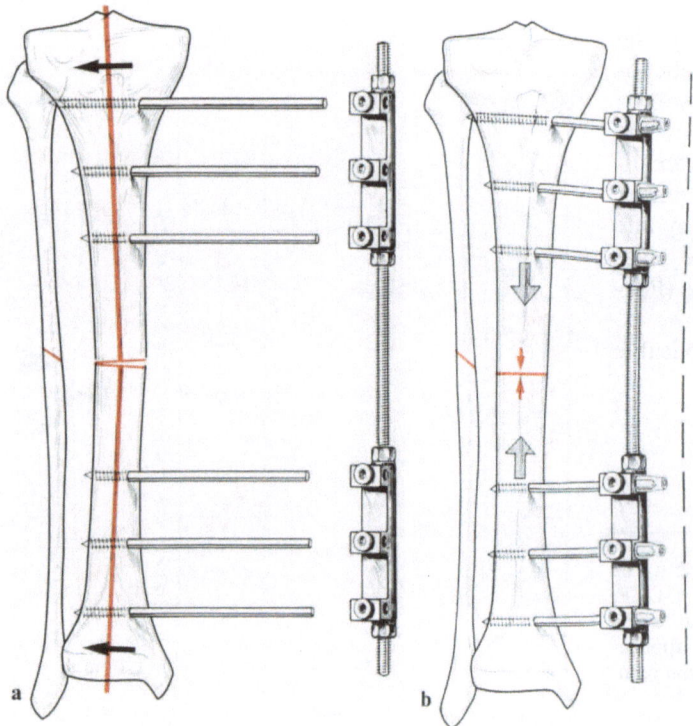

**Fig. 39 a, b.** "Prebending" of the bone for unilateral external fixation. **a** With the fragments angulated slightly, all the screws are inserted in a parallel array. **b** When interfragmental compression is applied with the frame, the axis of the bone straightens, and the gap adjacent to the rod is closed. Pressure is distributed evenly over the fracture cross-section. The rod is slightly elastically deformed

With the fragments reduced, the Schanz screws (threaded half pins) are inserted parallel and at right angles to the long axis of the bone. Before the rod is mounted, it is prebent to a 5° angle. When the rod is mounted the fracture line near the rod will gape initially, but it will close as the clamps and screws are approximated. The associated elastic deformation of the rod will ensure compression of the opposite cortex.

### 3.2.2.2 "Prebending" of the Bone (Fig. 39)

With the fragments held in slight angulation, the Schanz screws are inserted parallel to one another such that the fracture gapes adjacent to the rod. When compression is initiated, the rod is straight. But as compression is increased, the rod will bend, the bone axis straighten, closing the fracture line adjacent to the rod. As a result, the entire fracture surface is brought under axial compression.

### 3.2.2.3 Axial Compression with a "Spreading Rod" (Fig. 40)

With the fragments reduced, the Schanz screws are inserted parallel and at right angles to the long axis of the bone. One rod is mounted near the skin and exerts no compression; it serves only to maintain apposition of the fragments. Interfragmental compression is provided by a second rod mounted farther outward from the bone. This rod is used to apply a distracting force to the protruding ends of the screws. This causes an elastic deformation of the screws, whose spring tension exerts compression across the fracture site.

All of these methods are equally effective in ensuring uniform compression across a fracture.

The "spreading rod" technique is the simplest of the three. The reduction of the fragments is not disturbed during construction of the frame. The main disadvantage is the need for a second rod, which increases the overall size of the frame and thus may prove more objectionable to the patient.

The techniques involving "prebending" of the rod or bone are more difficult, because accurate reduction of the fragments is temporarily lost during erection of the frame. The advantage is that only one rod is required, and so the overall frame size is kept to a minimum.

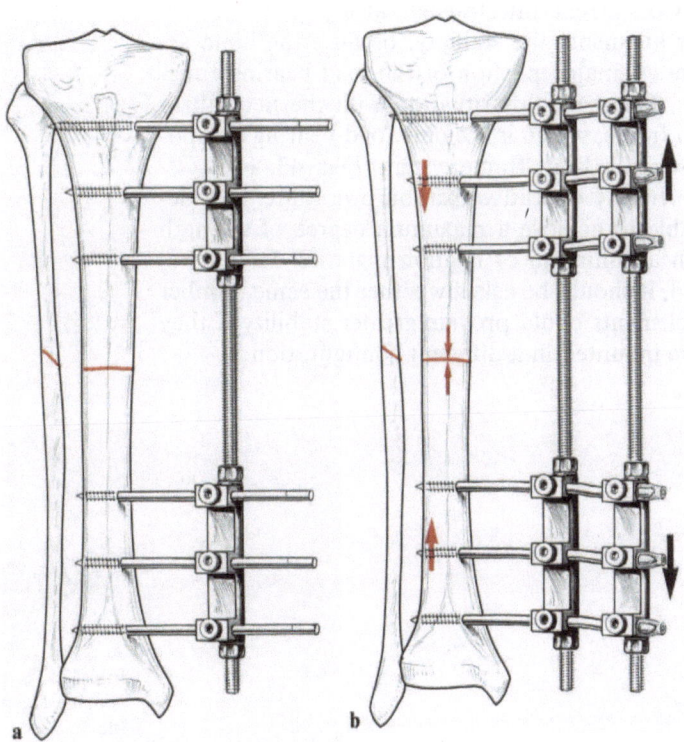

**Fig. 40 a, b.** The use of a spreading rod on a unilateral frame. **a** With the fragments anatomically reduced, the unilateral frame is erected without compression. **b** Interfragmental compression is produced by mounting a 2nd rod which distracts the ends of the screws

# 4 Means of Augmenting the Stability of the External Fixator

### 4.1 Increasing the Number of Pins or Screws

The placement of multiple pins or screws in each fragment increases the resistance of the bone-frame system to AP angulation. This resistance is equivalent to the bending strength of the external rods. Hence, the bilateral frame, with its pair of rods, is always superior to the single-rod unilateral frame.

### 4.2 Placement of the Pins and Screws
(Figs. 41, 42)

Poor stability results if the pins or screws are placed too far from the fracture site and are clustered too close together. A stable fixation results when the pins in each fragment are spaced as far apart as possible.

### 4.3 Increasing the Number of Rods

By increasing the number of rods comprising the frame, the total stability of the bone-frame system is increased, especially in terms of AP angulation. The frame also becomes more resistant to torsion, thus increasing the interfragmental torsion strength.

Concurrent interfragmental compression further augments the stability, because the bone assumes a major portion of the load-bearing function. Compare this situation with the neutralization frame, which is the only load-bearing component of the bone-frame system (Figs. 43, 44).

In any operative fixation procedure, it is desirable to achieve a maximum degree of strength with a minimum of fixation material. In that regard, it should be asked whether the same number of elements could provide greater stability if they were mounted in a different configuration.

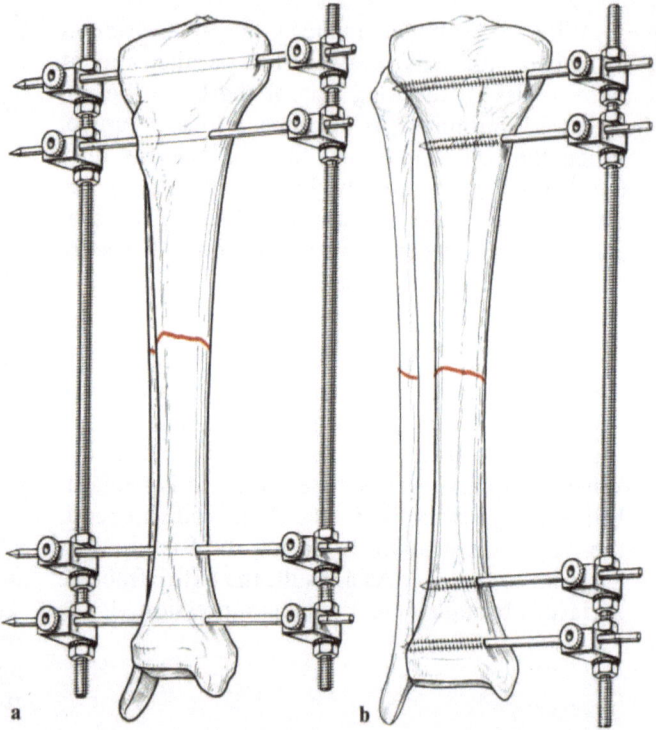

**Fig. 41 a, b.** Unstable pin placement. The farther the pins are placed from the fracture site, and the closer they are clustered together, the less stable the fracture

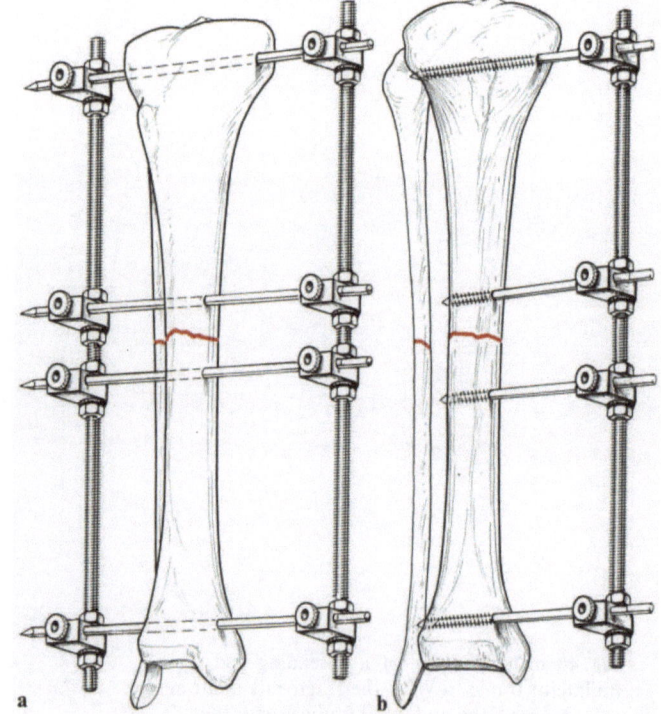

**Fig. 42 a, b.** Stable pin placement. Stability is enhanced by spacing the pins within each fragment as far apart as possible

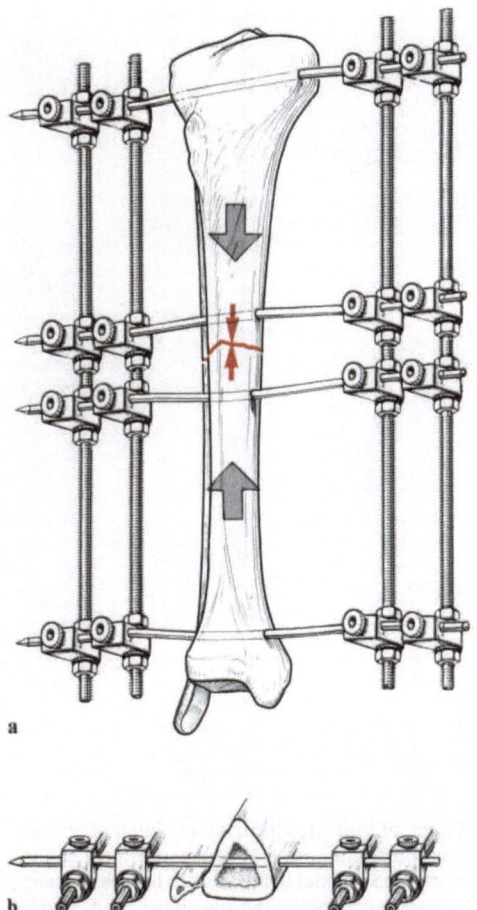

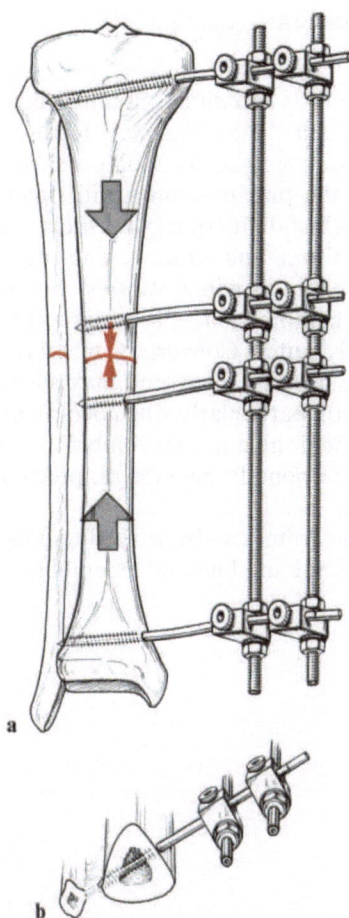

**Fig. 43 a, b.** Effect of rod number on bilateral frame stability. **a** The greater the number of rods, the greater the stability. **b** Sample arrangement of 4 rods in a common plane

**Fig. 44 a, b.** Effect of rod number of unilateral frame stability. **a** The greater the number of rods, the greater the stability. **b** Sample arrangement of 2 rods in one plane

## 4.4 The Double-Frame Configuration
(Figs. 45, 46)

Two or more rods can all be mounted in a single plane to create a "stiffer frame." Rods that are mounted in mirror-image fashion on each side of the plane of the pins or screws will significantly enhance the AP stability of the assembly ("double cadre" after VIDAL and ADREY). The rods are no longer exposed to bending stresses, but only to tension and compression – a pattern for which metal is ideally suited. Conversely, metal is vulnerable to cyclic bending loads and may succumb to fatigue fracture, particularly when bent in opposite directions. The double frame, combined with prestressing of the bone-frame system, precludes this complication.

The double frame can be utilized to good effect in both unilateral and bilateral assemblies.

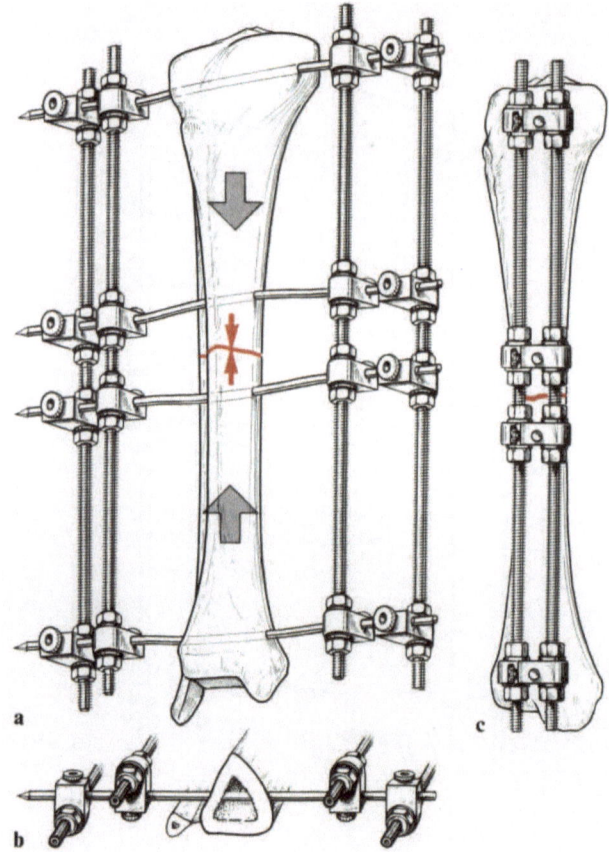

**Fig. 45 a–c.** Effect of rod arrangement on bilateral frame stability. **a** Four-rod frame with a biomechanically ideal pin placement, prestressed in axial compression. **b** Arrangement of the rods: 2 rods anterior to the pin plane, and 2 rods posterior to the pin plane. **c** Viewed from the side, the two rods form a second frame. The whole assembly is called a "double frame," therefore

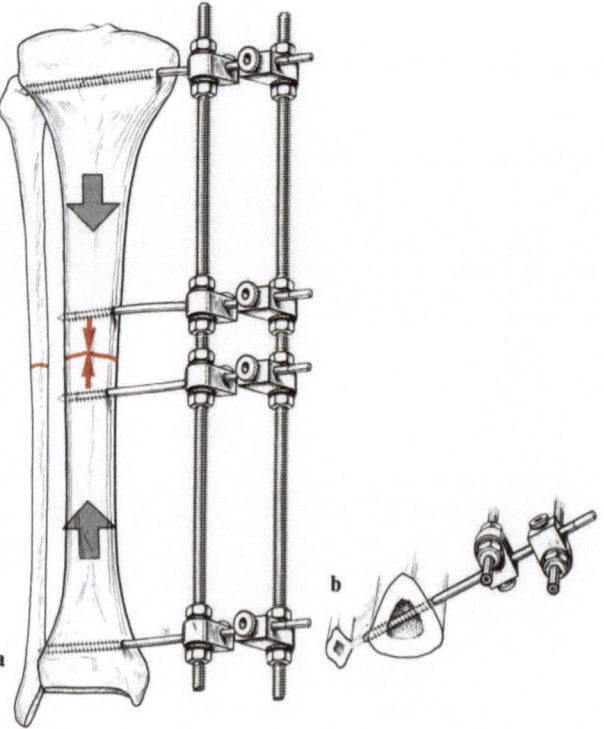

**Fig. 46 a, b.** Effect of rod arrangement on unilateral frame stability. **a** Two-rod frame with a biomechanically ideal screw placement, prestressed in axial compression. **b** Arrangement of the rods: 1 rod anterior, 1 rod posterior to the screw plane, analogous to Fig. 45 b

### 4.5 The Biplanar Frame (Figs. 47, 48)

We have seen that one means of preventing AP angulation of the bone-frame system is by fortifying the frame itself. Another method is to mount a second frame perpendicular to the first to create a "biplanar" configuration. This could be done, for example, by combining a unilateral and bilateral frame on the tibia, or two unilateral frames on the femur (WEBER and CECH).

The unilateral and bilateral frame configurations presented above are only a sample of the designs that can be created. In every case it should be possible to construct a framework that will provide the desired degree of stability, assuming that the pins or screws can gain adequate purchase in the bone. Bone purchase is not a major concern in situations where the bone ends are well apposed or fixed under axial compression, for in this case the metal is not the only load-bearing member of the bone-frame system. Indeed, the bone bears the major portion of the loads, while the fixator serves only to neutralize disruptive forces (bending, angulation, shear, torsion).

The biomechanical situation is far less favorable in the lengthening and neutralization modes. Here stresses are not transferred directly from one fragment to the next, but only indirectly through the external frame. Stress transfer from bone to metal occurs only at bone-pin interfaces. These points represent sites of extreme stress concentration, and thus form sites of predilection for loosening. This is why the pin anchorage in the bone is so crucial to the success of the fixation.

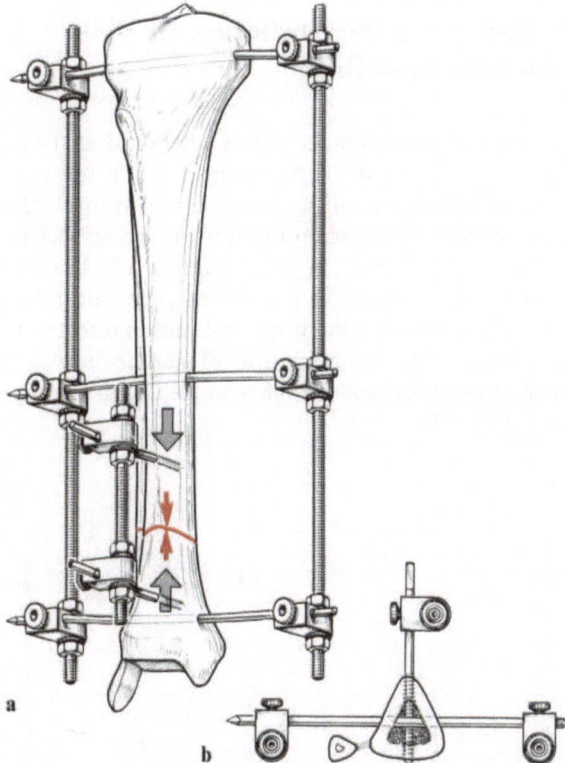

**Fig. 47 a, b.** Combination of two frames on the tibia. **a** The integration of a short fragment into the bone-frame system is ensured by erecting two frames in a biplanar array. **b** A cross-sectional view shows the mutually perpendicular arrangement of the bilateral and unilateral frames

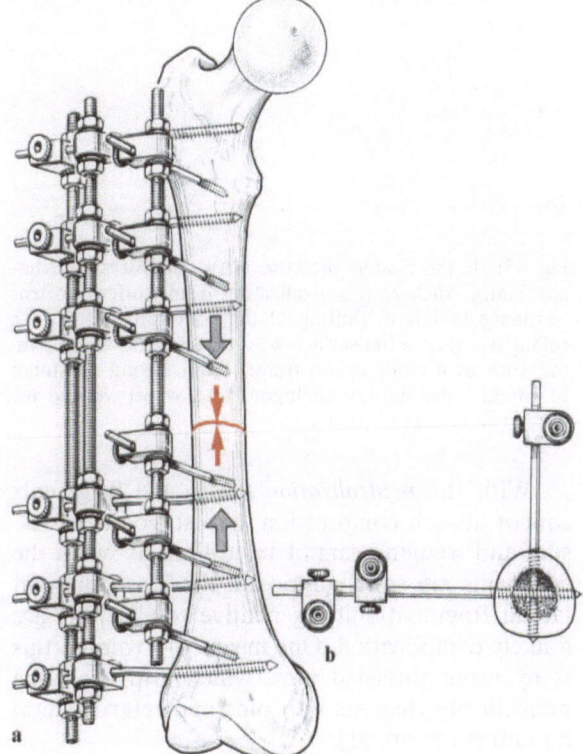

**Fig. 48 a, b.** Combination of two frames on the femur. **a** Two unilateral frames erected on the femur. The lateral frame mounted in the frontal plane has a second rod to augment stability. **b** In cross-section the mutually perpendicular arrangement of the unilateral frames is seen

## 5 Improving the Anchorage of Pins and Screws in Bone

Steinmann pins remain firmly anchored in bone as long as pressure is maintained along the pin-bone interface, as in the compression frame. The contact pressure is manifested by an elastic deformation of the pins. In this situation the bone is "wedged" between the transfixing pins, and lateral motion between the bone and pins is effectively prevented. This combination of *contact pressure and wedging* provides a highly stable frame anchorage (Fig. 49).

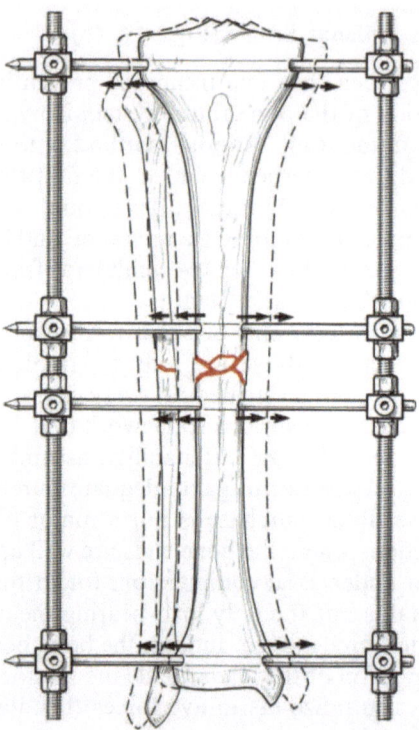

**Fig. 50.** Absence of contact pressure in a neutralization frame. The main fragments can shift back and forth on the parallel "rails," the transfixing pins

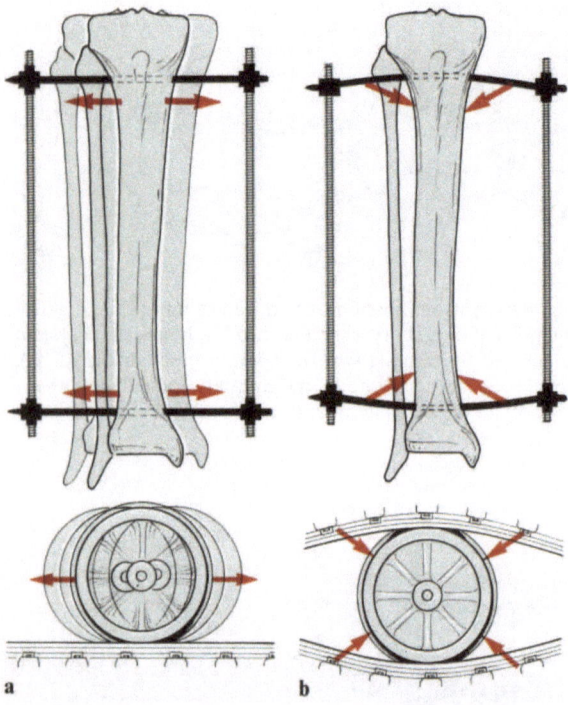

**Fig. 49 a, b.** Pin contact pressure. **a** An unprestressed external fixator, such as a neutralization frame, offers no true resistance to lateral shifting of the bone, analogous to a rolling wheel on a flat surface. **b** A prestressed external fixator, such as a compression frame, offers strong resistance to lateral bone shifting analogous to a wheel wedged between two concave surfaces

With the *neutralization frame*, the fragments cannot absorb compression, and so contact pressure and wedging cannot be utilized as when the fragments are solidly apposed. Pin loosening and lateral fragment shifting relative to the pins are a likely complication. One means of avoiding this is by using threaded pins, which grip the bone more firmly than smooth pins and retard lateral motion (Figs. 50, 51).

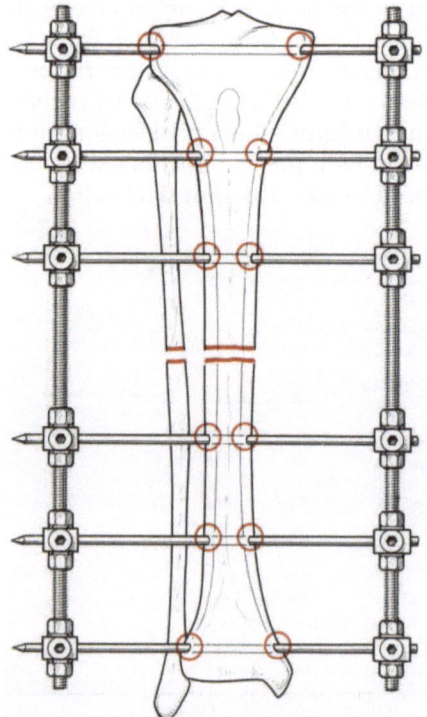

**Fig. 51.** Absence of contact pressure and pin number. Increasing the number of transfixing pins does not alter the fact that contact pressure is absent, and will not prevent lateral shifting of the fragments

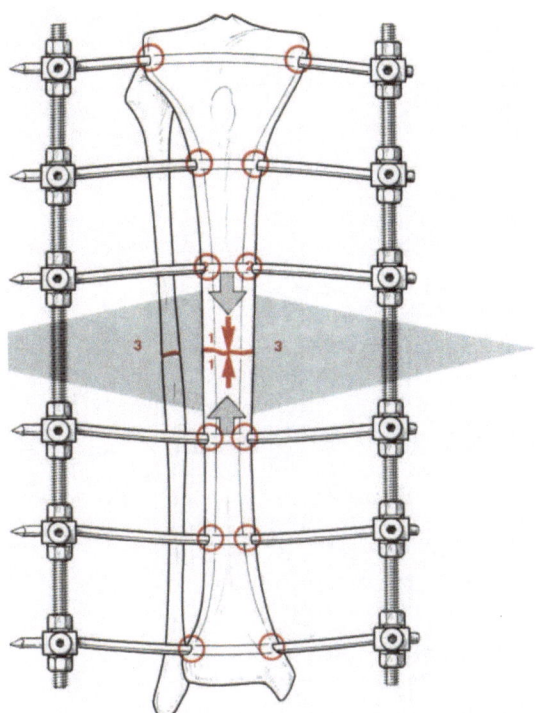

**Fig. 52.** Pin contact pressure and wedging of the fragments in a compression frame. Prestressing of the bilateral frame creates the following stabilizing factors: *1* interfragmental compression; *2* pin contact pressure; *3* wedging of the fragments

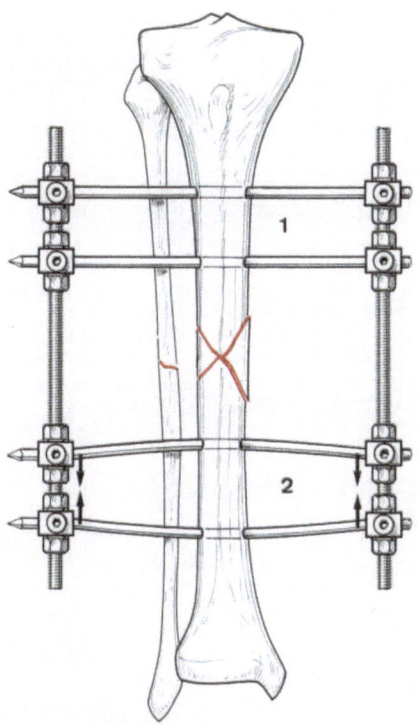

**Fig. 53.** Prestressing the pins within a fragment. *1* The pins in the proximal fragment are parallel, and there is no contact pressure at the bone-pin interface. Lateral shifting of the fragment is a real danger. *2* The pins in the distal fragment are prestressed relative to each other. Contact pressure and wedging prevent lateral fragment shifting

Both *contact pressure and wedging,* which automatically are present in the compression mode (Fig. 52), can also be utilized in the *neutralization mode.* In this case, however, the contact pressure and wedging are produced not across the fracture site, but *within the individual fragments* (Fig. 53).

The compressive strength of the individual fragments is exploited by *prestressing* adjacent pins relative to each other. This produces a contact pressure and pin deformation which inhibit pin shifting and loosening in the involved fragment and stabilize the anchorage. Prestressing is done by moving the ends of adjacent pins either toward or away from each other. In terms of stabilizing effect, it does not matter whether the *pins are prestressed in compression or distraction* (Fig. 54). We have encountered no clinical problems with either method, and each is equally satisfactory.

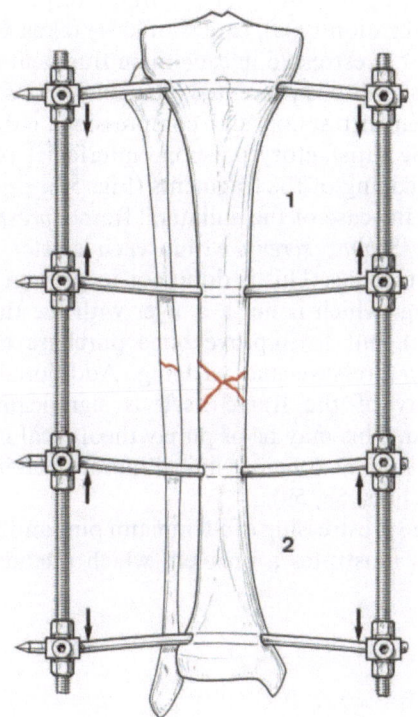

**Fig. 54.** Prestressing of pins by compression or distraction. *1* The proximal pair of pins is prestressed in compression. *2* The distal pair of pins is prestressed in distraction. Both techniques produce stabilizing contact pressure and wedging

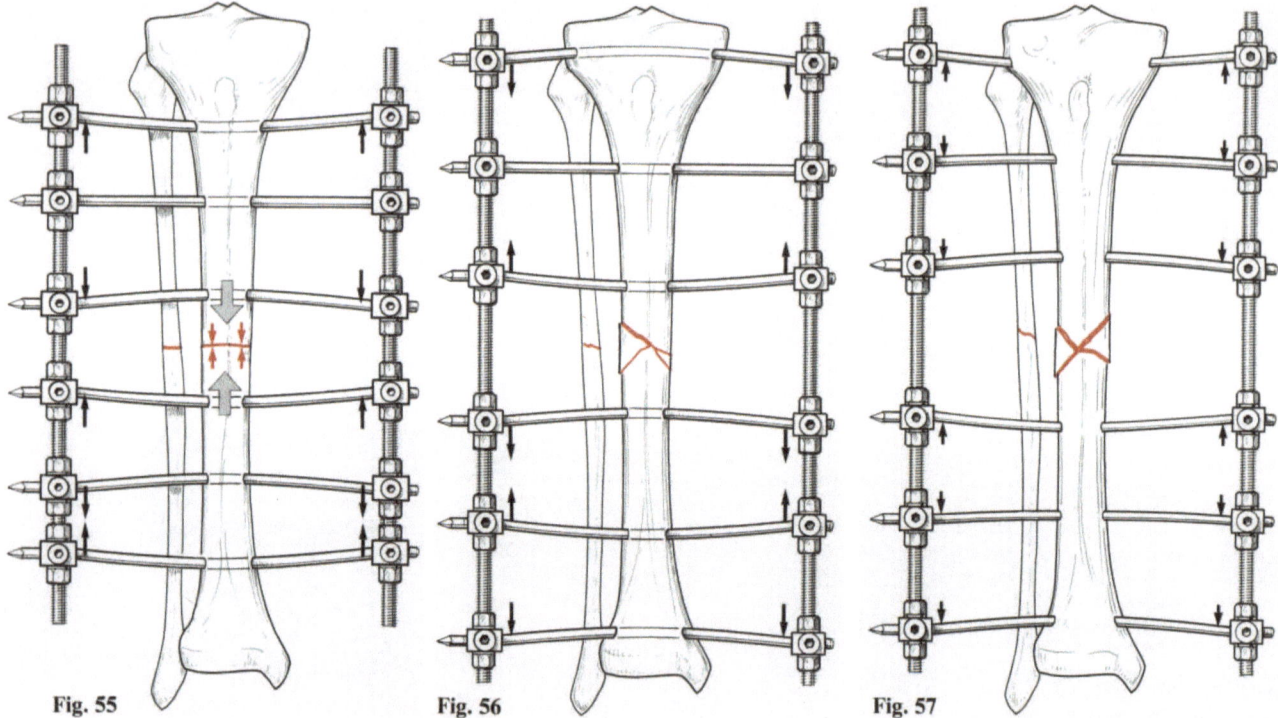

Fig. 55                          Fig. 56                          Fig. 57

*Pin stabilization by prestressing* is not only recommended for the neutralization frame, but is also advantageous for the compression frame (Fig. 55).

In clusters of more than two pins, it is sufficient to prestress one pair of adjacent pins in compression or distraction (Fig. 56).

During mounting of the frame (especially the neutralization type), care should be taken that the pins are prestressed in each main fragment so that pin instability is prevented. One may choose freely between distraction and compression; either will provide satisfactory pin-bone interfacial pressure and wedging of the fragments (Fig. 57).

In the case of the unilateral frame, *prestressing of the Schanz screws* within each cluster is also advantageous. This is done not to prevent lateral shifting (which is not a danger with the threaded screws), but to improve bone purchase through contact pressure and wedging. Additionally, the stability of the frame itself is significantly enhanced. This may be of purely theoretical interest, but it may also be of clinical importance in some cases (Figs. 58, 59).

The prestressing of Steinmann pins and Schanz screws illustrates a problem which attends every

**Fig. 55.** Prestressing the pins in a compression frame. The pins in each cluster are prestressed in compression or distraction so as to exert pressure across the fracture site

**Fig. 56.** Prestressing the pins in a neutralization frame. The pins in each cluster are prestressed in compression or distraction

**Fig. 57.** Prestressing the pins in a neutralization frame. The individual prestressing of adjacent pins (in compression or distraction) is utilized to protect the fracture from axial displacement

operative fixation: the implant itself is far less important than the manner in which the implant performs its function. An attempt should be made to utilize every implant to its fullest capacity so that a minimum of material can be used. This reflects the fundamental biomechanical principle of Wolff and Pauwels – that of maximum material economy, as we observe in living bone. We speak of the "minimax" principle: *minimum* input for *maximum* effect.

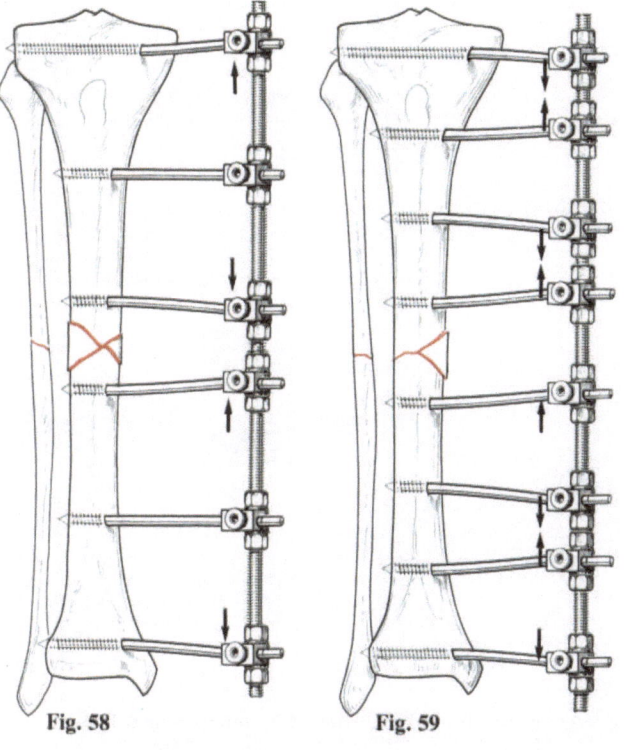

Fig. 58                              Fig. 59

**Fig. 58.** Prestressing the screws in a unilateral neutralization frame. The pins in each cluster are prestressed so as to maintain the position of the fragments

**Fig. 59.** Prestressing the screws in a unilateral neutralization frame in compression or distraction. The screws in the proximal and distal fragments are moved toward or away from each other to prestress the system

# 6 Restoring the Compressive Strength of Bone in the Absence of Interfragmental Contact

As we said earlier, interfragmental contact is favorable for external fixation, for it permits the creation of a prestressed, highly stable system in which a minimum amount of metal is used. Also, consolidation of the discontinuity is less problematic than when the bone ends are unapposed. Cases of the latter type require a more complex frame for their stabilization, and secondary procedures (cancellous bone grafting) are generally needed to bridge the bone defect. Fragments that are apposed heal more rapidly than fragments that are displaced or separated by a true defect. It is essential, therefore, that bone contact be restored without delay.

## 6.1 Restoring Bone Contact by Shortening
(Figs. 60–63)

In many arthrodeses, osteotomies and acute fractures with a short comminuted zone, a mild degree of shortening is tolerated in the interest of restoring bone contact. The same applies to certain septic nonunions in which length-preserving surgery has been unsuccessful.

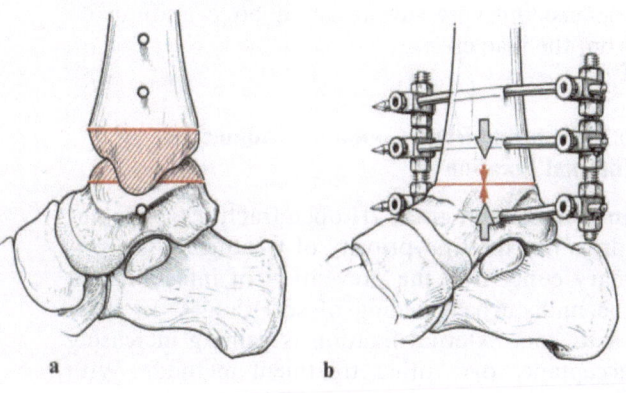

**Fig. 60 a, b.** Bone contact in an arthrodesis. **a** Extent of ankle joint resection. **b** Compression of the arthrodesis with a bilateral compression frame

**Fig. 61 a, b.** Restoring bone contact in an osteotomy by shortening. **a** Varus intertrochanteric osteotomy with wedge resection in a child. **b** Compression of the osteotomy with a unilateral compression frame

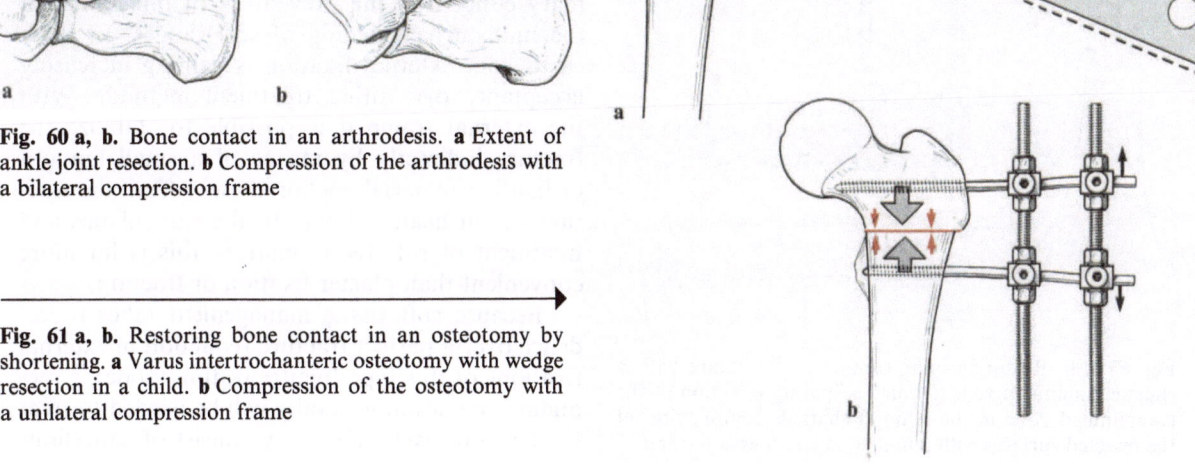

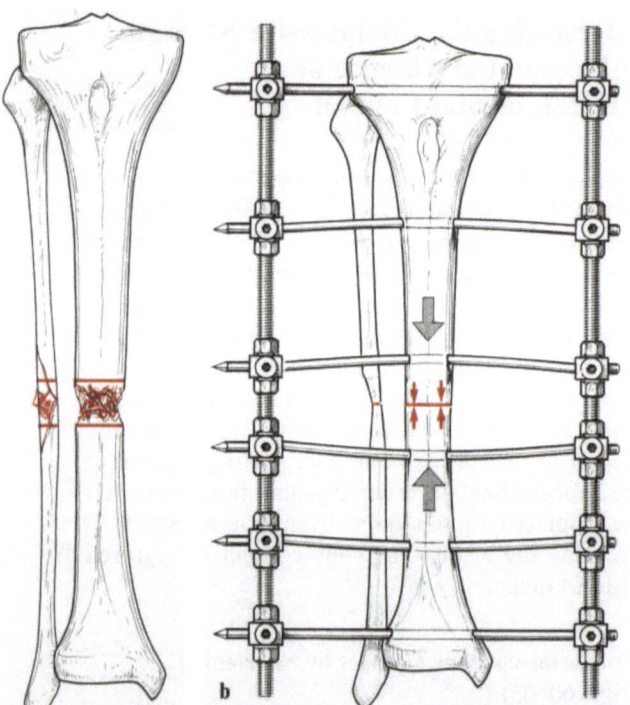

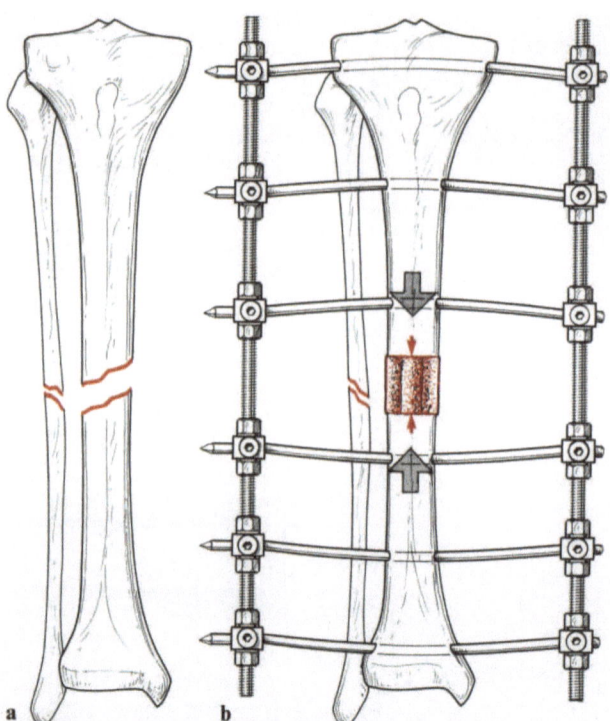

Fig. 62 a, b. Restoring bone contact in a fracture with a short comminuted zone (tibia). a Sparing resection of the comminuted zone in the tibial shaft. b Compression of the resected surfaces with a bilateral compression frame. A mild degree of limb shortening results

Fig. 64 a, b. Restoring bone contact by interposing a bone graft. a Nonunion associated with an osseous defect. b Managed by sparing transverse resection of the bone ends and interposition of pressure-resistant grafts. Compression with a bilateral frame

### 6.2 Restoring Bone Contact by Interposing a Pressure-Resistant Bone Graft (Fig. 64)

The gap is bridged by the interposition of a corticocancellous, pressure-resistant bone graft taken from the iliac crest.

### 6.3 Restoring Bone Contact by Adjunctive Internal Fixation

In grade II and grade III open fractures, bone union is not the first priority of treatment. The primary concern is the prevention of infection and the undisturbed healing of soft tissues. In these cases, too, external fixation is gaining increasing acceptance over other treatment methods. With the external frame it is possible to stabilize the fracture indirectly by means of a small amount of fixation material anchored away from the fracture site in healthy bone. In the surveillance and treatment of soft tissue injuries, this is far more convenient than plaster fixation or traction.

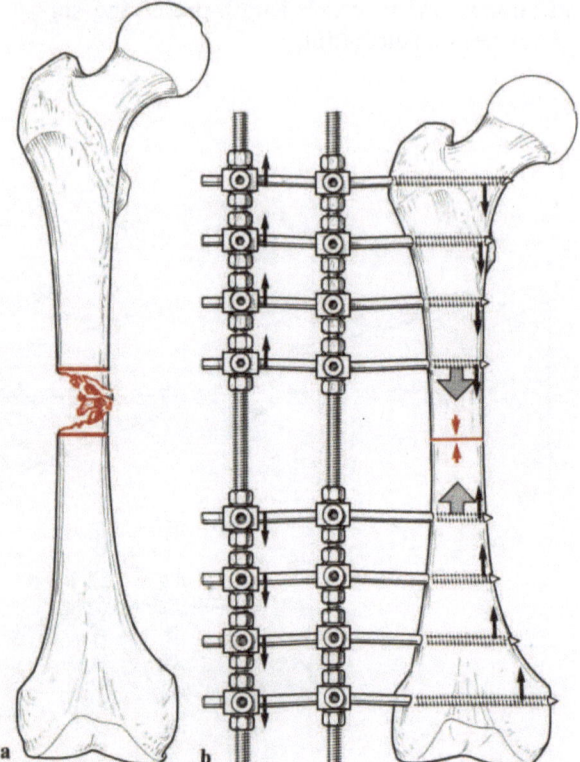

Fig. 63 a, b. Restoring bone contact in a fracture with a short comminuted zone (femur). a Sparing resection of the comminuted zone in the femoral shaft. b Compression of the resected surfaces with a unilateral compression frame

Because soft tissue management takes precedence over a perfect fracture reduction in external fixations of this type (neutralization mode), a secondary operation generally will be needed to treat the fracture itself. This may consist of cancellous bone grafting or secondary internal fixation with a plate or intramedullary nail. But could secondary procedures be avoided through improved primary fracture care? We share the view of BURNY that the combination of external fixation and internal fixation is beneficial in many cases (BRUNNER and WEBER). After more than 10 years' experience with *minimal internal fixation and external fixation*, three pertinent observations can be made:

a) An anatomic *reduction of the fragments decreases troublesome "dead space"* and therefore aids in the *prevention of infection*.

b) An accurate fixation ensures a more rapid *vascularization of the fragments from the medullary cavity* than when the fragments are displaced. This also helps to *prevent infection* by permitting antibiotics to reach the endangered area from the medullary cavity.

c) *Bony union of the fracture is facilitated* by apposition of the fragments. While all fracture gaps cannot be closed at first attempt, secondary operations are needed less frequently, and when required, they generally are less involved. This shortens the time to healing.

On the negative side, internal fixation in unskilled hands can easily compound the traumatic insult to soft tissues and bone. The advantages of minimal internal fixation can be realized only through *extreme caution* and a *meticulous technique*. The *minimal internal fixations* described below have proved highly beneficial for restoring the *compressive strength* of a fracture primarily. It must be understood, however, that none of these internal fixations would be sufficient in and of itself and that each must be *"neutralized" by an external frame*.

### 6.3.1 Lag Screw plus External Fixation
### (Figs. 65, 66)

Interfragmental compression with a lag screw is appropriate only for large fragments that can be reduced and fixed without additional stripping of their periosteum. Small fragments that retain soft-tissue attachments are best left alone; as healing progresses they will behave as pedicle grafts and will help to stabilize the fracture. Conversely, fragments in an open fracture that have been denuded of periosteum are potential sequestra. They should be removed and replaced with autogenous cancellous bone, which is far more receptive to vascular ingrowth and can survive an infection.

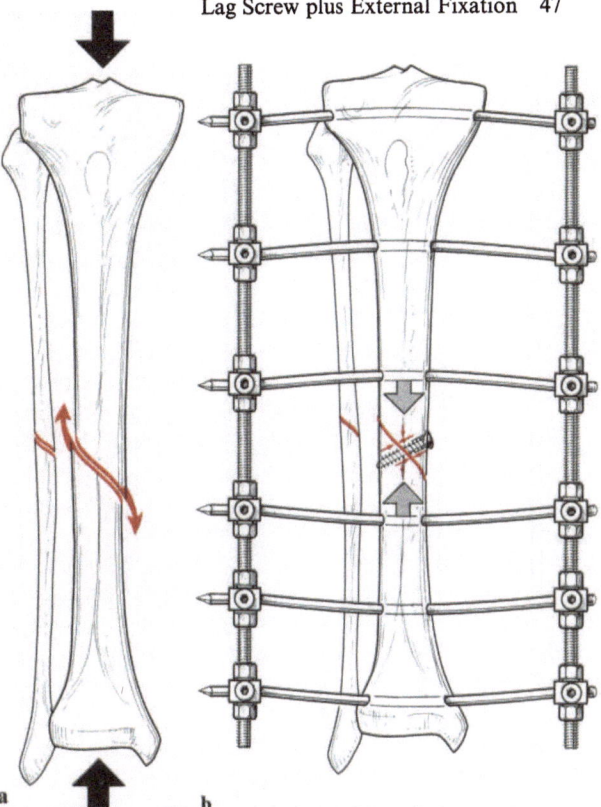

**Fig. 65 a, b.** Minimal internal fixation as a supplement to external fixation. **a** Tibial fracture with a tendency to override. **b** Fracture fixed with a lag screw and neutralized with a bilateral compression frame

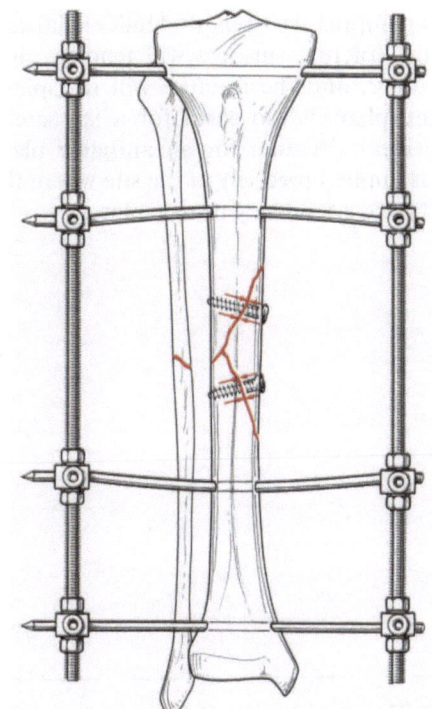

**Fig. 66.** Minimal internal fixation as a supplement to external fixation. Spiral fracture with a butterfly fragment. The fragment is fixed with lag screws, and the fracture is neutralized with a bilateral compression frame

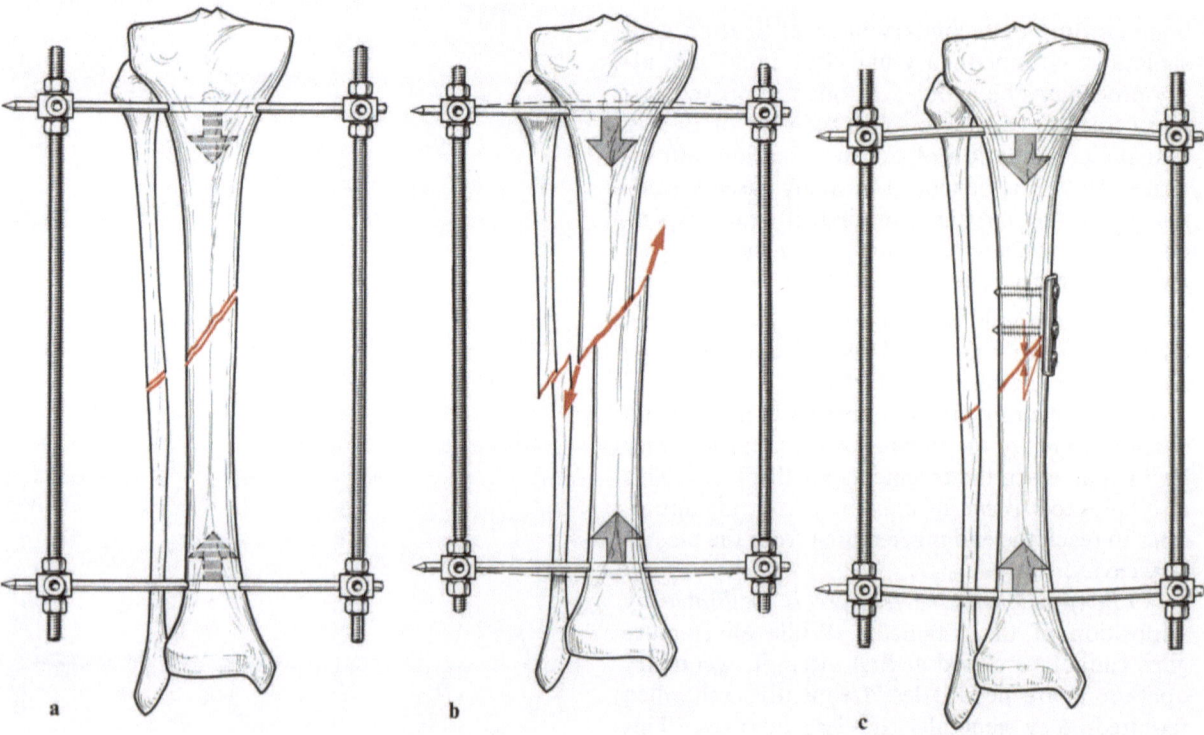

a                              b                              c

### 6.3.2 Antiglide Plate plus External Fixation (Figs. 67, 68)

With a short oblique fracture, reduction can restore contact between the bone ends, but it cannot afford compressive strength. Under axial compression the fracture surfaces will tend to glide past each other, and the fracture will redisplace. The fracture plane is too short for a lag screw. This is the ideal situation for an antiglide plate. The plate is applied precisely at the site where the fragments have a tendency to redisplace.

**Fig. 67 a–c.** The antiglide plate as an adjunct to external fixation. **a** The oblique fracture is reduced and "held" with a bilateral neutralizing frame. **b** If compression is applied in this situation, the fragments will tend to redisplace. **c** This is prevented by attaching a small "antiglide" plate across the fracture. Now it is possible to apply stabilizing compression

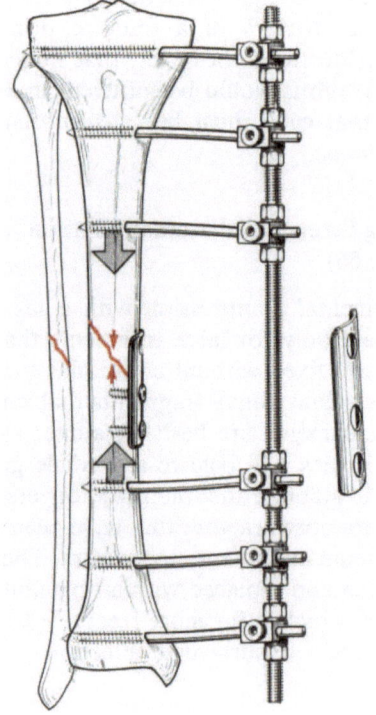

**Fig. 68.** The antiglide plate and type of frame. Owing to the presence of the antiglide plate, the oblique fracture is able to withstand compressive loading. This makes a bilateral frame unnecessary, and a unilateral frame will suffice

## 6.4 Restoring Bone Contact by Cancellous Bone Grafting

Losses of bone substance that would create an unacceptable degree of shortening are replaced by autogenous cancellous bone grafting. Under aseptic conditions (lengthening, tumor resection, resolved infection), internal fixation is carried out concurrently with the grafting (Fig. 69). In the presence of a septic defect, external fixation is required (Fig. 70).

While infection does not contraindicate bone grafting, it does make it more problematic. Occasionally the grafting will have to be repeated. The *success of the bone graft* depends almost entirely on whether it acquires a blood supply. This in turn is contingent on a *well perfused recipient bed* and an *absence of motion*. Thus, poorly perfused scar tissue and necrotic bone ends should be resected so that the graft will have an opportunity for vascular ingrowth from surrounding tissue.

Systematic, progressive loading of the operated extremity at 3–6 weeks after grafting is also important to the survival of the cancellous graft. Loading is essential to a favorable functional remodeling of the vascularized cancellous bone. Without this loading the grafts would be gradually resorbed (disuse atrophy or PAUWELS' principle of material economy).

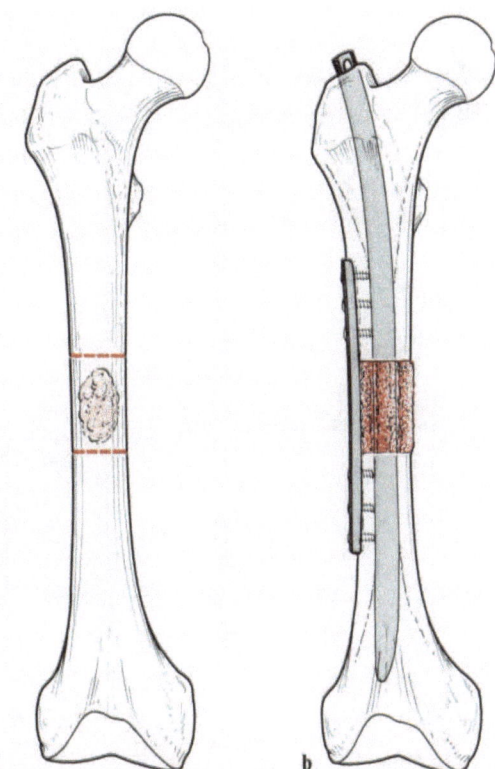

**Fig. 69 a, b.** Restoring bone contact by cancellous bone grafting and internal fixation. **a** Tumor (metastasis from hypernephroma) and extent of resection. **b** Intramedullary nail for rigidity, plate for neutralization, and cancellous bone for replacement of stock

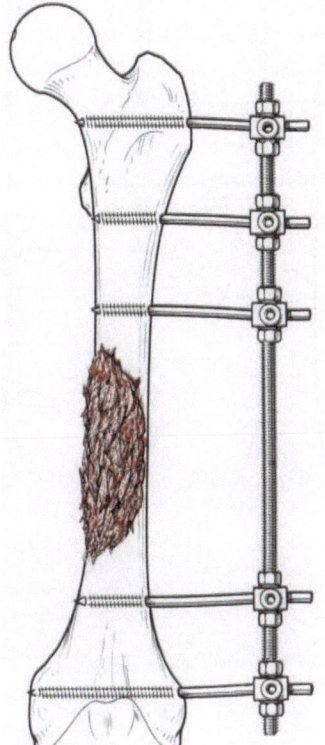

**Fig. 70.** Restoring bone contact by cancellous bone grafting and external fixation. Here an osteitis has been managed by sequestrectomy, cancellous bone grafting, and stabilization with an external frame

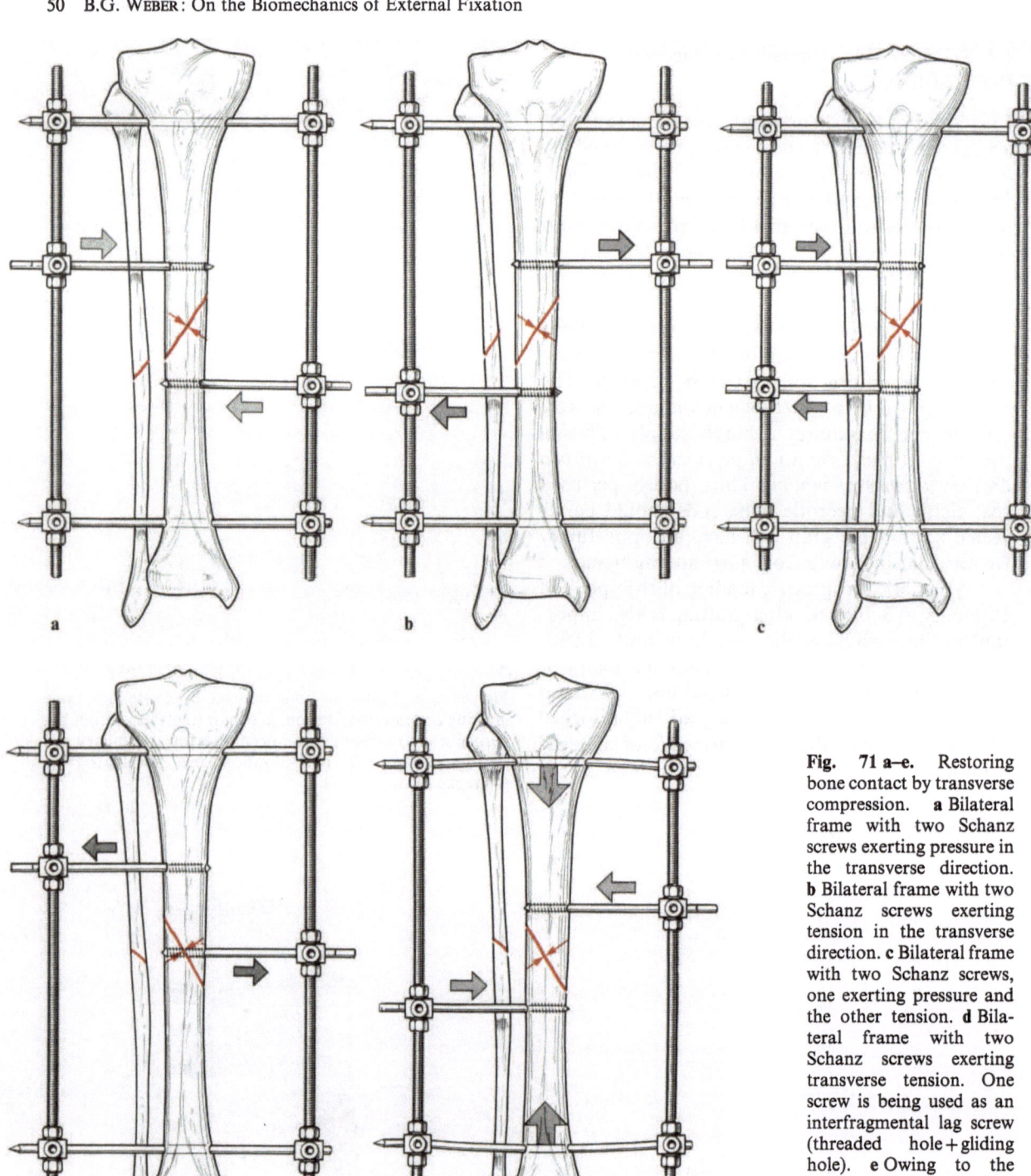

**Fig. 71 a–e.** Restoring bone contact by transverse compression. **a** Bilateral frame with two Schanz screws exerting pressure in the transverse direction. **b** Bilateral frame with two Schanz screws exerting tension in the transverse direction. **c** Bilateral frame with two Schanz screws, one exerting pressure and the other tension. **d** Bilateral frame with two Schanz screws exerting transverse tension. One screw is being used as an interfragmental lag screw (threaded hole + gliding hole). **e** Owing to the transverse compression, the bilateral frame can be utilized in the compression mode

## 6.5 Restoring Bone Contact by Transverse Compression

As we have seen, the classic pattern of interfragmental compression by an external frame is across a transverse discontinuity such as a transverse fracture, arthrodesis, osteotomy or nonunion.

With an oblique fragment plane, axial compression alone would cause the fragments to override. Frequently this can be prevented by adjunctive minimal internal fixation, usually with an antiglide plate. But if internal fixation cannot be used, external transverse compression offers an effective alternative (Fig. 71):

Compression across the oblique fragment plane is produced by means of supplementary Schanz screws which apply pressure or tension to one or both fragments. Contact is improved, and the bone-metal system is reinforced.

## 6.6 Restoring Bone Contact by Fragment Manipulation (Fig. 72)

In fractures with multiple fragments, minimal internal fixation is not always capable of restoring bony contact. Reduction is accomplished by engaging both the principal fragments and the larger interposed fragments with Steinmann pins or Schanz screws and manipulating them into alignment so that satisfactory bone contact is obtained.

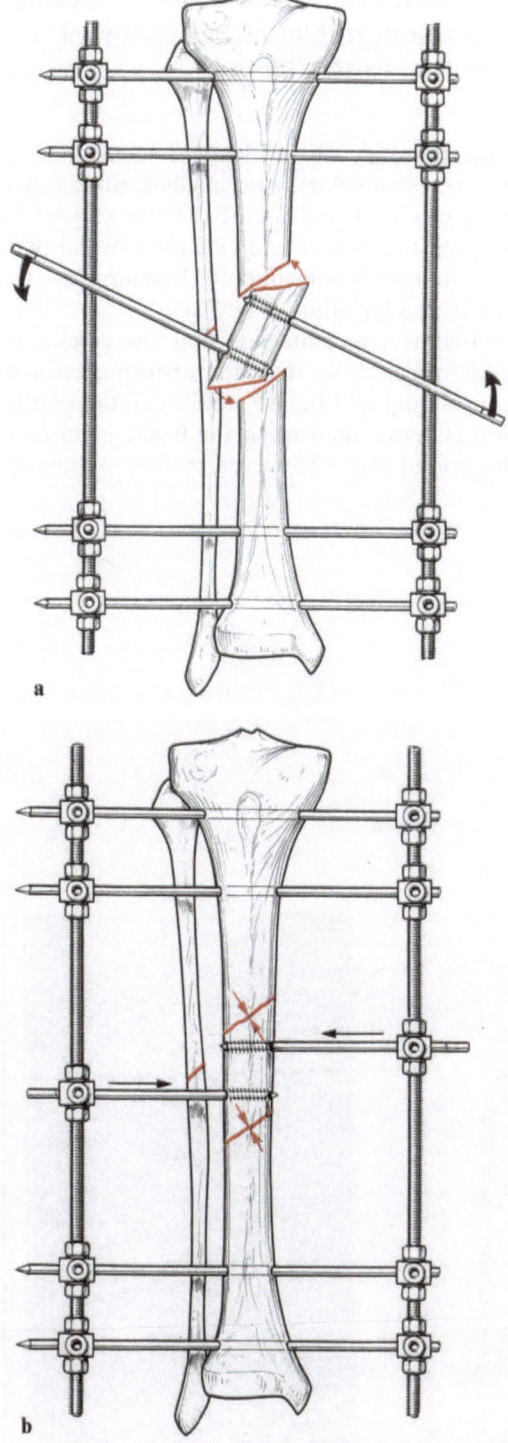

**Fig. 72 a, b.** Restoring bone contact by fragment manipulation. **a** The intercalary fragments in a segmental fracture can be manipulated by means of Schanz screws. **b** Stabilizing interfragmental pressure through transverse compression

# 7 Sagittal or "Intermediate" Screw Placement in Unilateral External Fixation of the Tibia

The advantage of the classic Schanz screw insertion perpendicular to the medial, proximal tibial surface is that the tips of the screws pass safely between the flexors and extensors in the plane of the interosseous membrane, lessening the risk of neurovascular injury (Fig. 73).

BEHRENS recommends that the screws be inserted precisely in the anterior-to-posterior direction, stating that the AP stability of this configuration is better than when the frame is mounted in the frontal plane. However, this reasoning neglects the resultant sacrifice of varus and valgus stability, and the risk that the screw tips, as they emerge from the posterior tibial surface, may damage the posterior tibial artery and nerve. In addition, this placement weakens the mechanically important anterior tibial crest, which I feel is a significant concern with regard to the subsequent risk of tibial stress fracture. For these reasons I would reserve the sagittal frame mounting for special indications (Fig. 74).

The "standard" orientation of the unilateral frame on the tibia appears to be biomechanically correct: The "intermediate" position between the frontal plane and sagittal plane (BEHRENS) protects the tibia from angulation in all directions, particularly when the frame itself is reinforced.

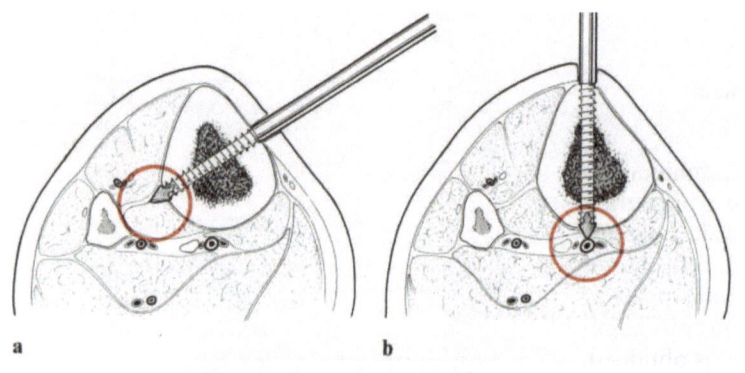

a                                            b

**Fig. 73 a, b.** Risk of injury with a unilateral frame. **a** With an intermediate screw placement between the sagittal and frontal planes, the screw tips lie on the plane of the interosseous membrane. **b** With a sagittal screw insertion, the posterior tibial artery and nerve are vulnerable to injury

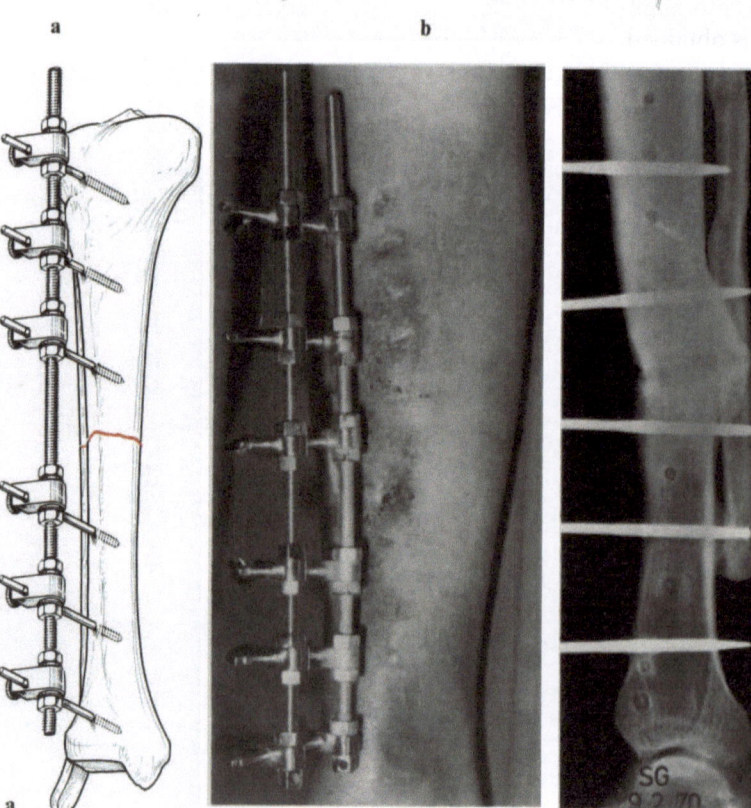

a                    b                    c

**Fig. 74 a–c.** The sagittal unilateral frame. **a** The screws are inserted through the anterior tibial crest in an anterior-to-posterior direction. **b** Clinical example. **c** The sagittal frame is justified in cases where a previous bilateral frame had to be removed due to loosening and multiple pin tract infection. The new screw placement does not violate the old pin tracts

# 8 Summary of the Biomechanics of External Fixation

## 8.1 The External Fixator and Bone

Whenever possible, the external fixator should not be the solitary load-bearing member, or at least should perform that function only for a limited time during neutralization and lengthening. *Interfragmental contact* and a *bony buttress* should be established as soon as possible so that the bone can contribute to load bearing.

## 8.2 Unilateral or Bilateral Frame

When an external fixator is in place, *stress transfer* from one main fragment to the next must always occur through at least *two columns*.

If *there is no interfragmental contact* (or bony buttress), then the two rods of the *bilateral frame* or the two rods of two *unilateral frames* (femur) constitute the load-bearing columns.

If *interfragmental contact is present,* then a *unilateral frame* will suffice, with the bone serving as one column and the rod as the other.

## 8.3 Elasticity of the External Fixator

In every case the external fixator should be removed as soon as possible to encourage *secondary bone healing with callus formation*. While rigid frames retard the formation of an irritation and fixation callus, *stable, elastic frames* promote it. The goal is to employ frame designs which fully utilize the elastic forces of the fixation apparatus, and also enable the bone to participate in load bearing so that a prestressed bone-frame system is obtained.

# C The Threaded External Fixator. Instrumentation

B.G. WEBER

## 1 Introduction

If external fixation is to achieve the desired result, the plan of operation must be based upon clear biomechanical concepts, and the procedure must be carried out strictly according to plan. Planning and execution are the responsibility of the surgeon.

Success and failure depend primarily on the knowledge and skills of the physician, and only secondarily on instrumentation. Nevertheless, a workable plan can be executed only with the aid of workable instrumentation which satisfies stringent criteria.

### 1.1 Requirements of the External Fixator

The same *metal* must be used for all elements of the external fixator, and it must be of the same high quality that is required for internal plates and screws. The external fixators of the ASIF are made of AISI 316 L stainless chromium-nickel-molybdenum steel (POHLER, STRAUMANN).

The frame assembly must be stable enough for *postoperative mobilization* of the stabilized extremity not to cause loosening or failure of the device. This goal depends on the holding power of the pins and screws, i.e., on the design and mode of application of the external fixator and the quality of the involved bone. The inherent stability of the tubular external fixator (BOLTZE, CHIQUET, NIEDERER) is identical to that of the threaded fixator (JÖRG). In the compression mode, however, the threaded fixator is far superior to systems that have swiveling clamps (CHARNLEY).

It should be possible to modify the *elasticity* or *rigidity* of the external fixator by altering its configuration. To achieve this adaptability, it must be possible to satisfy all conceivable requirements using the same modular elements.

The external fixator should be *acceptable to the patient*. That is, its design should be such that it does not degrade the patient's self-image nor unduly restrict his movements. From this standpoint a great many external fixation systems are in urgent need of *"humanization,"* and their indi-

cations should be limited in favor of less psychologically invasive forms of treatment.

### 1.2 The External Fixator of the ASIF

The first external fixation device of the ASIF, the threaded external fixator, was developed by MÜLLER in 1952.

In 1976 MÜLLER developed the *tubular system,* which today is more widely used than the older threaded device.

Only in recent years has the threaded fixator been modified somewhat, less for the purpose of improving it than to facilitate its handling. Special attention was given to the standardization of its elements. Several new elements were also added, such as a double clamp, triple clamp and two-piece clamp. Nevertheless, the goal still is to cope with all situations using the smallest number of elements possible.

A particular innovation, based on a suggestion by the authors, is the capability to bend the threaded rods as needed to eliminate the need for universal joints. It was felt that swivel clamps (universal clamps) would compromise the superior stability of the threaded fixator as demonstrated by CHARNLEY and MATHESON.

## 2 The Elements of the Threaded External Fixator

### 2.1 Steinmann Pins (Fig. 75)

Steinmann pins are available in two diameters and the following lengths:

4.5 mm diam.: 150 mm, 180 mm, 200 mm
5.0 mm diam.: 180 mm, 200 mm, 250 mm.

The points are of the trocar type, with three cutting edges capable of reaming out a predrilled hole to the diameter of the pin. The actual point of the pin is "broken" as a safeguard against neurovascular injury.

### 2.2 Schanz Screws (Fig. 76)

The shorter Schanz screws are available in two diameters, 4.5 and 5.0 mm, and all are 9 cm long, excluding the thread. Available thread lengths are 30, 34, 38, 42 and 46 mm.

The long screws are 22 cm in length and 5 mm in diameter. All have a 50-mm thread.

The screw points have the same trocar shape as the Steinmann pins. The screws are self-tapping when driven into a predrilled hole.

Because the pitch of the thread corresponds to that of the 4.5-mm cortex screw, the hole may be prethreaded with the 4.5-mm tap if desired.

The Schanz screw has a somewhat shallower thread than the 4.5-mm cortex screw. This was done to increase its mechanical strength.

The pilot holes for the pins and screws are predrilled with the standard 3.2- and 3.5-mm ASIF drill bits. The smaller bit is used for the 4.5-mm pins and screws, and the larger bit for the 5-mm pins and screws.

### 2.3 The 4.5-mm and 3.5-mm Cortex Screws (Fig. 77)

For external fixations of the forearm and wrist, Steinmann pins and Schanz screws are replaced with 4.5-mm cortex screws up to 70 mm long, and with 3.5-mm cortex screws up to 50 mm long. Threads for the cortex screws are precut with special taps that have a trocar point. The 3.5-mm and 2.7-mm cortex screws and a corresponding threaded minifixator (see Sect. 3) are used for external fixations of the hand and fingers.

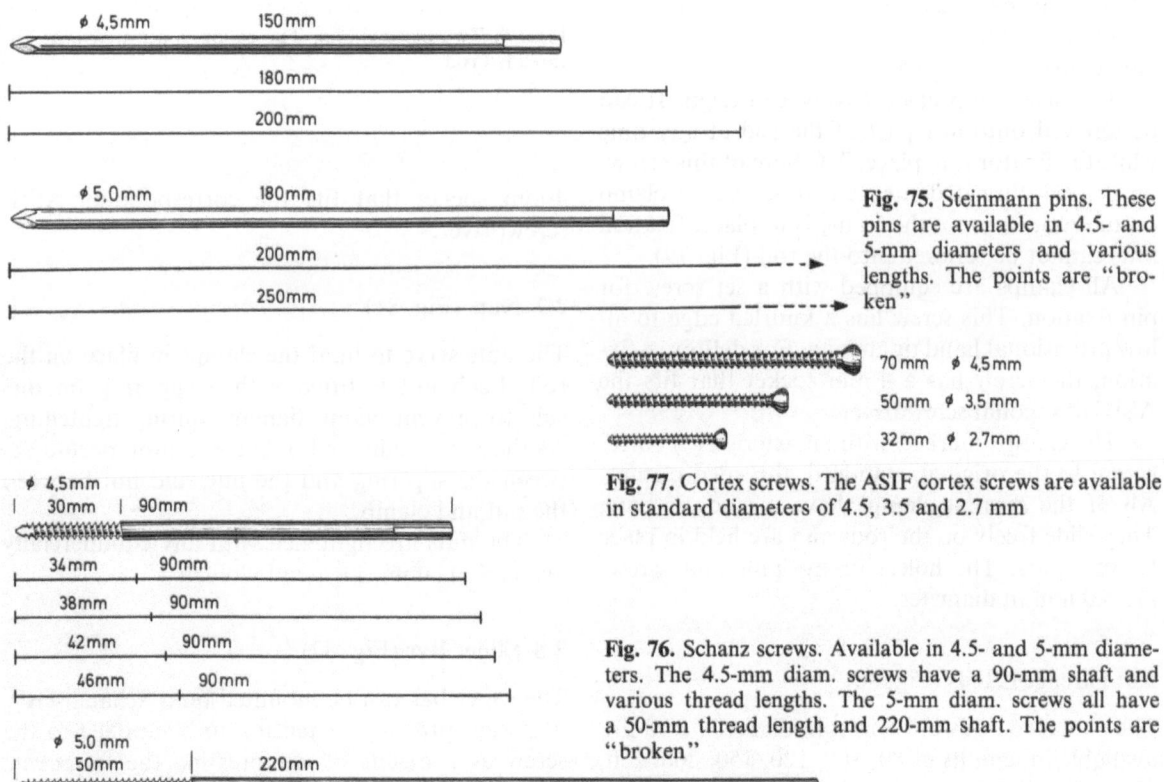

**Fig. 75.** Steinmann pins. These pins are available in 4.5- and 5-mm diameters and various lengths. The points are "broken"

**Fig. 77.** Cortex screws. The ASIF cortex screws are available in standard diameters of 4.5, 3.5 and 2.7 mm

**Fig. 76.** Schanz screws. Available in 4.5- and 5-mm diameters. The 4.5-mm diam. screws have a 90-mm shaft and various thread lengths. The 5-mm diam. screws all have a 50-mm thread length and 220-mm shaft. The points are "broken"

## 2.4 Drill Bits, Drill Sleeves and Taps

2.5-mm  Drill bit and drill sleeve: predrilling of distal radius and second metacarpal for 3.5-mm cortex screws.

3.2-mm  Drill bit and drill sleeve: predrilling for 4.5-mm Steinmann pins, Schanz screws and for 4.5 mm cortex screws.

3.5-mm  Drill bit and drill sleeve: predrilling for 5.0-mm Steinmann pins and Schanz screws.

4.5-mm  Tap with tap sleeve: optional tapping for 4.5-mm and 5.-0-mm Schanz screws.

3.5-mm  Tap: sleeveless tapping for 3.5-mm cortex screws (see Chap. D).

4.5-mm  Tap: sleeveless tapping for 4.5-mm cortex screws (see Chap. D).

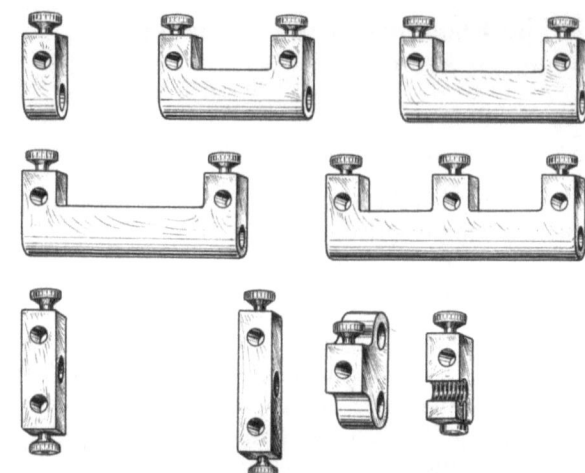

**Fig. 78.** Clamps. Single and multiple clamps; clamps for 2 pins or 2 rods; two-piece clamp for secondary mounting

## 2.5 Clamps for Steinmann Pins, Schanz Screws, 4.5-mm and 3.5-mm Cortex Screws
(Fig. 78)

* Single clamp for 1 rod
Double clamp, 30 mm, for 1 rod
Double clamp, 40 mm, for 1 rod
Double clamp, 50 mm, for 1 rod
Triple clamp, 60 mm, for 1 rod
* Double transverse clamp, 18 mm, for 1 rod
* Double transverse clamp, 24 mm, for 1 rod
Single clamp for 2 rods
Single open clamp for 1 rod.

The last clamp has a two-piece design. It can be screwed onto any part of the rod at any time while the fixator is in place. The bore of this screw-on clamp is threaded internally to secure the clamp on the rod, for once the frame is in place, fixation nuts cannot be screwed into the rod (Fig. 79).

All clamps are equipped with a set screw for pin fixation. This screw has a knurled edge to allow provisional hand tightening. For definitive fixation, the screw has a 4-mm socket that fits the ASIF hexagonal screwdriver.

The clamps marked with an asterisk (*) correspond to the original, standard, threaded clamps. All of the current clamps have a smooth bore. They slide freely on the rods and are held in place by two nuts. The holes for the pins and screws are 5.0 mm in diameter.

## 2.6 Threaded Rods (Fig. 80)

The threaded rods are 8 mm in diameter and are available in lengths of 80, 100, 120, 150, 200, 250, 300, 350, 400 and 450 mm. Each end carries a

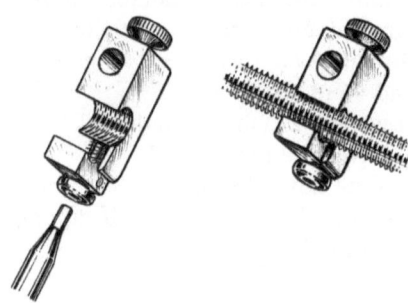

**Fig. 79.** Two-piece clamp. The clamp is screwed onto the threaded rod

4-mm socket that fits the corresponding ASIF screwdriver.

## 2.7 Nuts (Fig. 81)

The nuts serve to hold the clamps in place on the rod. Each nut is fitted with a slip ring on one side to prevent clamp damage during tightening. As the nut is tightened, relative motion occurs between the slip ring and the nut, and not between the nut and clamp.

The nuts are tightened with any commercially available 11-mm open-end wrench.

## 2.8 Slider Bar (Fig. 82)

The slider bar can be mounted on a Schanz screw to permit pressure or tension to be applied to the screw as a means of compressing the fragments in the transverse direction.

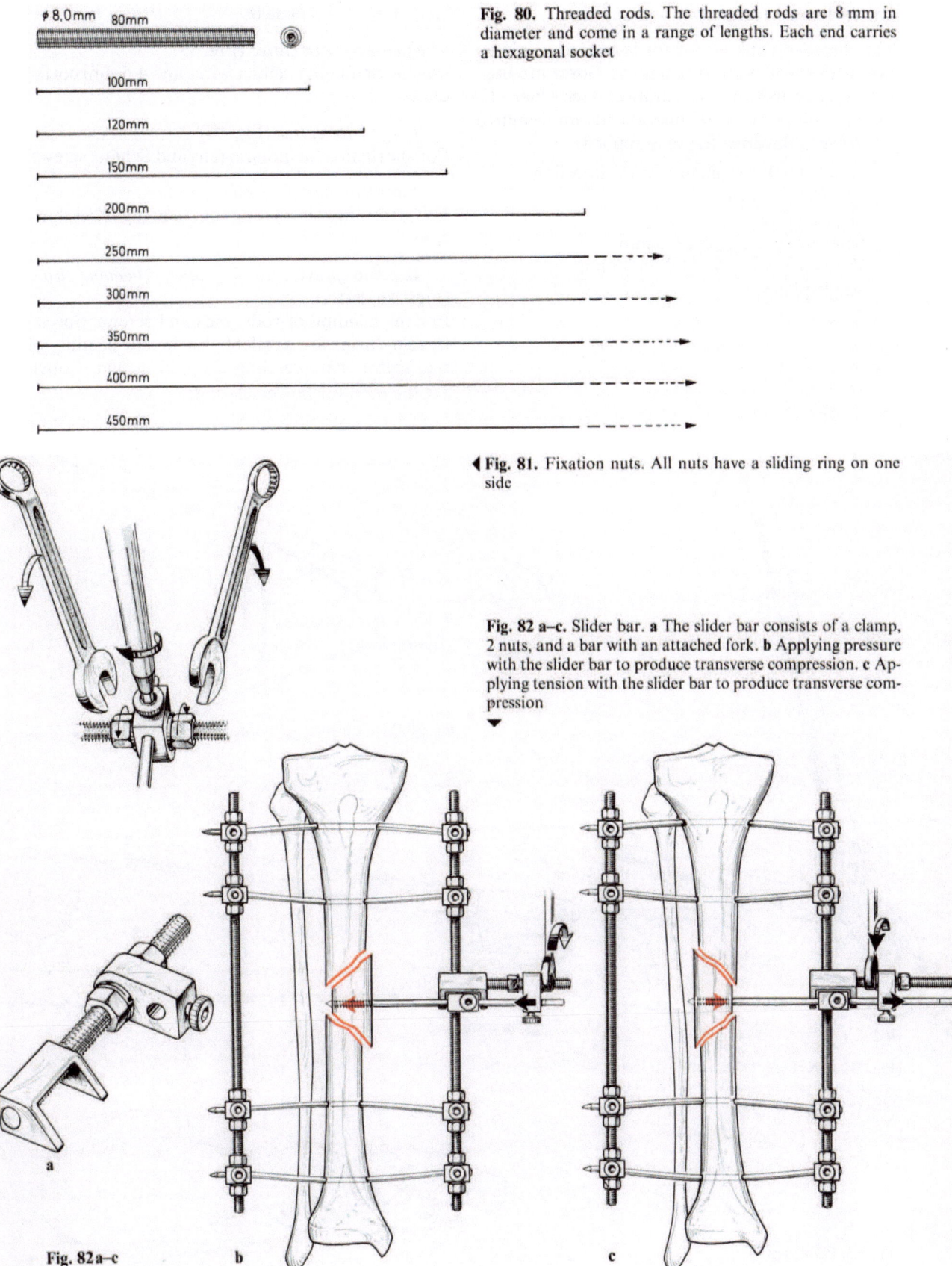

**Fig. 80.** Threaded rods. The threaded rods are 8 mm in diameter and come in a range of lengths. Each end carries a hexagonal socket

◄ **Fig. 81.** Fixation nuts. All nuts have a sliding ring on one side

**Fig. 82 a–c.** Slider bar. **a** The slider bar consists of a clamp, 2 nuts, and a bar with an attached fork. **b** Applying pressure with the slider bar to produce transverse compression. **c** Applying tension with the slider bar to produce transverse compression

▼

Fig. 82 a–c

## 2.9 Additional Instruments and Implants

The threaded external fixator is used in conjunction with other ASIF instruments. Some are used with special fixator configurations (see Chap. K, 2). The following ASIF instruments are required whenever a threaded frame is applied:

Hand chuck for pin and screw insertion
ASIF power drill
Depth gauge
Screwdrivers, 3.5 and 4.5 mm
Kirschner wires, 0.8–1.2 and 3 mm
Angle plates.

## 2.10 Special Instruments

*Medium-size wire cutter* (Fig. 83)
For shortening Kirschner wires and 4.5-mm cortex screws.

*Large wire cutter* (Fig. 84)
For shortening Steinmann pins and Schanz screws.

*Parallel pliers* (Fig. 85)
For grasping, extracting or bending Kirschner wires.

*Bending press, bending pliers, bending irons* (Figs. 86, 87)
For the bending of rods, pins and screws. Special bending irons are available for in-situ bending of the fixator. Rod bending is useful in that it obviates the need for universal joints.

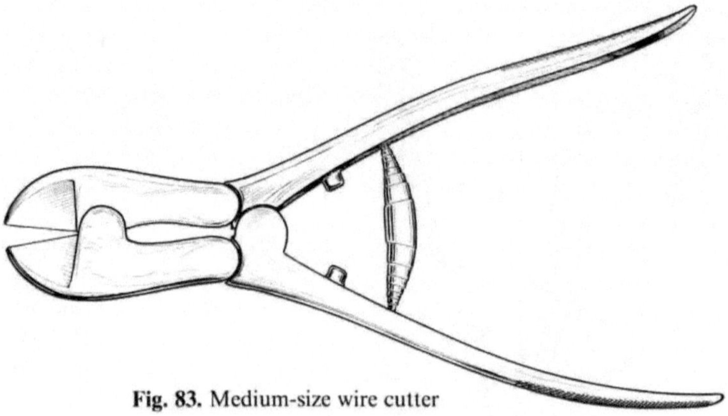

**Fig. 83.** Medium-size wire cutter

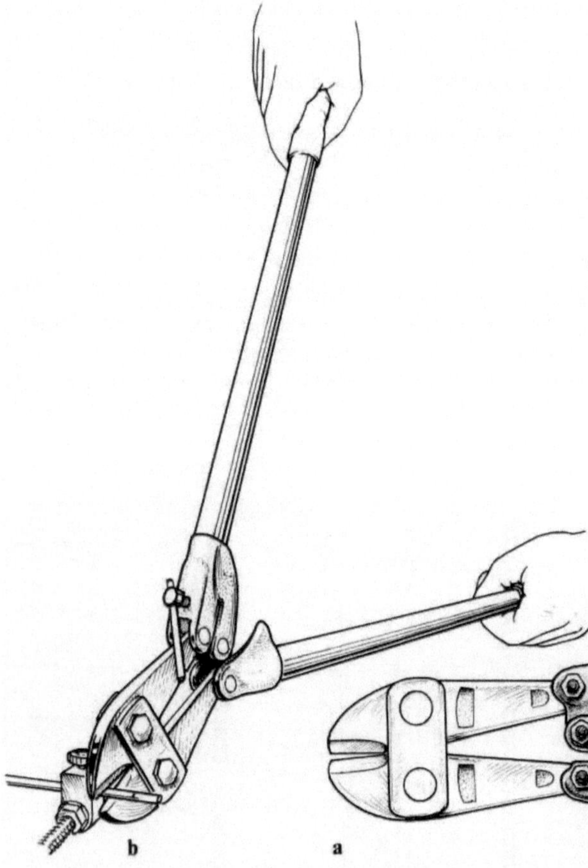

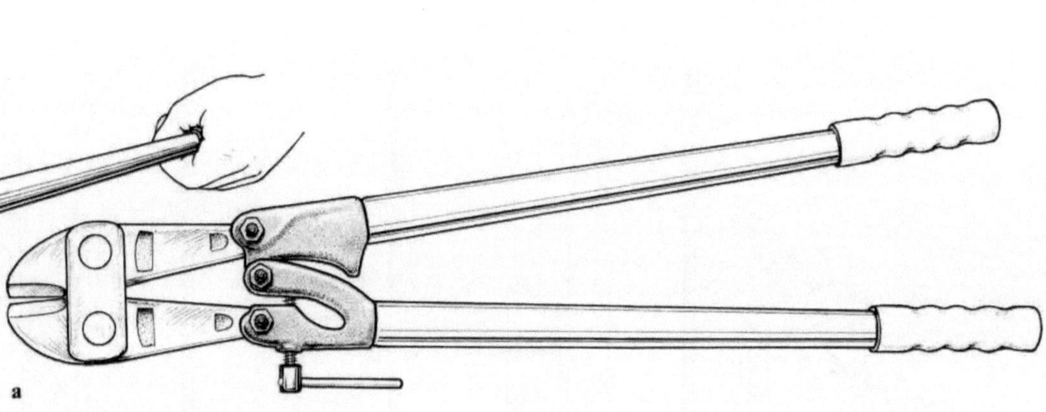

**Fig. 84 a, b.** Large wire cutter. **a** Large wire cutter with a reduction gear for added leverage. **b** Cutting of Steinmann pins or Schanz screws

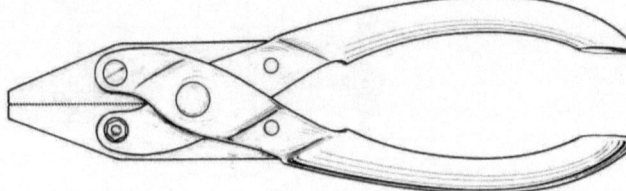

**Fig. 85.** Parallel pliers

## 3 The Threaded Minifixator (Fig. 88)

For two years a miniature version of the threaded external fixator has been available for use on the hand and especially the fingers. The rods are 5 mm in diameter, and 3.5-mm and 2.7-mm cortex screws are used in place of Steinmann pins and Schanz screws.

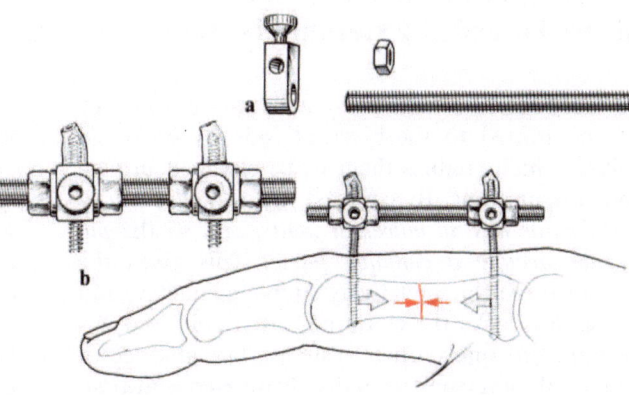

**Fig. 88 a, b.** The threaded minifixator. **a** The miniature elements are analogous to those of the full-size device: clamp, threaded rod, nut. **b** Size comparison: *Top:* The standard threaded fixator. *Bottom:* The minifixator, used here to treat a transverse fracture through the proximal phalanx of a finger

**Fig. 86.** Bending pliers

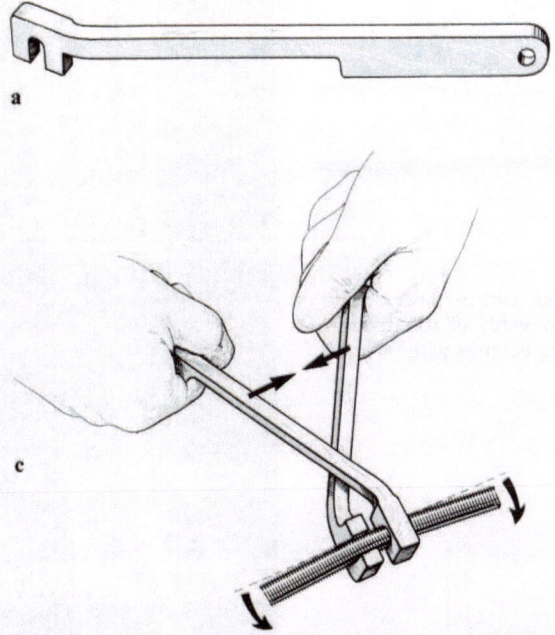

**Fig. 87 a–d.** Bending irons for the threaded rods. **a** Both bending irons have the same 40° angulation. **b** Applied in an uncrossed fashion, the irons are used to bend the rod away from the operator. **c** They are applied in a crossed fashion to bend the rod toward the operator. **d** Bending a Schanz screw

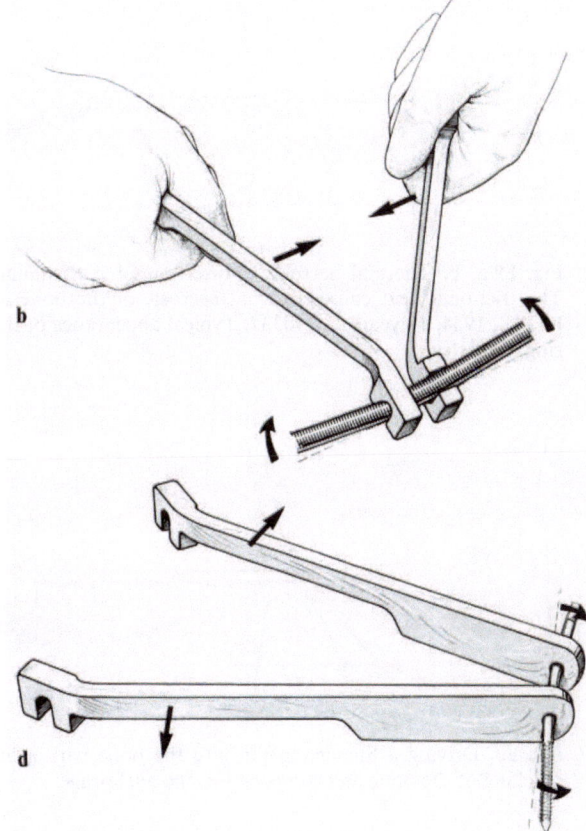

# D Operative Technique for the Threaded External Fixator

B.G. Weber

## 1 The Special Characteristics of the Threaded External Fixator

In most external fixation systems, the pin groups are connected to the external rods by universal joints, which enables them to be clamped in various orientations. By contrast, the *threaded external fixator has no universal joints,* and so the *pin groups occupy a common plane.* This gives the threaded fixator a relatively simple geometry, and the device lacks the cluttered, often confused appearance of many other systems. The absence of universal joints may seem disadvantageous at first, but this is offset by the advantages of enhanced stability and a clear operative concept.

## 2 Errors of Pin and Screw Insertion

To achieve a long-term anchorage of pins and screws in bone, it is important to avoid the following errors of insertion:
- A pin or screw should never be inserted directly with a *power drill.* The resulting heat would cause thermal necrosis of bone with a high risk of pin tract infection, pin loosening and ring sequestrum (Fig. 89).
- Pins and screws should never be driven into the bone with a *hammer.* This would *fracture the bone* and prevent a stable pin anchorage (Fig. 90).

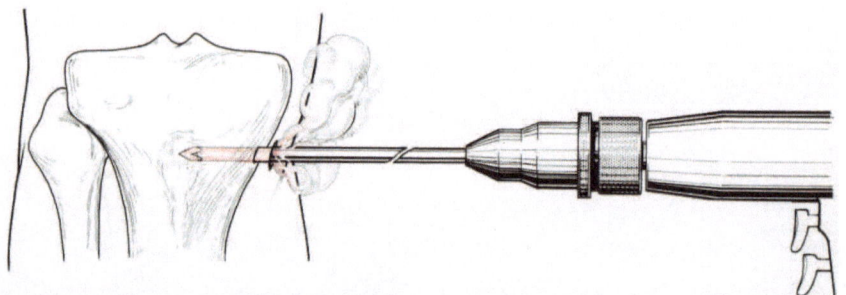

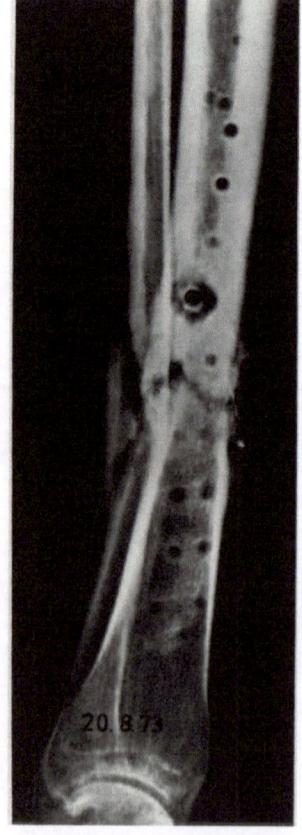

**Fig. 89 a, b.** Thermal necrosis. **a** Insertion of a Steinmann pin with a power drill: The frictional heat causes thermal necrosis of the bone and possibly of soft tissues. **b** H.H., 1954, 19 years, ♀, 170337. Typical appearance of thermal necrosis with infected ring sequestrum

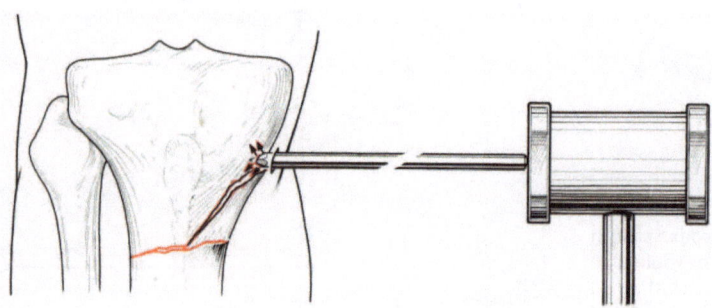

**Fig. 90.** Driving a Steinmann pin into the bone with a hammer causes cracking of the bone and compromises the anchorage

– Pins and screws should not puncture the skin
during insertion, as this would cause *skin necrosis* and *infection* at the puncture site (Fig. 91).

## 2.1 Technique for Steinmann Pins (Fig. 92)

– *Cutaneous stab incision.* Two stab incisions are
made for each Steinmann pin – one each at the
entry and exit sites. These incisions should be
long enough to *prevent skin tension and pressure*
around the pin. An incision that is tense or too
small will predispose to skin necrosis and infection. If too long, the incision should be sutured
so that a seal can develop.
– *Predrilling the pilot hole.* Predrilling facilitates
pin insertion. The drill bit should be large enough that the pin can be advanced by hand without undue difficulty. If too much resistance is
felt, the hole should be redrilled with the next
larger bit size. Predrilling is always done
through a suitable *drill sleeve* so that soft tissues
between the skin and bone (fascia, muscle, vessels, nerves) are protected from damage by the
bit. The 3.2-mm drill bit is used for 4.5-mm pins,
and the 3.5-mm bit for 5-mm pins.
– *Pin insertion.* The pins are clamped into the universal hand chuck and driven through the pilot
hole with a back-and-forth twisting motion.
When the pin raises the skin on the opposite
side, a stab incision is made at that site and
the insertion is continued.
– *Pin site corrections.* If slight skin tension is
found at any of the pin sites, an incision is made
into the tight skin. Incisions found to be too
large are sutured to reduce their size.
  If a pin is found to exit the skin at the wrong
location, as evidenced by extreme skin tension,
the pin is withdrawn with the hand chuck until
it just disappears beneath the skin. A new stab
incision is made at the correct site, and the pin
is brought out through the new incision
(Fig. 93).
– *Erecting the bilateral frame.* Single, double or
triple clamps are attached with set screws to the
exposed ends of the pins. Each clamp is fixed
to the threaded rod with two nuts.
  In the *compression mode* the pin groups are prestressed by compressing them toward one another.
  In the *neutralization mode* the pins within each
cluster are prestressed toward or away from one
another to retard lateral shifting.

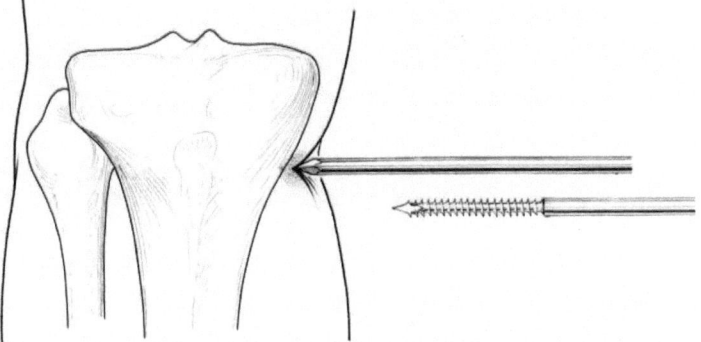

**Fig. 91.** Skin perforation by a pin or screw. The point of
the pin or screw causes pressure necrosis of the skin

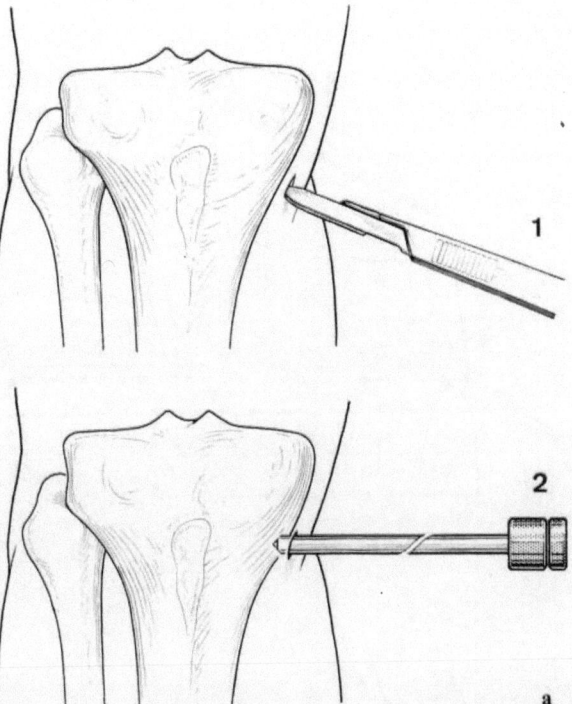

**Fig. 92 a–c.** The technique of Steinmann pin insertion. **a** A
stab incision is made (*1*), and the drill sleeve with stylet
(or drill bit) is introduced (*2*). **b** When the drill sleeve abuts
against the bone, the stylet is withdrawn (*3*) and a 3.2-mm
pilot hole is drilled (*4*). **c** The Steinmann pin is inserted
(*5*), and a counterincision is made (*6*). The stab incision
may require extension to release skin tension and obtain
a seal (*7*)

**Fig. 92b. c**
Legend see p. 61

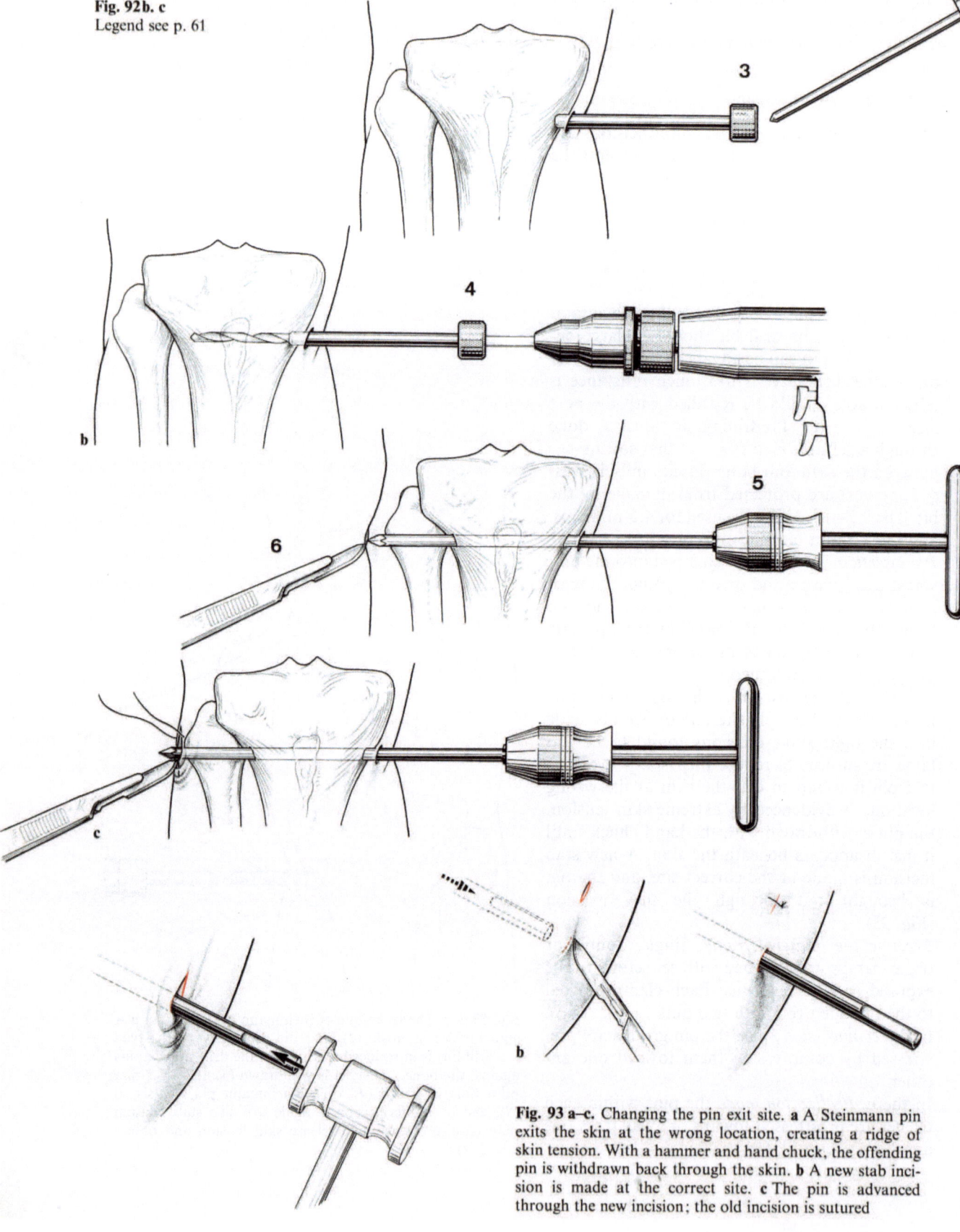

**Fig. 93 a–c.** Changing the pin exit site. **a** A Steinmann pin exits the skin at the wrong location, creating a ridge of skin tension. With a hammer and hand chuck, the offending pin is withdrawn back through the skin. **b** A new stab incision is made at the correct site. **c** The pin is advanced through the new incision; the old incision is sutured

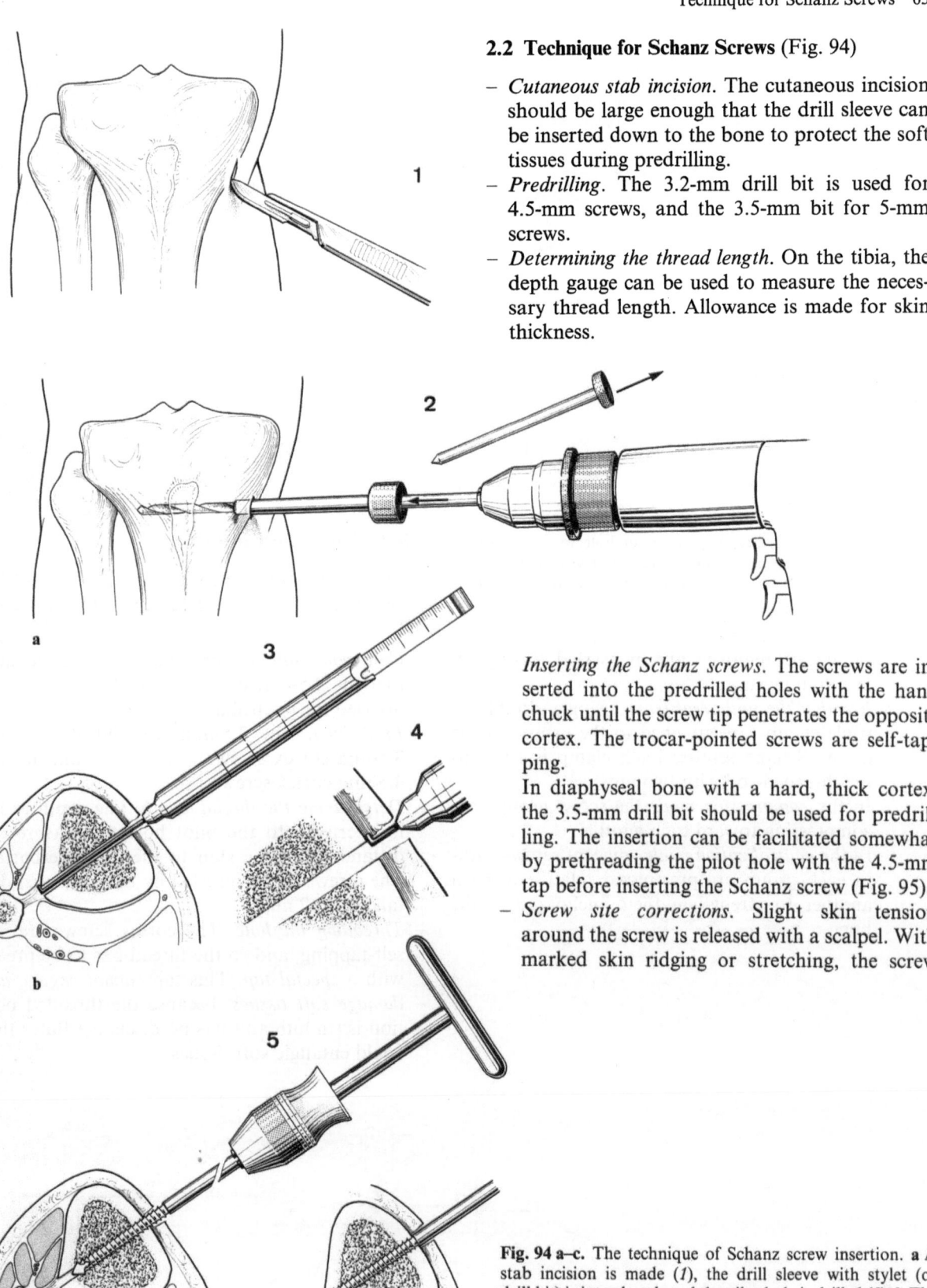

## 2.2 Technique for Schanz Screws (Fig. 94)

- *Cutaneous stab incision.* The cutaneous incision should be large enough that the drill sleeve can be inserted down to the bone to protect the soft tissues during predrilling.
- *Predrilling.* The 3.2-mm drill bit is used for 4.5-mm screws, and the 3.5-mm bit for 5-mm screws.
- *Determining the thread length.* On the tibia, the depth gauge can be used to measure the necessary thread length. Allowance is made for skin thickness.

*Inserting the Schanz screws.* The screws are inserted into the predrilled holes with the hand chuck until the screw tip penetrates the opposite cortex. The trocar-pointed screws are self-tapping.

In diaphyseal bone with a hard, thick cortex, the 3.5-mm drill bit should be used for predrilling. The insertion can be facilitated somewhat by prethreading the pilot hole with the 4.5-mm tap before inserting the Schanz screw (Fig. 95).

- *Screw site corrections.* Slight skin tension around the screw is released with a scalpel. With marked skin ridging or stretching, the screw

**Fig. 94 a–c.** The technique of Schanz screw insertion. **a** A stab incision is made (*1*), the drill sleeve with stylet (or drill bit) is introduced, and the pilot hole is drilled (*2*). **b** The thread length (*3*) and skin thickness are measured (*4*). **c** The Schanz screw is driven in until the end of the thread engages against the cortex (*5*)

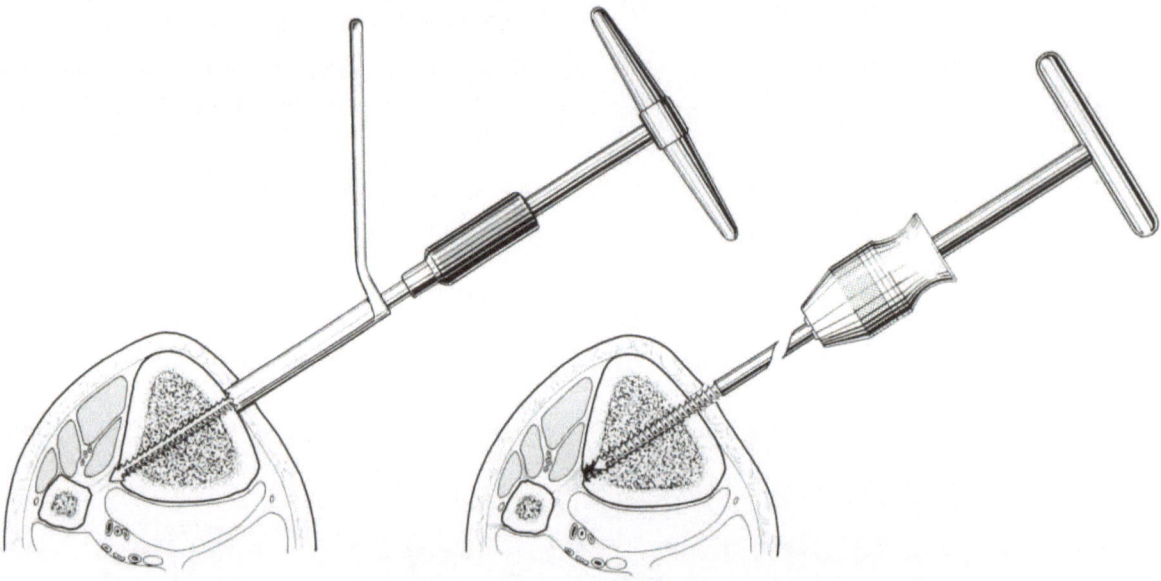

**Fig. 95 a, b.** Prethreading the pilot hole in hard cortical bone and for 5-mm diam. Schanz screws. **a** Cutting the thread through the tap sleeve. **b** Insertion of the screw

should be removed and reinserted through a new stab incision.
- *Erecting the unilateral frame.* Single, double or triple clamps are attached to the exposed ends of the Schanz screws. Each clamp is fixed to the threaded rod with two nuts.
  In the *compression mode* the screw groups are compressing toward each another.
  In the *neutralization mode* adjacent screws within each group are prestressed relative to each another to strengthen their anchorage in the bone.

## 2.3 Technique for Cortex Screws

Cortex screws are used for unilateral external fixations of the forearm and juvenile tibia (Figs. 96, 97).

- *Cutaneous stab incision.* The skin is incised such that the 2.5-mm or 3.2-mm drill sleeve can be inserted for predrilling.
- *Predrilling.* The 2.5-mm drill bit is used for 3.5-mm cortex screws, and the 3.2-mm bit for 4.5-mm cortex screws.
- *Determining the thread length.* The depth gauge is inserted into the pilot hole to measure the distance from the skin to the opposite cortex. The screw will be inserted by the measured distance plus 2 mm.
- *Threading the hole.* The cortex screws are not self-tapping, and so the thread has to be precut with a *special tap.* This tap *cannot engage and damage soft tissues,* because the threaded portion is smooth and has no discharge flutes that could entangle soft tissues.

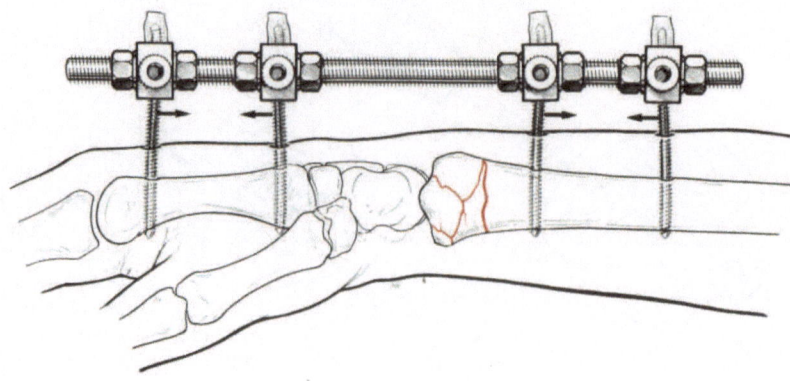

**Fig. 96.** Cortex screws in the external frame. Here cortical screws are used in a small unilateral frame applied to a distal radial fracture

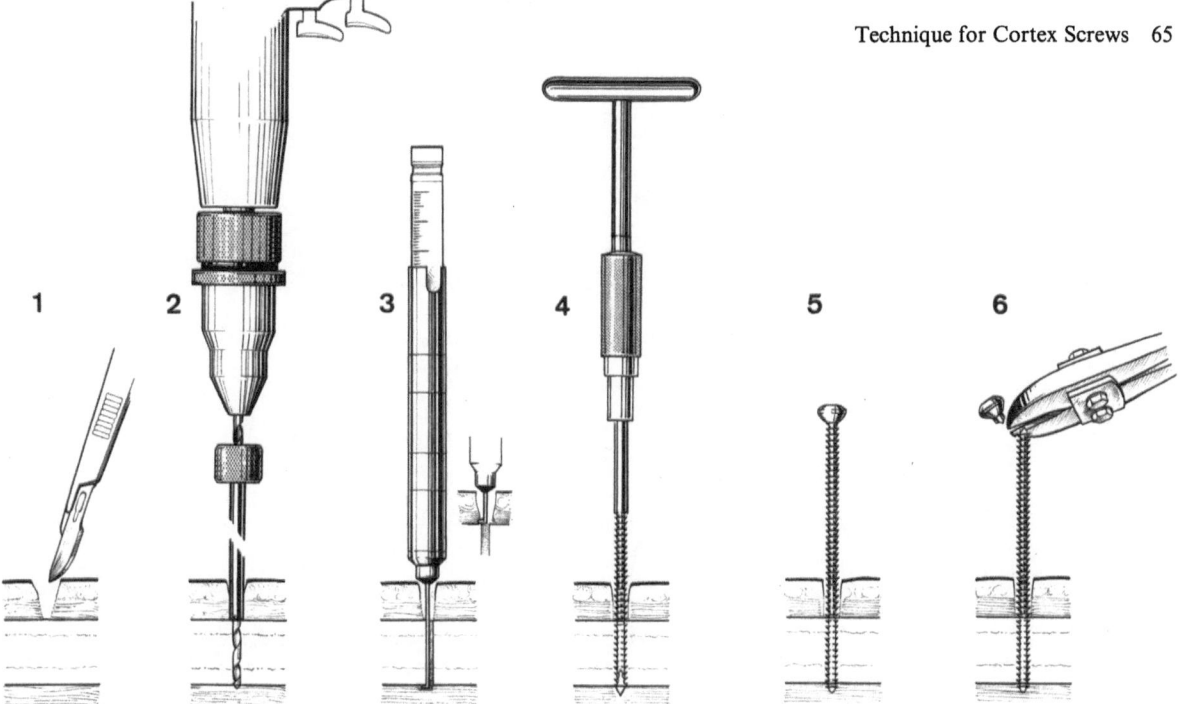

**Fig. 97.** The technique of cortex screw insertion. Through a stab incision (*1*) the bone is predrilled through the drill sleeve (*2*), the length is measured with the depth gauge (*3*), the drill hole is threaded with the special tap (*4*), a long cortex screw is inserted (*5*), and the screw head is cut off (*6*)

- *Inserting the cortex screws*. The screws are inserted through the stab incision into the predrilled hole.
- *Erecting the unilateral frame* (Fig. 96). The *screw heads* must be *cut off* with the wire cutter before the clamps can be attached to the cortex screws. Each clamp is fixed to the threaded rod with two nuts in the distraction, neutralization or compression mode, as required.

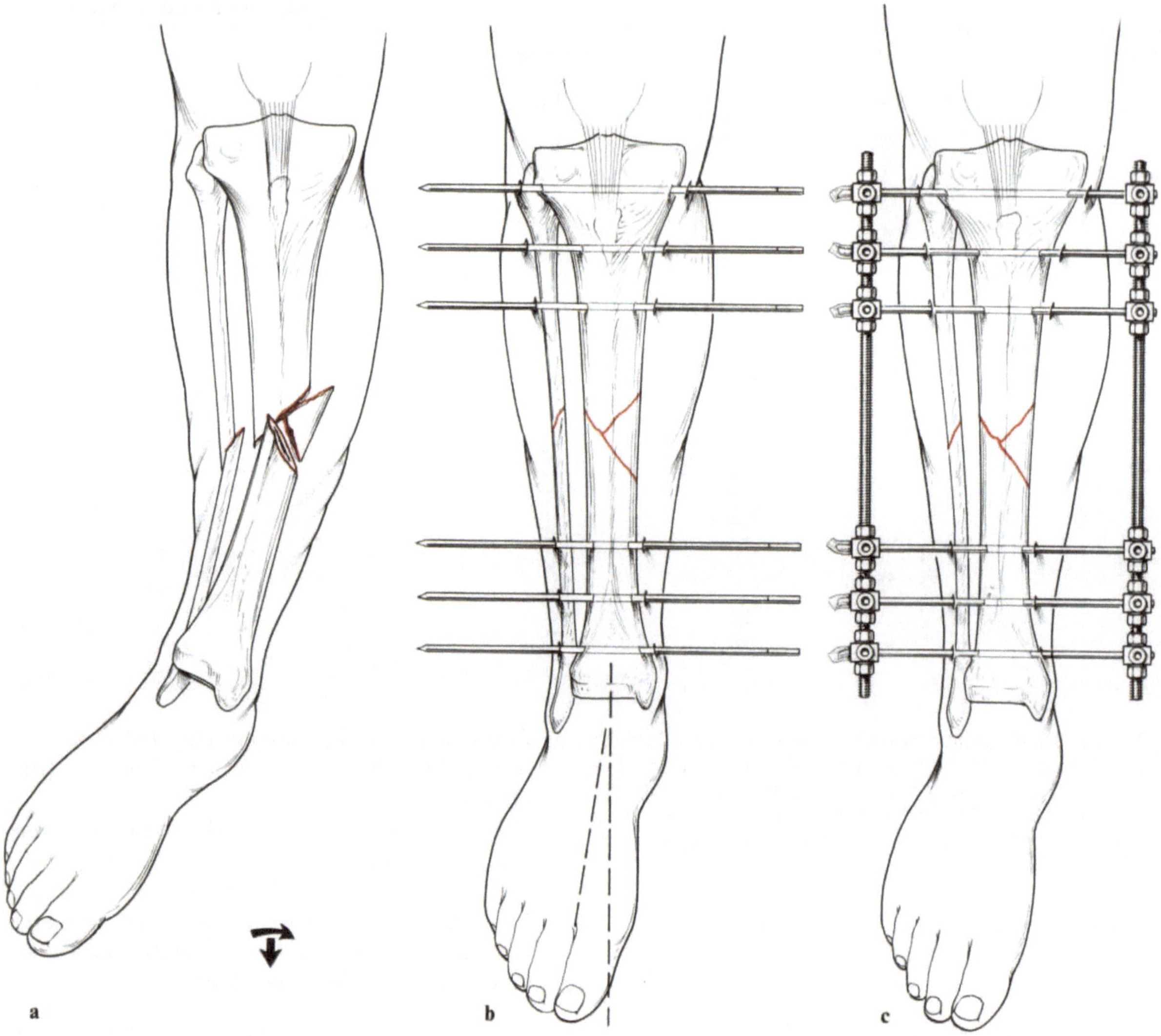

Fig. 98 a–c. Concept of the threaded external fixator. a The primary step is reduction. b Then the pins (or screws) are inserted. c All pins (or screws) in the frame lie on the same plane

# 3 Reduction

## 3.1 Concept

The threaded external fixator has no need for universal joints, because with this device the pins are inserted into the fragments to form a parallel, uniplanar array only *after* the fragments have been reduced. With this sequencing of pin placement, nonarticulated clamps may be used to construct the frame (Fig. 98). This distinguishes the threaded fixator from other devices in which the pins are inserted prior to reduction and then are used to manipulate the fragments into alignment. Frequently this creates a disordered array of protruding pins which can be interconnected only by means of universal joints and rods. This often results in large, complex frameworks whose sheer size and volume make them difficult for the patient to tolerate (Fig. 99).

By employing a strategy of "reduction first," it is possible to achieve a maximum degree of material economy. The assemblies are simpler, less cumbersome, and far more acceptable to the patient.

*Principle No. 1 for the threaded external fixator:*
*The fragments are reduced before the pins are inserted.*

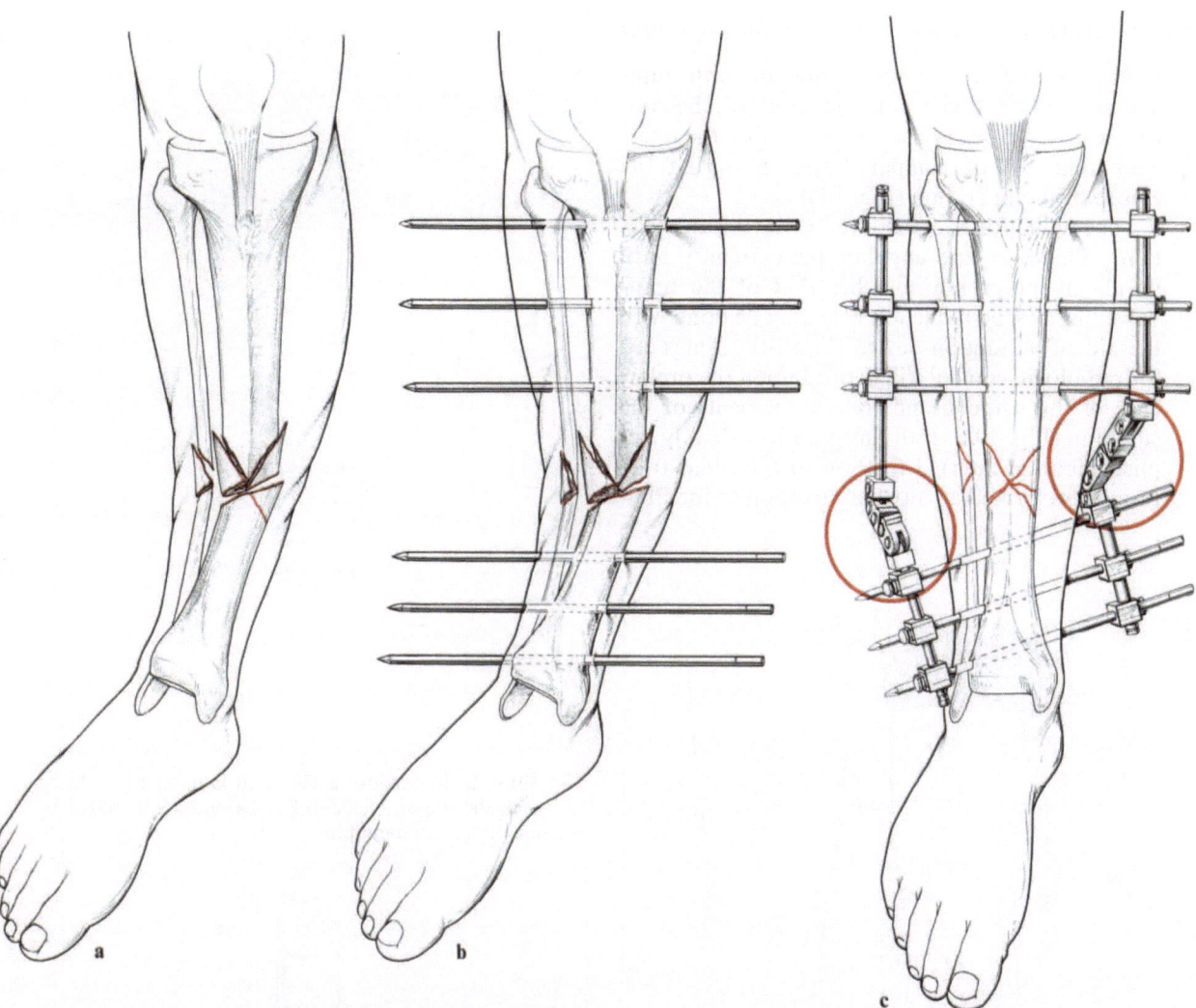

**Fig. 99 a–c.** The usual concept of other external fixation systems. **a** An accurate reduction is deferred. **b** The pin groups are inserted. **c** Only now are the fragments reduced. Universal joints are needed to erect the frame

### 3.2 Technique (described here for a tibial fracture)

In cases where an anatomic reduction with minimal internal fixation is not contemplated, the contralateral lower leg is also draped so that the operated tibia can be compared with it during the course of the operation (Fig. 100).

The reduction is carried out by having an assistant pull, rotate and angulate the extremity until its alignment grossly matches that of the uninvolved limb. The reduction also may be done with the aid of a traction device (Fig. 101). The need for radiologic control will depend upon the preference of the surgeon and the requirements of the situation (Fig. 102). If the surgeon has already applied minimal internal fixation to the tibial fracture or performed an auxiliary fixation of the fibu-

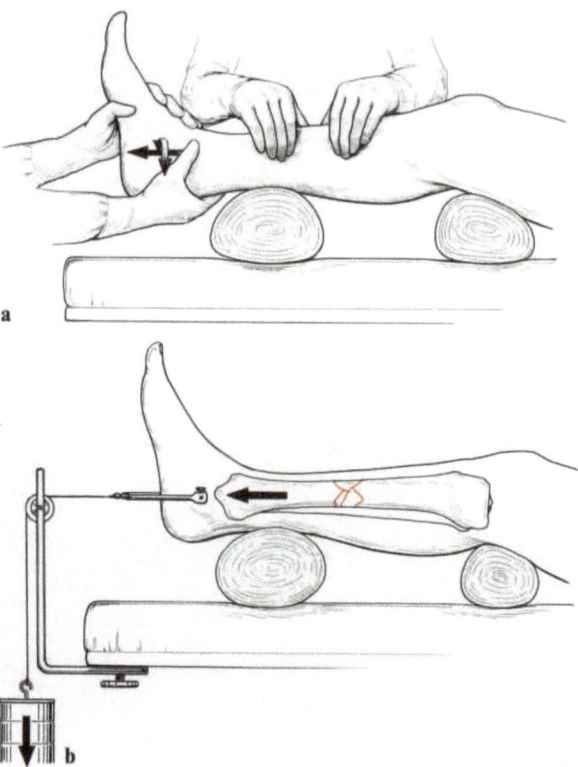

**Fig. 101 a, b.** Reduction. **a** The limb is manually reduced to match the opposite side. **b** Reduction may be aided by traction on a Steinmann pin

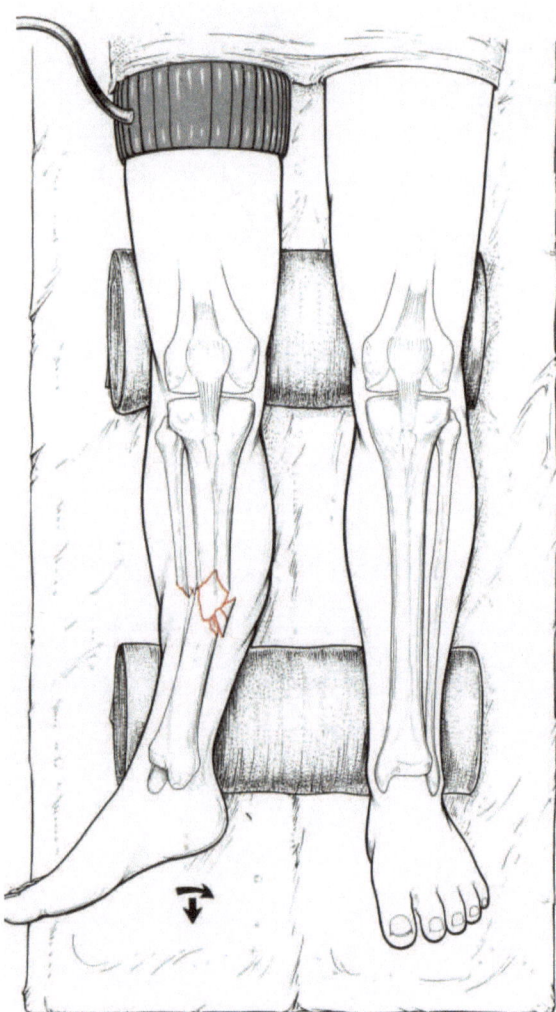

**Fig. 100.** Asepsis, draping, positioning. Both legs are prepared and draped to permit comparision with the healthy side. A tourniquet is placed on the injured leg

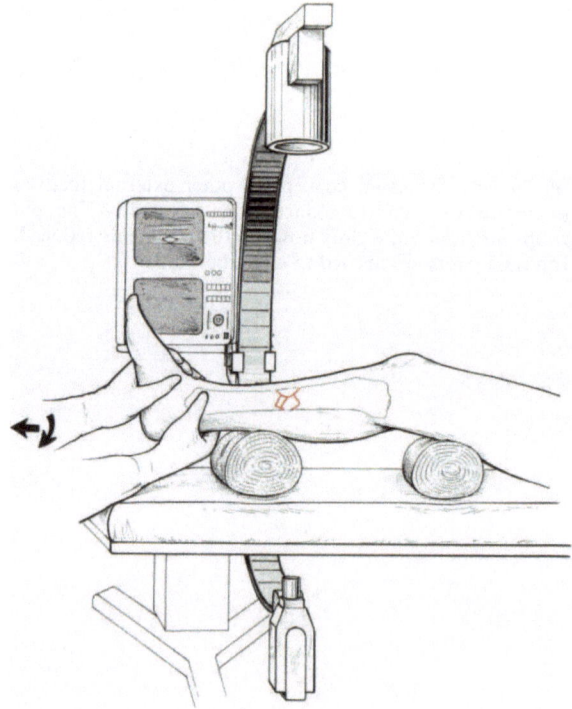

**Fig. 102.** Radiologic assessment of the fracture. The reduction may be carried out under image intensifier control

la, reduction will be obtained automatically. In any case, the external fixator is not applied until axial alignment of the tibia is satisfactory. At this time the choice for a unilateral or bilateral frame is made.

# 4 The Application of a Bilateral Frame

## 4.1 Pin Placement

With the aid of radiographs or an image intensifier, the proposed sites of pin placement in the reduced tibia are ascertained and marked. This is done by inserting thin Kirschner wires (0.8 mm diam.) laterally through the skin over the anterior tibial border (Fig. 103). A radiologic check is made to determine whether the proposed levels of pin insertion are appropriate. All the Kirschner wires should occupy the same, frontal plane, and this plane should coincide with that of the knee joint axis. It is important to remember that the ankle joint and foot show 20–25° of lateral rotation relative to this plane owing to the anatomic torsion of the tibia. The exact degree of tibial torsion is easily assessed by comparison with the opposite side.

Viewed in cross-section, the pins should traverse the tibia at a point midway between the anterior tibial border and posterior tibial surface (Fig. 104). The anterior tibial border already has been "probed" with the Kirschner guide wires. Additional Kirschner wires are used to probe the posteromedial border and posterior surface. Once all Kirschner wires are in place, the pins should traverse the bone midway between each pair of wires (Fig. 105).

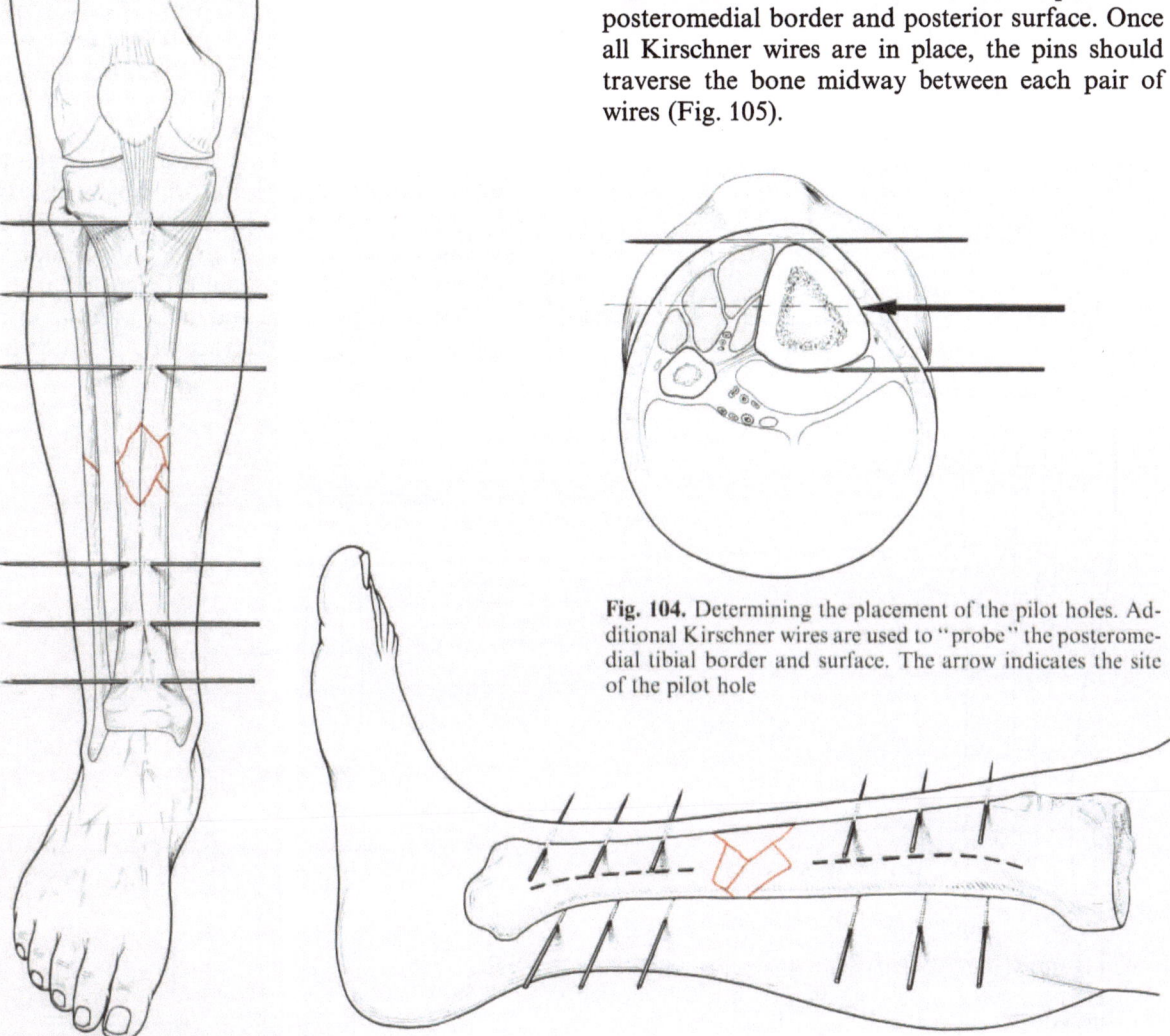

**Fig. 104.** Determining the placement of the pilot holes. Additional Kirschner wires are used to "probe" the posteromedial tibial border and surface. The arrow indicates the site of the pilot hole

**Fig. 103.** Determining pin placement. The proposed levels of pin placement are marked with thin Kirschner wires inserted percutaneously over the anterior tibial border

**Fig. 105.** The Kirschner wires mark the sites for the Steinmann pins

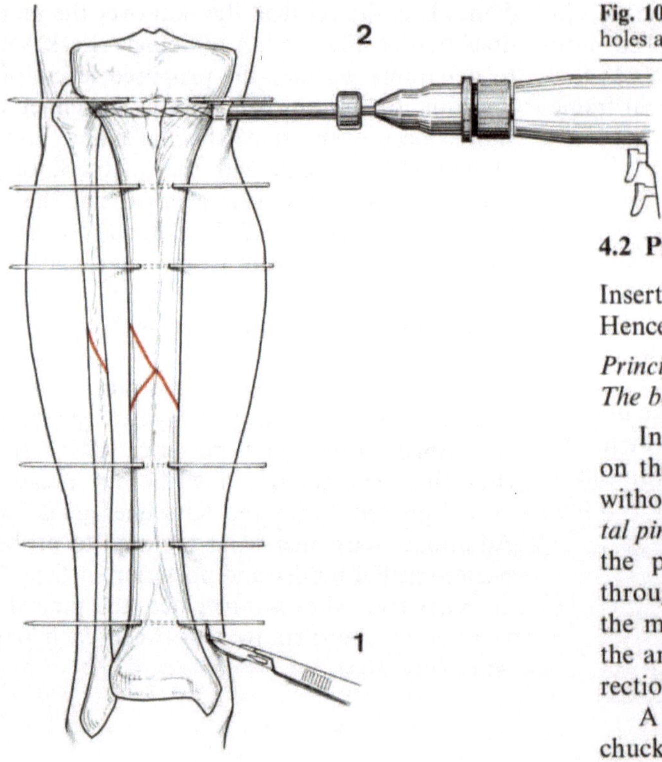

**Fig. 106.** Predrilling. Stab incisions are made (*1*), and pilot holes are drilled for the uppermost and lowermost pins (*2*)

## 4.2 Pin Insertion

Insertion of the pins should not damage the bone. Hence:

*Principle No. 2 for the threaded external fixator:*
*The bone is predrilled before the pins are inserted.*

In the reduced tibia, all pin entrance sites lie on the same line; i.e., the fragments are aligned without AP angulation. *The most proximal and distal pins are inserted first:* Through a stab incision, the pilot hole is drilled with the 3.2-mm bit through a protective sleeve, taking care to drill the medial and lateral cortices exactly parallel to the anterior Kirschner wire, which serves as a directional guide (Fig. 106).

A 4.5-mm Steinmann pin locked in the hand chuck is driven through the drill hole with a twisting motion until the tip elevates the lateral skin, at which point an exit stab incision is made and pin advancement is continued (Fig. 107).

The most proximal and distal pins are inserted first, placing each a distance of 2–3 cm from the

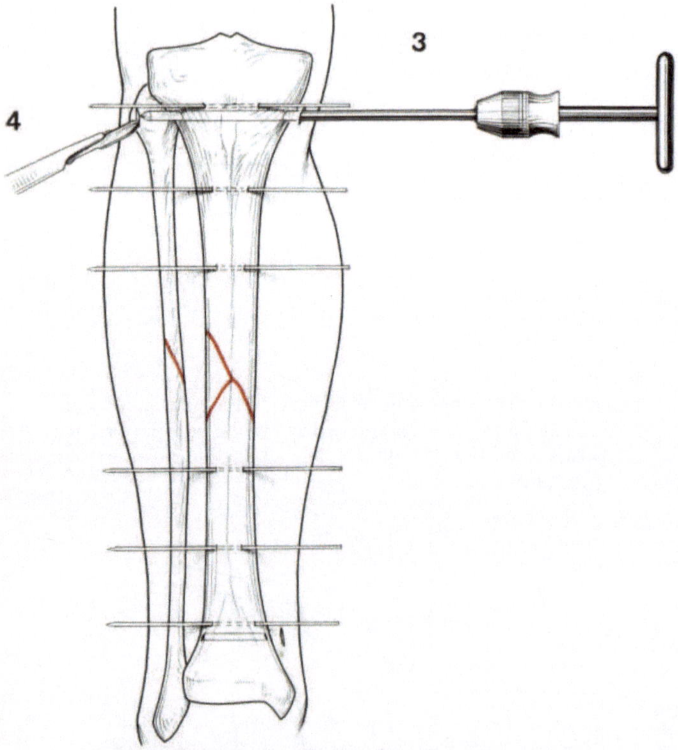

**Fig. 107.** Insertion of the pins. The pin is driven through the pilot hole (*3*) and exits through a counterincision in the skin (*4*)

**Fig. 108.** Location of the outermost pins. With the fracture reduced, the two pins should be parallel, uniplanar, and perpendicular to the long axis of the tibia

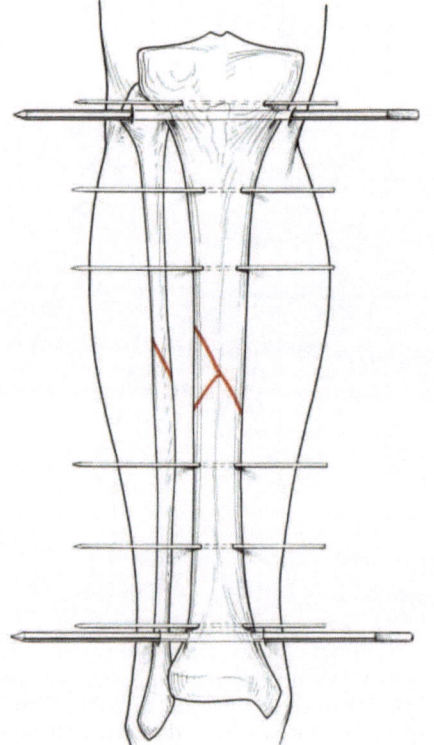

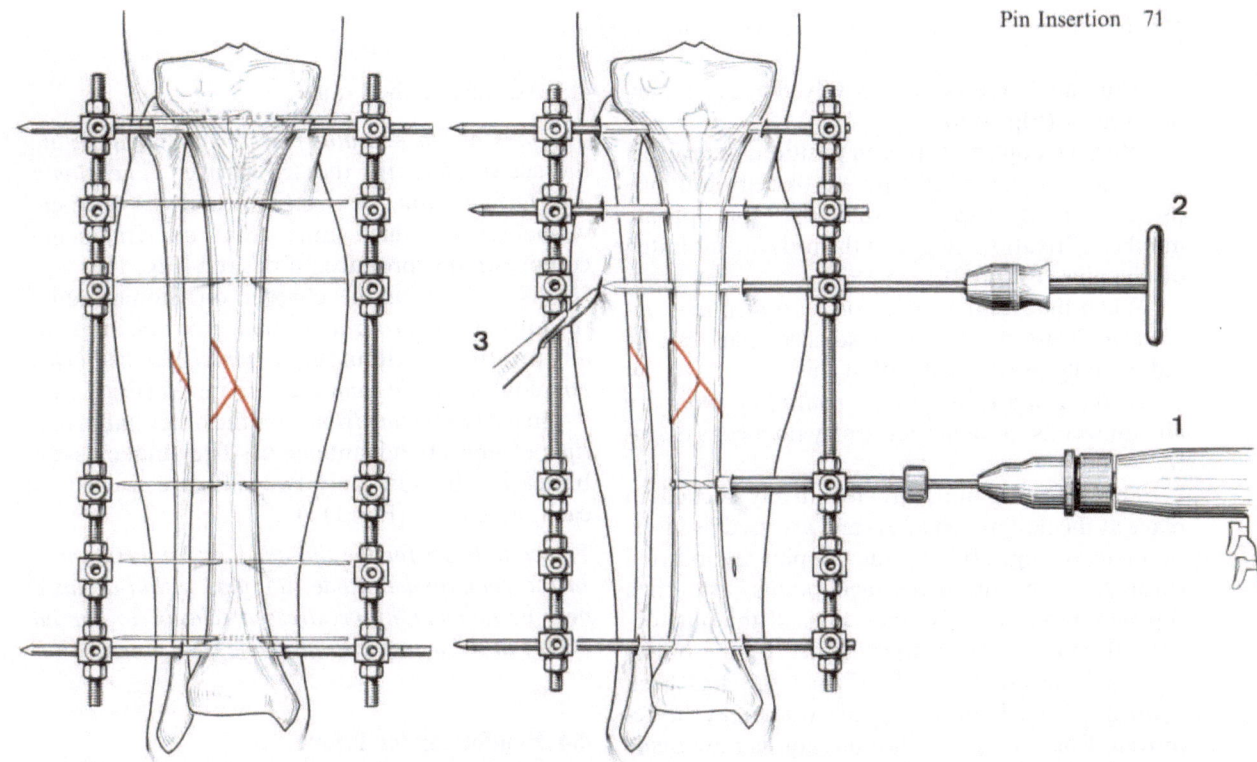

**Fig. 109.** Mounting the threaded rods with empty clamps. The two rods and associated clamps are provisionally mounted

**Fig. 111.** Using the clamps as guides. The drill sleeve and bit are introduced through the clamps, and the pilot holes are drilled (*1*); the pins are inserted (*2*); counterincisions are made (*3*); and the pins are moved forward into the opposite clamps

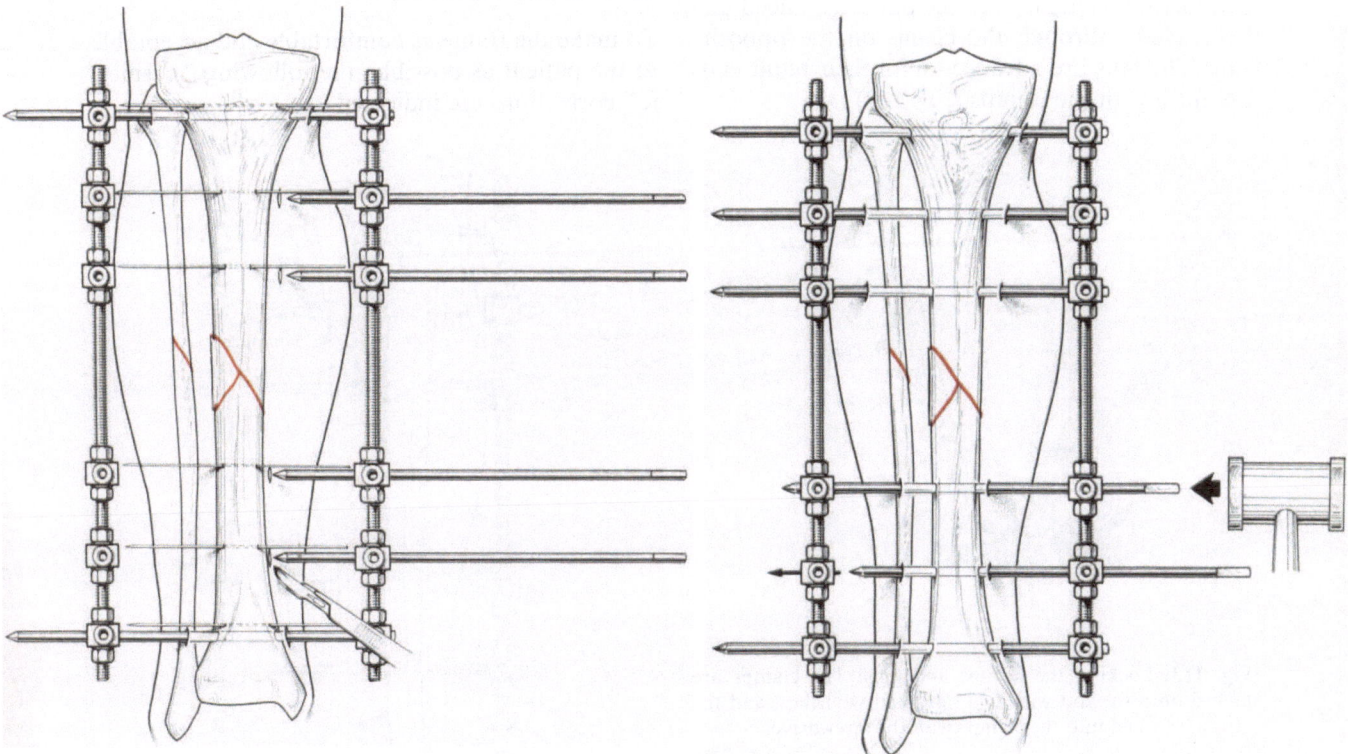

**Fig. 110.** Using the clamps as guides. The pins are introduced through the clamps, and stab incisions are made

**Fig. 112.** Advancing the pins. The pins are advanced using the hand chuck and hammer

knee and ankle joints, respectively. The remaining pins follow (Fig. 108).

With the outermost pins in position, the correct type and number of clamps are placed onto two threaded rods, together with the approproate number of fixation nuts, and the rods are mounted on the pins (Fig. 109).

When the frame is used for *neutralization, single clamps* are used so that adjacent pins can be individually prestressed within clusters.

In the *compression mode, multiple clamps* are advantageous, though they are by no means essential.

The empty clamps are tentatively locked in place at the designated levels and are used as insertion guides (Fig. 110). Steinmann pins are inserted through the clamps until their points just touch the skin. Great care is taken that all the pins occupy the same plane – that defined by the outermost pins inserted initially. When this has been confirmed, the Kirschner guide wires may be removed. For each pin a stab incision is now made opposite the pin point, the pin is withdrawn from its clamp, the drill sleeve is introduced through the clamp and soft tissue, and the 3.2-mm pilot hole is drilled. Then the pin is reinserted through its clamp and driven into the bone (Fig. 111). The exit incision is made, and the pin is advanced and "threaded" through the clamp on the opposite side. The pins are advanced until their blunt ends are flush with the clamps (Fig. 112).

## 4.3 Assembling the Frame

*The pins are locked into the clamps* by tightening the set screws with the screwdriver. *The clamps are locked onto the rods* with two open-end wrenches, at which time axial interfragmental compression is produced if desired (Fig. 113).

As we saw in the chapter on Biomechanics, the pins in a *neutralization frame* must be individually prestressed within the *proximal and distal clusters,* and so *single clamps* are required (Fig. 114).

In a *compression frame,* on the other hand, *multiple clamps* are advantageous. They make assembly easier, because only two nuts are needed for each pin cluster (Fig. 115).

*Principle No. 3 for the threaded external fixator: In the compression mode, the pins within a cluster may be individually prestressed relative to one another; in the neutralization mode, they must be.*

## 4.4 Reinforcing the Frame

The frame can be reinforced by erecting additional external rods.

## 4.5 Finishing the Frame

To make the frame as comfortable and acceptable to the patient as possible, the following "cosmetic" corrections are indicated:

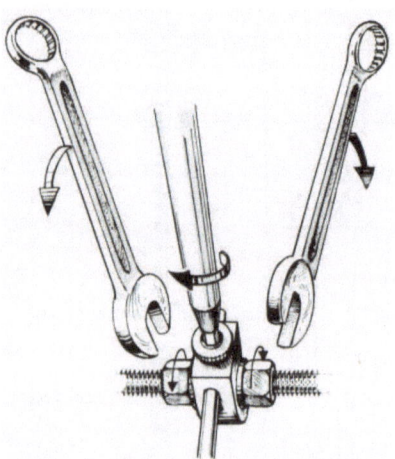

**Fig. 113.** Locking the clamps and pins. The clamps are locked onto the rod with two open-end wrenches, and the pins are locked into the clamps with the screwdriver

**Fig. 114.** Prestressing the pins in a neutralization frame. Single clamps are required for individual pin prestressing

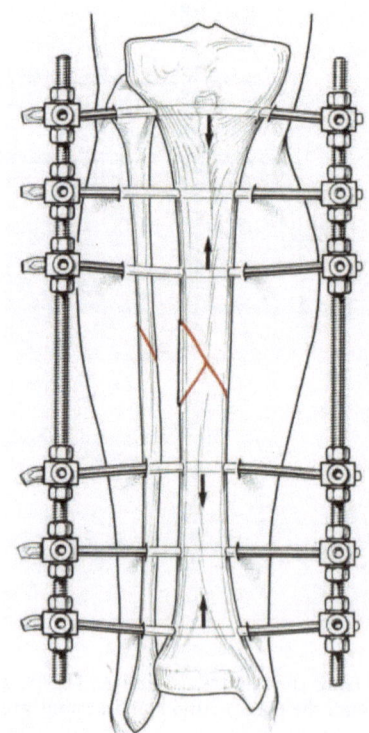

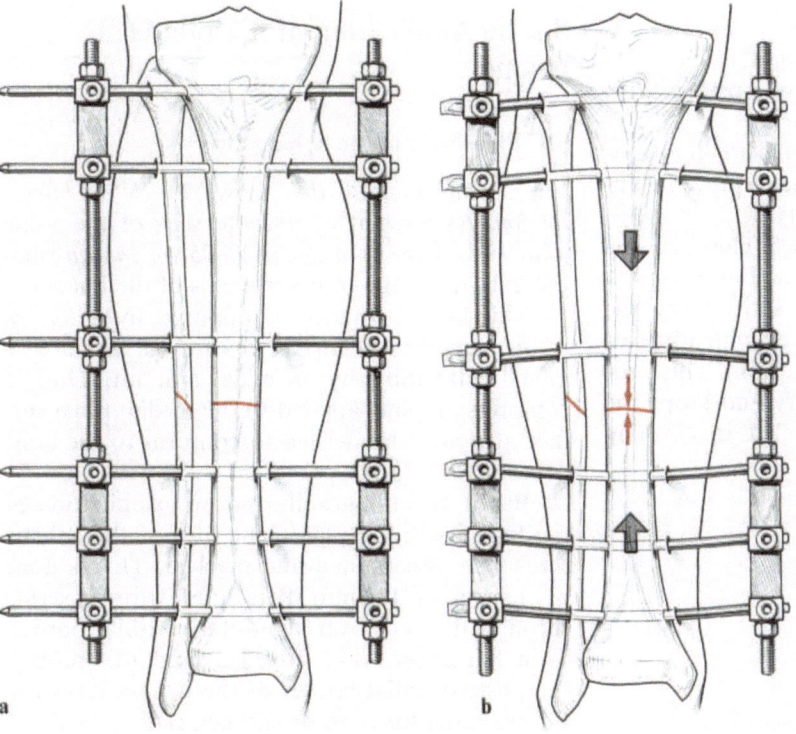

**Fig. 115 a, b.** Multiple clamps in a compression frame. **a** In the compression frame, multiple-pin clamps may be used. All pins are parallel before compression is applied. **b** After compression is applied, the two pin groups are bowed toward each other

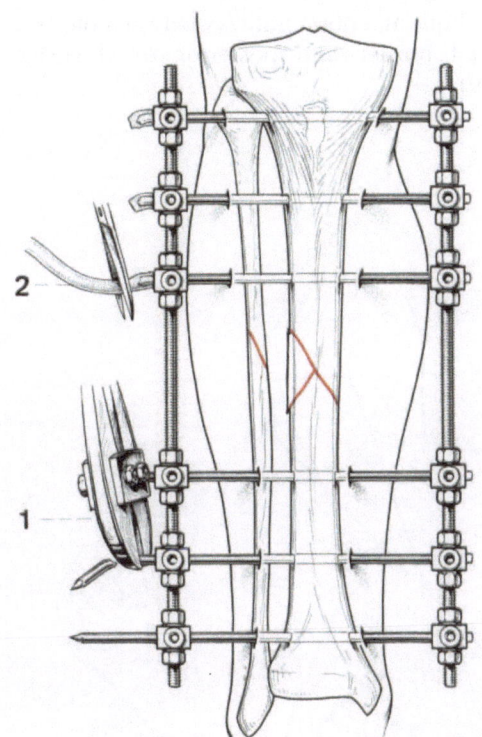

**Fig. 116.** Shortening the pins. The sharp points of the pins are snipped off with the large wire cutter (*1*). The sharp ends are covered with rubber drains (*2*)

**Fig. 117.** The finished bilateral frame. The frame does not encumber the patient during walking

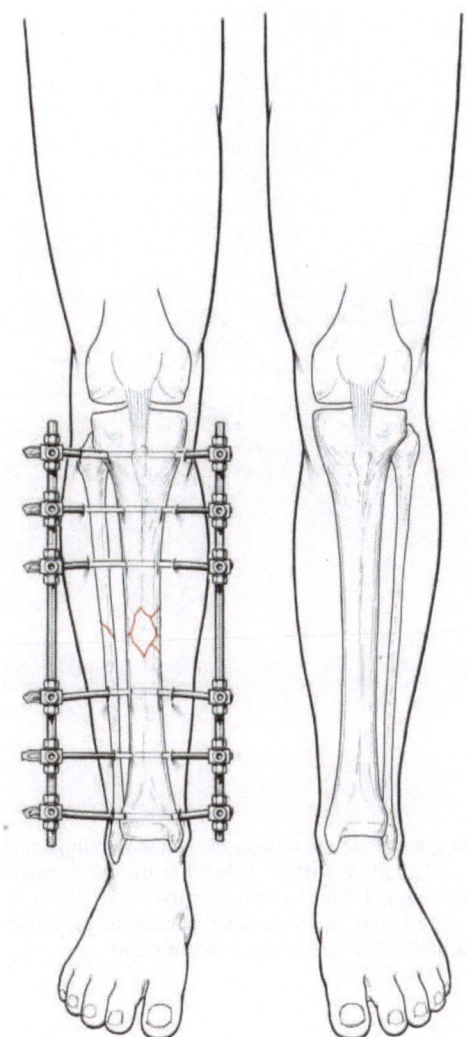

– The clamps should be mounted as close to the skin as possible without touching it. Some clearance should be left to allow for postoperative swelling.
– All fixation nuts should be tested for tightness and given a firm, final tightening to prevent subsequent loosening and instability.
– All projecting pins are clipped close to the clamps with the large wire cutter (Fig. 116).
– When all frame adjustments are satisfactory, the sharp ends of the pins are covered with adhesive tape or a small piece of rubber drain. This protects the patient from self-injury and keeps the fixator from becoming entangled in clothing (Fig. 117).

# 5 The Application of a Unilateral Frame

### 5.1 Placement of the Schanz Screws

The normal human *tibia* shows 20–25° of *lateral torsion*. As a result of this, the axis of the ankle joint and of the foot show *20–25° of lateral rotation* relative to the transverse axis of the knee.

This lateral rotation is opposed by a *torsion of the medial tibial surface toward the medial side* in its distal third by an equal amount. Thus, a compression plate applied to the medial tibial surface also must be twisted to conform to the bone contour (Fig. 118).

Based on radiographs and an examination of the limb itself, the placement sites of the Schanz screws are ascertained and marked. This is done by means of 0.8-mm Kirschner wires inserted through the skin over the anterior tibial border. Thin Kirschner wires are also used to "probe" the posteromedial border of the tibia. Marked in this way, the sites can be checked radiologically.

Viewed in cross-section, the screws should traverse the bone at a point midway between the anterior tibial border and posterior tibial surface (Fig. 119).

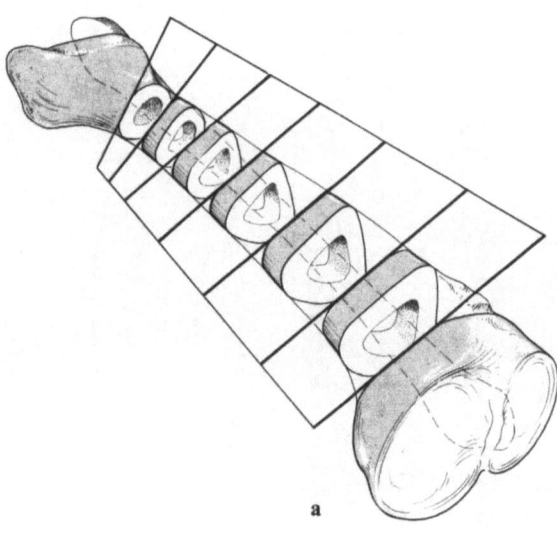

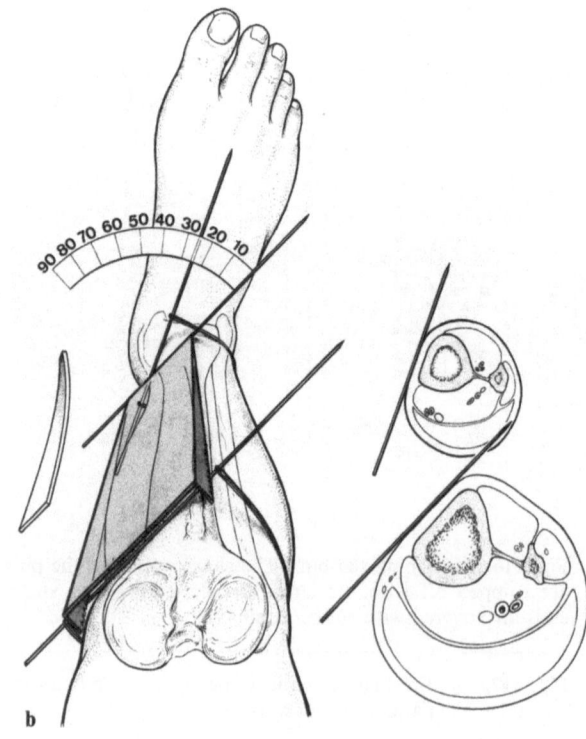

**Fig. 118a, b.** Anatomic torsion of the medial tibial surface. **a** The medial tibial surface twists toward the medial side as its descends. **b** This torsion is equal to 20–30° and can be measured with a torsiometer consisting of Kirschner wires, a protractor and a base (after Weber)

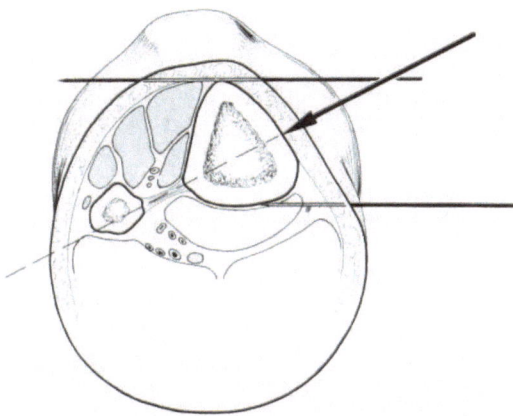

**Fig. 119.** Determining the placement of Schanz screws. The future sites of screw placement (*arrow*) are marked with percutaneous Kirschner wires

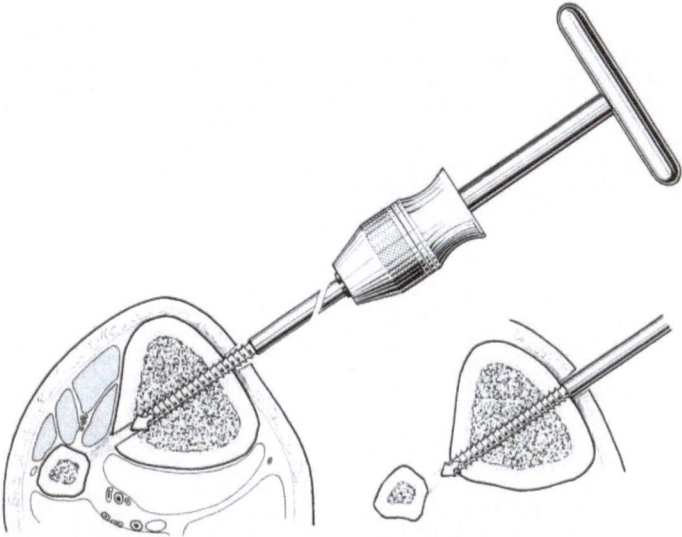

**Fig. 120.** Location and direction of the Schanz screws. The screws should traverse the bone midway between the anterior and posterior tibial borders, perpendicular to the medial tibial surface

The Schanz screws are inserted from the medial aspect such that they do not violate the anterior or posterior compartments. The proximal *Schanz screws* are inserted *perpendicular to the medial tibial surface* so that their tips engage the lateral tibial border (Fig. 120). The distal Schanz screws are on the same plane as the proximal screws. Owing to the anatomic torsion of the medial tibial surface however, the distal screws are not perpendicular to the bone at that location, but are oriented at a 20–25° angle.

### 5.2 Screw Insertion

Insertion of the screws should not damage the bone. Hence:

*Principle No. 2 for the threaded external fixator:*
*The bone is predrilled before the screws are inserted.*

With the fracture reduced, the most proximal and distal screws are inserted first, making certain that they occupy the same plane at right angles to the tibia long axis (Fig. 121): The 3.2-mm drill bit and protective sleeve are introduced through a stab incision. A pilot hole is drilled through the medial cortex perpendicular to the medial tibial surface and is carried through the opposite cortex in the direction of the interosseous membrane and fibula.

The depth gauge is inserted to measure the length of the pilot hole, skin thickness included. Subtracting the skin thickness gives the necessary thread length for the Schanz screw (Fig. 122).

The Schanz screw is driven through the predrilled hole until the "shoulder" of the screw abuts against the medial cortex. The sharp, three-

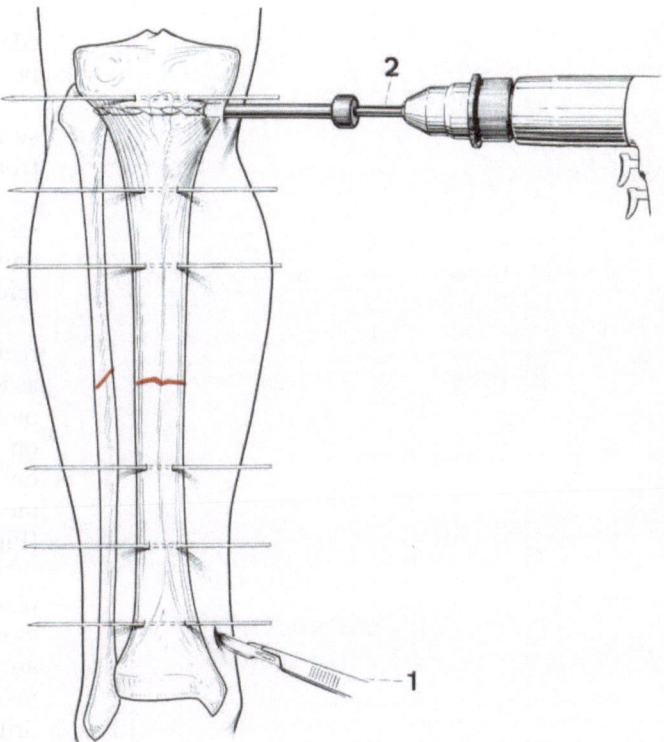

**Fig. 121.** Predrilling. Stab incisions are made (*1*), and pilot holes are drilled (*2*) for the uppermost and lowermost screws

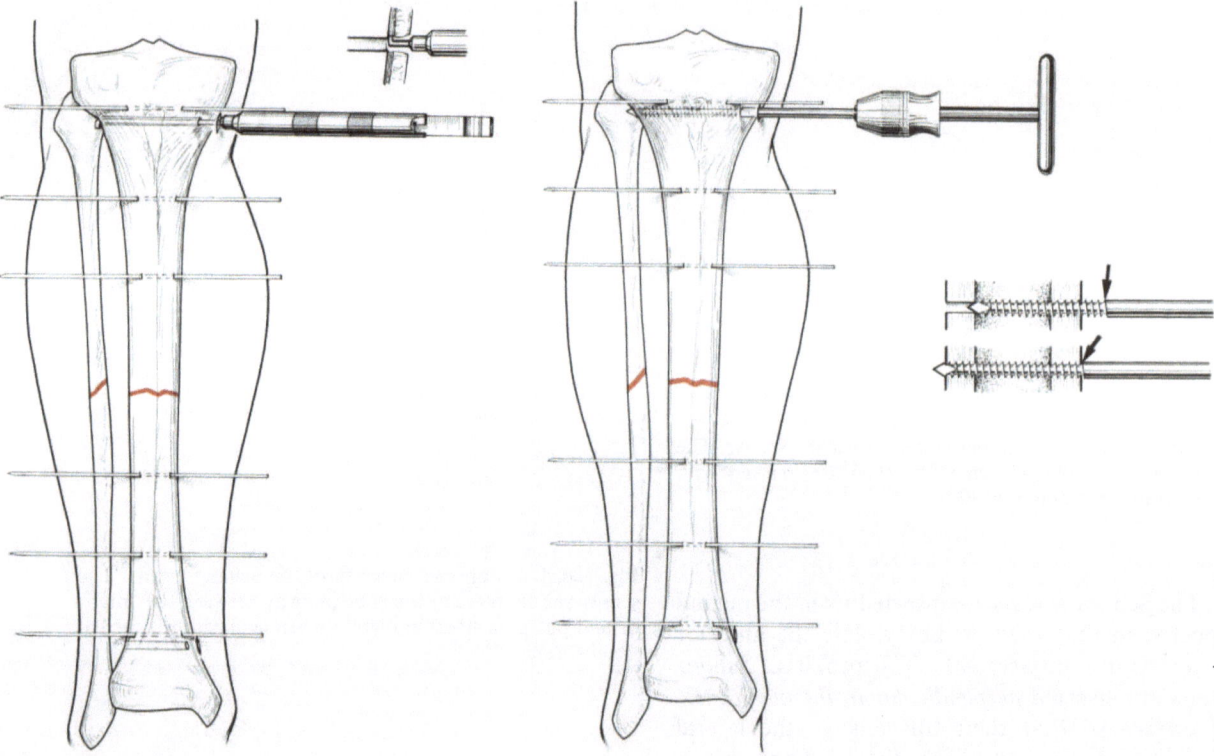

**Fig. 122.** Measuring the thread length. The necessary thread length is measured with the depth gauge

**Fig. 123.** Inserting the screws. The two screws are driven in until their shoulders engage on the cortex

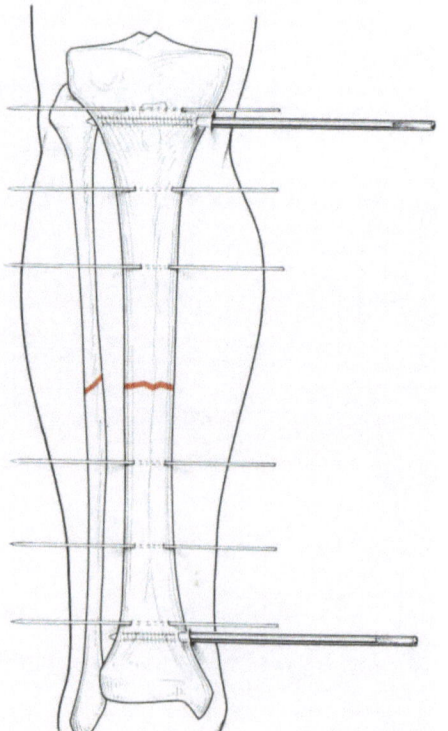

**Fig. 124.** Location of the outermost screws. With the fracture reduced, the two outermost screws are parallel, uniplanar, and perpendicular to the tibial long axis

edged point of the screw provides a good self-tapping action during insertion (Fig. 123).

The screw point cannot injure lateral soft tissues, because the shoulder of the screw stops it from advancing past the opposite cortex.

The most proximal and distal screws are inserted first, placing each one 2–3 cm from the knee and ankle joints, respectively. The remaining screws follow (Fig. 124).

With the outermost screws in position, the correct type and number of clamps are placed onto a threaded rod, together with the appropriate number of fixation nuts, and the rod is mounted on the inserted screws. Because a unilateral frame on the tibia should be used in the compression mode only, multiple clamps are advantageous (Fig. 125).

The empty clamps are tentatively locked in place at the designated levels. Using the clamps as guides, the 3.2-mm drill bit and protective sleeve are introduced through stab incisions, and the remaining pilot holes are drilled. Care is taken to drill the holes such that parallelism is maintained between the screws of the proximal and distal clusters. The Schanz screws are inserted through the mounted clamps (Figs. 126 and 127).

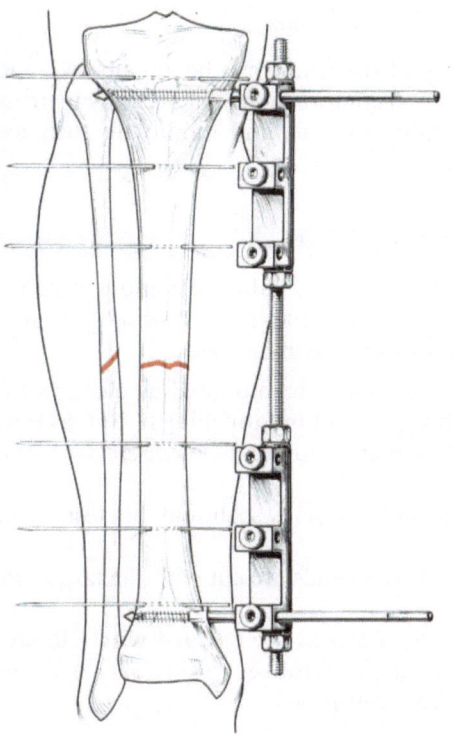

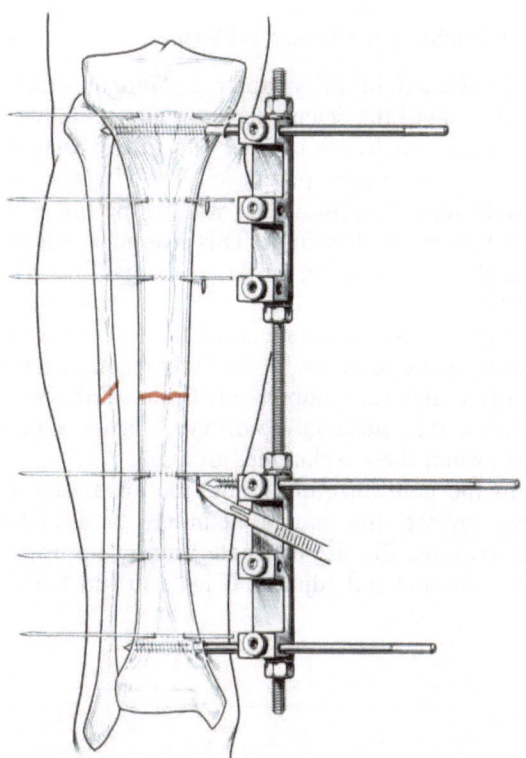

**Fig. 125.** Mounting the threaded rod with empty clamps. The rod with associated clamps is provisionally mounted

**Fig. 126.** Using the clamps as guides. The screws are introduced through the clamps, and stab incisions are made

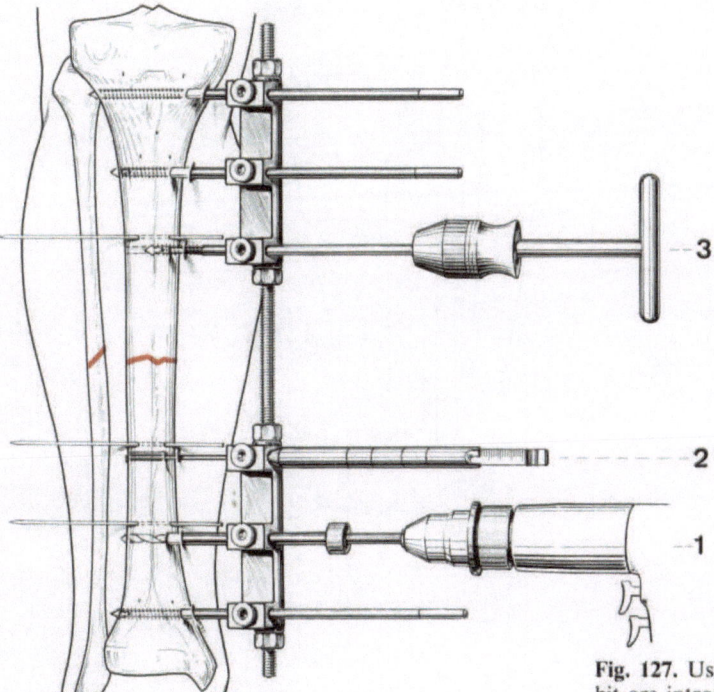

**Fig. 127.** Using the clamps as guides. The drill sleeve and bit are introduced through the clamps and pilot holes are drilled (*1*). The thread length is measured and calculated (*2*), and the screws are inserted (*3*)

## 5.3 Assembling the Unilateral Frame

As mentioned in the chapter on Biomechanics, prestressing of the Schanz screws is not mandatory in a unilateral frame because the thread ensures an adequate bone purchase. The fracture is brought under compression by adjusting the position of the multiple clamps. This is done by adjusting and then tightening the fixation nuts (Figs. 128 and 129).

The technique of prebending the rod or screws or using a spreading rod is strongly recommended for the unilateral compression frame. Care must be taken that no axial deformity (varus) is produced when these techniques are used.

In the neutralization mode, the advantage of screw prestressing should definitely be utilized. This requires the use of single clamps, appropriately mounted and adjusted (Figs. 130 and 131).

## 5.4 Reinforcing the Frame

The stability of the frame can be augmented, and interfragmental compression enhanced, by increasing the number of rods and modifying their arrangement.

## 5.5 Finishing the Frame

To make the frame as comfortable and acceptable to the patient as possible, the following "cosmetic" corrections are recommended:

- The clamps should be mounted as close to the skin as possible without touching it. Some clearance is left to accommodate postoperative swelling.
- All nuts and set screws should be tested for tightness.
- Projecting screw ends are cut with the large wire cutter.
- Sharp ends of screws are covered with adhesive tape or a piece of rubber drain to protect the patient from self-injury.

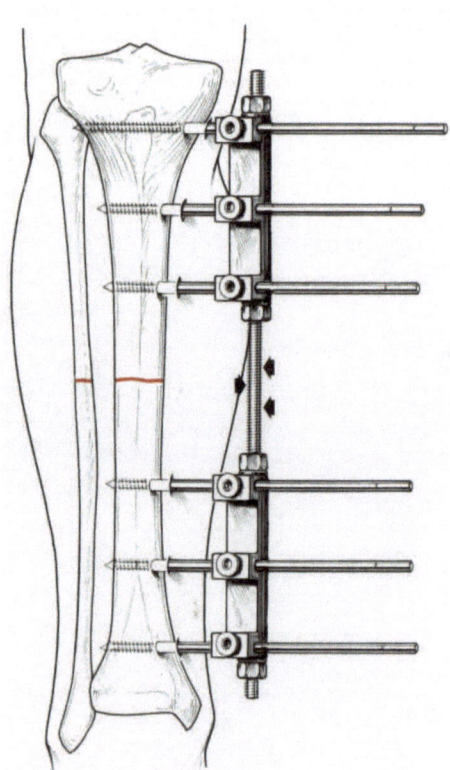

**Fig. 128.** The unilateral frame before compression is applied. The Schanz screws are parallel and locked within their clamps. The rod may be prebent as required (*arrows*)

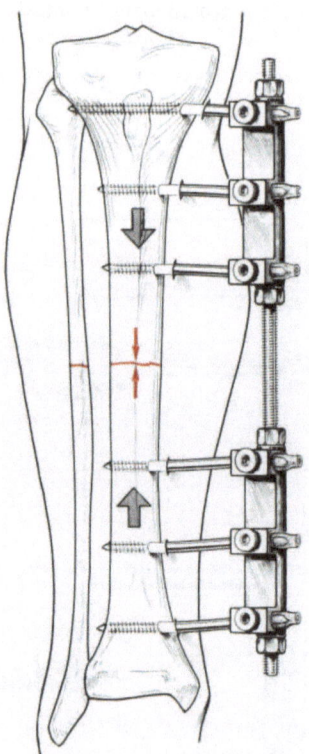

**Fig. 129.** The unilateral compression frame. Interfragmental compression can be applied with the aid of multiple clamps (or groups of single clamps)

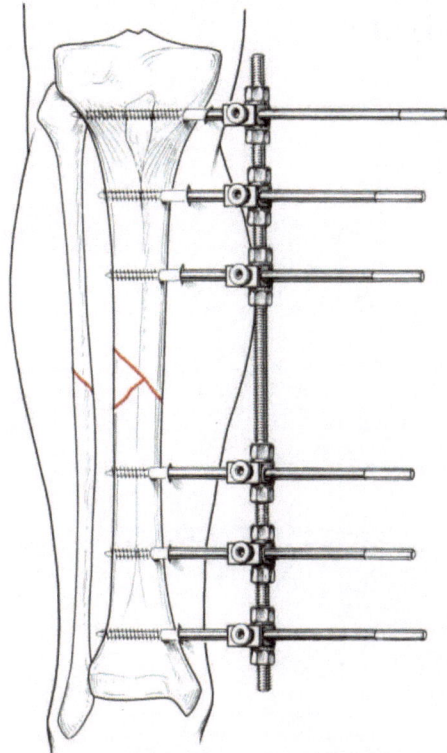 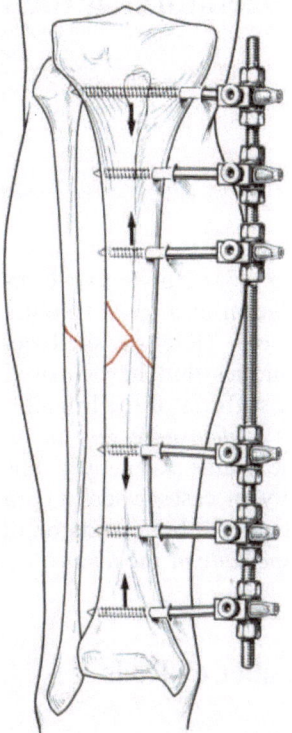

**Fig. 130.** The unilateral neutralization frame. Single clamps are used to permit individual prestressing of the screws

**Fig. 131.** Prestressing the screws in a unilateral neutralization frame. The screws within the two groups are prestressed relative to each other with the aid of single clamps

# E Techniques for Reinforcing the External Fixator

B.G. Weber

We have discussed the standard operative technique for the external fixation of a tibial fracture under normal circumstances. Here we shall describe some special techniques that have proved useful for augmenting the stiffness of the frame.

In my experience it is *seldom necessary to increase the rigidity* of the frame. Generally this should be considered only in cases where a gap or defect is present between the bone ends or in instances of nonunion, *especially of the femur.*

## 1 Increasing the Number of Rods
(Fig. 132)

In both the unilateral and bilateral frames, extra rods can be applied in addition to the minimum number required. The clamp-rod unit can be doubled or even trebled while maintaining a uniplanar configuration.

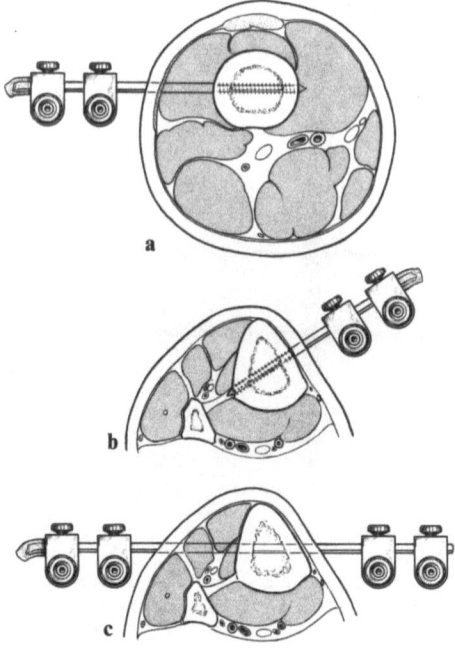

**Fig. 132 a–c.** Rods in a common plane. All rods are mounted on the pins or screws in the same plane. **a** Unilateral frame on the femur. **b** Unilateral frame on the tibia. **c** Bilateral frame on the tibia

## 2 Mounting Additional Rods in a Perpendicular Configuration (Fig. 133)

If extra rods are to be applied, it is most effective to mount them in a perpendicular or "mirror image" configuration, as this will provide enhanced stability at no additional expense. This corresponds to the "double frame" principle of Adrey and Vidal. The AP stability of this configuration is excellent.

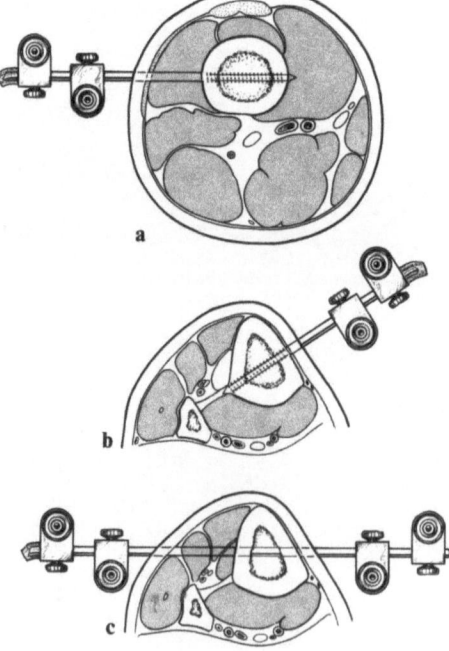

**Fig. 133 a–c.** Rods in mirror-image planes. The rods are mounted on the pins or screws in mirror-image arrays, producing a double-frame effect. **a** Unilateral frame on the femur. **b** Unilateral frame on the tibia. **c** Bilateral frame on the tibia

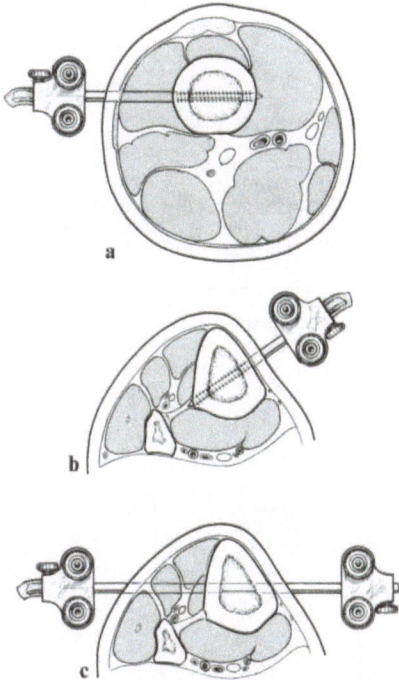

**Fig. 134 a–c.** Double clamps for two rods. Instead of two single clamps mounted in mirror-image fashion, analogous double clamps can be used to create a double-frame effect. **a** Unilateral frame on the femur. **b** Unilateral frame on the tibia. **c** Bilateral frame on the tibia

A similar effect can be achieved by using double clamps for two rods. Either a unilateral or bilateral double-frame assembly can be created by the use of these clamps (Fig. 134).

# 3 Stability of the Unilateral Frame

Because the unilateral frame is intrinsically less stable than the bilateral frame, its use on the femur calls for special reinforcing measures. The most favorable situation for a unilateral frame is one in which the bone ends are well apposed and can transmit compressive loads. Various methods are available for increasing the stabilizing interfragmental pressure:

### 3.1 Increasing Stability in the Presence of Bone Contact (Fig. 135)

A second rod, called the "spreading rod," is mounted external to the fixation rod. When the

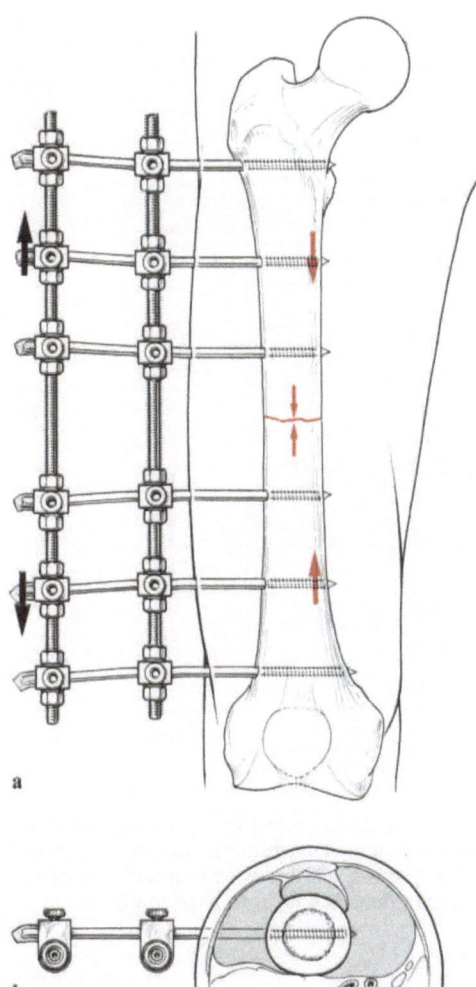

**Fig. 135 a, b.** Use of a "spreading rod" in the presence of bone contact. **a** The spreading action of the lateral rod produces interfragmental compression. **b** Cross-section: The distance between the two rods is large to ensure greater interfragmental pressure

clamps on the spreading rod are moved apart, the Schanz screws come under a bending stress which causes their points to deflect toward the fracture line. In this way the screws can exert a sustained compression across the fracture site on the order of 10 kg per screw.

### 3.2 Increasing Stability in the Absence of Bone Contact

If bone contact is absent and the use of a bilateral frame is not feasible (e.g., on the femur), it is imperative that measures be taken to fortify the unilateral frame.

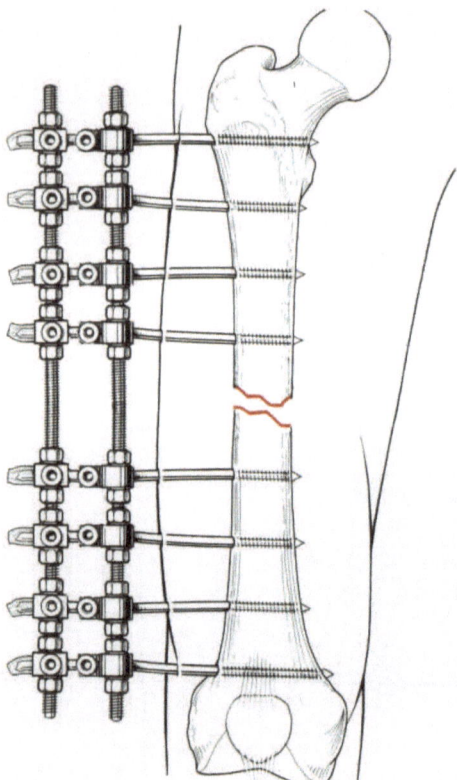

**Fig. 136.** Reinforcing the frame in the absence of bone contact. This can be done by increasing the number of screws and their primary stress, and by increasing the number of rods and mounting them in a mirror-image configuration

### 3.2.1 Increasing the Number of Schanz Screws (Fig. 136)

The screws are prestressed within clusters. Supporting double rods are mounted near the skin to resist compression and thus prevent possible varus angulation associated with partial weight bearing or muscular tension. A single, tension-resistant retaining rod is mounted farther out from the skin to maintain the position of the screw ends. It is advantageous to prestress the system in valgus as a safeguard against tension-compression cycling and fatigue fracturing of the device.

### 3.2.2 Applying Two Unilateral Frames in Two Planes (Fig. 137)

On occasions where a single, reinforced unilateral frame on the femur cannot provide adequate stability, a second, anterior unilateral frame may be applied.

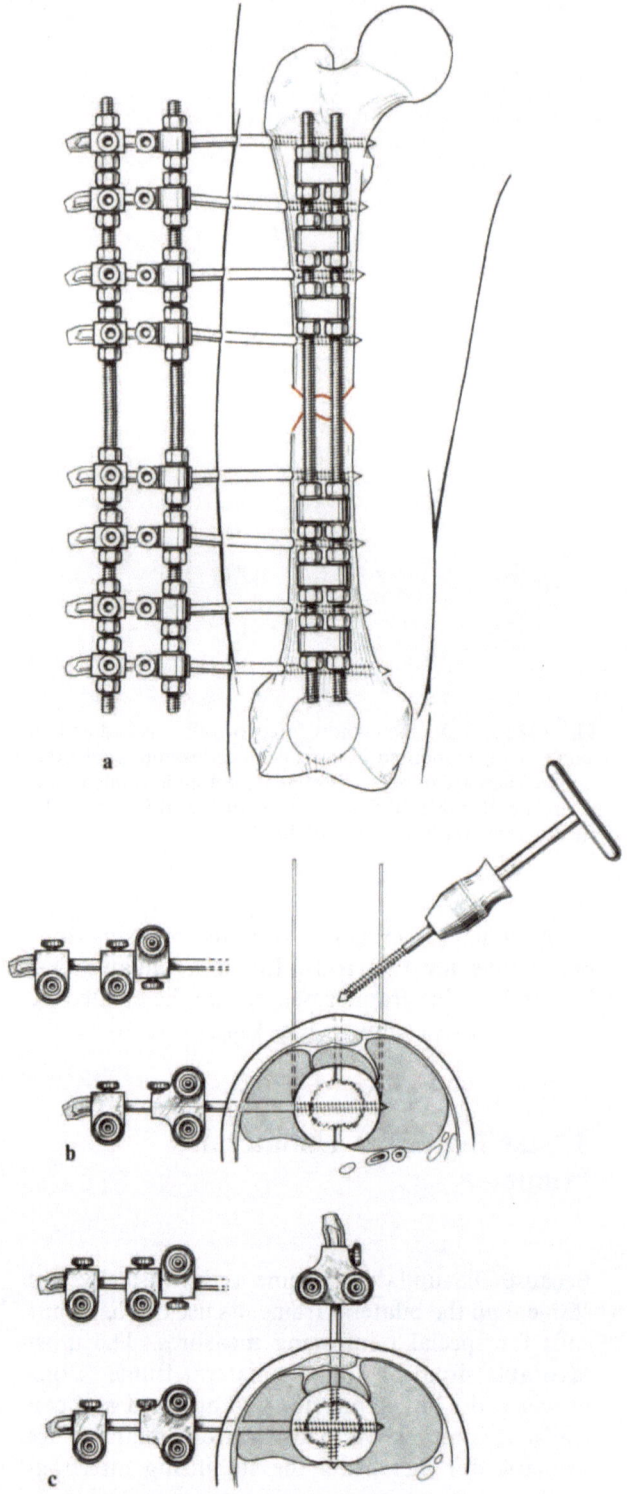

**Fig. 137 a–c.** Two unilateral frames in two planes. **a** Two unilateral frames are mounted at right angles to each other. The mirror-image arrangement of the rods provides a double-frame effect. **b** Cross-section: The location of the drill holes is marked on the femur (and elsewhere) with Kirschner wires. **c** Cross-section: The clamps can be used in various ways to fortify the fixation

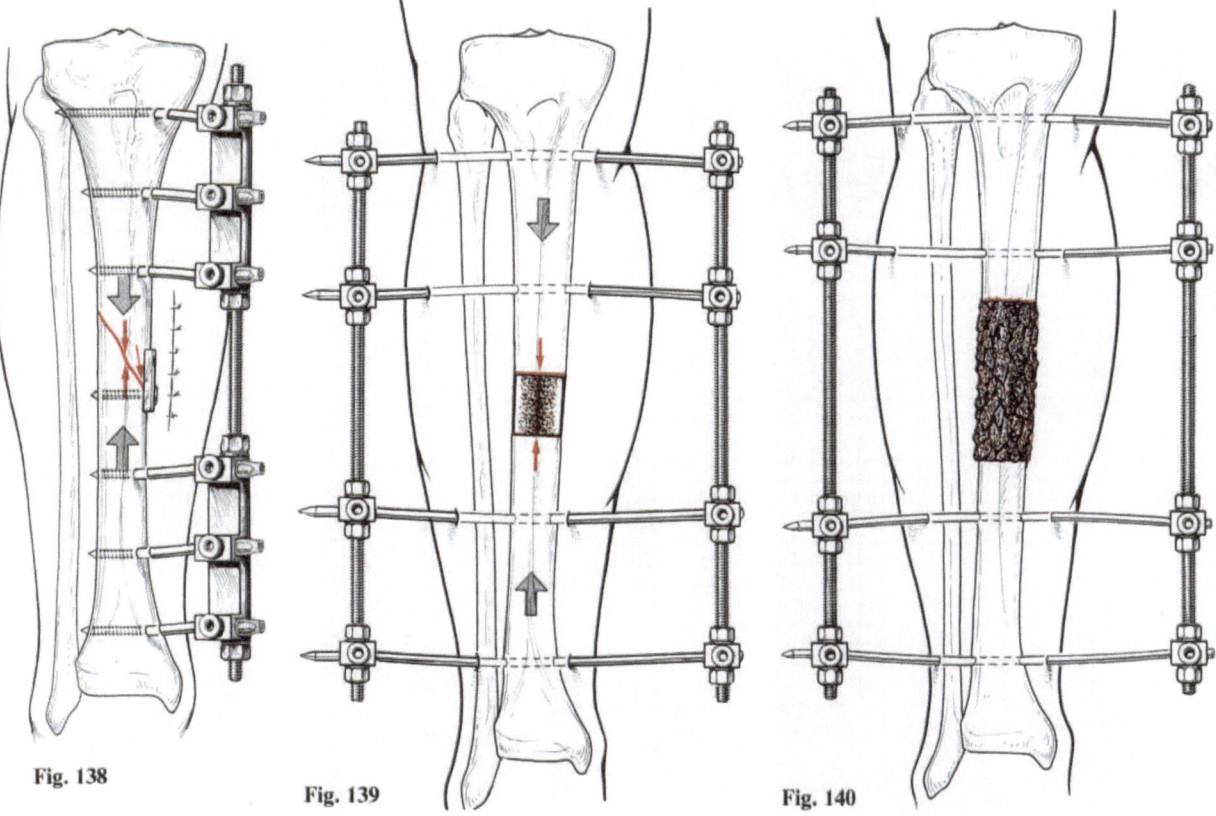

Fig. 138

Fig. 139

Fig. 140

**Fig. 138.** Minimal internal fixation plus external fixation. Minimal internal fixation (e.g., an antiglide plate) is applied to restore compressive strength to the fracture. In this situation a unilateral frame is adequate

**Fig. 139.** Pressure-competent bone grafts plus external fixation. The defect is bridged with pressure-resistant bone grafts so that a compression frame may be applied

**Fig. 140.** Autogenous cancellous bone grafts. Large defects are bridged with pieces of autogenous cancellous bone, whereupon a neutralization frame is applied

# 4 Restoring Bone Contact

The restoration of bone contact is important, as it improves stability and promotes ossification.

## 4.1 Minimal Internal Fixation (Fig. 138)

Minimal internal fixation converts on otherwise unstable fracture into a pressure-resistant fracture, and thus permits the use of a compression frame.

## 4.2 Pressure-Resistant Corticocancellous Bone Grafts (Fig. 139)

Small comminuted zones or nonunions associated with small osseous defects can be bridged with autogenous, pressure-competent corticocancellous bone taken from the iliac crest.

## 4.3 Autogenous Cancellous Bone (Fig. 140)

Even large diaphyseal defects can be obliterated by interposing autogenous cancellous bone grafts between the bone ends in the presence of a good recipient bed (with a well perfused soft-tissue envelope).

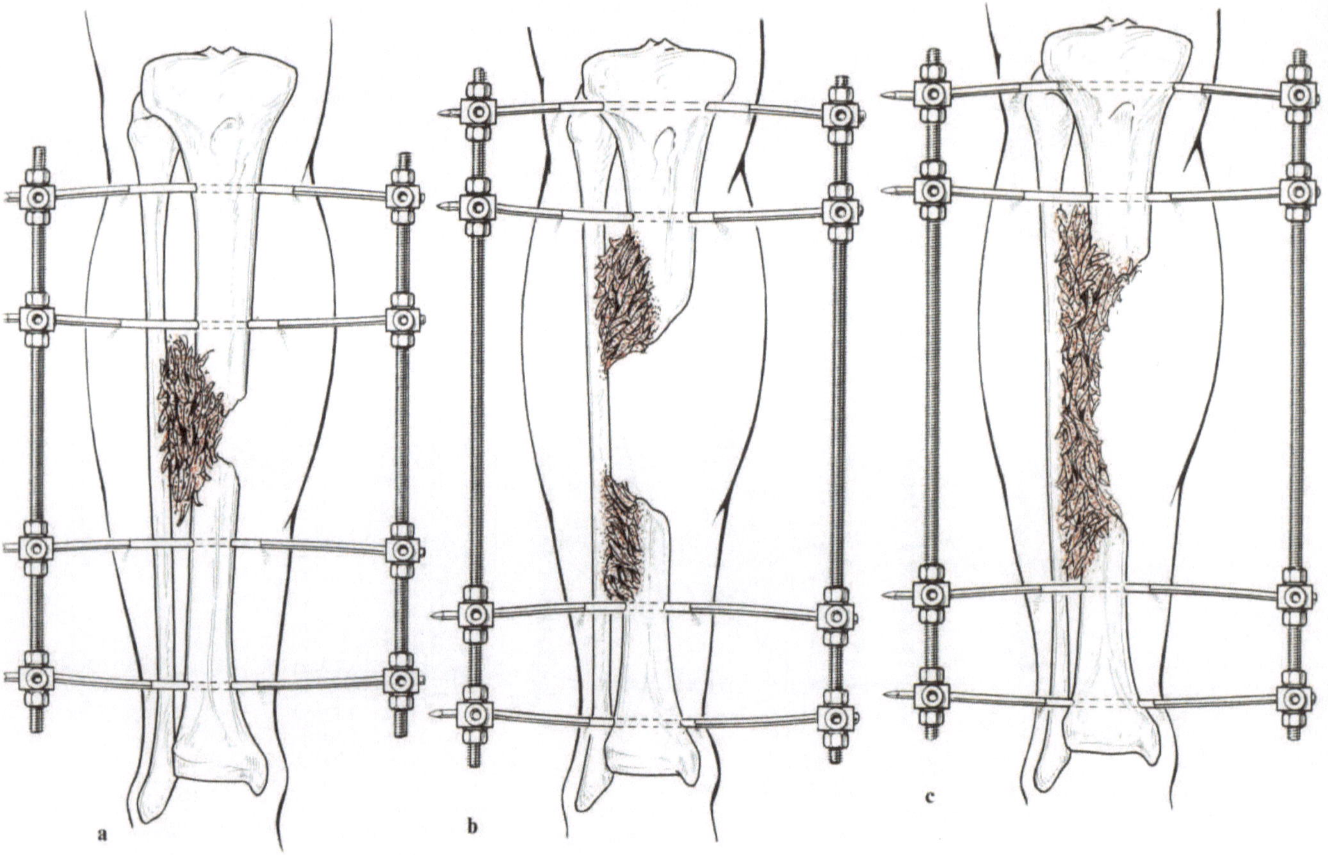

Fig. 141 a–c. Fibula-pro-tibia grafting (creation of tibiofibular synostosis). **a** The cancellous bone is introduced from the lateral side, anterior or posterior to the interosseous membrane, and a neutralization frame is erected. **b** With major loss of bone substance, **a** grafting is done in a first step. **c** The bone grafting is completed in a second step

## 4.4 Cancellous Bone Grafting via an Uninfected Route (Fig. 141)

In a septic nonunion of the tibia accompanied by bone loss, the cancellous bone is applied through an uninfected route. The defect is approached along the interosseous membrane from the anterolateral or posterolateral side. A tibiofibular synostosis is created to stabilize the tibia ("fibula-pro-tibia" graft).

In some cases the cancellous bone is applied to the posterior tibial surface through a posteromedial approach (Fig. 142).

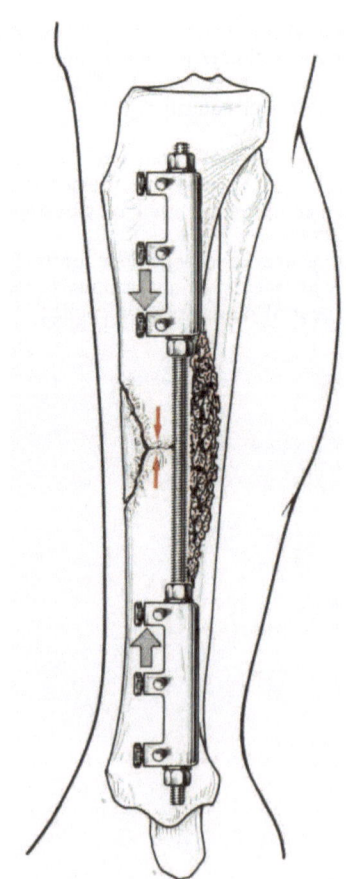

Fig. 142. Posteromedial cancellous bone grafting. The bone grafts are applied through a posteromedial approach, parallel to the posteromedial border of the tibia

### 4.5 Decortication and Cancellous Bone Grafting (Fig. 143)

In nonreactive nonunions that are accompanied by bone loss, decortication combined with cancellous bone grafting is an effective means of replacing lost osseous substance, stimulating osteogenesis and promoting ossification.

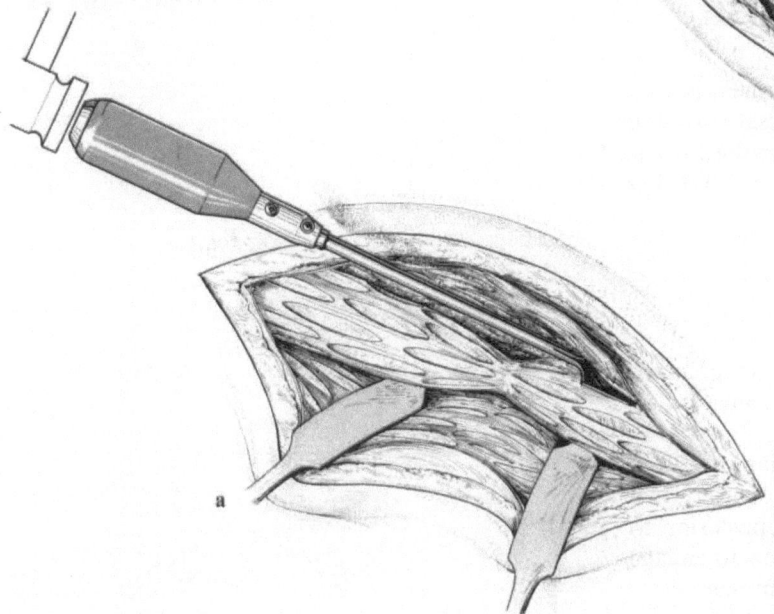

**Fig. 143 a, b.** Decortication and cancellous bone grafting. **a** In decortication, a hammer and chisel are used to raise slivers of cortical bone which retain soft tissue attachments. **b** The harvested cancellous bone is then applied to the decorticated area

## 5 Stability Enhancement and Frame Design

Pins and screws which impale muscles are a hindrance to postoperative exercise. Therefore we favor frame designs that are free of this disadvantage. Owing to the various techniques available for reinforcing the threaded external fixator by modifying its design, we find that a greater number of tibial fractures, osteotomies and nonunions are amenable to treatment with a unilateral frame than ever before. Even on the femur, a single unilateral frame applied in the frontal plane frequently is sufficient and need not be supplemented by a second, anterior frame. This brings us to:

*Principle No. 4 for the threaded external fixator:*
*If at all possible, a unilateral fixator should be used in preference to a bilateral or biplanar frame.*

This preference is largely a result of an increasing reliance on minimal or appositional internal fixation in the management of open fractures. With these internal appliances in place, a unilateral frame may be used in cases where otherwise a bilateral configuration would be needed.

On the other hand, the surgeon should not hesitate to use a bilateral frame on the tibia, or two unilateral frames on the femur, whenever such devices would stabilize the limb better than other methods. The stability necessary for consolidation is a far more important concern than unrestricted mobility, for once the bone continuity has been restored, any losses of mobility generally are relieved quickly by appropriate therapeutic exercises.

# F Situations Requiring a Special Operative Technique

B.G. WEBER

## 1 Stabilization of Short Fragments

There may be cases in which one fragment is very short and lacks the substance necessary for the anchorage of multiple fixation pins. On these occasions several options are available for stabilizing the short fragment.

### 1.1 Stabilization with the Double Transverse Clamp (Fig. 144)

The distal tibial fragment is too short to accommodate more than one pin and will be prone to malalignment.

By using a double transverse clamp with a 1.8-cm hole spacing, it is possible to insert two pins that are situated anterior and posterior to the rod, rather than "in line," and thus to engage the fragment with two pins rather than one.

A double transverse clamp with a 2.4-cm hole spacing is available for use on the proximal tibia.

### 1.2 Stabilization with Single Clamps

The problem of the distal tibia can be solved as follows:

In addition to the normal pin, a second pin is inserted through the short fragment and attached to the primary frame by two short, separate rods (Fig. 145).

In other situations a second pin can be stabilized by means of two clamps that are mounted on the rod in mirror-image fashion (Fig. 146).

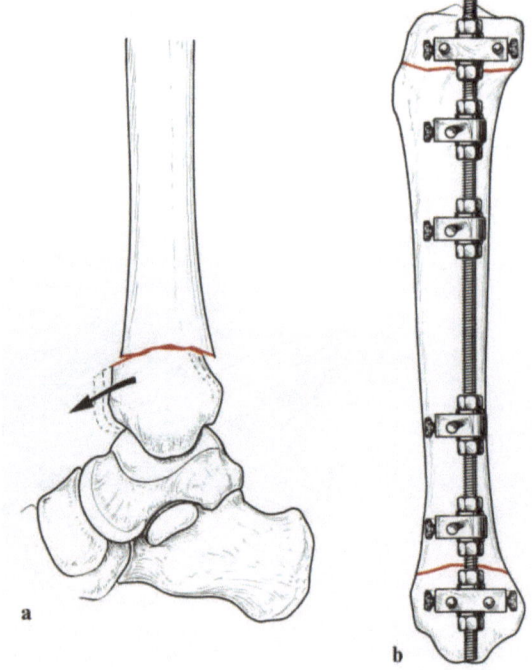

**Fig. 144 a, b.** The double transverse clamps for short fragments. **a** Short distal fragment. **b** Distal double clamp: 18 mm; proximal double clamp: 24 mm

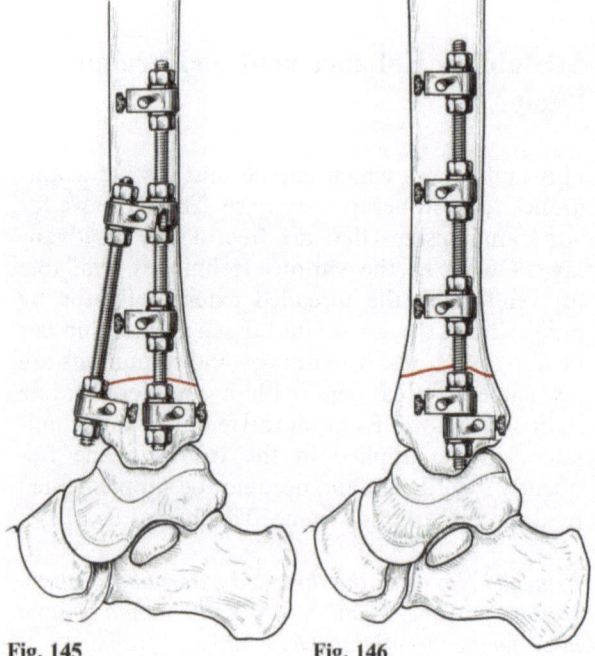

**Fig. 145.** A second frame for short fragments. The short fragment is engaged with a second pin that is connected to the main frame by 2 short rods

**Fig. 146.** Single, mirror-image clamps for short fragments. The single clamps, mounted in mirror-image fashion, produce the same effect as double transverse clamps

Fig. 145          Fig. 146

## 1.3 Stabilization with a Second Frame
(Fig. 147)

One method of "gripping" the small fragment is to erect a small unilateral frame perpendicular to the bilateral frame or 2 half-frames at a right angle.

## 1.4 The Joint-Spanning Frame (Fig. 148)

A fragment located near a joint may be so short as to preclude a stable immobilization by internal fixation, and the minimal internal fixation will require neutralization by an external device. In this case a bilateral frame may be applied in a transarticular configuration to span the adjacent joint. This has three advantages:

    a) It neutralizes the minimal internal fixation;

    b) It permits suspension of the extremity for wound care;

    c) It prevents joint deformity, such as talipes equinovarus.

## 2 Diagonal Bracing Rod (Fig. 149)

In fractures with bone loss, nonunions with bone loss or infected fractures of the tibia, there may be only enough room for two Steinmann pins in the two peripheral fragments. The resultant frame stability is poor, especially in the AP direction, on account of the long segment of diaphysis that must be bridged by the device. It is beneficial in such cases to erect a diagonal bracing rod, which is bent as needed with the bending iron and held in place by a pair of supplemental clamps. In essence, this third rod creates a "double frame" effect of the ADREY and VIDAL type.

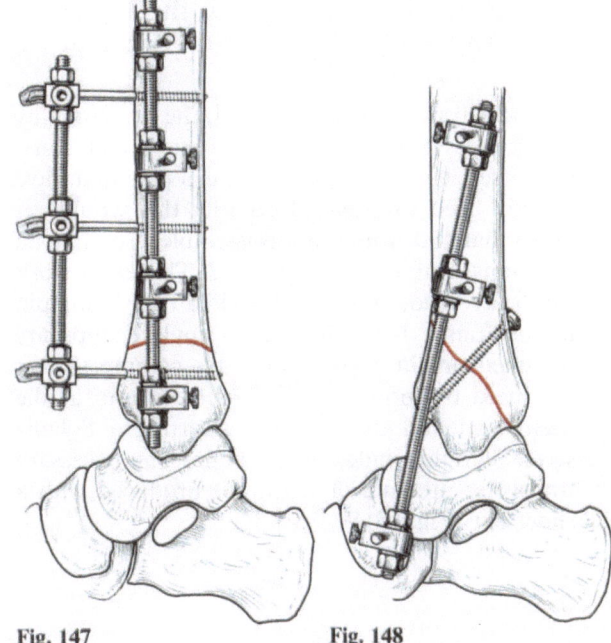

**Fig. 147**                    **Fig. 148**

**Fig. 147.** Two perpendicular frames for short fragments. The short fragment is immobilized by means of one frontal, uni- or bilateral frame and one sagittal, unilateral frame

**Fig. 148.** The transarticular frame. Minimal internal fixation is applied to the very short distal fragment. The fixation is neutralized with a bilateral frame which spans the joint

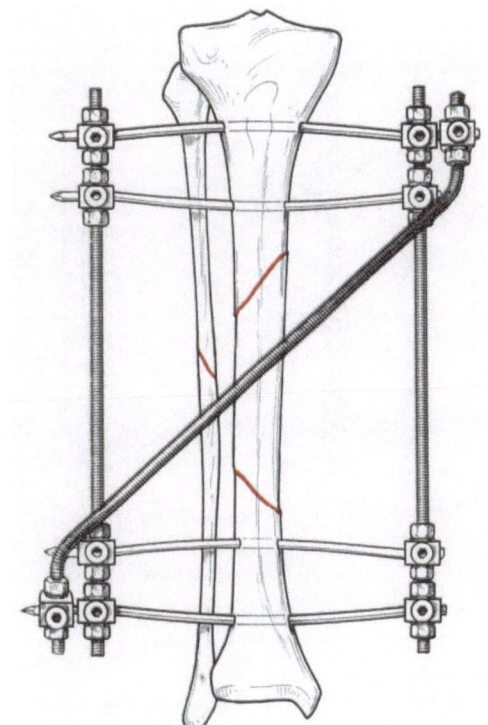

**Fig. 149.** Diagonal bracing rod. The diagonal bracing of a bilateral frame with highly peripheral screws "neutralizes" against AP displacement, creating a double-frame effect

## 3 Adding Single Clamps to the Frame, and Transverse Compression (Fig. 150)

After the frame has been erected, the surgeon may find it necessary or desirable to place an additional pin or screw at some point between pins that have already been inserted. Ordinarily this would require that the frame be disassembled so that an additional clamp can be installed. This extra work can be avoided, however. To add a transfixing pin to the frame, two self-locking single clamps are mounted on the rods. Transverse compression is produced by mounting a two-piece clamp at the desired site on the rod and inserting a Schanz screw at right angles to the bone. The necessary transverse pressure or tension is produced with a slider bar (Fig. 151).

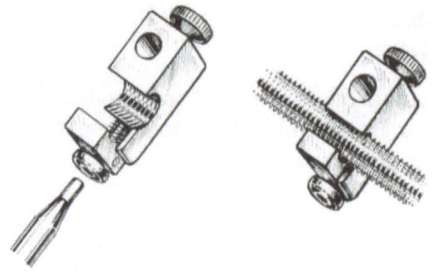

**Fig. 150.** Addition of single clamps. A supplemental two-piece clamp can be added to the frame between clamps that are already in place

**Fig. 151 a–c.** Supplementary single clamp and transverse compression. **a** A Schanz screw held by a supplementary single clamp can be used to restore apposition of the middle fragment and exert transverse compression. **b** The Schanz screw is locked into the clamp. **c** The unilateral frame is stressed so that it functions in the compression mode
▼

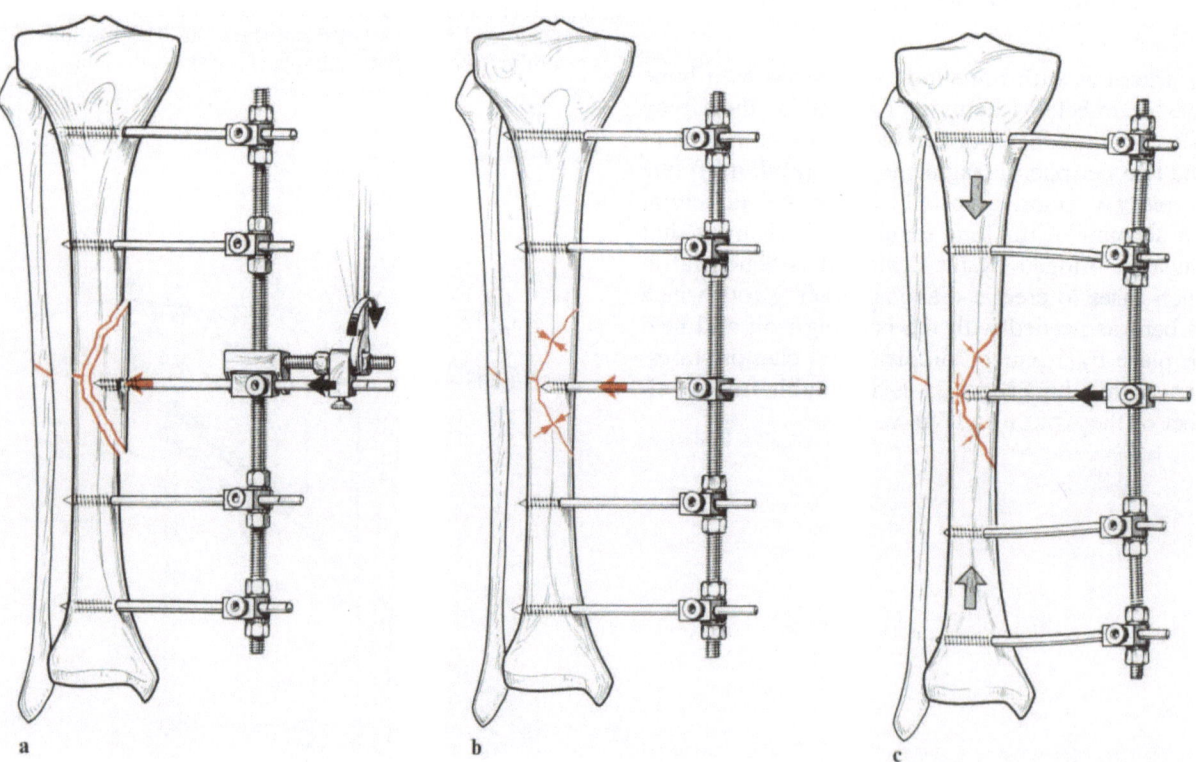

a

b

c

# G  Axial Corrections

B.G. WEBER

If the "reduction first" strategy is followed when applying the threaded external fixator, there will seldom be problems of axial malalignment once the frame has been assembled. However, in the event that a minor error of axial alignment is recognized after the frame is erected, it may be possible to correct the error without dismantling the device.

## 1  Axial Corrections in the Bilateral Frame

Slight axial malalignments can be corrected by bending the rods in situ (Fig. 152).

*Valgus or varus angulation* is corrected by bending the rods and then moving the clamps as required by means of the fixation nuts (Figs. 153 and 154).

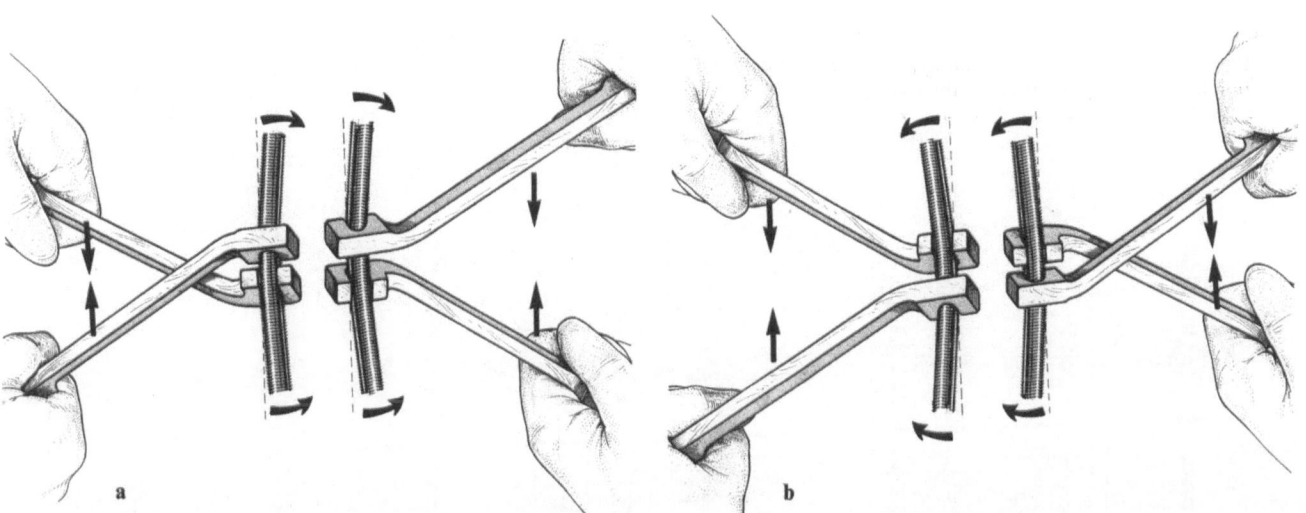

**Fig. 152 a, b.** Bending the rods in situ. The clamps on one rod must be loosened before the correction is carried out. Using two bending irons, the rods are bent (angled) in the desired direction. Then the clamps are adjusted and fastened in place. **a** Handling of the bending irons for one direction; **b** handling of the irons for the opposite direction

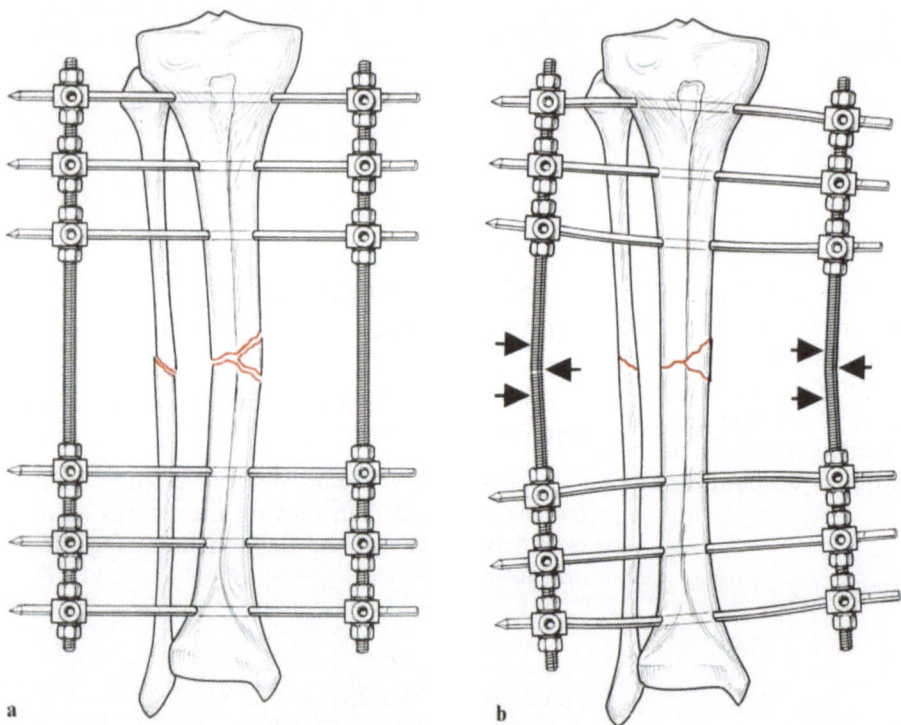

**Fig. 153 a, b.** Correction of valgus. **a** A valgus angulation.
**b** Valgus corrected by bending the rods

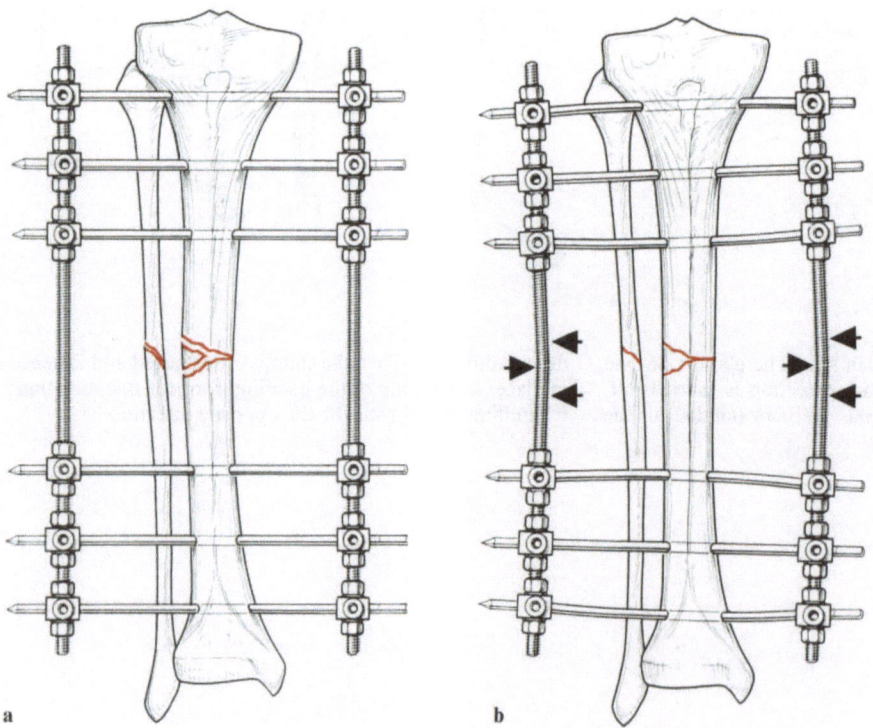

**Fig. 154 a, b.** Correction of varus. **a** A varus angulation.
**b** Varus corrected by bending the rods

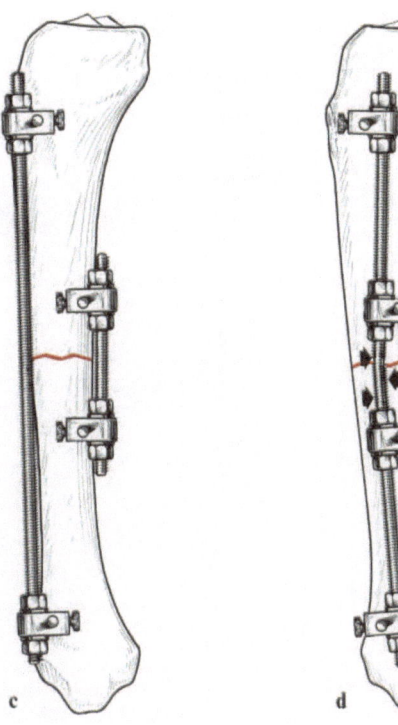

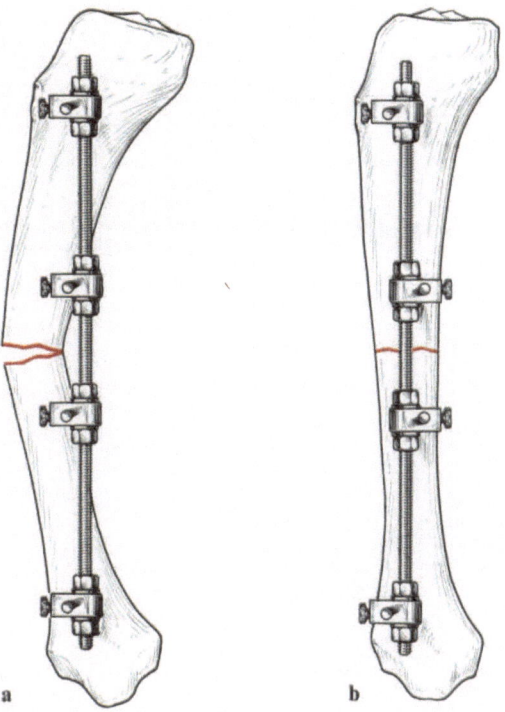

**Fig. 155 a–d.** Correction of AP angulation. **a** Example of anterior angulation. **b** Corrected by turning the clamps near the fracture. **c** Corrected by erecting two separate frames. **d** Corrected by turning the clamps near the fracture and bending the rod

*AP angulation* can be corrected by various means (Fig. 155):

– by turning the clamps near the fracture so that some pins are anterior to the rods and the rest are posterior to the rods;
– by erecting separate frames for the pins close to and distant from the fracture site;
– by turning the clamps near the fracture and, if this is not adequate, by also bending the rods with the bending irons.

*Malrotation* not exceeding 20° is corrected by bending the rods in situ with the bending irons.

In some cases it may be sufficient to turn the clamps over one or both fragments, depending on the amount of correction needed (Fig. 156).

With gross rotational malalignment, the frame should be disassembled, the faulty pin cluster removed and correctly reinserted, and the frame reassembled.

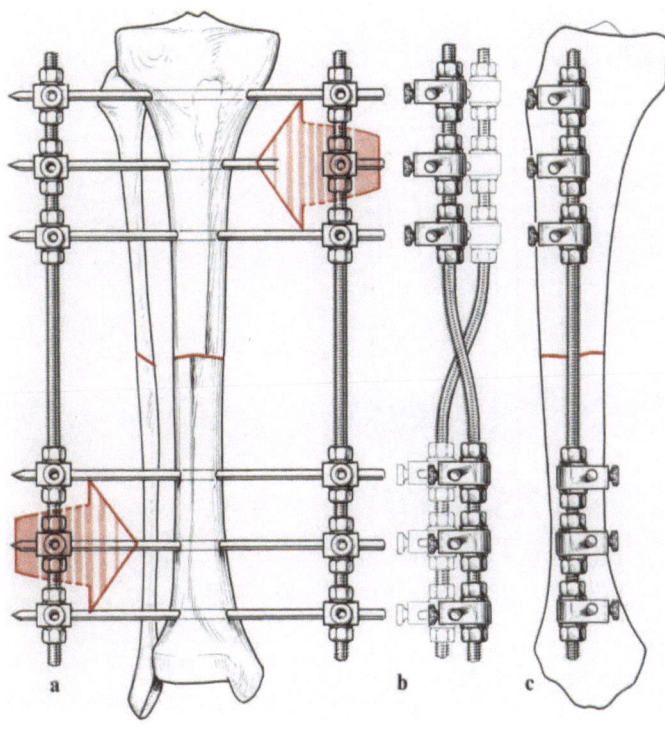

**Fig. 156 a–c.** Correction of malrotation. **a** Malrotation not exceeding 20°. **b** Corrected by bending the rods with the bending irons. **c** Corrected by turning the clamps in a reciprocal, diagonal fashion

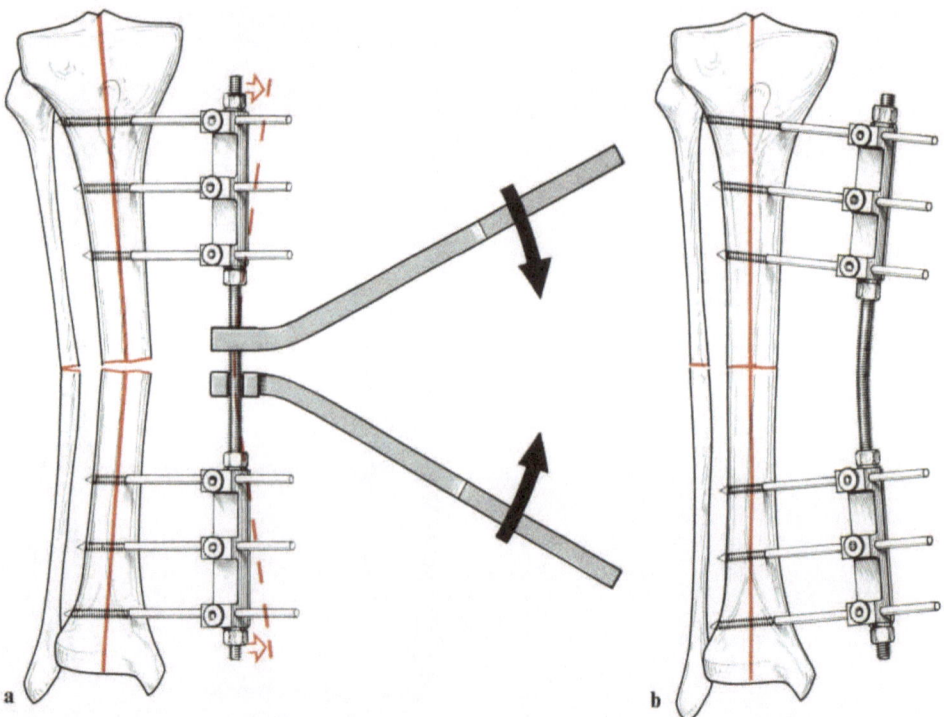

**Fig. 157 a, b.** Correction of valgus. **a** One clamp is loosened, and the rod is bent. **b** The clamp is locked in place following the correction

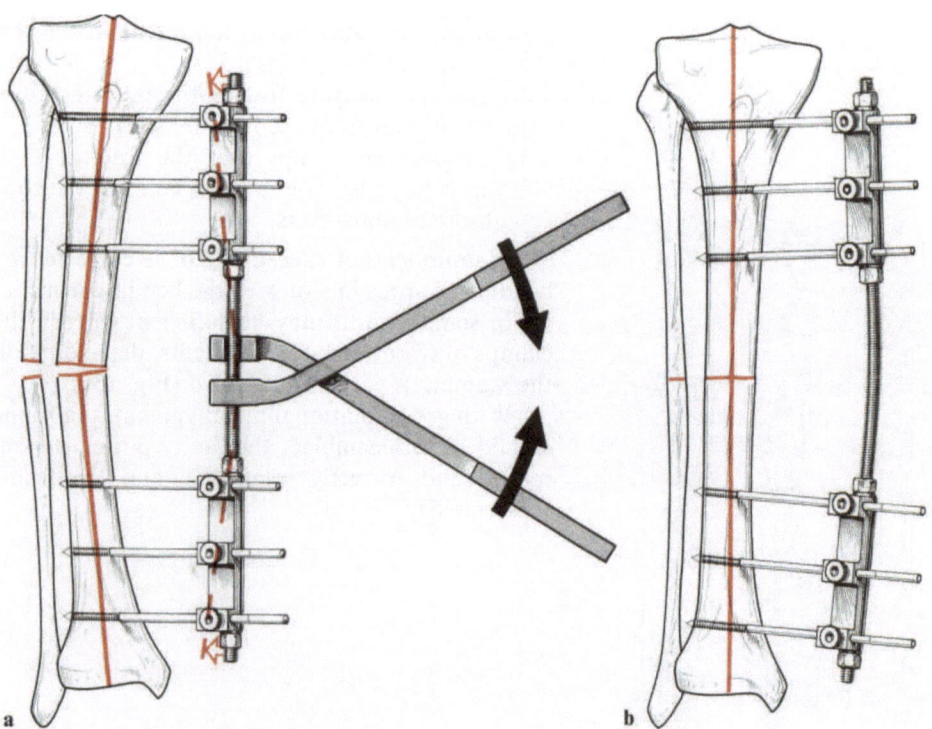

**Fig. 158 a, b.** Correction of varus. **a** One clamp is loosened, and the rod is bent. **b** The clamp is locked in place following the correction

## 2  Axial Corrections in the Unilateral Frame

A *valgus angulation* is easily corrected by placing the rod under tension. If this does not suffice, the rod may be bent with the bending irons (Fig. 157).

A *varus angulation* is corrected in an analogous manner by bending the rod (Fig. 158).

*AP angulation* is managed in the same way as in the bilateral frame. The same applies to *rotational malalignment*.

With gross malrotation, the frame must be partially or completely disassembled and reapplied.

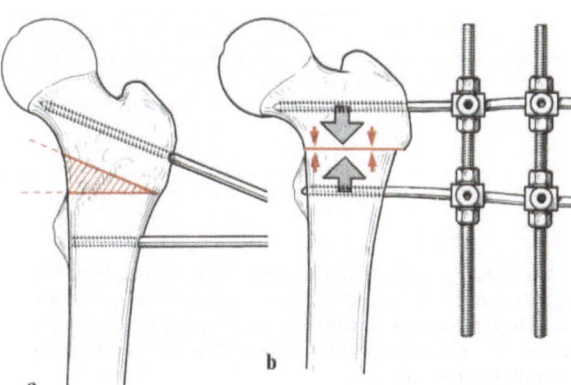

## 3  Axial Corrections with the Aid of an External Frame

In osteotomies, arthrodeses and firm nonunions where an axial correction is proposed, the first step is to insert a pair of Steinmann pins or Schanz screws at an angle to each other which corresponds to the proposed angle of the correction. Following the osteotomy, the mobile fragment is tipped until the pins are parallel, indicating that the desired amount of correction has been achieved. This is the accepted technique for correcting varus, valgus and malrotation (Fig. 159).

Occasionally the correction is carried out in a staged fashion by turning the clamp-holding nuts by a small amount each day, as in the case of a firm nonunion (Fig. 160). Staged corrections of this type are usually reserved for major axial deformities in adolescents. An analogous procedure is used for lengthening osteotomies, in which a 2- to 3-mm length gain per day is the rule.

**Fig. 159 a, b.** External fixation of an osteotomy. **a** The screws are inserted at the desired angle of the correction, and a wedge osteotomy is performed. **b** The correction is made, at which point the screws are parallel

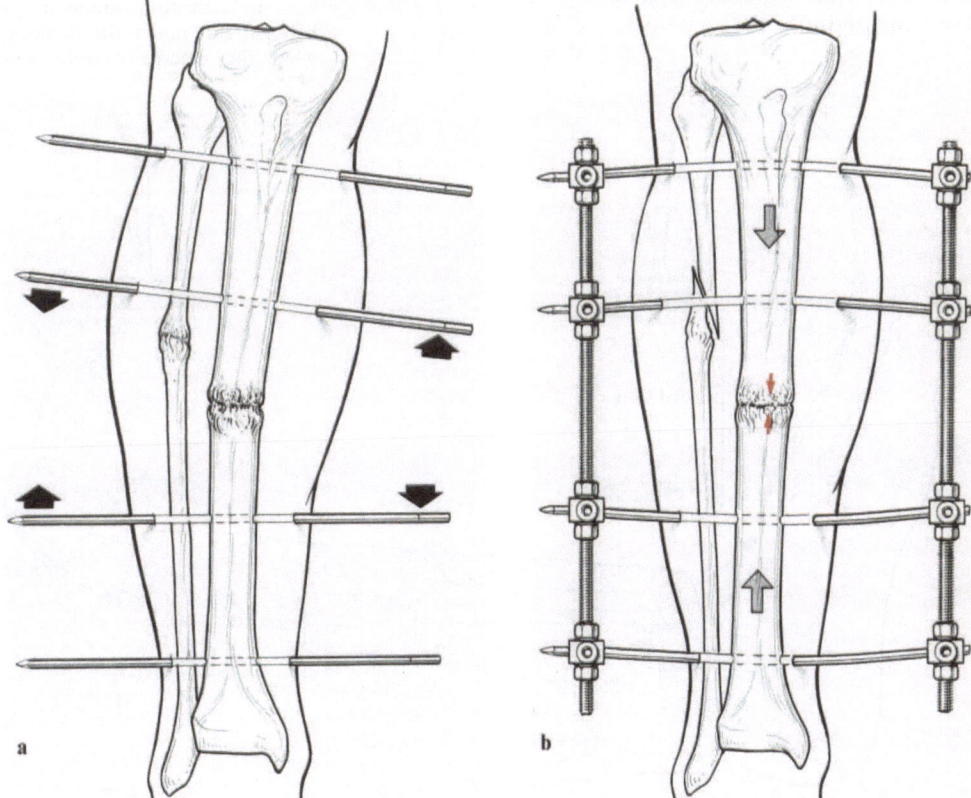

**Fig. 160 a, b.** External fixation for staged correction. **a** Example of a firm nonunion. The pins are inserted at the desired angle of correction. The lateral rod exerts tension initially, and the medial rod exerts distraction. A small amount of correction is made daily. **b** End result of the staged correction

# H Local Care Following Frame Application

B.G. WEBER

The sites at which the pins exit from the skin require systematic care.

## 1 Postoperative Care

The immediate *postoperative dressing* must absorb extruded blood, must be able to dry continuously so that moist chambers do not form, and must be easily changed (Fig. 161).

The "dead spaces" between the skin, pins, clamps and rods are loosely filled with a bulky gauze dressing. The pin sites are overlaid with separate gauze pads on the anterior and posterior sides of the rods, and a layer of sterile cottonoid is wrapped over the gauze. The entire absorbent pack is held in place with an elastic bandage.

Strict care must be taken that the dressing material does not exert pressure on the heel, patella or olecranon. It is best to leave these critical pressure sites exposed so that they are accessible to inspection.

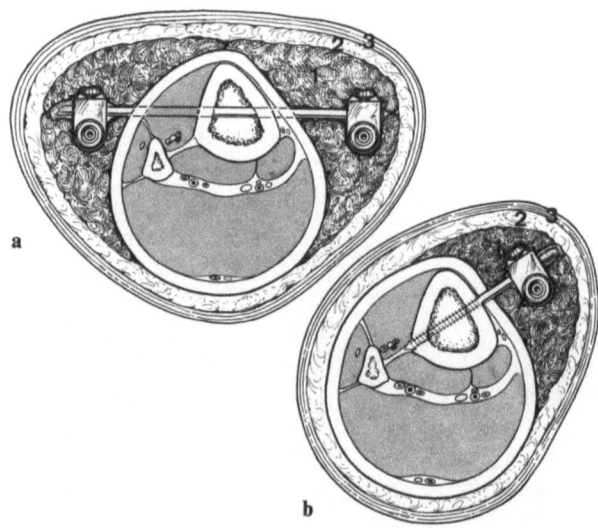

**Fig. 161 a, b.** Postoperative dressing. Bulky gauze pads (*1*) are applied over the pin sites on the anterior and posterior sides. They are covered with cottonoid (*2*) and an elastic bandage (*3*). **a** Dressing for a bilateral frame. **b** Dressing for a unilateral frame

**Fig. 162.** Suction drainage. Redon suction drains are brought out under the dressing in the same direction in which they emerge from the wound and skin
▼

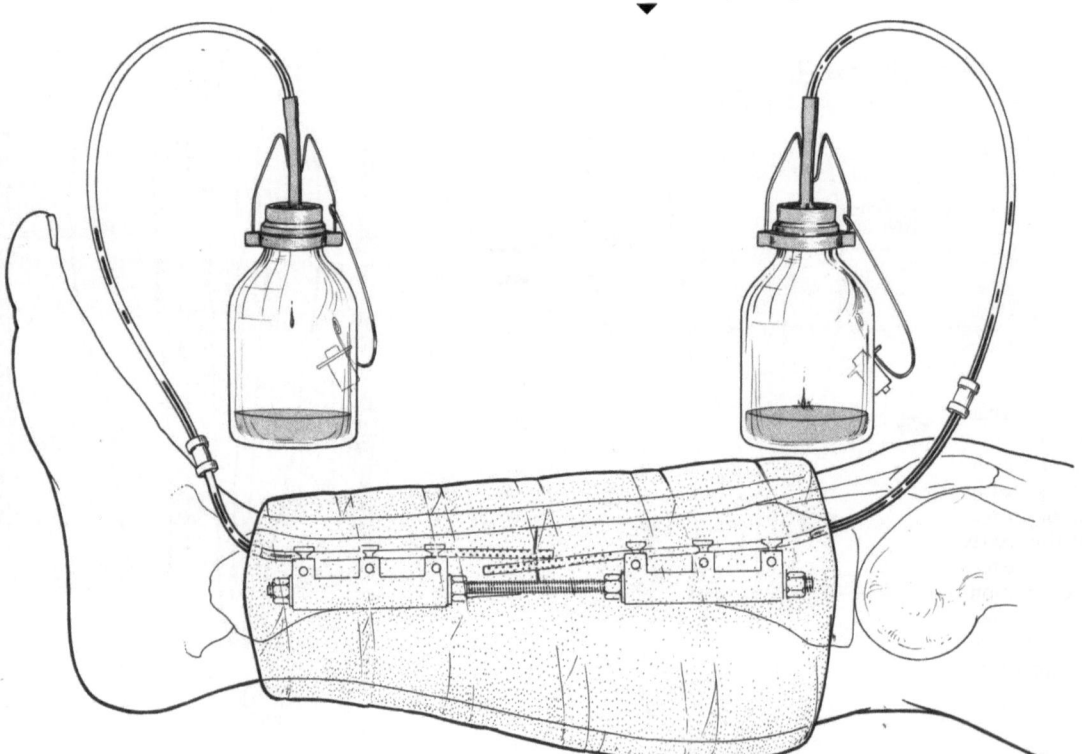

*Suction drains* are brought out through or under the dressing in the same direction they exit the skin. Only in this way can the drains be easily extracted from the wound 1–3 days later without having to remove the dressing (Fig. 162).

Barring complications, the *first dressing change* is made 3–6 days after the frame is applied. Until that time the extremity has been kept elevated, and swelling will have subsided. Since the gauze dressing has been applied over the pin sites from the anterior and posterior sides, the two halves of the dressing can be peeled apart like the halves of a sandwich without causing any pain (Fig. 163).

An identical dressing is applied for the second and usually the last time, for the pin sites should be completely dry by the 6th–8th postoperative day.

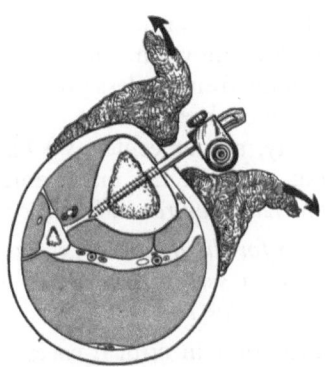

**Fig. 163.** The first dressing change. The two gauze pads are easily and painlessly separated anteriorly and posteriorly

## 2 Further Supervision

The *pin sites* are free of tension and irritation owing to the small stab incisions that were made. At one week postoperatively there should be no evidence of hematoma or swelling owing to the absorbent dressing, suction drains and limb elevation. At this point the patient himself can take over the routine tasks of pin care. The ward nurse teaches him the technique of *daily antiseptic swabbing* of the pin sites (Fig. 164):

The pins and skin are cleansed twice daily with ordinary cotton swabs soaked in a solution of hydrogen peroxide and 2% colorless merphene, taking care to clean away any crusts of fibrin or dried blood that have formed. This local care is continued after the patient has been discharged. The dressing is removed after swelling has subsided, usually between 10 and 20 days postoperatively.

The patient returns to the clinic for weekly or biweekly *follow-up examinations by his surgeon*. It is important to remember that the injured extremity is exercise-competent while the external fixator is in place, and that *partial use of the limb* is both possible and beneficial.

Active exercises, performed if necessary under the guidance of a physical therapist, are the only postoperative therapy that is required.

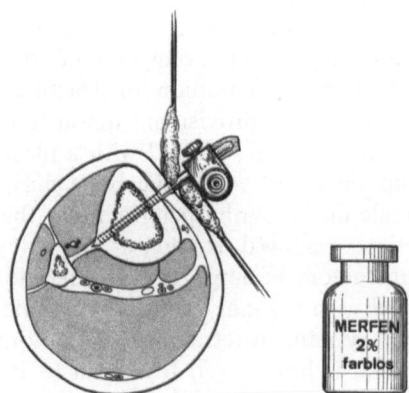

**Fig. 164.** Pin care. The pin or screw sites are cleansed and swabbed twice daily with antiseptic solution.

# I Duration of External Fixation, and Removal of the External Fixator

B.G. WEBER

## 1 General Duration of External Fixation

The time an external fixator remains in place is standardized for *elective orthopedic procedures*, e.g.:

- Intertrochanteric osteotomies in children: $4^1/_2$ weeks, followed by hip spica for $4^1/_2$ weeks.
- Arthrodeses of the knee joint: $4^1/_2$ weeks, followed by knee cast for $4^1/_2$ weeks.
- Arthrodeses of the ankle joint: $4^1/_2$ weeks, followed by walking cast for $4^1/_2$ weeks.

For *acute fractures*, the time the fixator remains in place will vary with the patient's progress. In the most favorable case, the fixator is left on for only 6 weeks. If secondary operations are required, up to 20 weeks of external fixation may be necessary.

When used for *nonunions*, the fixator should remain in place between 12 and 16 weeks.

As a general rule, an external fixator remains in place no longer than is absolutely necessary. As long as the fixator remains on the limb, secondary pin track infection is a danger. Once the osteotomy, arthrodesis, nonunion or fracture shows definite evidence of provisional union, the frame may be removed and replaced with a plaster cast or similar device in which the bone may go on to complete union. With open fractures, the frame is sometimes removed as soon as the soft tissues show satisfactory healing. At that time the device is replaced with internal fixation by a plate or intramedullary nail. In refractory septic nonunions of the tibia, it has proved beneficial to have the patient wear an articulated cast brace for 6–12 months after discontinuance of the frame. It has been found that functional remodeling of bone progresses well under the protection of such a device.

*Principle No. 5 for the threaded external fixator:*
*The fixator remains in place as long as necessary, and no longer.*

## 2 Early Removal of Individual Pins or Screws

*Pin track infection* is one of the most dreaded complications of external fixation. While the danger of pin track infection is slight when all technical details of the operation are carried out as described, and is practically nil in aseptic elective procedures, it may still occur in open fractures and is particularly common in infected fractures and septic nonunions. Incipient infections along a pin tract generally can be controlled simply by removing the offending pin. This will compromise the stability of the frame unless provisions for such an eventuality have been made.

That is why, at our center, we have adopted the following tactic in the management of *open fractures, infected fractures and infected nonunions*:

*Principle No. 6 for the threaded external fixator:*
*Use as few pins or screws as possible, but as many as are necessary, plus 1 reserve!*

This means that in critical cases each pin or screw cluster contains enough implants that one may be removed if necessary without significantly lessening the stability of the fixation. We recommended using 3–4 pins per main fragment on the tibia, and 4–5 on the femur.

In the example shown in Fig. 165, serous drainage from one screw track persisted for 3 weeks but resolved at once when the screw was removed.

A different situation is seen in Fig. 166: Here, for "simplicity," the Steinmann pins had been inserted directly by means of a power drill without the benefit of a pilot hole. The heat from the drilling caused bone necrosis with formation of a ring sequestrum, and the hot pin burned the skin. Tissue damage of this type is almost invariably followed by infection. Removal of the pin is not enough in such cases, and only a sequestrectomy and open cancellous bone grafting can eradicate the iatrogenic osteitis.

**Fig. 165 a, b.** "Innocent" screw track infection. Early removal of a screw. P.F., 1959, 22 years, ♂, 171508.

**a** Open fracture of the tibia. Minimal internal fixation and unilateral compression frame.

**b** The Schanz screw second from the top was removed prematurely, at 3 weeks postinjury, due to a persistent serous drainage. Prompt healing of the draining screw track and fracture ensued

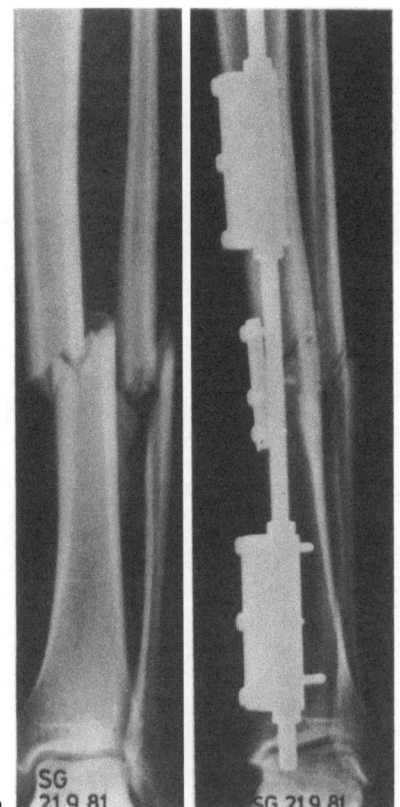

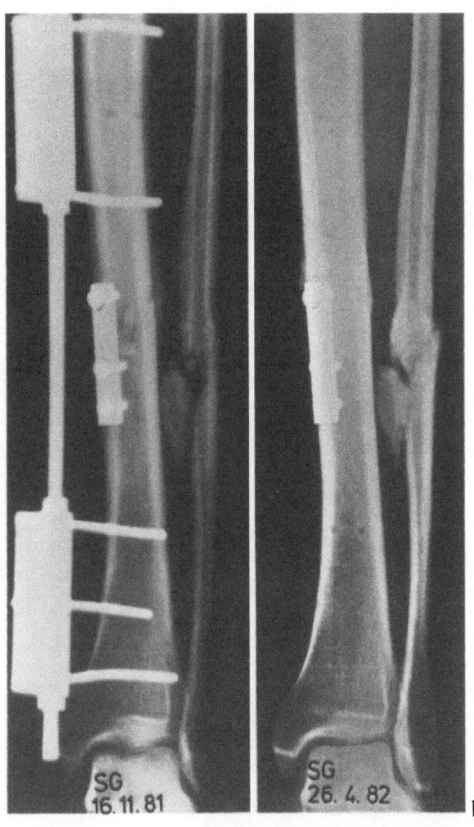

## 3 Staged Removal of Combined Frames

When two separate frames are combined on one limb – usually two unilateral frames on the femur – bony consolidation may progress so well that, by 2–3 months, one of the frames may be taken off. This is particularly important from the standpoint of therapeutic exercise, because the anterior frame "pins" the quadriceps muscle to the femur and prevents complete flexion of the knee.

**Fig. 166.** Severe pin track infection: skin necrosis, ring sequestrum. H.H., 1954, 19 years, ♂, 170337.

One year previously: open fracture, external fixation, infection, removal of extenal fixator (abroad). At presentation: ring sequestrum, osteitis, skin necrosis, infected nonunion

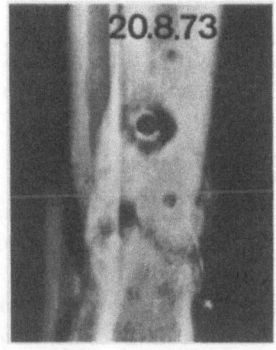

## 4 Removal of the External Fixator

The removal of fixation pins or screws from the bone can be a very painful procedure. This is especially true in the diaphysis, and less so in the epiphysis and metaphysis. Thus, we recommend that pin removal be carried out in an operating room under *brief general anesthesia.*

Before the fixator is removed, it must be ascertained whether or not the device is exerting compression, and whether stresses exist within the pin

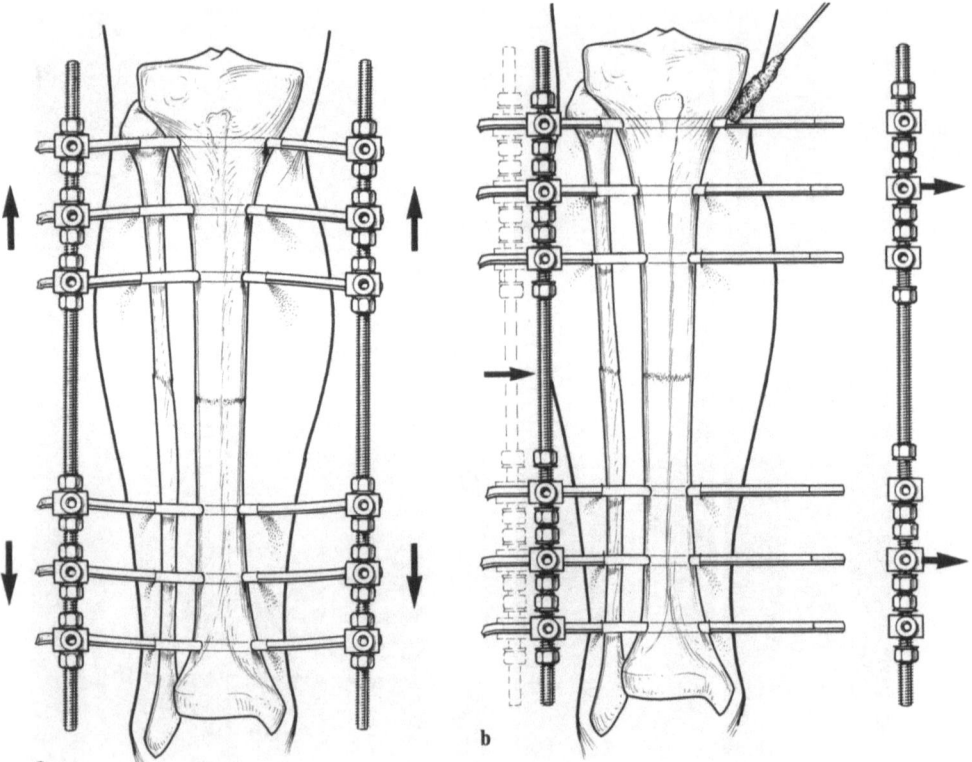

**Fig. 167 a–c.** Removal of a bilateral compression frame. **a** Release of axial compression (or individual pin stresses) by synchronous loosening of the clamps on each side. **b** After stresses are released, the medial clamps and rod are removed without disturbing the pins. **c** The pins are disinfected on the medial side, grasped by their lateral ends and twisted out through the clamps

or screw clusters. All stresses in the apparatus must be released before the pins or screws are removed from the bone.

In a *compression frame* the first step is to *release the axial compression* by loosening the clamp-holding nuts. As a nut on one side is loosened, its counterpart on the opposite side is loosened simultaneously. Both the loosening process and the initial application of compression are facilitated by the use of multiple-pin clamps.

### 4.1 Removal of a Bilateral Frame (Fig. 167)

*Pin stresses are released* by loosening the clamps within and between pin clusters, taking care that opposite clamps are loosened in synchrony. Once the pin stresses have been relieved, the clamps may be removed from the blunt, uncut ends of the pins. On the opposite side, however, it may not be possible to slide the clamps off the sheared ends due to the slight deformation occasioned by the cutting of the pins. This is especially true when 5-mm Steinmann pins are used. Thus, the recommended procedure for pin removal is first to disinfect the free ends of the pins with 2% colorless merphene solution, then grip the cut ends of the pins with the hand chuck and twist the pins out through the clamps, which are still in place.

### 4.2 Removal of a Unilateral Frame
(Fig. 168)

The stress in the frame is first released by loosening the clamp-holding nuts. If the Schanz screws were shortened with the large wire cutter during assembly, one should not try to pull the clamps over the cut ends, especially with 5-mm screws. Instead, the screws should be gripped with the hand chuck and removed with the clamps still in place.

### 4.3 Care of the Pinholes

It is normal for the pinholes to bleed for several minutes following pin removal. Therefore, these sites are covered with sterile gauze and lightly wrapped with an elastic bandage for 10 minutes. After that time the skin is cleansed with antiseptic, and the dressing is replaced.

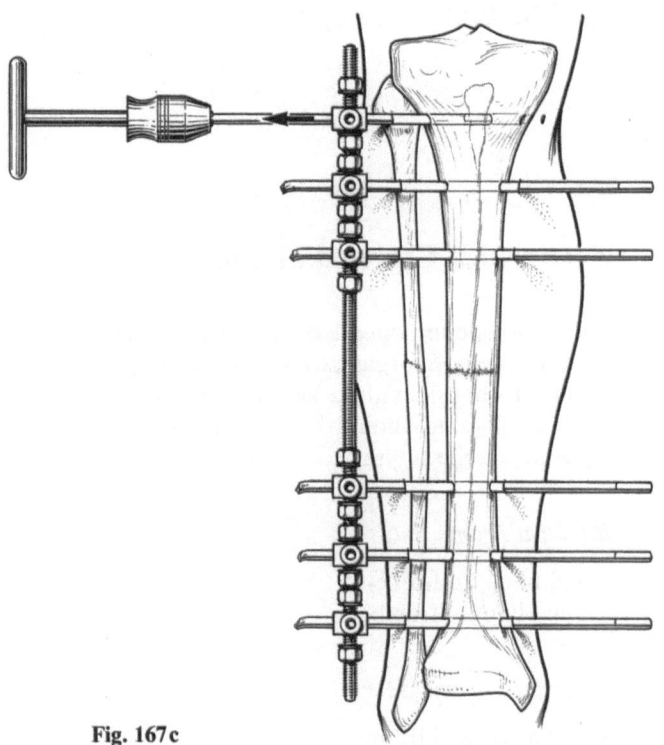

**Fig. 167c**

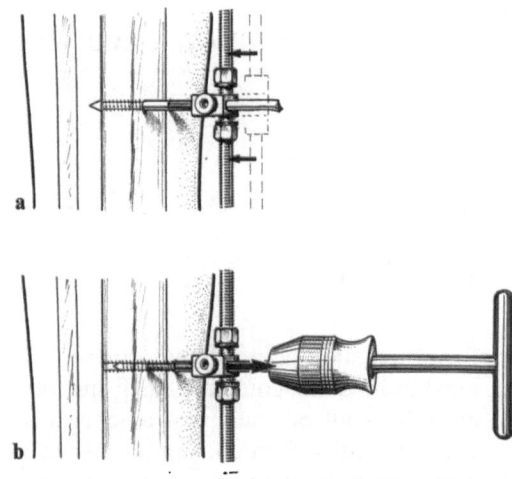

**Fig. 168 a, b.** Removal of a unilateral frame. **a** The clamps are loosened to release axial compression (or individual pin stresses). The clamps are pushed toward the tibia so that the screw ends can be grasped. **b** The screws are twisted out through the clamps

If a plaster cast is to be applied, this should be deferred for several hours until the pinholes have sealed. The dressing beneath the cast should be sterile and free of blood so that bacterial growth is not encouraged.

If plaster is not applied the wounds will become epithelialized in four days, at which time the dressing may be removed.

# 5 "Dynamization" of External Fixator Frames

As bone healing is in progress primarily stiff frames are to be "dynamized" by staged removal of supplementary rods. Due to the decrease of stress protection, ossification is stimulated and bony union accelerated.

Such "dynamization" is normally done 2–3 months after a compound fracture when the soft-tissue damage has healed and cancellous bone grafts are longer than 6 weeks in situ and therefore vascularised.

# K  Instrumentation Used with the Threaded External Fixator

B.G. WEBER

## 1  General

From the standpoint of the surgeon, it would be ideal to have the complete ASIF instrumentarium as well as all personal instruments available for every operative fixation. But, given the busy operating schedule of today's surgeons and the finite resources of the cost bearer, such a requirement is unrealistic.

It is a rule in surgery that certain instruments are indispensible for a particular operation, while others are necessary under certain circumstances, and others are entirely unnecessary. The same applies to external fixations: Certain instruments and components must be prepared for particular applications. It is safe to assume that many other instruments, such as intramedullary nails and angled-blade plates, will not be required. Of course, there will always be a need for general bone and soft-tissue instruments such as scalpels, forceps, periosteal elevators, suture material, etc.

## 2  Threaded External Fixator Sets

The various components of the threaded external fixator have been organized into the following sets, which are considered to be standard for current applications and should be kept ready for use in separate, sterile trays:

*Bilateral Frame Sets*

Small bilateral frame
Large bilateral frame

*Unilateral Frame Sets*

Small unilateral frame
Large unilateral frame

*Special Frame Sets*

External fixation device for the spine (MAGERL type)
Lengthening apparatus (WAGNER type)
    The indications for and components of the different frame sets are listed below:

### 2.1  Small Bilateral Frame (Fig. 169)

*Indications:* Arthrodesis of the knee, ankle, elbow. Supramalleolar or upper tibial osteotomy. Staged correction of equinus deformity. Supracondylar or supramalleolar traction.

*Components:*
12 Nuts
 3 Double clamps, 30 mm
 5 Double clamps, transverse, 24 mm
 3 Double clamps, transverse, 18 mm
 5 Single clamps
 2 Single clamps, open

 3 Steinmann pins, 4.5 mm diam., 180 mm long
 2 Steinmann pins, 5 mm diam., 180 mm long
 4 Steinmann pins, 5 mm diam., 200 mm long

 3 Threaded rods, 150 mm
 3 Threaded rods, 120 mm

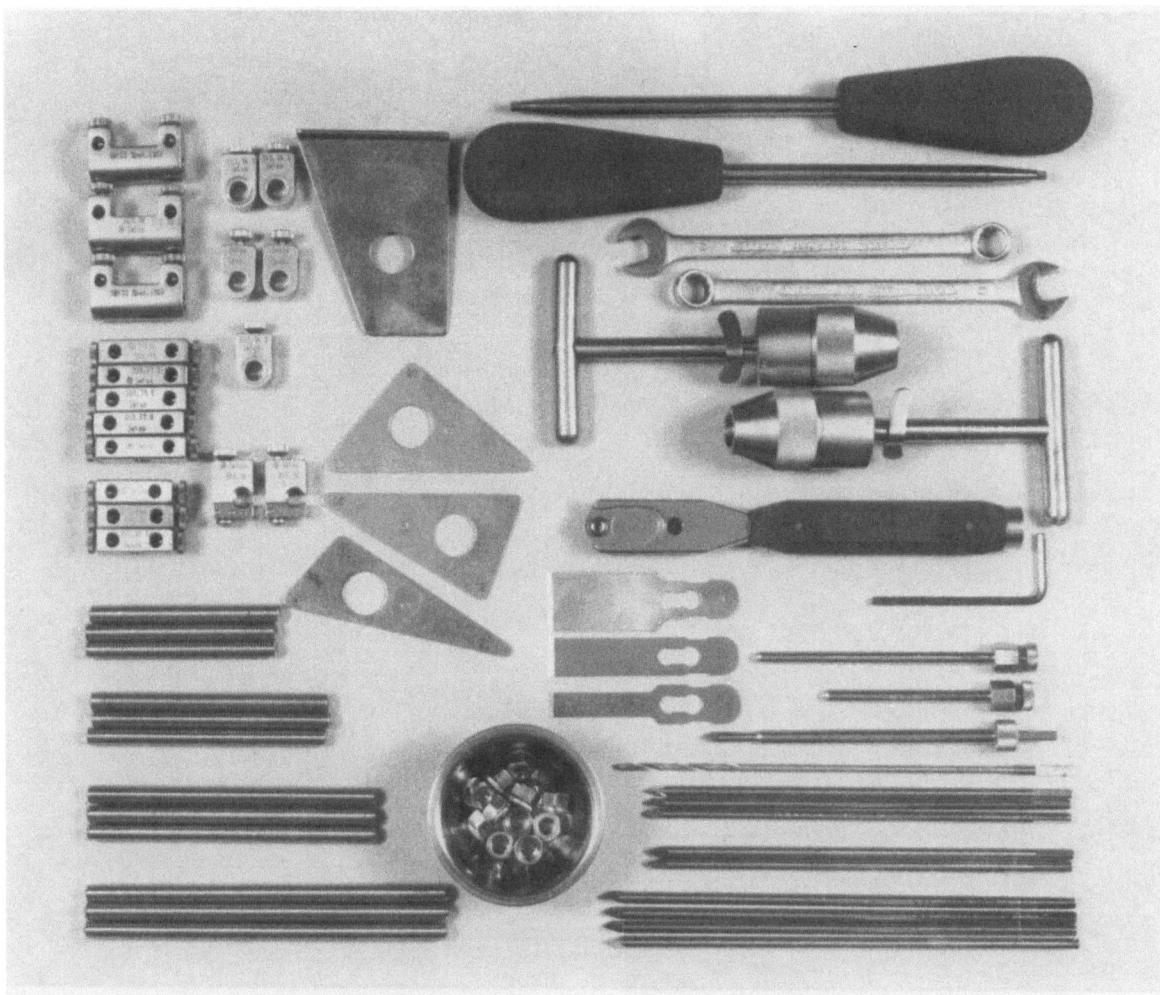

**Fig. 169.** Tray contents for the small bilateral frame

3 Threaded rods, 100 mm
3 Threaded rods, 80 mm

2 Combination wrenches
2 Hand chucks
2 Screwdrivers
1 Chisel with blades (3 pieces)
1 Set of angle plates (4 pieces)
1 Hexagonal socket wrench
1 Drill bit, 3.2 mm
3 Tap sleeves with trocar

## 2.2 Large Bilateral Frame (Fig. 170)

*Indications:* Open tibial fracture, infected fracture, tibial nonunion, lengthening osteotomy of the tibia.

*Components:*
20 Nuts
 8 Single clamps for 2 rods

3 Double clamps, 30 mm
3 Double clamps, 40 mm
3 Double clamps, 50 mm
5 Triple clamps
12 Single clamps
2 Single clamps, open

4 each Steinmann pins, 4.5 mm diam., 150, 180, 200 mm long
4 each Steinmann pins, 5 mm diam., 180, 200, 250 mm long

2 Threaded rods, 450 mm
2 Threaded rods, 400 mm
3 Threaded rods, 350 mm
3 Threaded rods, 300 mm
2 Threaded rods, 250 mm
2 Threaded rods, 200 mm

2 Combination wrenches
2 Hand chucks
2 Screwdrivers

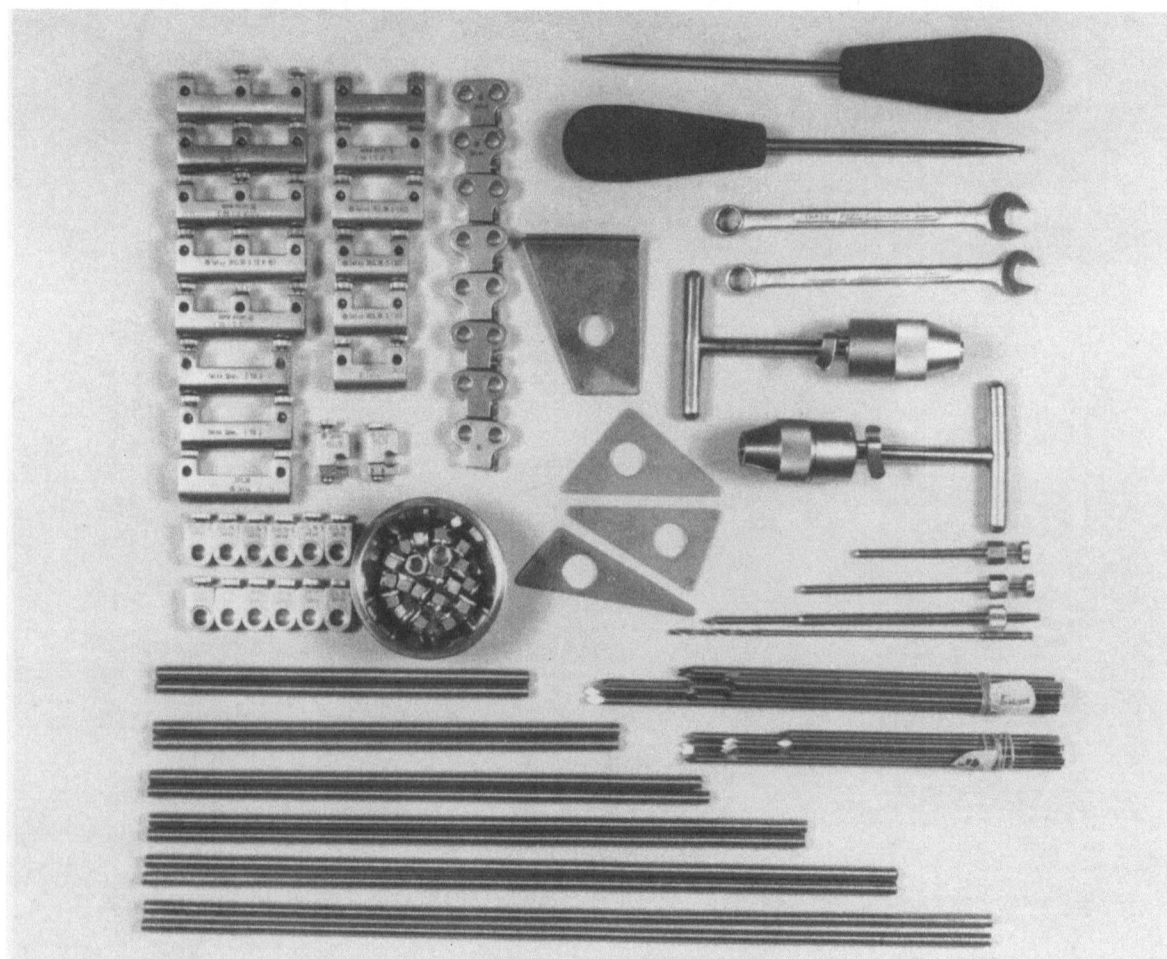

1 Set of angle plates (4 pieces)
1 Drill bit, 3.2 mm
3 Tap sleeves with trocar.

### 2.3 Small Unilateral Frame (Fig. 171)

*Indications:* Distal radial fracture, arthrodesis of the wrist, open tibial fracture in children.

*Components:*
10 Nuts
 2 Double clamps, 30 mm
 2 Double clamps, 40 mm
 2 Double clamps, 50 mm
 5 Single clamps
 2 Single clamps, open
 2 Threaded rods, 200 mm
 2 Threaded rods, 250 mm
 5 Cortex screws, 3.5 mm, 50 mm
 5 Cortex screws, 4.5 mm, 80 mm
 2 Combination wrenches
 2 Depth gauges, 4.5 and 3.5 mm
 4 Screwdrivers

▲
**Fig. 170.** Tray contents for the large bilateral frame

**Fig. 171.** Tray contents for the small unilateral frame ▶

**Fig. 172.** Tray contents for the large unilateral frame ▶

2 Special taps, 4.5 and 3.5 mm, with handle
2 Drill bits, 3.2 and 2.7 mm
1 Drill sleeve, 3.2 and 2.7 mm.

### 2.4 Large Unilateral Frame (Fig. 172)

*Indications:* Infected nonunion of the humerus, femur or tibia; open tibial fracture; pelvic fracture.

*Components:*
20 Nuts
 7 Single clamps for 2 rods
 3 Double clamps, 30 mm
 3 Double clamps, 40 mm
 3 Double clamps, 50 mm
 3 Triple clamps
 6 Single clamps
 2 Single clamps, open

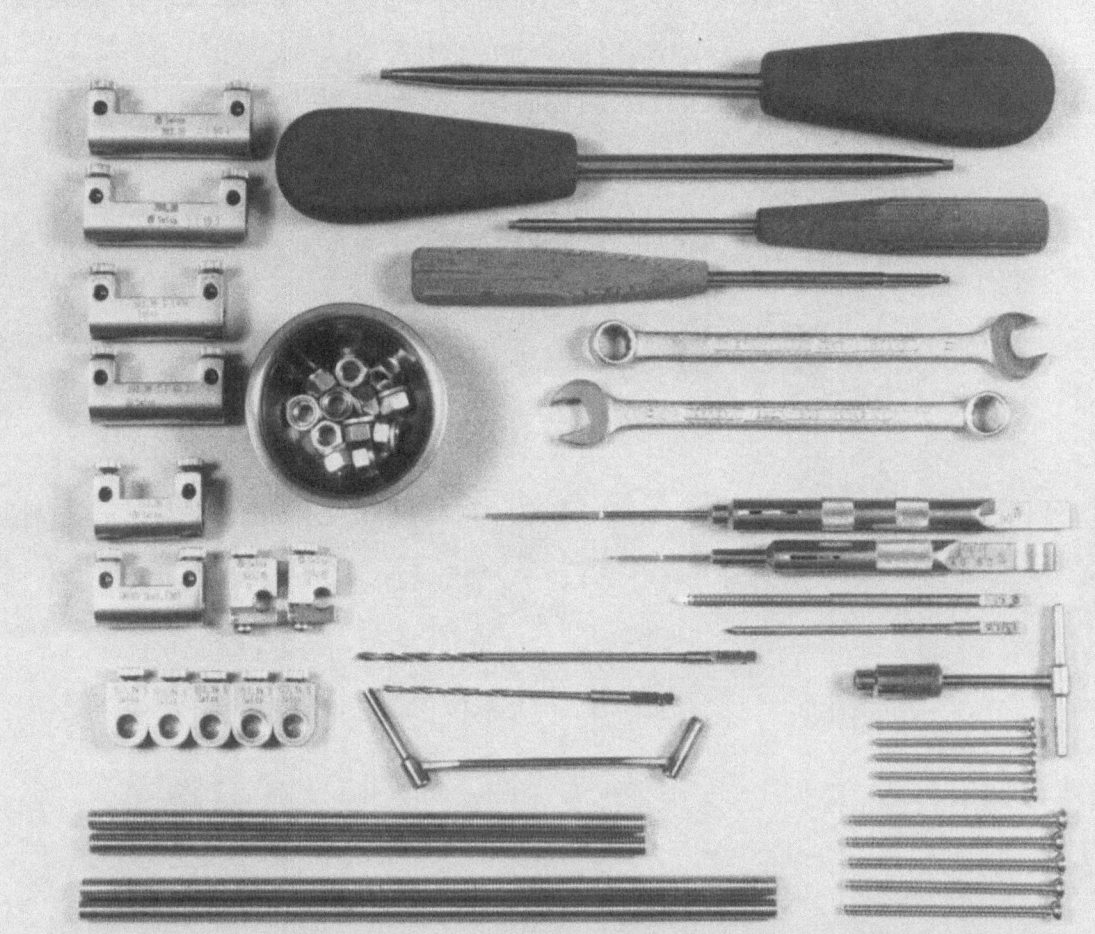

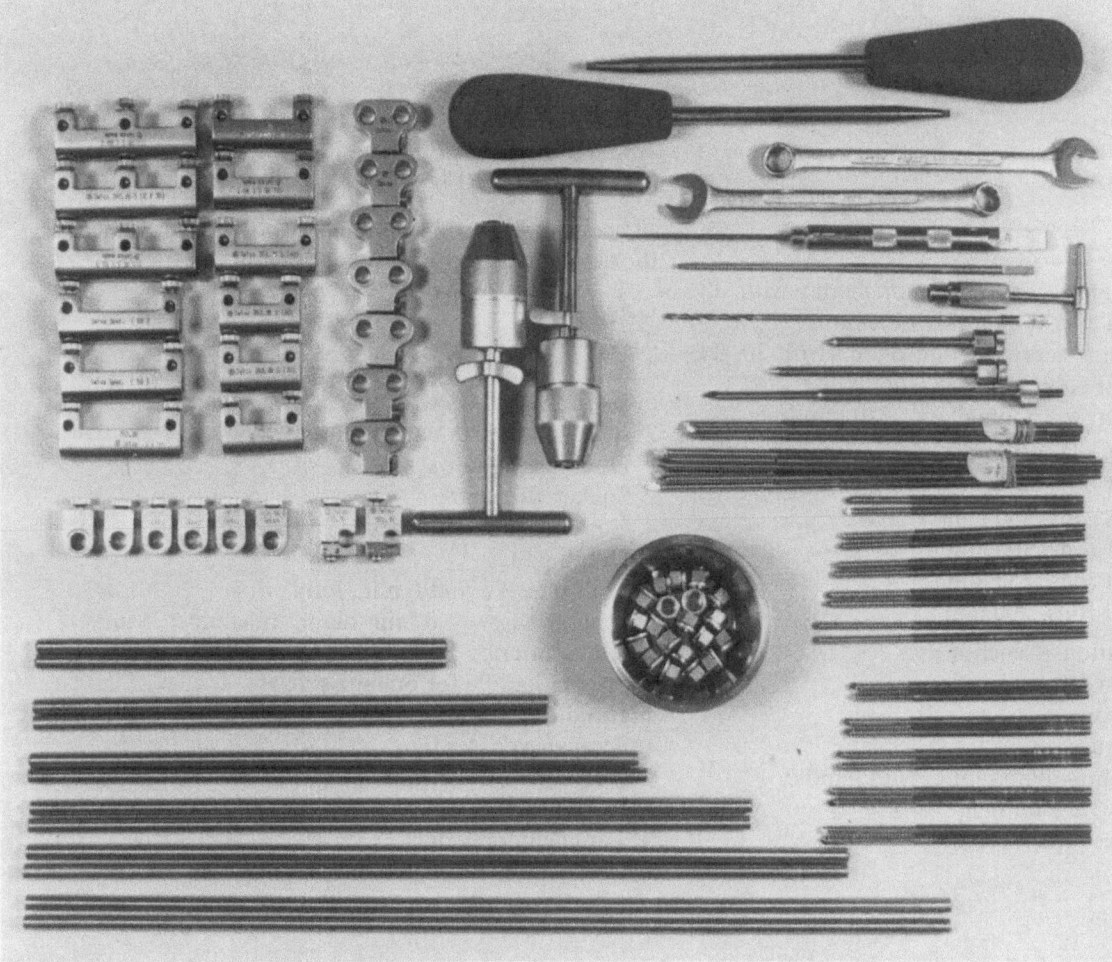

Fig. 171

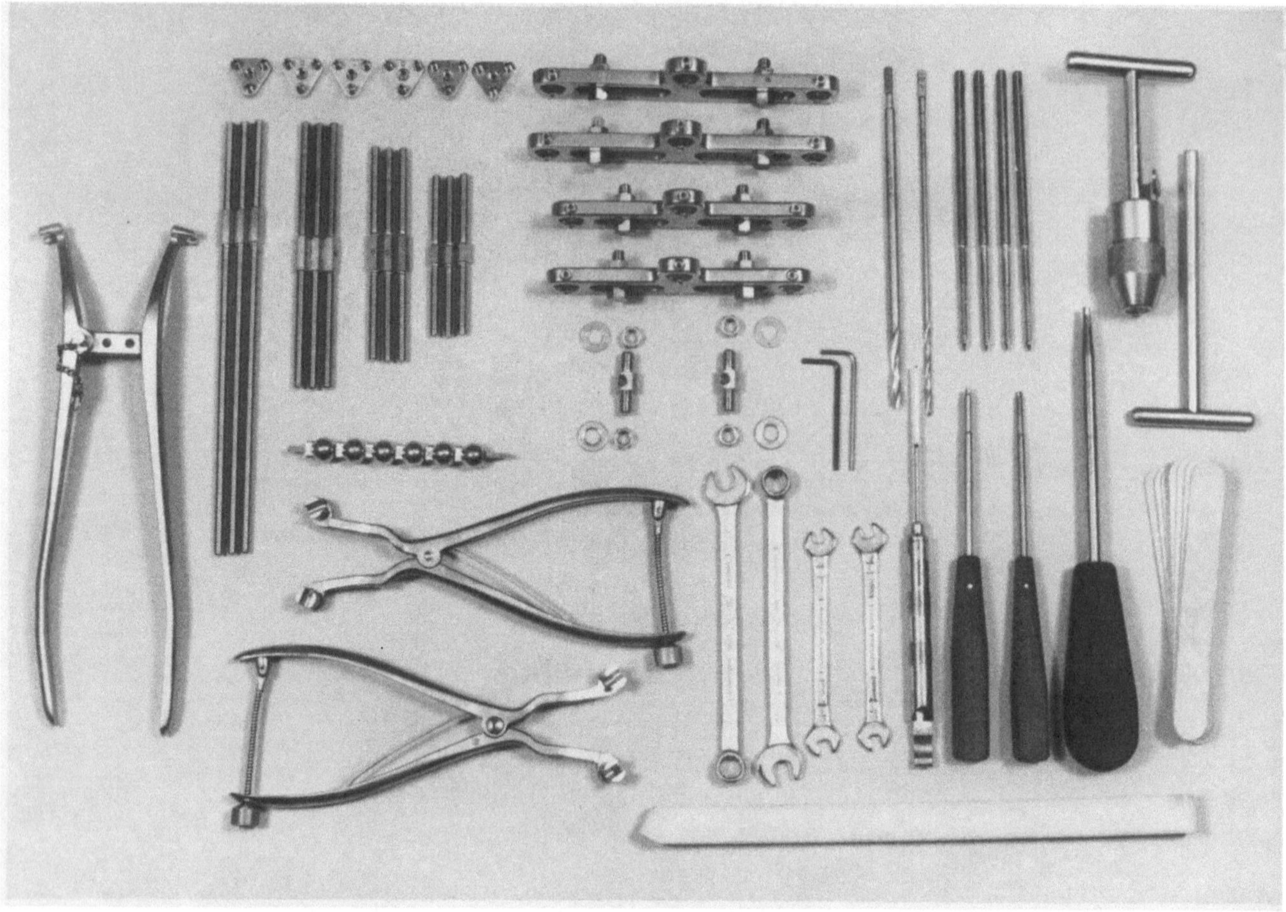

**Fig. 173.** Tray contents for the spinal external fixation device (Magerl type)

2 each Schanz screws, 4.5 mm diam., with 30, 34, 38, 42 and 46 mm thread lengths
2 each Schanz screws, 5 mm diam., with 30, 34, 38, 42 and 46 mm thread lengths
10 Schanz screws, 5 mm diam., 220 mm long

2 Threaded rods, 450 mm
2 Threaded rods, 400 mm
2 Threaded rods, 350 mm
2 Threaded rods, 300 mm
2 Threaded rods, 250 mm
2 Threaded rods, 200 mm

2 Combination wrenches
2 Hand chucks
2 Screwdrivers
1 Depth gauge
1 Tap, 4.5 mm diam., long, with handle
1 Drill bit, 3.2 mm, long
3 Tap sleeves with trocar

## 2.5 Spinal External Fixation Device (Magerl Type) (Fig. 173)

*Indications:* Unstable spinal fractures from the thoracolumbar to lumbosacral region.

*Components:*
3 Reduction forceps
3 each Threaded rods of different lengths
6 Retaining plates with set screws
2 each Transverse bars with set screws
2 Double set screws
2 Socket wrenches
4 Combination wrenches
1 Depth gauge
2 Drill bits, 3.5 and 6 mm, long
4 Schanz screws, 6 mm diam. posterior, 5 mm diam. anterior
1 Special handle for Schanz screws
1 Handle
1 Screwdriver, 4.5 mm
2 Screwdrivers, 3.5 mm
1 Plastic screw holder
8 Tongue depressors

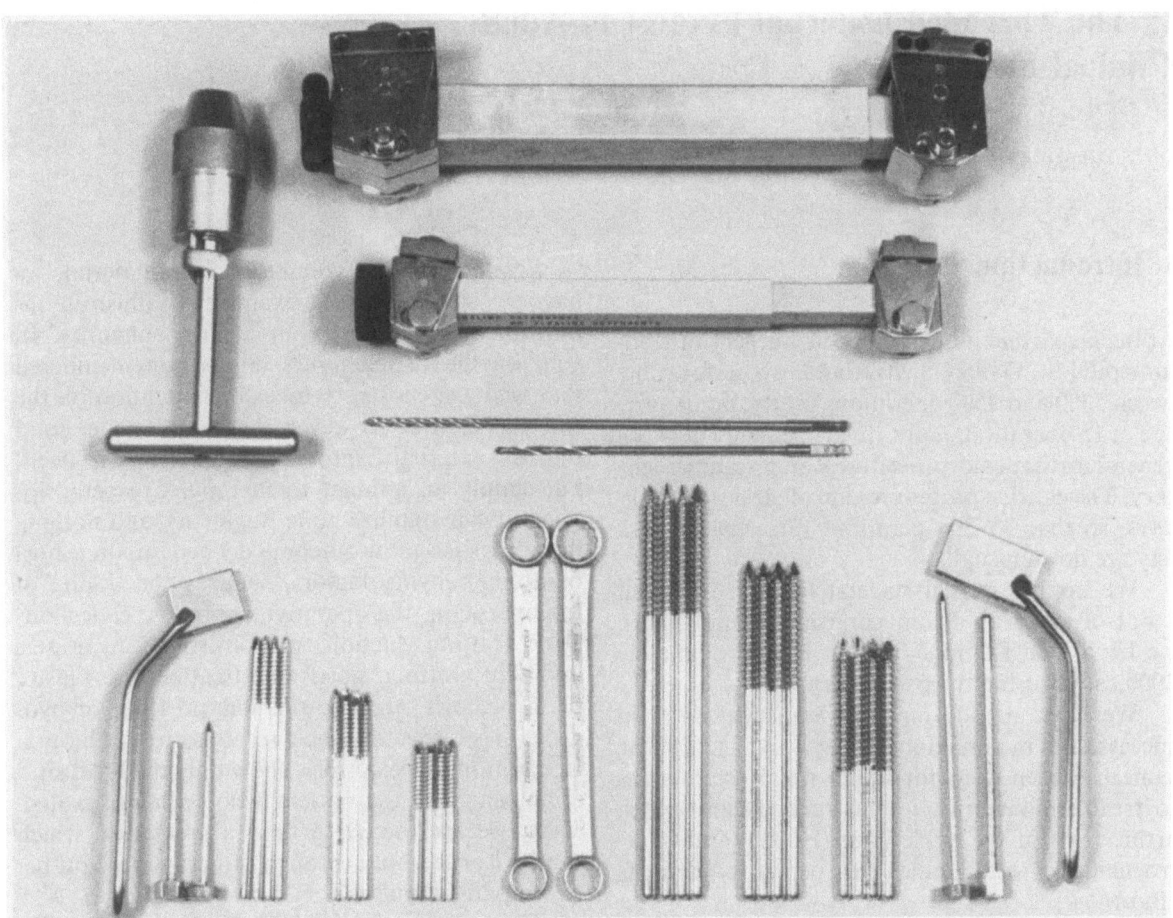

## 2.6 Lengthening Apparatus (WAGNER Type)
(Fig. 174)

**Fig. 174.** Tray contents for the lengthening apparatus (WAGNER type)

*Indications:* Lengthening of the humerus, forearm bones, femur or tibia, or shortening of these bones in some instances.

*Components:*
1 Lengthening telescope, large
1 Lengthening telescope, small
2 Drill bits, 3.2 mm
2 Special drill sleeves
2 Tap sleeves with trocar
2 Combination wrenches
3 each Schanz screws, 4 mm diam., 60, 80 and 100 mm long
3 each Schanz screws, 6 mm diam., 100, 130 and 160 mm long
1 Handle

The combination of *six different external fixator sets* may seem cumbersome, but it is not. The *rods and clamps* are *reusable*. On the other hand, *bent rods, Steinmann pins, Schanz screws, cortex screws* and *Kirschner wires* used with the threaded fixator are *nonreusable* and are in the same discardable category as other ASIF implants such as plates, screws and intramedullary nails.

Scrub nurses find that these *six functional units of the external fixator* are of considerable value in organizing and facilitating their work. The surgeon, moreover, is able to give highly specific orders as to which instruments are to be prepared for a particular operation.

# L The Threaded External Fixator in Adults. Clinical Examples

B.G. WEBER

## 1 Introduction

At the Department of Orthopedic Surgery of Kantonsspital St. Gallen, Switzerland, we perform between 5000 and 5500 operations yearly, or an average of 15 operations daily, divided equally between general orthopedic procedures and trauma surgery. The elective procedures are all done on weekdays, so that 25–30 operations on a given work day are not unusual.

We apply external skeletal fixation in about 1 out of every 25 of our surgical patients. Thus, we have used external fixation in approximately 3000 cases during the past 15 years.

We have already reported statistical data on success rates in nonunions (WEBER and CECH). The same has been done for upper tibial osteotomies to treat osetoarthritis of the knee (DEBRUNNER), arthrodeses of the ankle joint (PELET), and intertrochanteric osteotomies in pediatric patients (BRUNNER).

Statistical evaluations are more difficult for open fractures, because these cases represent a highly inhomogeneous body of material. Nevertheless, since 24 years we have followed and documented every case that has presented at our clinic. In the process, we have continually added to our knowledge, especially with regard to open fractures, and have witnessed the substantial benefits of minimal internal fixation combined with sparing, reinforced external fixation. By contrast, our techniques for osteotomies, arthrodeses and certain nonunions have changed relatively little over the past 20 years (Figs. 175–178).

Here we shall discuss the WAGNER apparatus only in very general terms, drawing on illustrative cases. The reader should refer directly to the author for more detailed information.

The use of the threaded external fixator in children and adolescents is discussed by BRUNNER in a separate chapter.

A true innovation is the spinal external fixation device designed by MAGERL. It is described in the second part of the book.

From our large volume of case material, we have selected instructive examples to illustrate indications, techniques, courses and outcomes. In studying the case examples, it must be remembered that we have chosen to focus our attention on the external fixator. However, it must be understood that the external fixator is not a therapy in itself, but simply an adjunct to therapy. Correctly applied, it can stabilize bone fragments, and nothing more. A successful outcome depends upon a host of accompanying factors, such as the timing of the operation, the operative approach, cancellous bone grafting, suction, suction-irrigation, muscle and skin grafting, postframe treatment in plaster or in orthosis, and the possible presence of pyogenic organisms and their response to antibiotics. In addition, the examples show only the local situation, and not the patient who is being treated. Thus, we are forced to omit a great deal which can be learned only through direct interaction between patient and physician.

The literature, and especially the American literature, tends to evaluate operative orthopedic procedures in terms of statistical data on success rates. This approach overlooks the fact that success or failure depends not on the procedure alone, but on a triad of factors:

1. The indication
2. The procedure
3. The execution of the procedure, i.e., the ability of the surgeon.

The third factor is the least discussed among surgeons. However, it is the most important in operative orthopedics, just as in any other human endeavor which relies on manual and physical skills. The best piano and sheet music or the most perfect slalom course and best skiing equipment will not help the untrained pianist or skier to master his specialty. The surgeon owes his patients training and mastery; he would expect no less of the pilot who flies him to a medical conference or resort. It is wrong to think that the only "good" techniques in orthopedic surgery are those that are technically easy to perform. Orthopedic surgery is not that simple, which is why the simplifying,

**Fig. 175 a–c.** Tibial osteotomy performed in 1959. H.E., 1934, 25 years, ♀, BZH.

**a** Valgus deformity secondary to nonunion of a tibial fracture.
**b** Two months after corrective osteotomy, fixation with small bilateral compression frame.
**c** 4 $^1/_2$ months postoperatively: osteotomy is solid

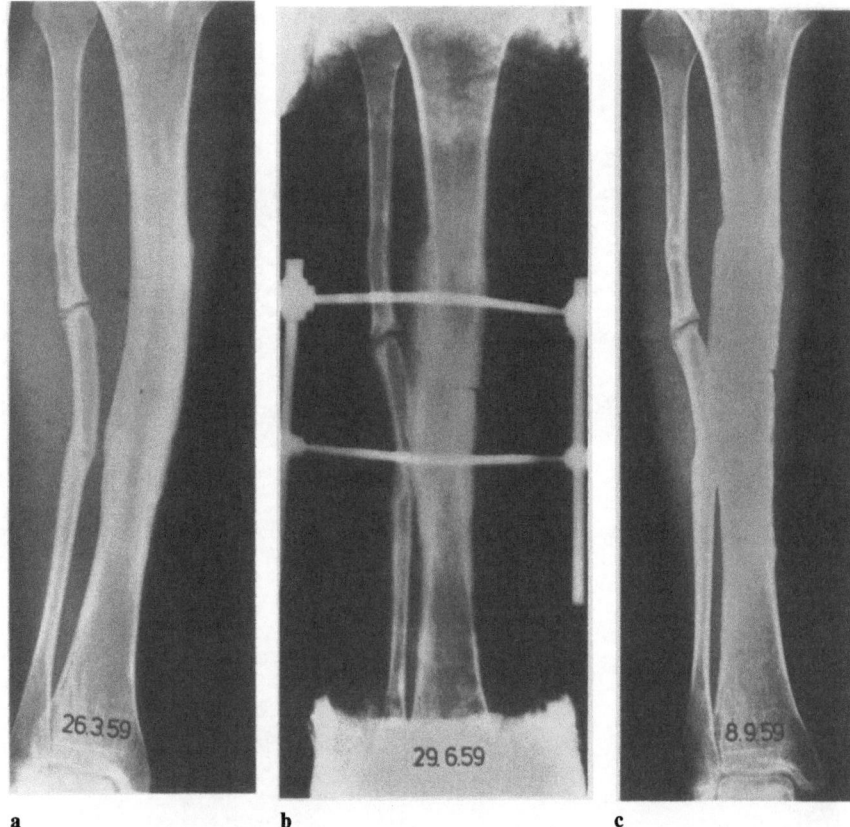

a                    b                    c

inflationist views expressed by some authors (such as ALLAN Jr.) should, at least in Europe, be given little serious attention. Orthopedic surgery is a medical specialty which cannot be mastered in a few years of training, and which additionally requires a high degree of manual talent (CHARNLEY's "mechanical feeling") on the part of the surgeon. The purpose of our clinical examples, then, is to illustrate what we have been able to accomplish at our clinic with the aid of the threaded external fixator. For the experienced surgeon, the examples will provide a self-confirmation; for the novice, we hope they will provide a stimulus for personal experimentation, always adhering to the basic pedagogic rules of working from the simple to the complex, and from the known to the unknown.

Viewed in these terms, the examples represent the personal experience of particular orthopedic surgeons – an experience which is transferable only to a limited degree and ultimately must be gained through personal effort.

Case examples can be organized and presented according to various criteria, such as indication, technique, or anatomic localization. We have organized our material according to the skeletal region involved, citing indications which we feel best illustrate the application of the method.

In the outline of each patient's history, it is stated whether primary treatment was instituted outside our clinic (abroad).

On the X-ray pictures, the dates are written: day, month, year

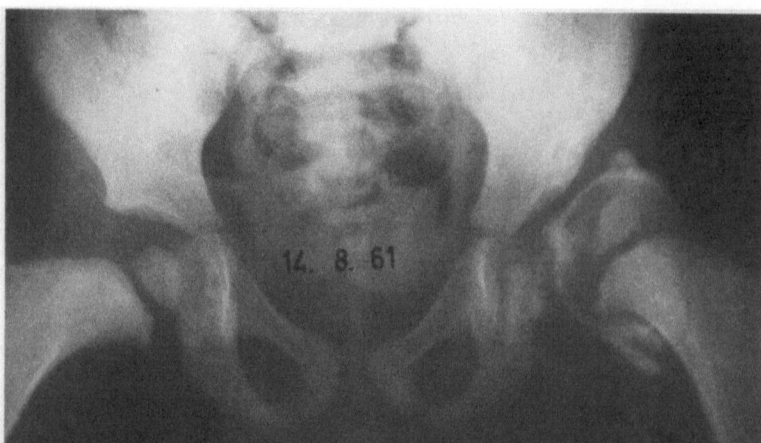

a

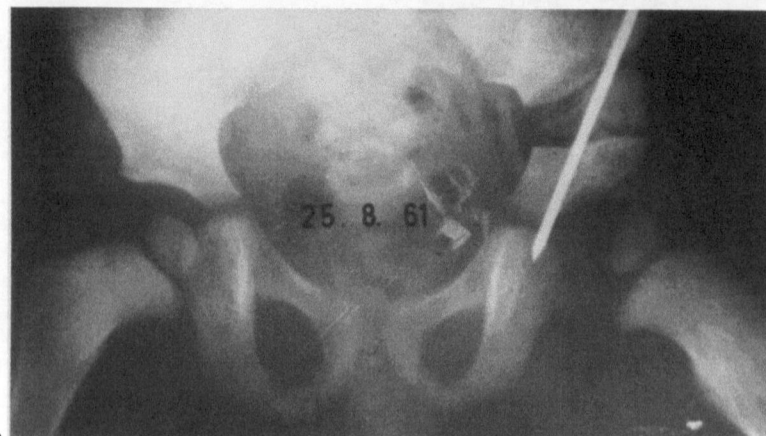

b

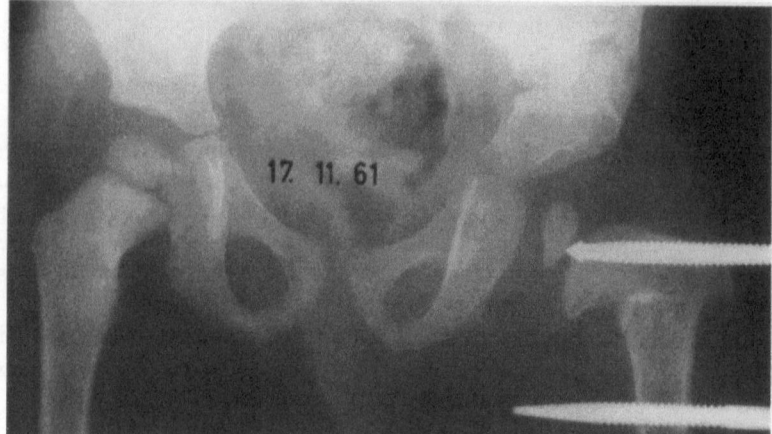

c

**Fig. 176 a–d.** Intertrochanteric osteotomy of the femur in a small child, performed in 1961. A.J., 1958, 3 years, ♂, BZH.

**a** Congenital dislocation of the hip, arthrography.
**b** Salter osteotomy, head fails to seat in acetabulum.
**c** Six weeks after intertrochanteric varus derotation osteotomy, fixation with unilateral compression frame.
**d** 3¹/₂ years later: complete recovery

**Fig. 177 a, b.** Arthrodesis of the ankle joint performed in 1958. H.M., 1913, 45 years, ♀, BZH.

**a** Arthrodesis for osteoarthritis, immobilized with small bilateral compression frame.
**b** Follow-up at 12¹/₂ years postoperatively

**Fig. 176d**

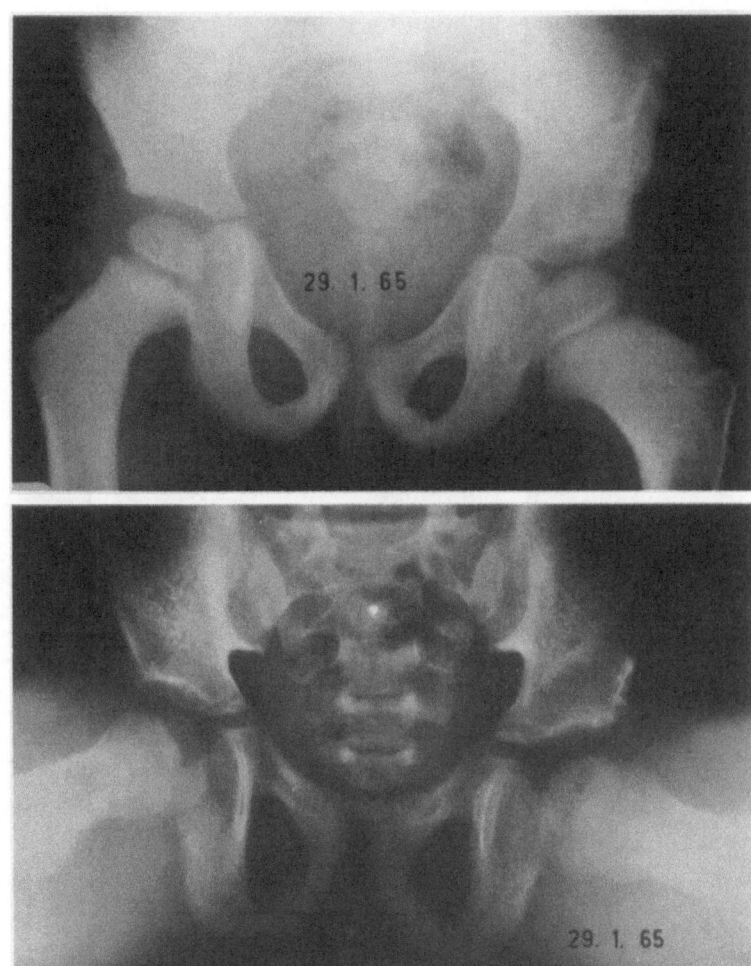

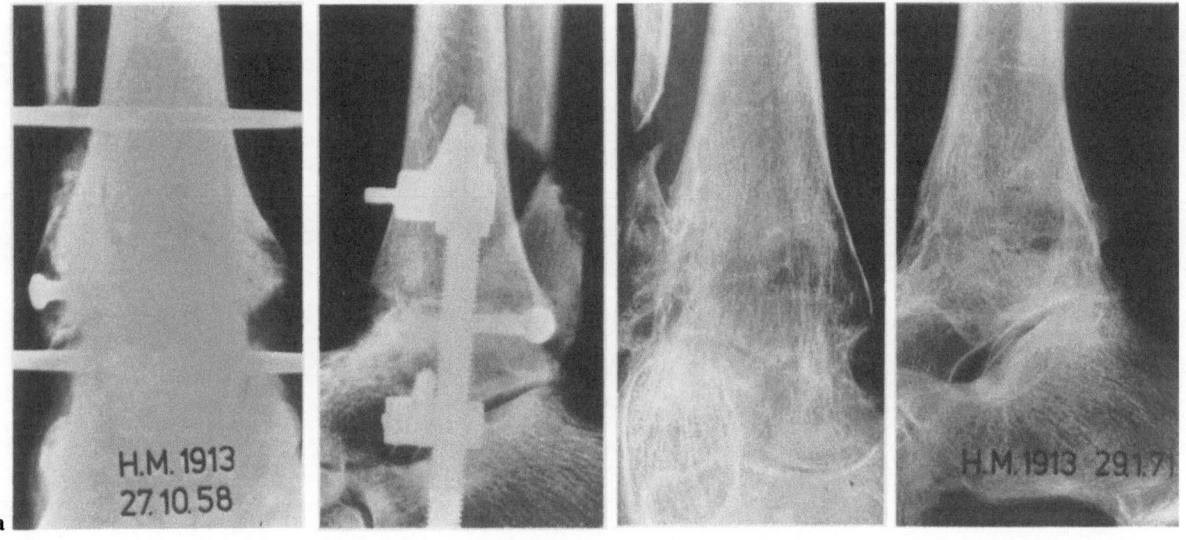

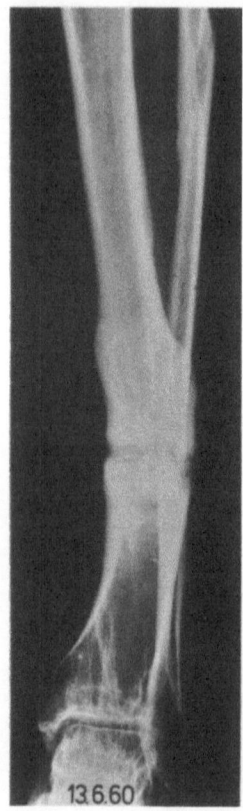

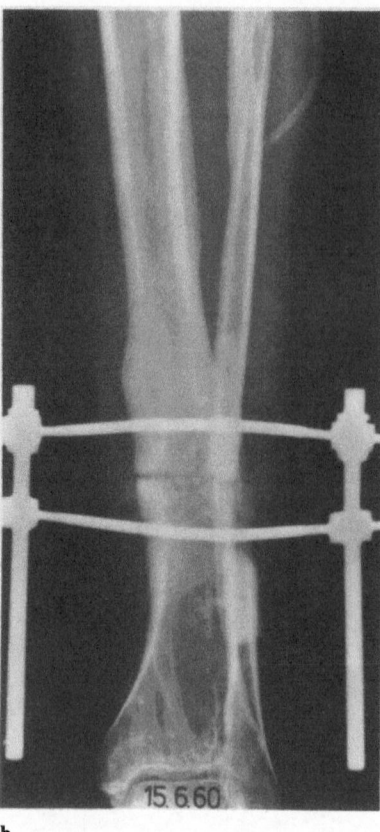

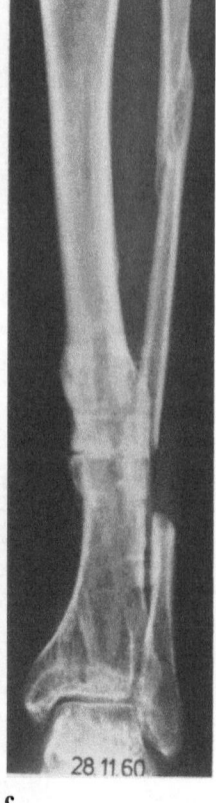

a                    b                    c

**Fig. 178 a–c.** Compression plating of a tibial nonunion performed in 1960. S.A., 1926, 34 years, ♂, BZH.

**a** Tibial nonunion with varus deformity.
**b** Corrective osteotomy of the nonunion. Fixation with small bilateral compression frame.
**c** Five months after osteotomy: nonunion is solid

## 2  Humerus (Figs. 179–181)

### Examples:

**Fig. 179 a–c.** Open fracture of the humerus with radial nerve paralysis. Unilateral frame. S.D., 1939, 42 years, ♂, 252268.

**a** Grade II open humeral fracture with radial nerve paralysis. Debridement, incision of intraneural radial nerve hematoma. Unilateral neutralization frame for 10 weeks.
**b** 4¹/₂ months postinjury: soft tissues and fracture are healed, paralysis is resolving.
**c** One year after fracture: complete recovery

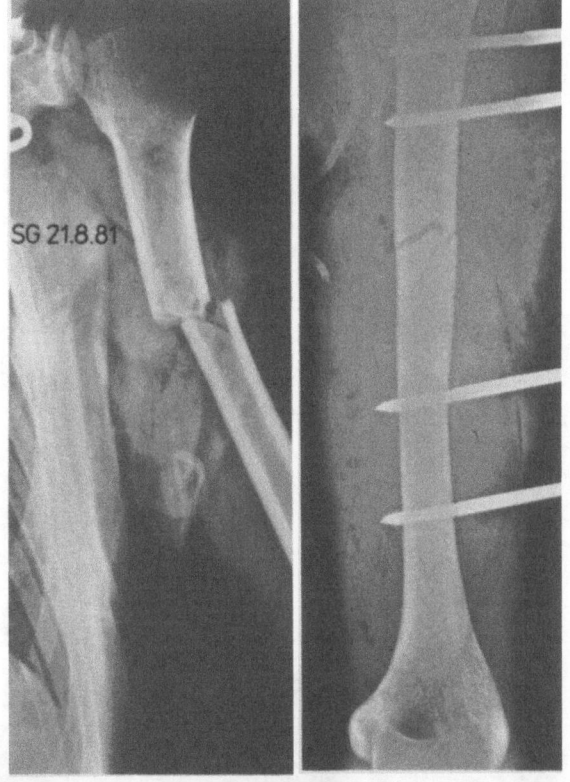

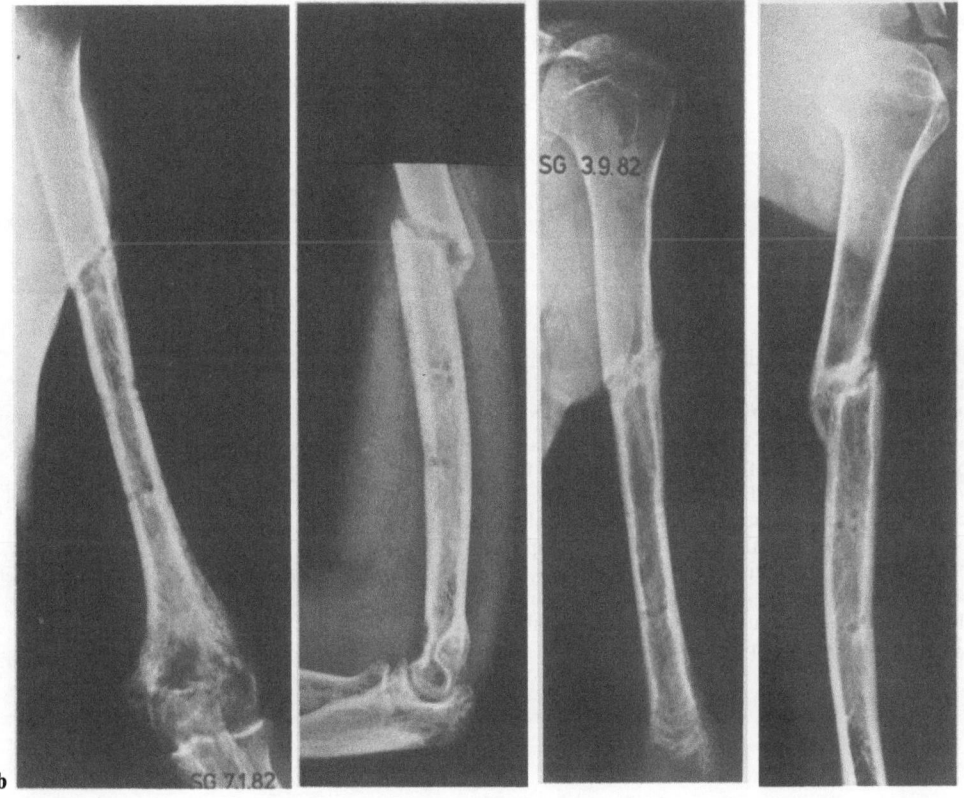

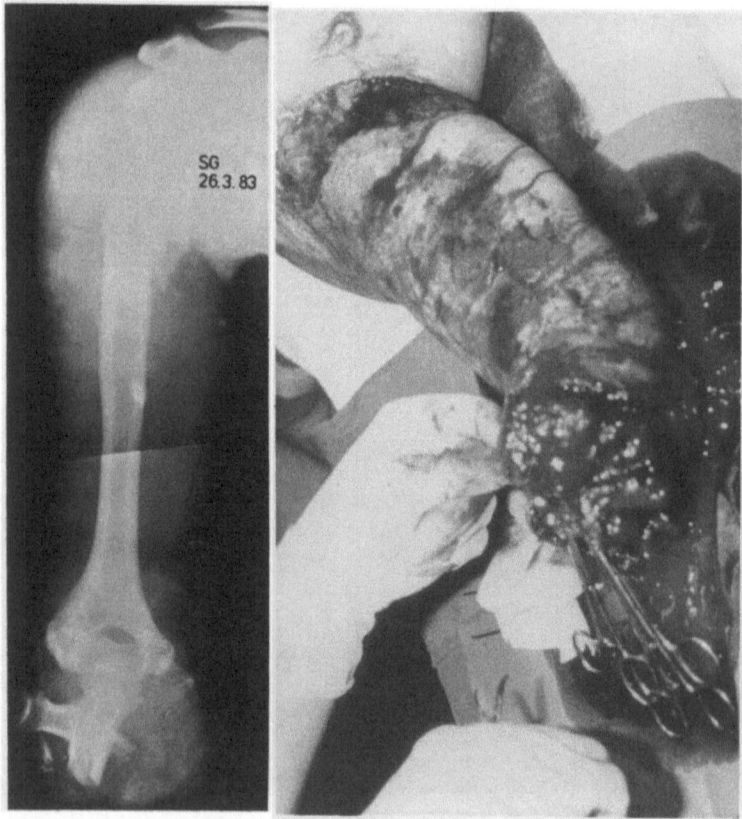

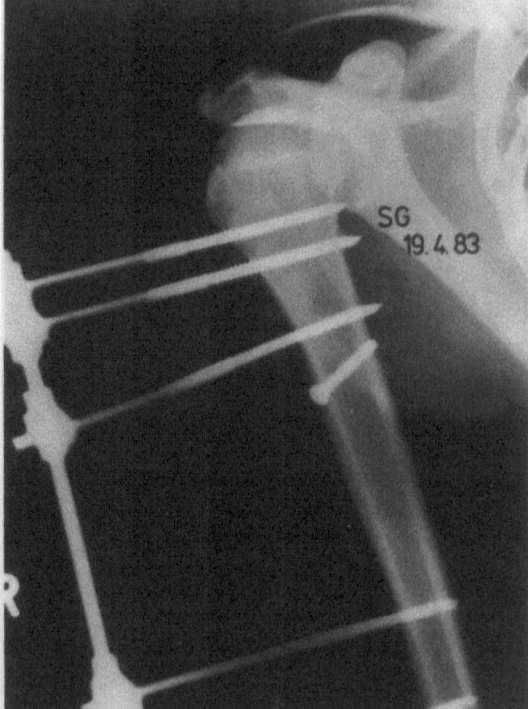

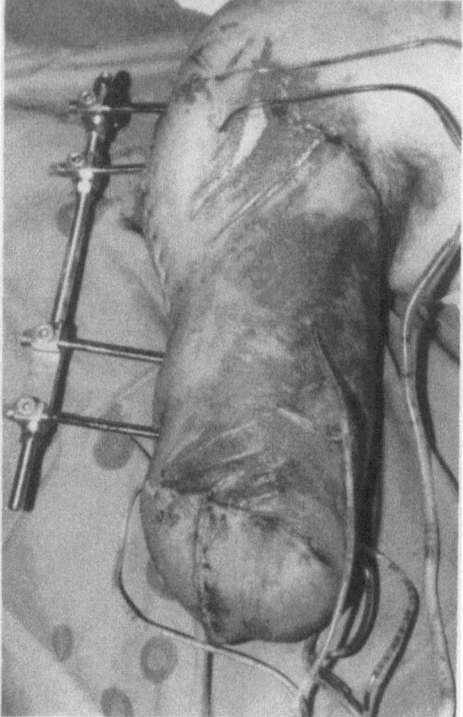

**Fig. 180 a–d.** Traumatic amputation of the proximal forearm with crushing of soft tissues and humeral fracture. Unilateral frame. M.U., 1964, 19 years, ♂, 269456.

**a** Patient was run over by an automobile, sustaining an amputation at the level of the elbow, a humeral fracture, and a severe crush injury of the forearm.
**b** Open minimal internal fixation of humeral shaft and unilateral neutralization frame for 8 weeks. Stump care.
**c** Two months postinjury: humeral fracture is healing well, soft tissues are healed.
**d** Five months postinjury: complete functional recovery of the humerus (forearm prosthesis)

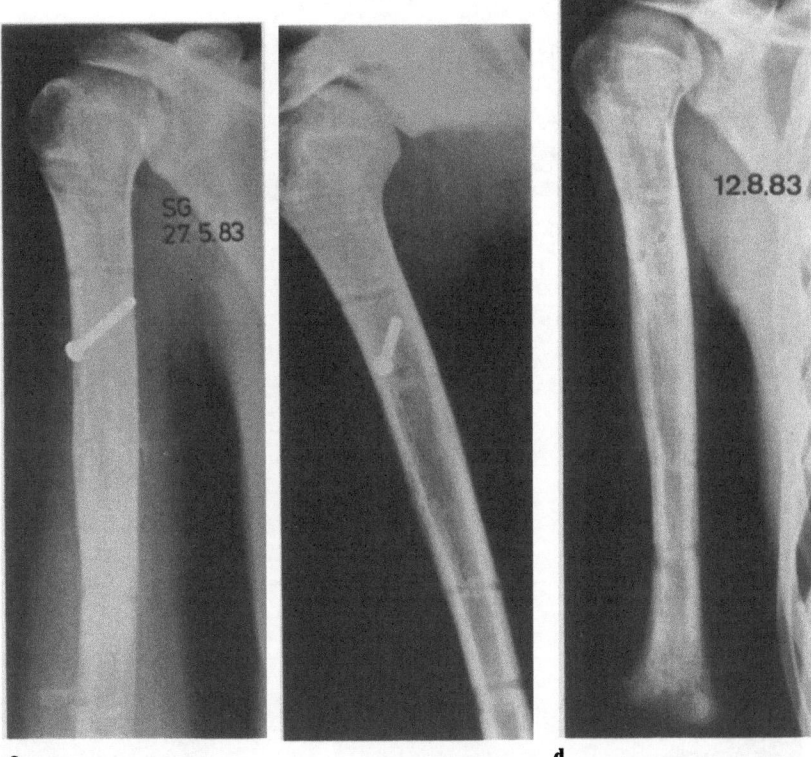

Fig. 180c, d

c                                                    d

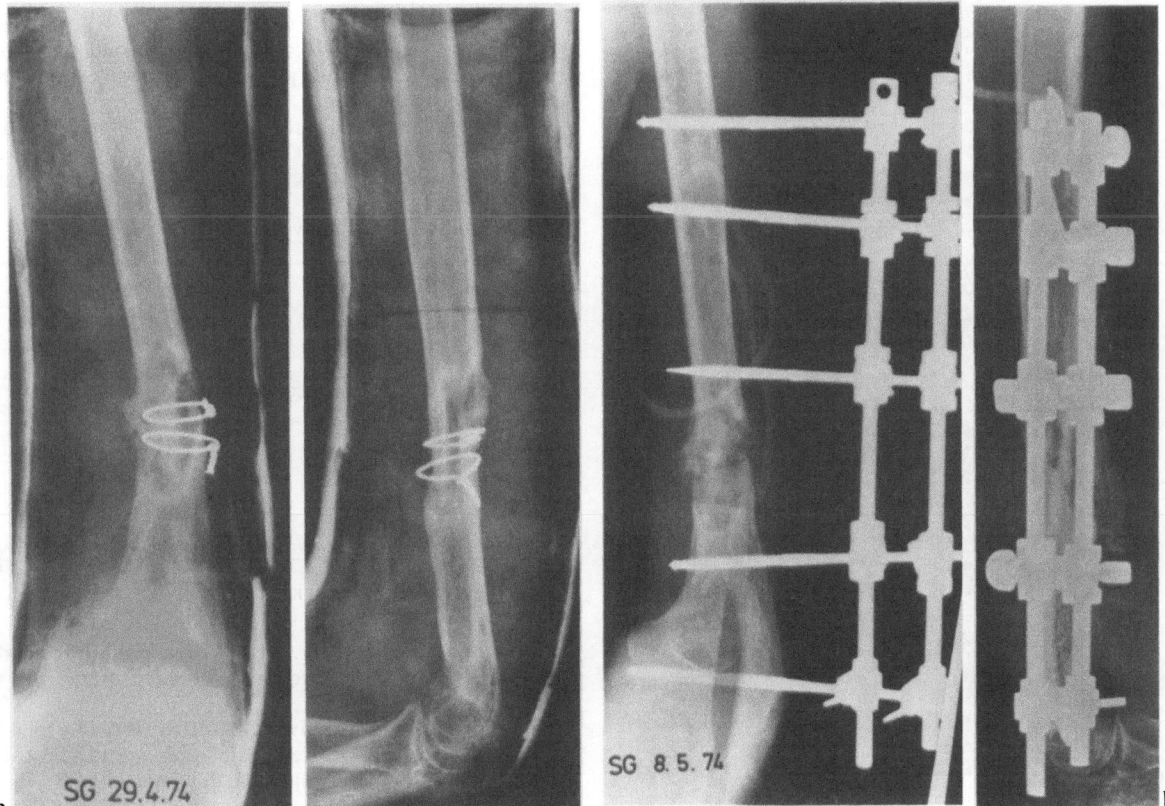

a    SG 29.4.74

b

Fig. 181a, b. Legend see p. 114

z. 181c, d

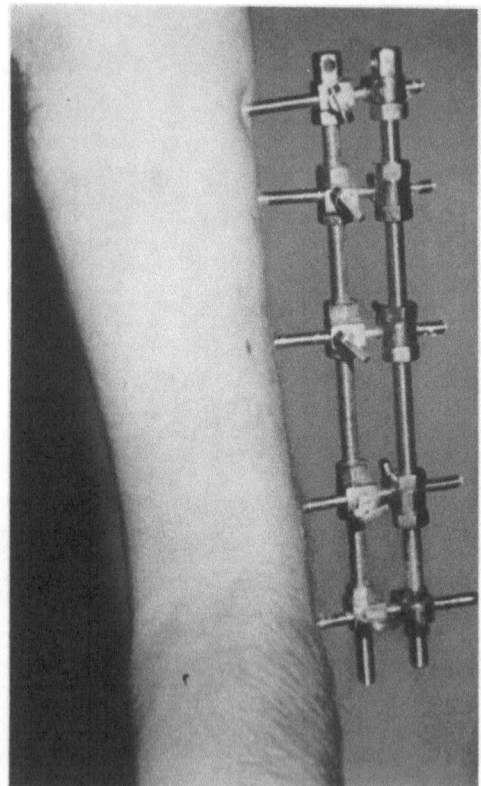

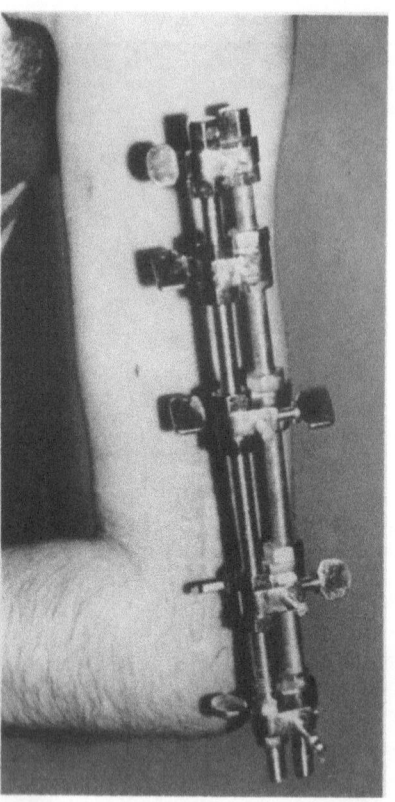

c

d

**Fig. 181 a–d.** Infected nonunion of the humerus. Unilateral frame. A.L., 1949, 25 years, ♂, 177317.

**a** Eight months previously: fracture, intramedullary nailing and cerclage. Infection and pin removal (abroad). At presentation: infected nonunion.

**b** Sequestrectomy, unilateral compression frame for 12 weeks. Cancellous bone grafting.

**c** Eight weeks postoperatively: initiation of therapeutic exercises.

**d** Five months postoperatively: union

**Fig. 182 a–c.** Supracondylar osteotomy of the humerus. Unilateral frame. T.M., 1944, 18 years, ♀, 72810.

**a** Cubitus varus secondary to elbow fracture in childhood. Valgus osteotomy, unilateral compression frame for 6 weeks, then plaster for 6 weeks.

**b** Four months postoperatively: osteotomy is finally solid.

**c** $10^1/_2$ years postoperatively: joint axes are identical on both sides, function is comparable to uninjured limb

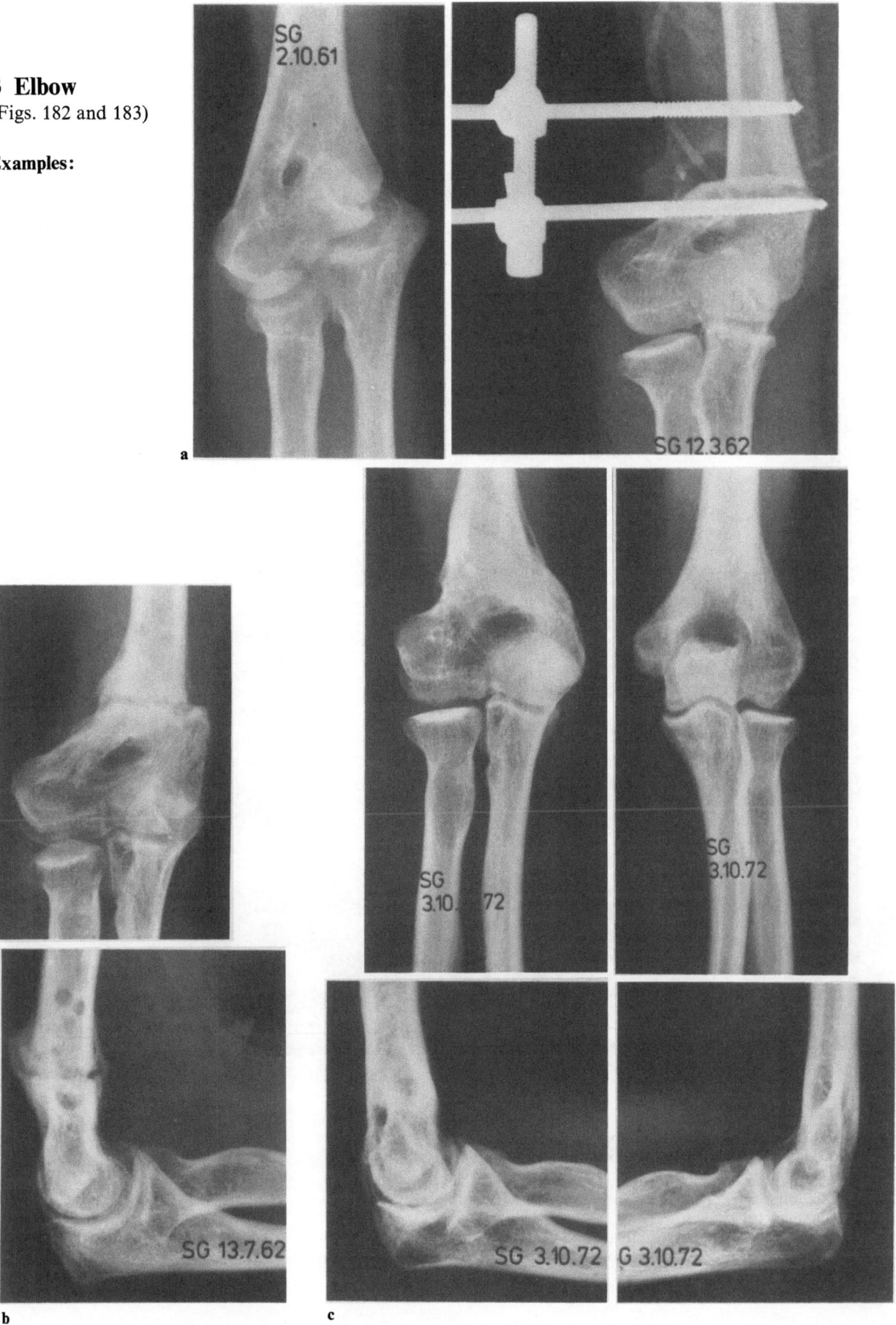

## 3 Elbow
(Figs. 182 and 183)

**Examples:**

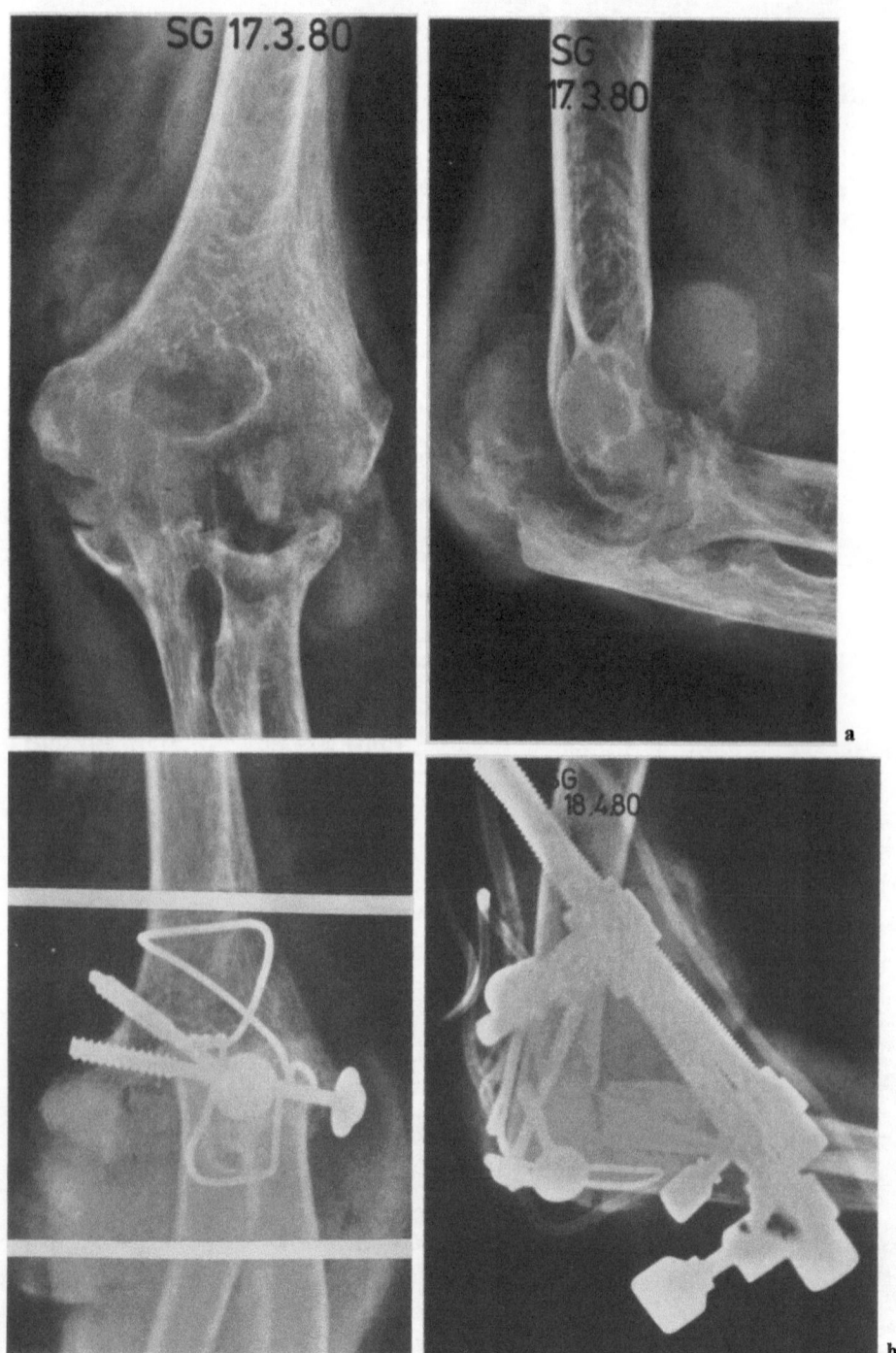

**Fig. 183 a–d.** Arthrodesis of the elbow for tuberculous arthritis. Bilateral frame. B.G., 1926, 54 years, ♀, 237595.

**a** Tuberculous arthritis of the elbow.
**b** Resection + lag screw + tension band + bilateral neutralization frame for 7 weeks.
**c** Seven weeks postoperatively, plaster for 6 weeks.
**d** Six months postoperatively: arthrodesis is consolidated

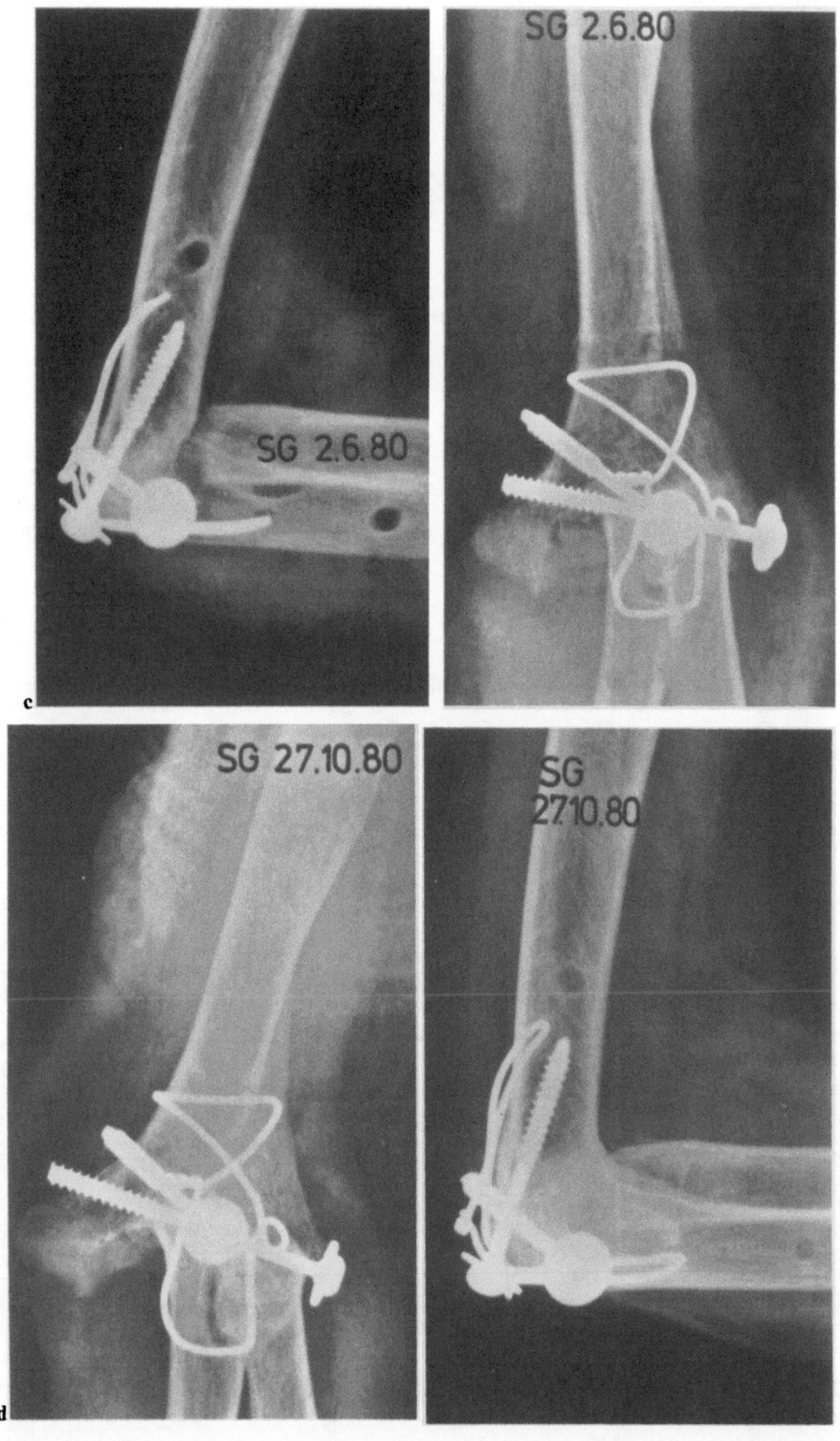

**Fig. 183c, d**

## 4 Wrist (Figs. 184–188)

**Examples:**

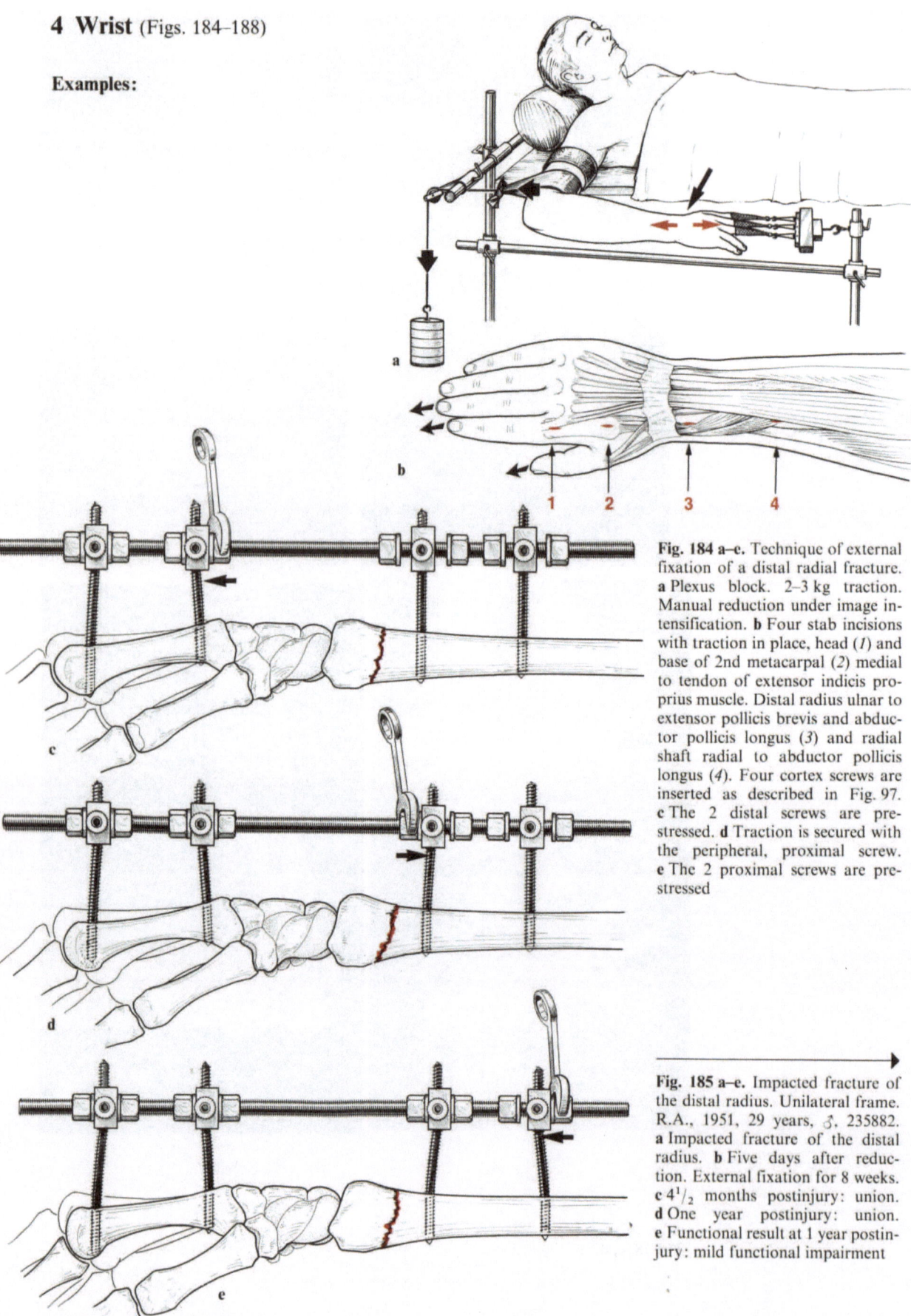

**Fig. 184 a–e.** Technique of external fixation of a distal radial fracture. **a** Plexus block. 2–3 kg traction. Manual reduction under image intensification. **b** Four stab incisions with traction in place, head (*1*) and base of 2nd metacarpal (*2*) medial to tendon of extensor indicis proprius muscle. Distal radius ulnar to extensor pollicis brevis and abductor pollicis longus (*3*) and radial shaft radial to abductor pollicis longus (*4*). Four cortex screws are inserted as described in Fig. 97. **c** The 2 distal screws are prestressed. **d** Traction is secured with the peripheral, proximal screw. **e** The 2 proximal screws are prestressed

**Fig. 185 a–e.** Impacted fracture of the distal radius. Unilateral frame. R.A., 1951, 29 years, ♂. 235882. **a** Impacted fracture of the distal radius. **b** Five days after reduction. External fixation for 8 weeks. **c** $4^1/_2$ months postinjury: union. **d** One year postinjury: union. **e** Functional result at 1 year postinjury: mild functional impairment

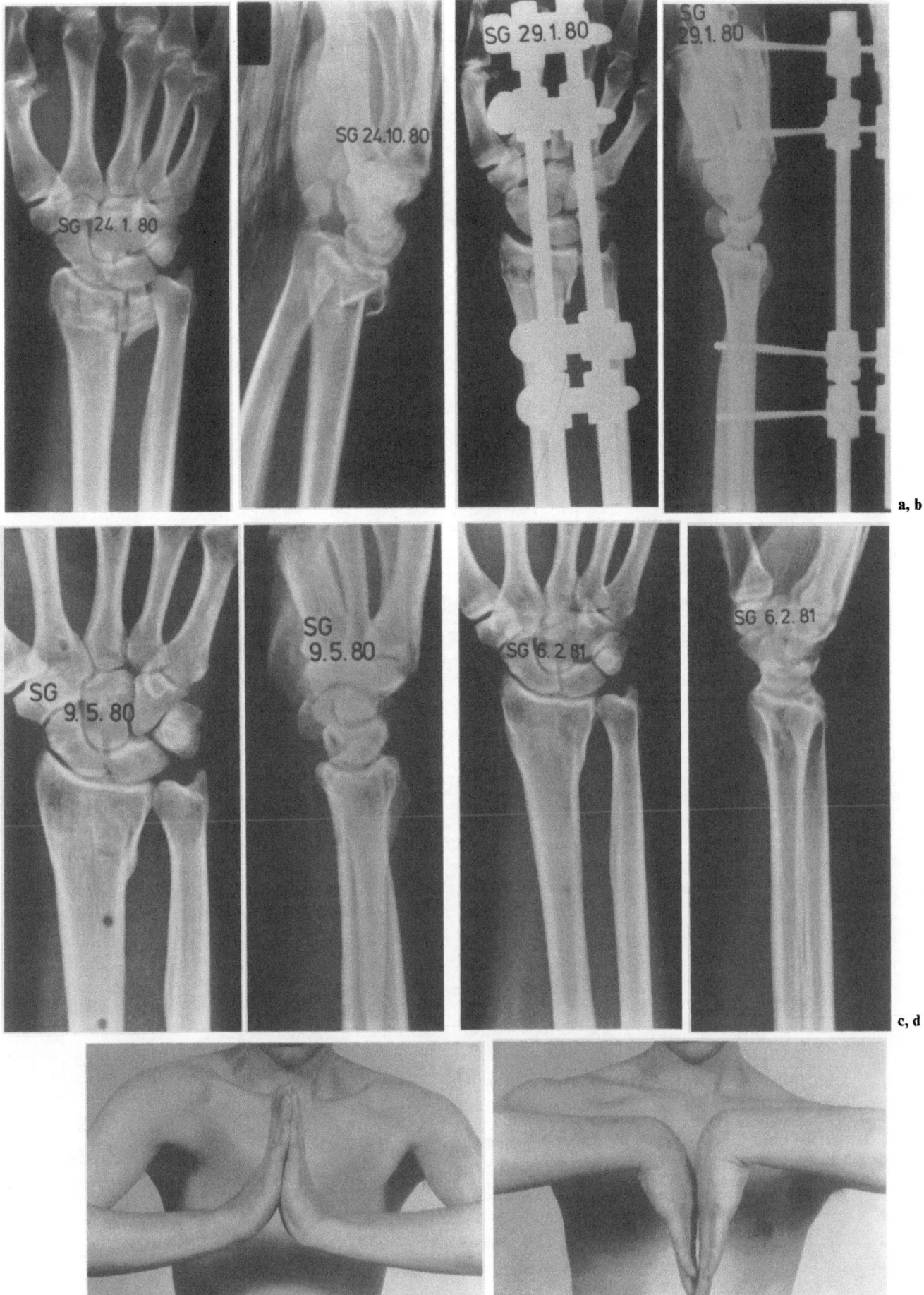

a, b

c, d

e

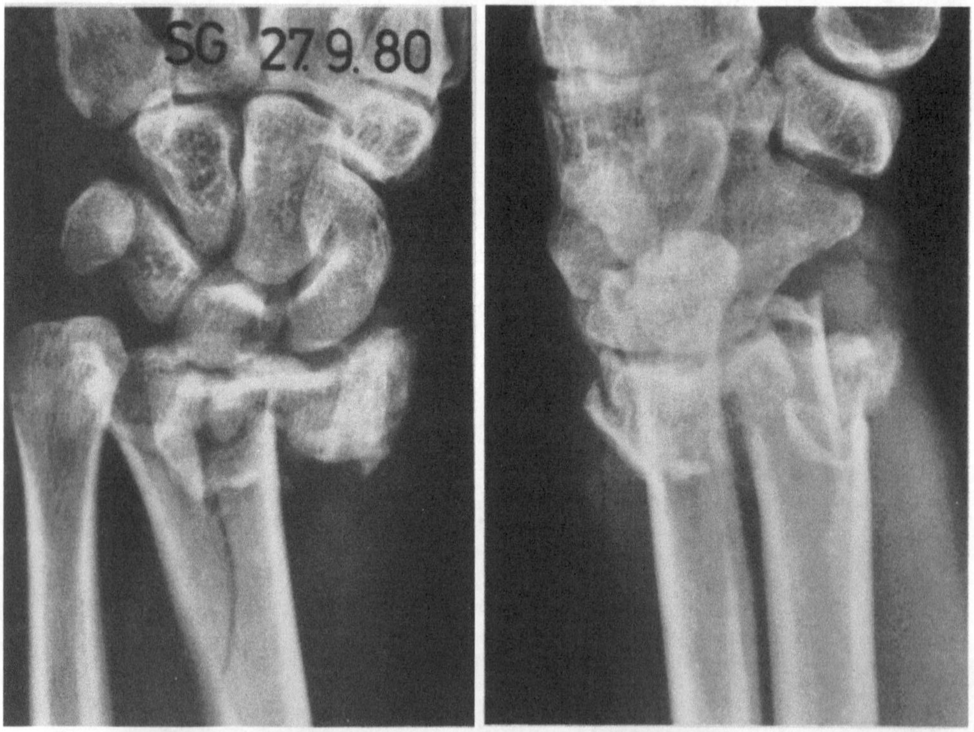

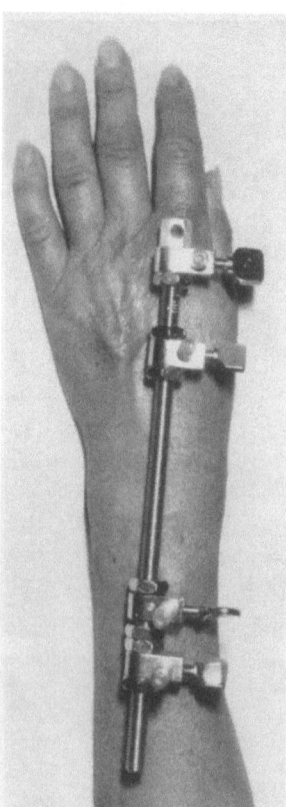

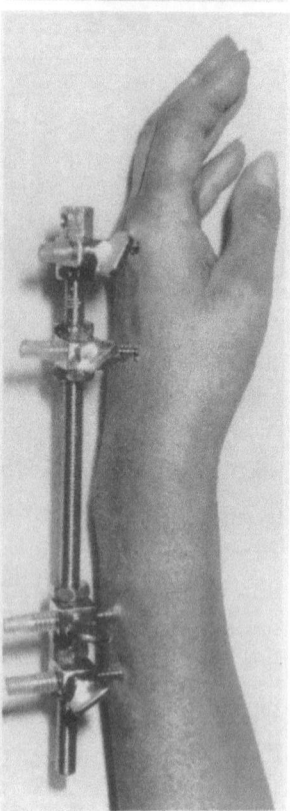

**Fig. 186 a–f.** Comminuted fracture of the distal radius. Unilateral frame. S.C., 39 years, ♀, 190867.

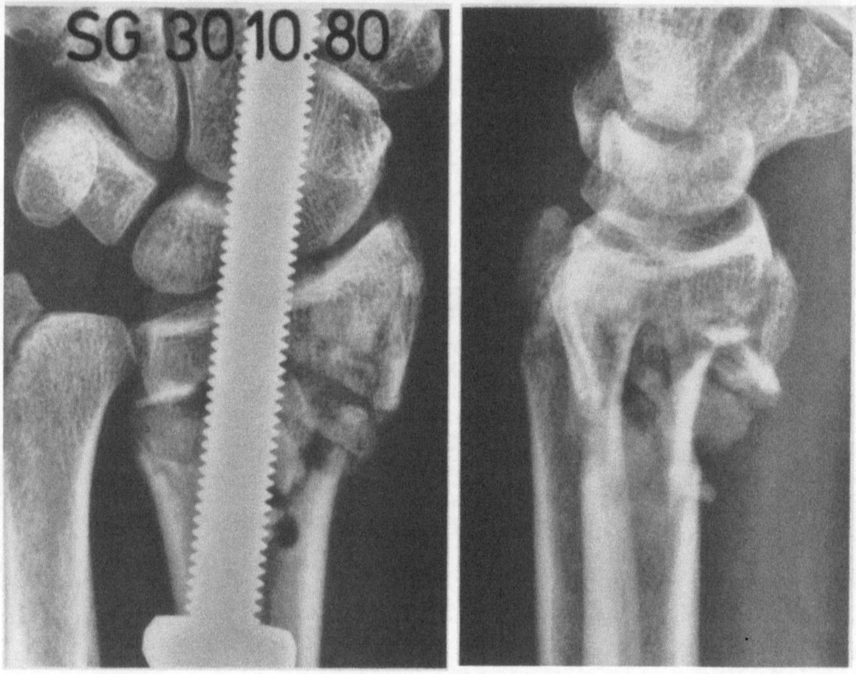

**a** Comminuted distal radial fracture.
**b** One month after reduction and external fixation for 8 weeks.
**c** External fixator in place, 1 month postinjury.
**d** Three years postinjury: radiographs identical on both sides.
**e** Three years postinjury: complete recovery
**f** Symmetrical function

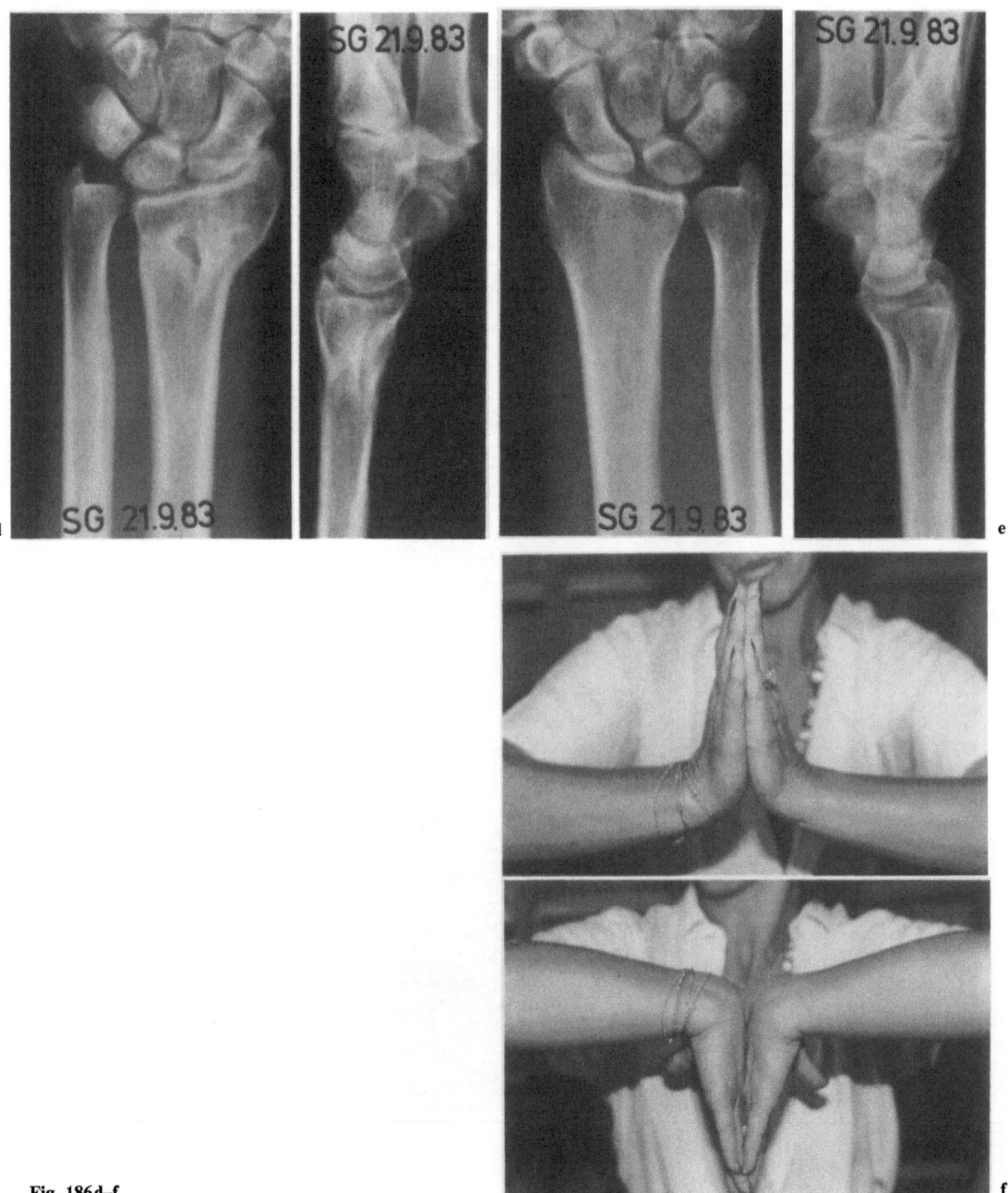

d

e

**Fig. 186d–f**

f

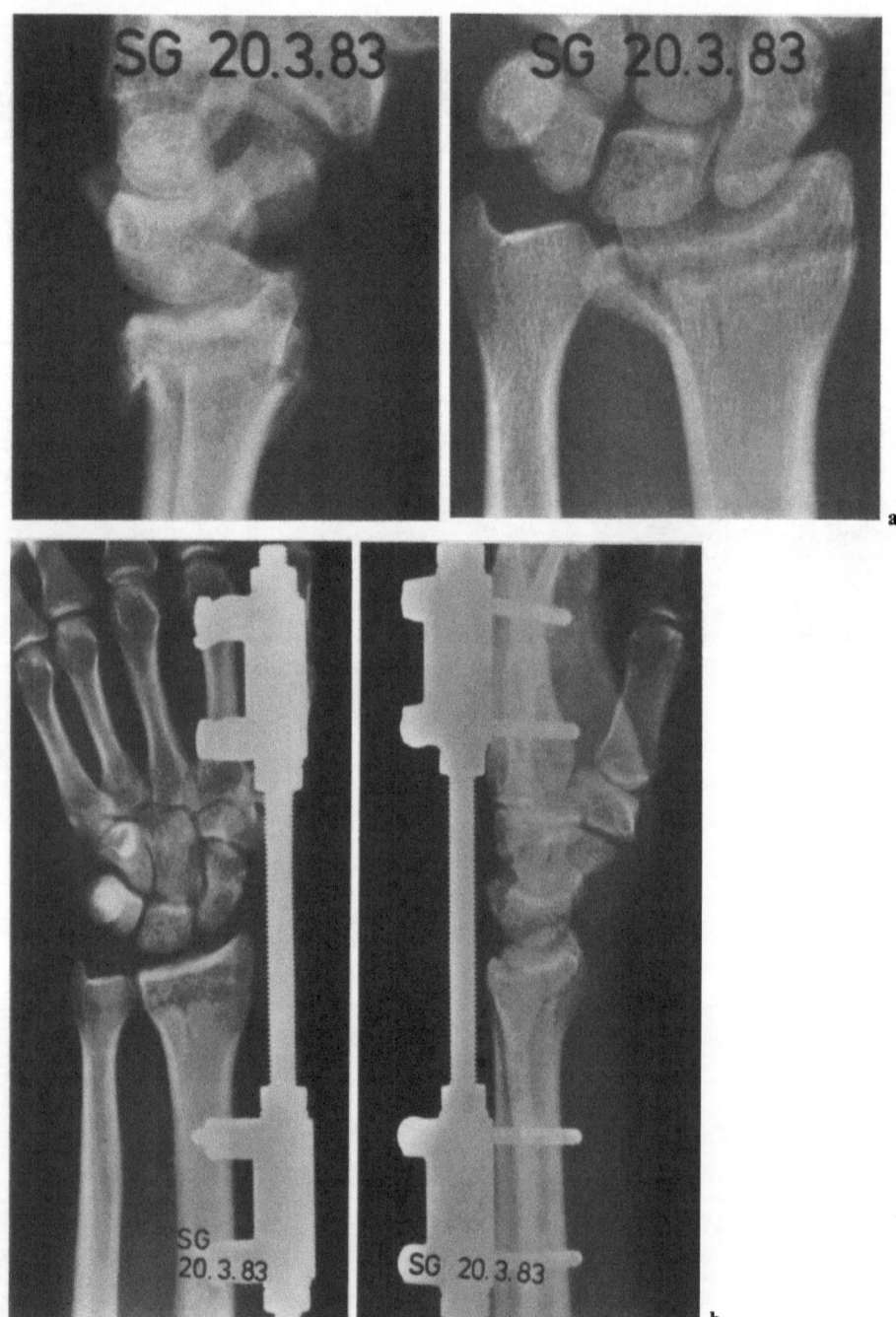

**Fig. 187 a–g.** Bilateral fracture of the distal radius and navicular bone. Unilateral frame. F.E., 1949, 34 years, ♂, 190359.

**a** Distal fracture of the left radius.
**b** Reduction and external fixation for 6 weeks.
**c** Eight months postinjury: complete recovery.
**d** Right navicular fracture.
**e** External fixation for 8 weeks.
**f** Eight weeks postinjury: fracture is united.
**g** Eight months postinjury: complete recovery

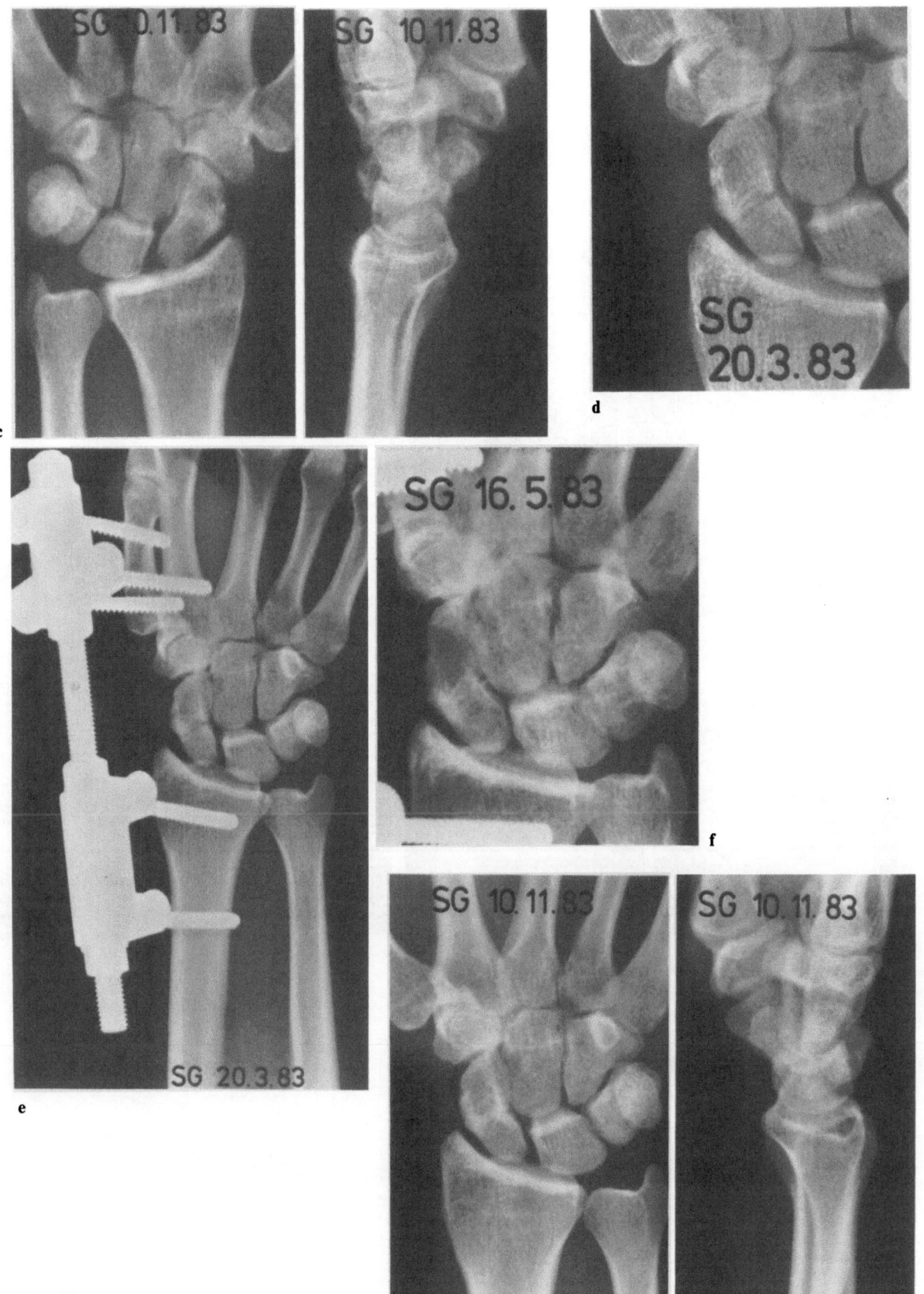

Fig. 187 c–g

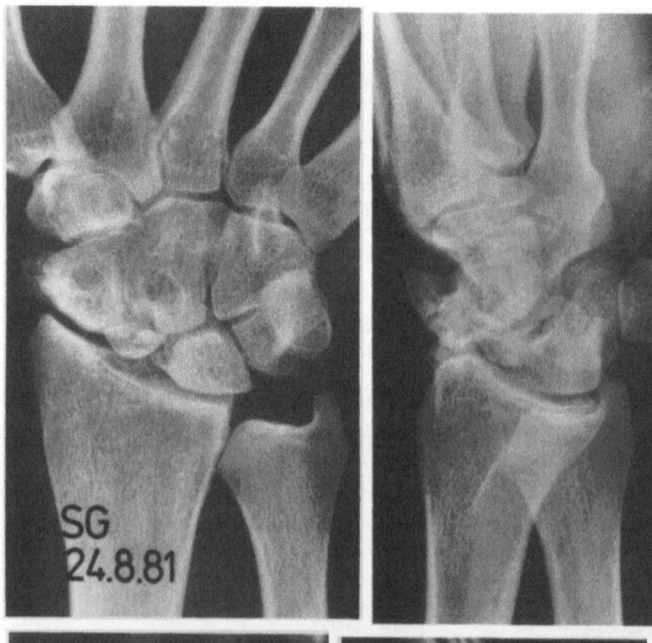

**Fig. 188 a–c.** Radiocarpal arthrodesis. Unilateral frame. N.J., 1936, 46 years, ♂, 259830.

**a** Post-traumatic osteoarthritis with nonunion of the navicular bone.

**b** Four weeks after freshening of radiocarpal joint and interposition of corticocancellous iliac bone graft between radius and trapezium. External fixation for 8 weeks. Plaster for 4 weeks.

**c** Seven months postoperatively: arthrodesis is consolidated

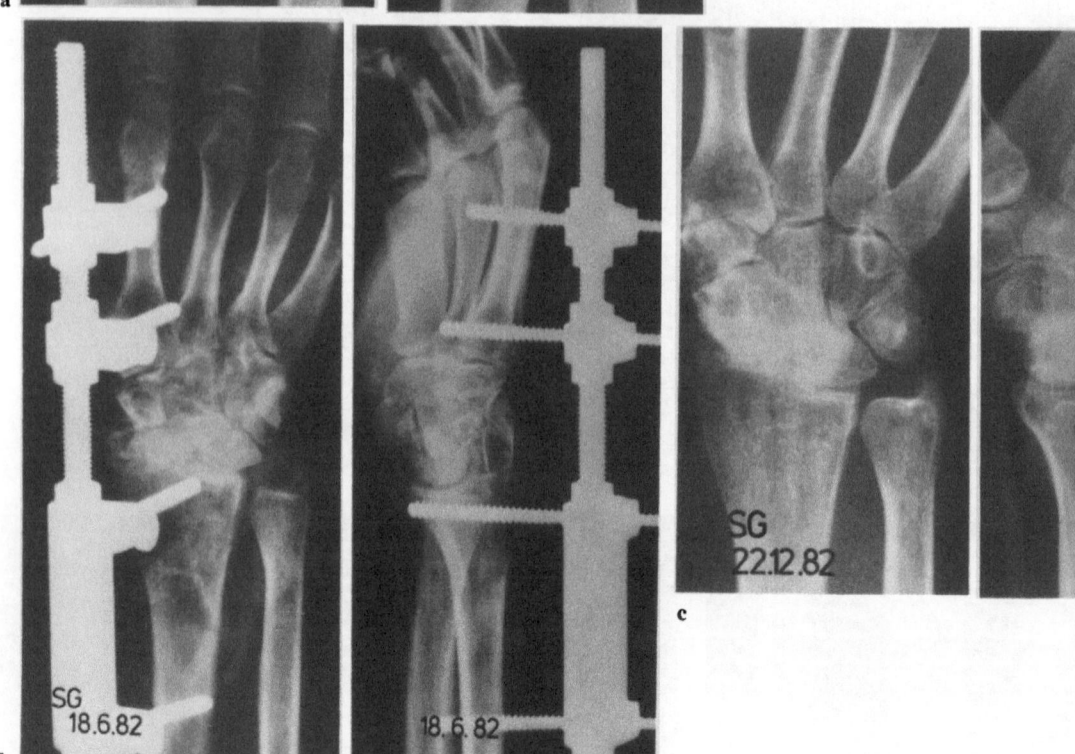

# 5 Pelvis (Fig. 189)

**Example:**

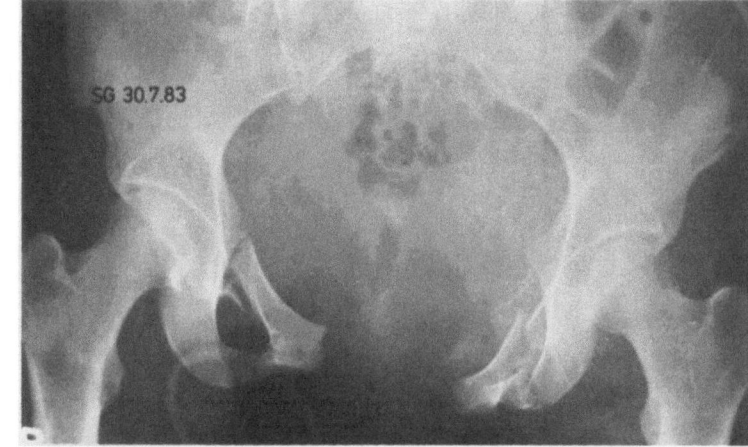

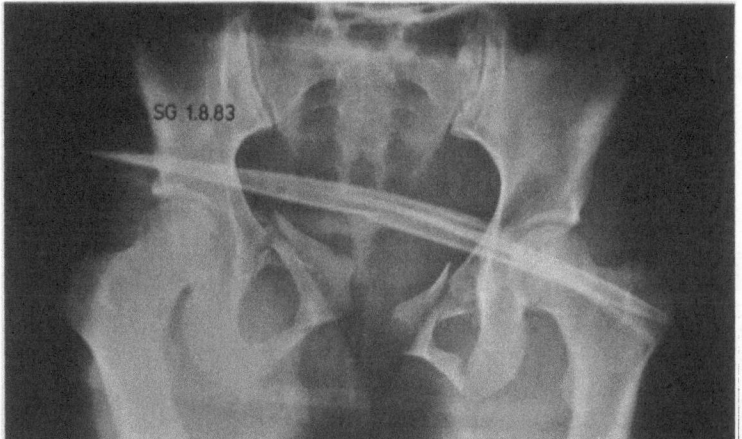

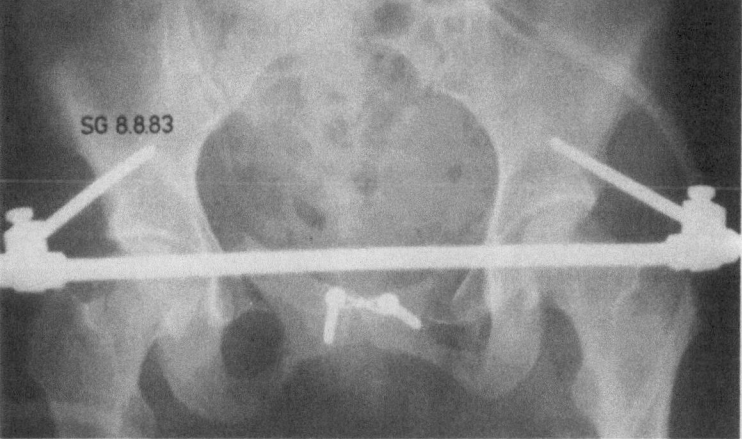

**Fig. 189 a–c.** Pelvic ring fracture. Unilateral frame. S.M., 1961, 22 years, ♀, 205238.

**a** Postinjury radiograph shows five-part disruption of pelvic ring with dislocation of right sacroiliac joint, rupture of symphysis, and butterfly fractures of both rami.

**b** After one week: tension banding of symphysis + unilateral compression frame for 7 weeks. Schanz screws through inferior iliac spine.

**c** Two months postinjury: Patient has been ambulating on crutches for 2 weeks and is hampered little by the frame (= "humane" design). Radiograph in right one-legged stance shows that the fractures and disruptions are stable. Removal of frame.

**d** 1 year 2 months postinjury: Pelvic ring is stable. Metal removal is provided

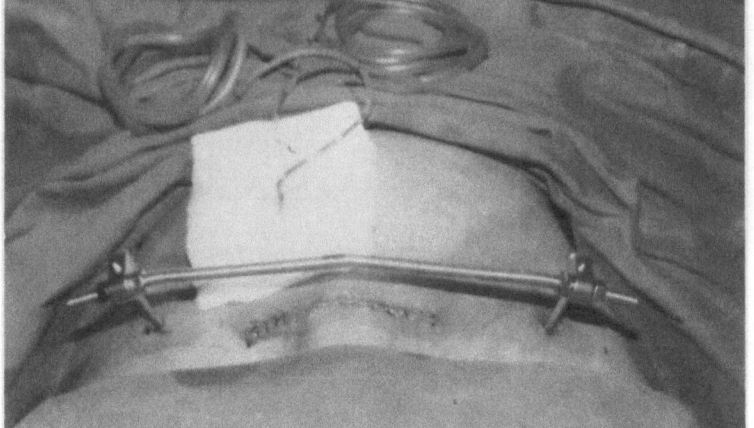

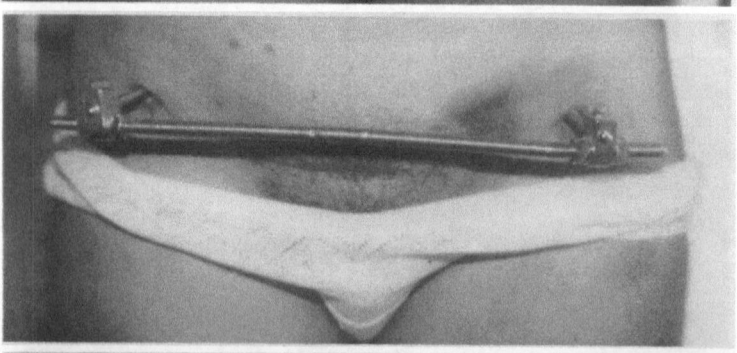
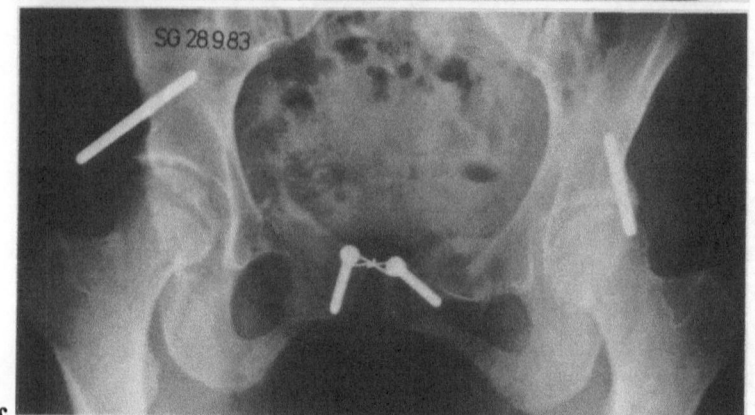
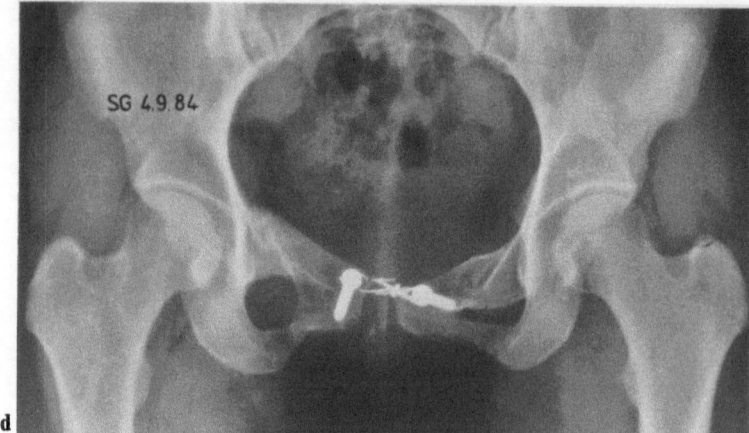

**Fig. 189c, d.** Legend see p. 125

# 6 Femur
(Figs. 190–197)

**Examples:**

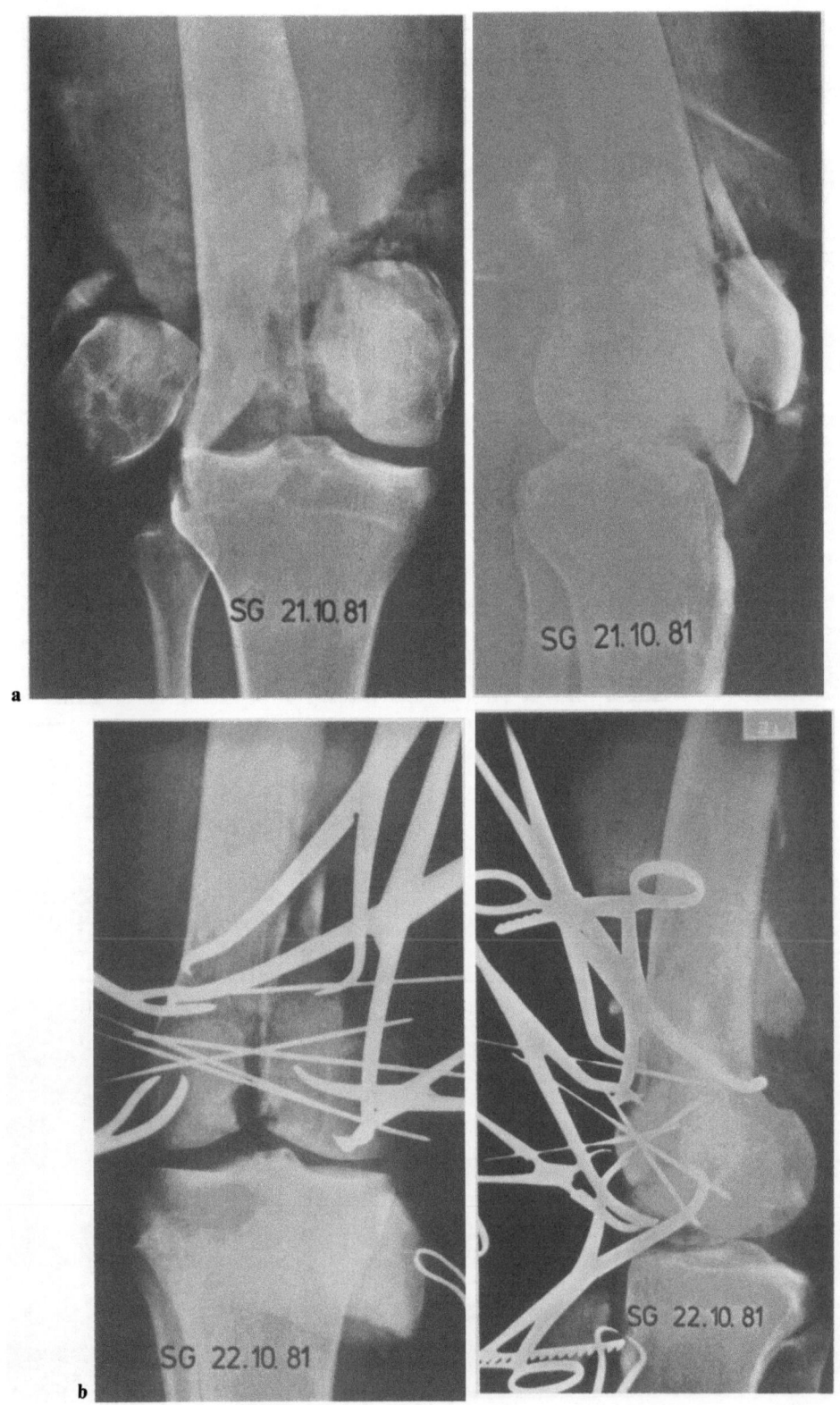

**Fig. 190a, b.** Legend see p. 129

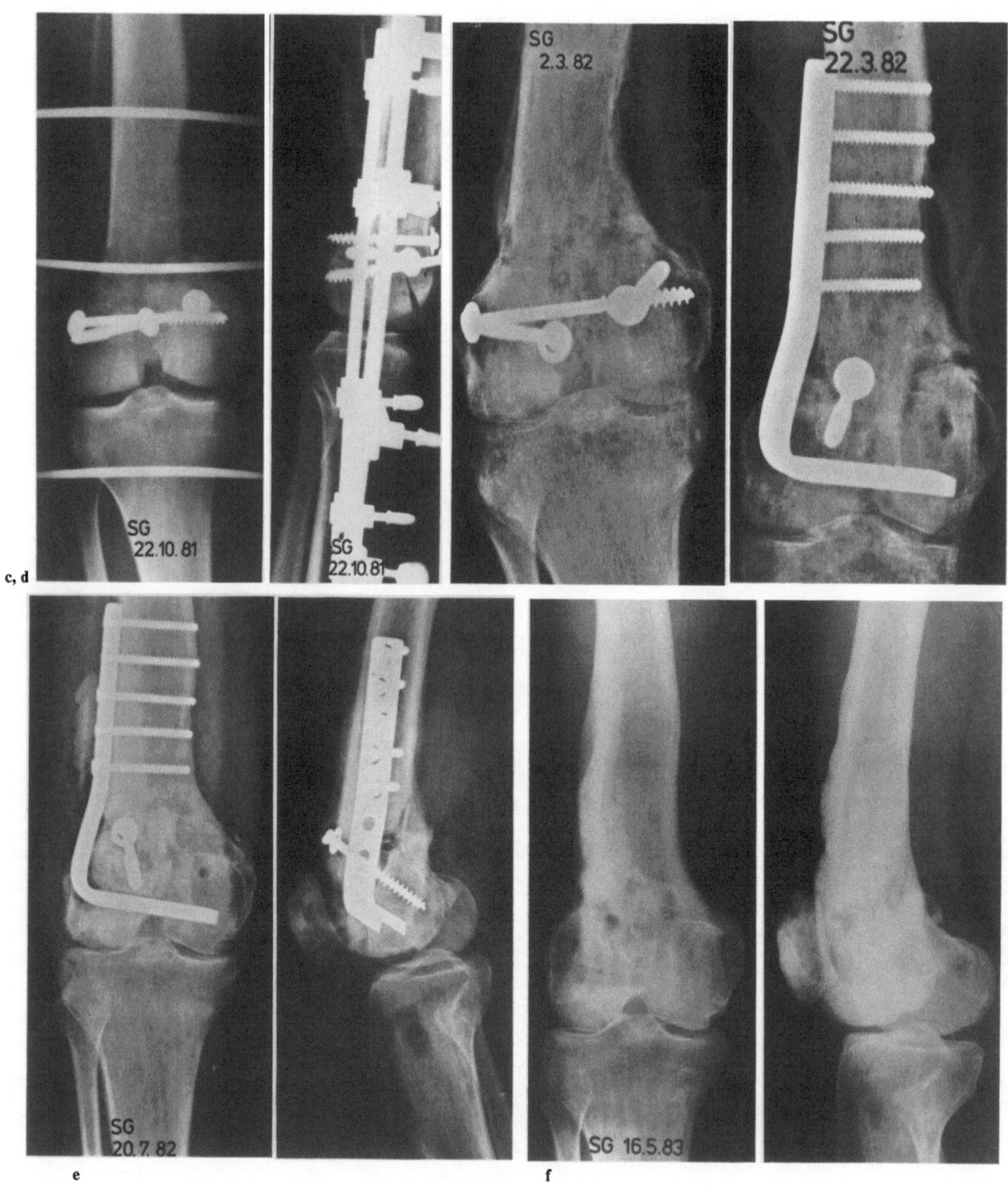

c, d

e

f

Fig. 190c–f

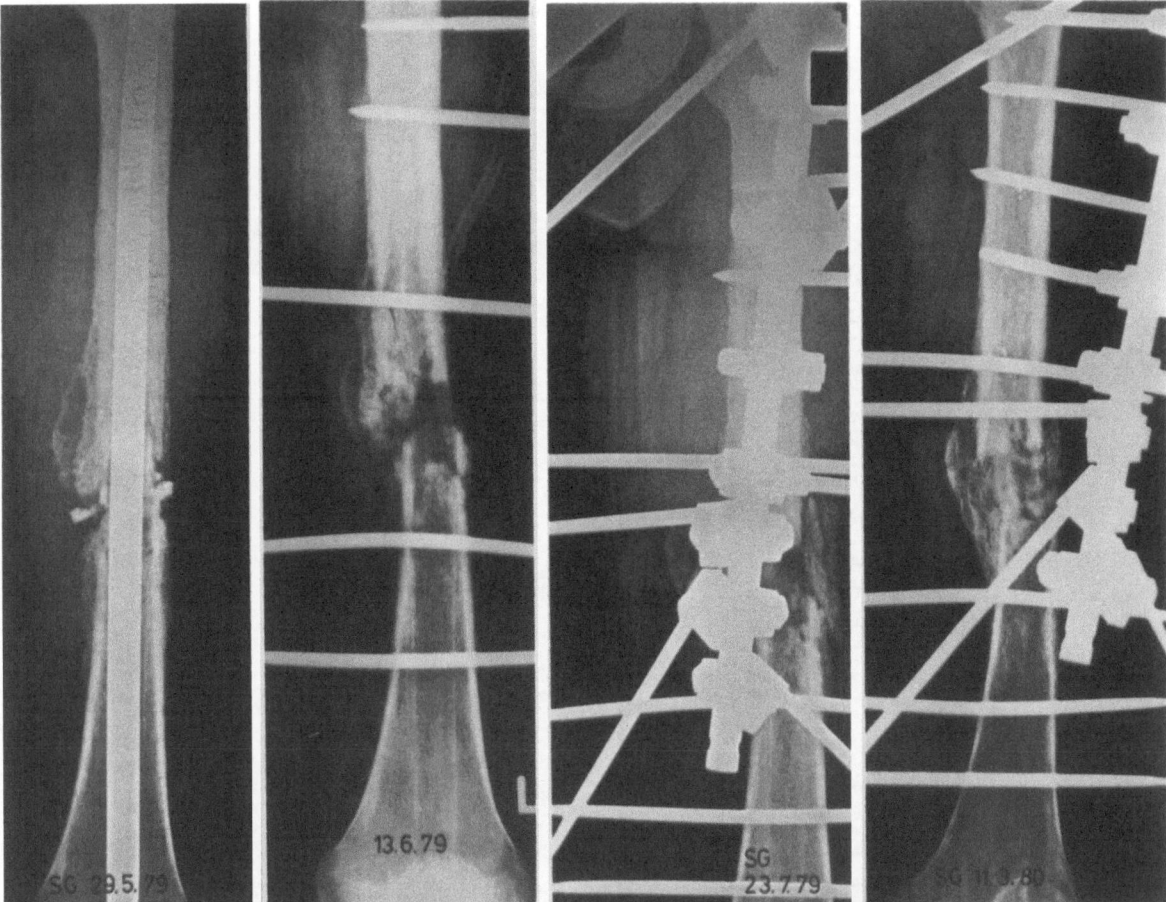

a       b

**Fig. 191 a–c.** Infected femoral fracture. Combined unilateral and bilateral frame. K.B., 1960, 19 years, ♀, 228 997.

**a** Four months previously: closed femoral fracture, intramedullary nailing, infection (abroad). At presentation: infection, sinus. Treatment: sequestrectomy, suction irrigation, combined unilateral and bilateral frame (combination of threaded and tubular rods).
**b** Cancellous bone grafting after 2 weeks. External fixation for 9 months until graft take.
**c** Forty months after external fixation: complete recovery

◄─────────────

**Fig. 190 a–f.** Open distal femoral fracture. Bilateral frame. A.E., 1962, 19 years, ♂, 149 740.

**a** Grade III open fracture of the distal femur.
**b** Radiograph at operation: reduction, preliminary fixation.
**c** Postoperative radiograph: internal fixation with 3 lag screws and cancellous bone graft. Knee-spanning bilateral frame for 10 weeks.
**d** Five months postinjury: fracture is united, but varus deformity is present, necessitating a valgus osteotomy.
**e** Four months postoperatively: osteotomy is solid.
**f** Twenty months postinjury: fracture is united, limb axis is good, knee flexion 70°

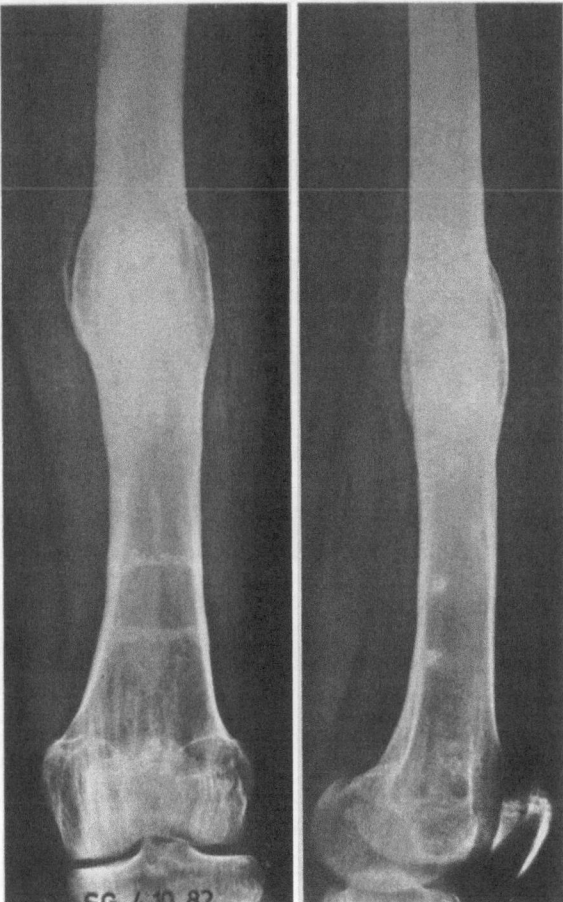

c

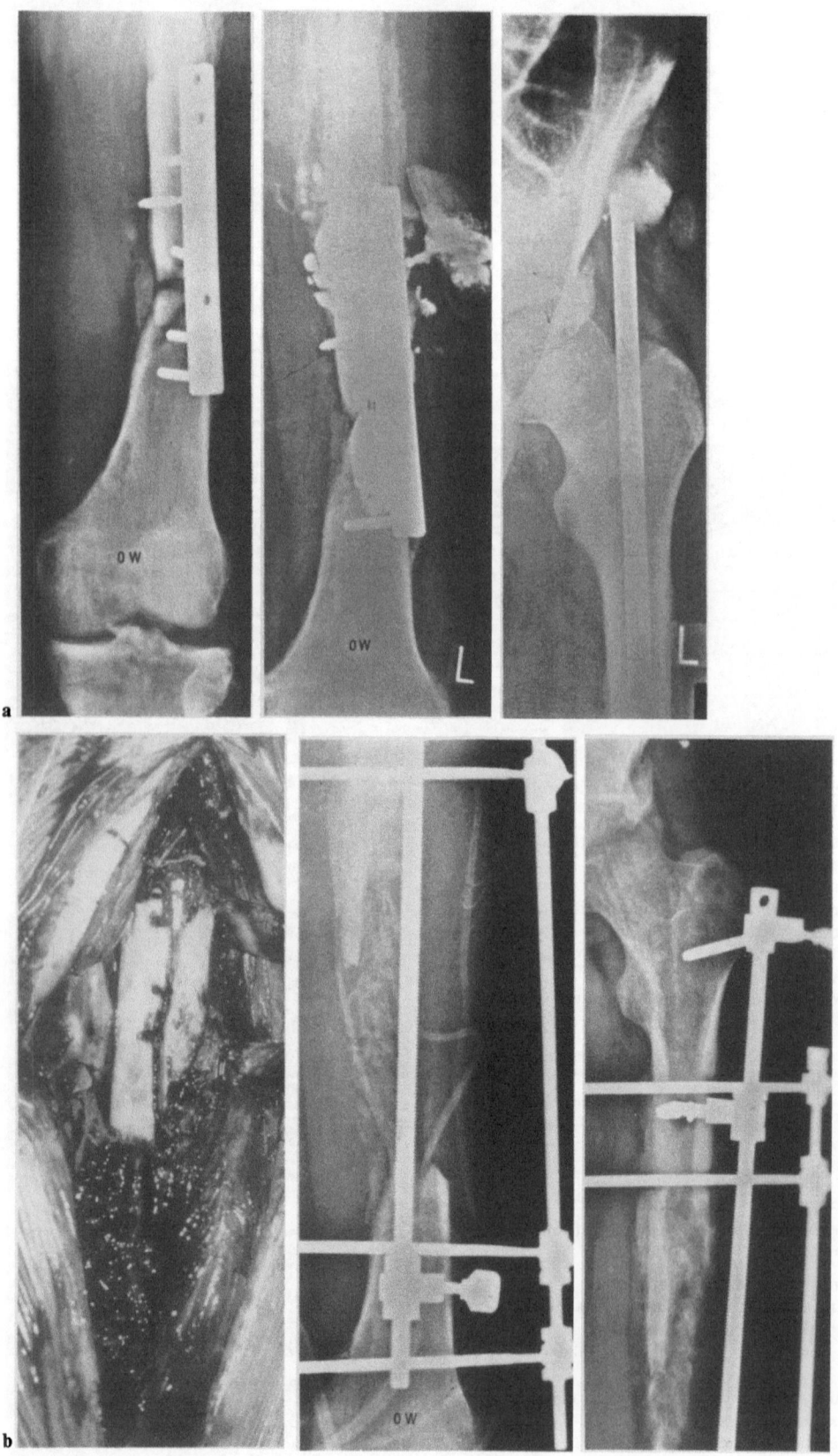

Fig. 192a, b

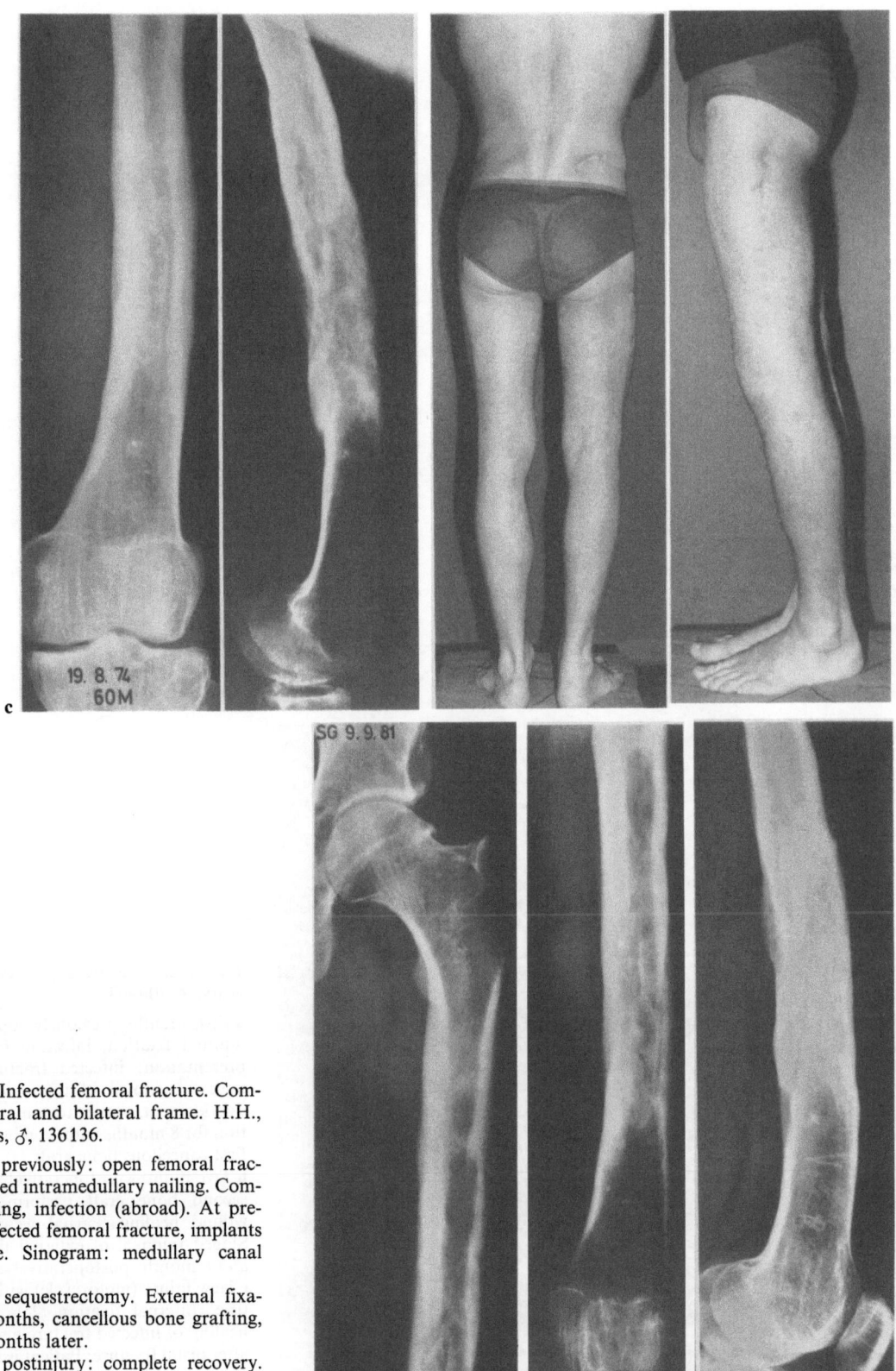

**Fig. 192 a–d.** Infected femoral fracture. Combined unilateral and bilateral frame. H.H., 1949, 22 years, ♂, 136136.

**a** Ten weeks previously: open femoral fracture. Attempted intramedullary nailing. Compression plating, infection (abroad). At presentation: infected femoral fracture, implants still in place. Sinogram: medullary canal phlegmon.
**b** Operation: sequestrectomy. External fixation for 5 months, cancellous bone grafting, repeated 3 months later.
**c** Five years postinjury: complete recovery. Knee flexion 110°.
**d** Twelve years postinjury: complete recovery

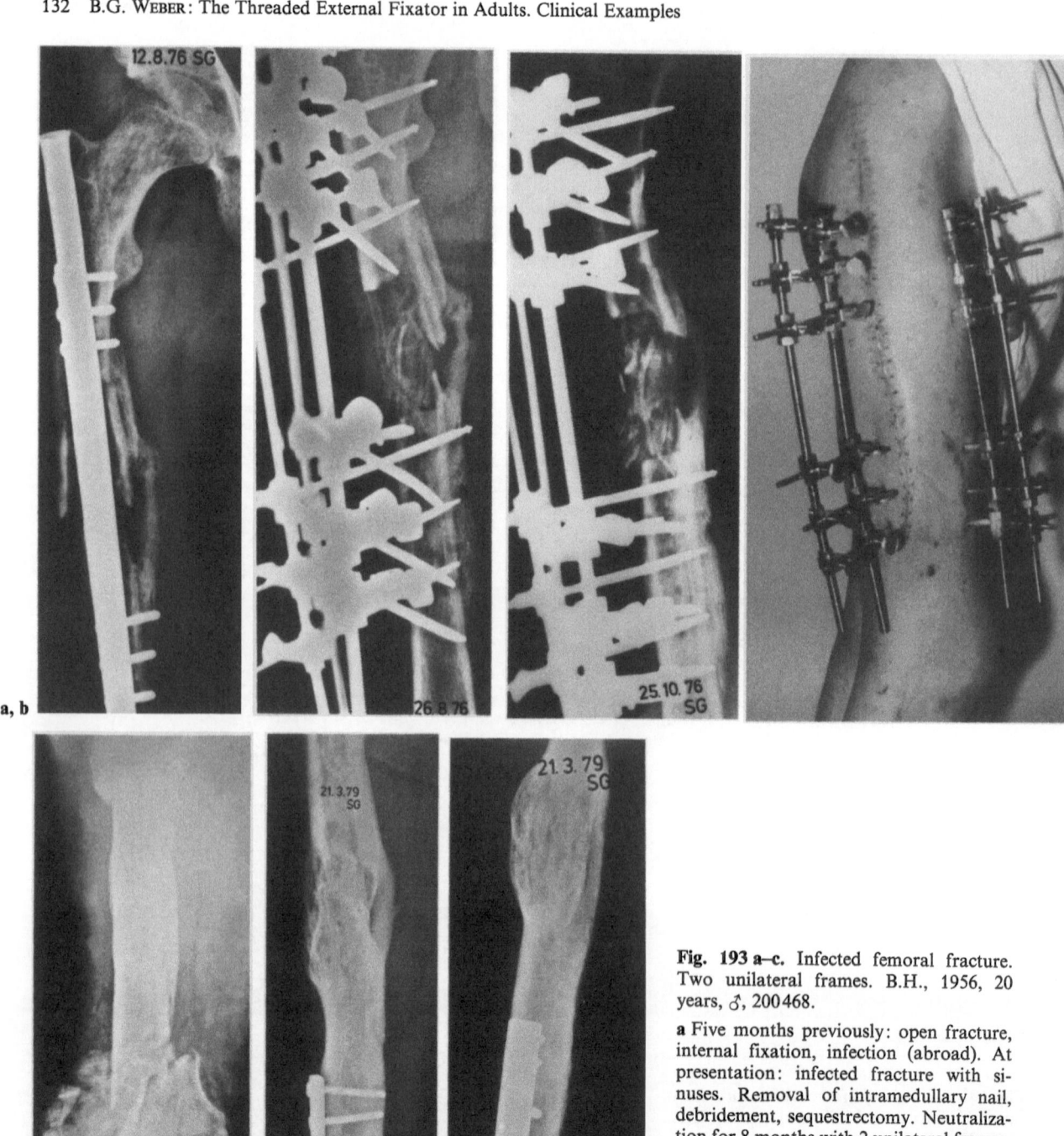

**Fig. 193 a–c.** Infected femoral fracture. Two unilateral frames. B.H., 1956, 20 years, ♂, 200468.

**a** Five months previously: open fracture, internal fixation, infection (abroad). At presentation: infected fracture with sinuses. Removal of intramedullary nail, debridement, sequestrectomy. Neutralization for 8 months with 2 unilateral frames, first cancellous bone graft.

**b** Two months postoperatively: graft take, second bone graft performed. Primary wound healing. Partial weight bearing. Staged removal of external fixation at 5 and 8 months postoperatively.

**c** New injury (motorcycle) with open fracture. Internal fixation. $2^1/_2$ years after healing of infected fracture and $1^3/_4$ years after distal fracture: Patient is free of complaints and has 90-0-5 range of knee motion with 3 cm shortening

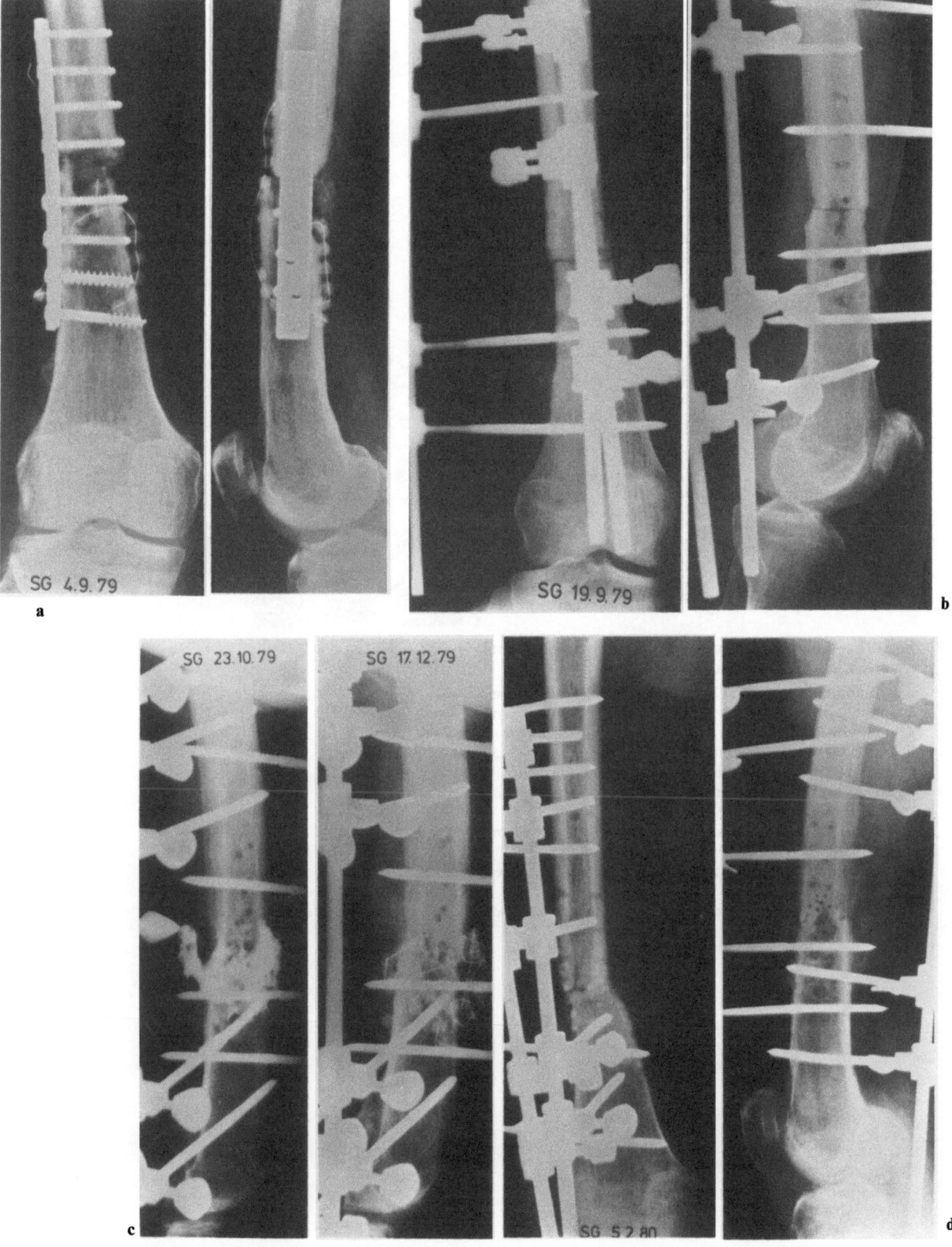

**Fig. 194a–d.** Legend see p. 134

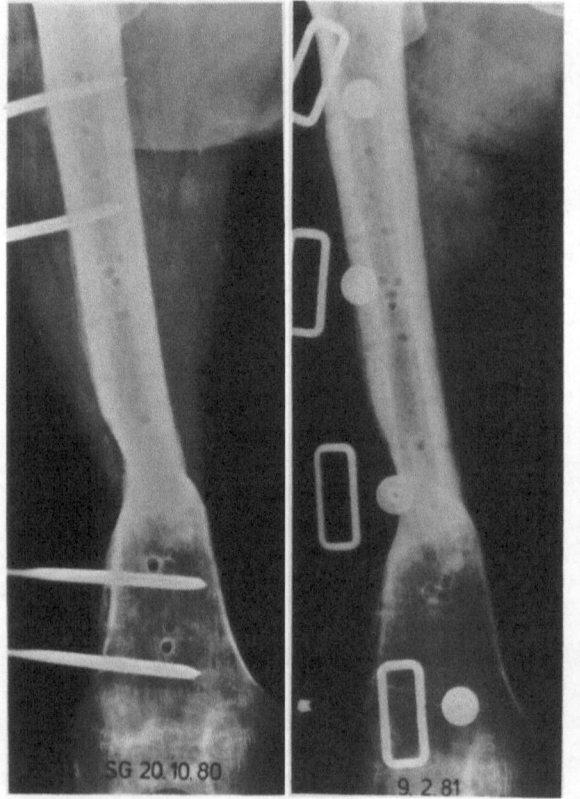
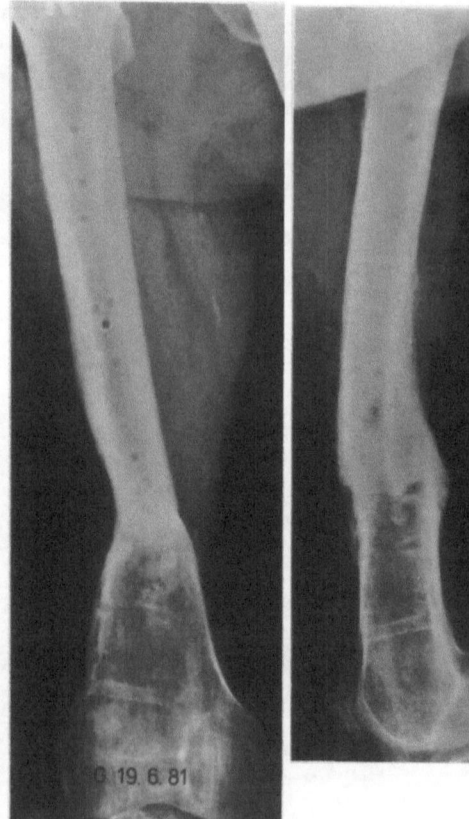

e

f

**Fig. 194 a–f.** Infected nonunion of the femur. Two unilateral frames. T.W., 1924, 55 years, ♂, 186039.

**a** Six months previously: closed fracture. Internal fixation, infection (abroad). At presentation: 4 sinuses, plate in situ, gentamycin-PMMA chains.
**b** Treatment: debridement + sequestrectomy with 2-cm shortening, cancellous bone graft, external fixation.
**c** Abscess formation, sinogram, evacuation of abscesses, insertion of gentamycin-PMMA chain.
**d** One month *later:* redebridement, removal of sequestra, drilling, cancellous bone graft.
**e** Twelve months after start of treatment: removal of external fixation.
**f** $1^3/_4$ years after start of treatment: nonunion and infection are healed

**Fig. 195 a–e.** Infected nonunion of the femur. Two unilateral frames. O.M., 1946, 33 years, ♂, 229056.

**a** Ten months after fracture, internal fixation, infection (abroad). At presentation: lateral sinus, instability. Treatment: tightening of loose screws, debridement, sequestrectomy, iliac bone graft, gentamycin-PMMA chains. Four weeks in external frame. Sinus.

**b** Plate removal, gentamycin-PMMA chain in plate bed, external fixation for 6 months. Third medial bone graft.

**c** Six months after start of treatment: fixator is partially dismantled, cast is applied.

**d** Fourteen months after start of treatment: infection is healed, but nonunion is not yet solid. Intramedullary nail.

**e** $2^1/_2$ years after start of treatment: nonunion is clinically solid and can bear weight normally. Infection healed, knee flexion 50°

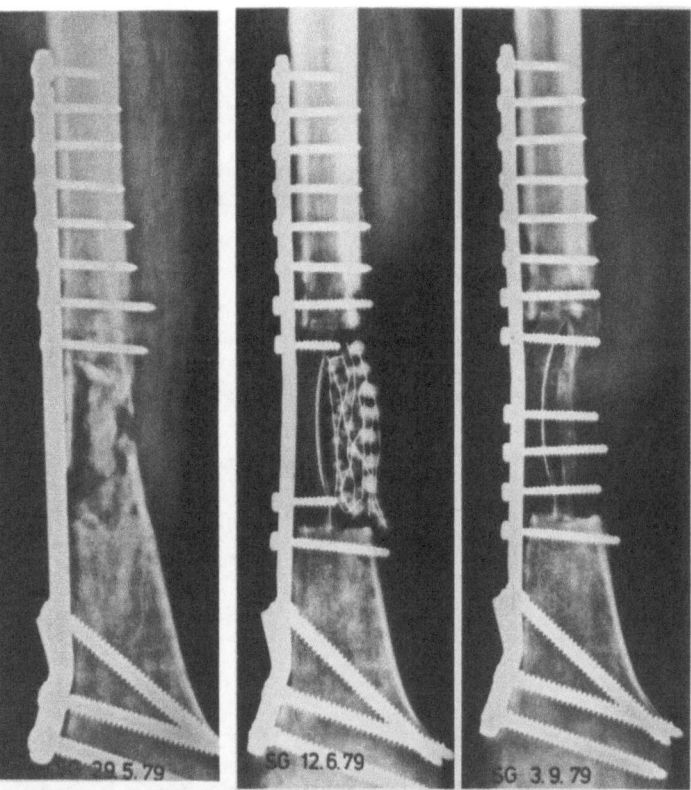

a

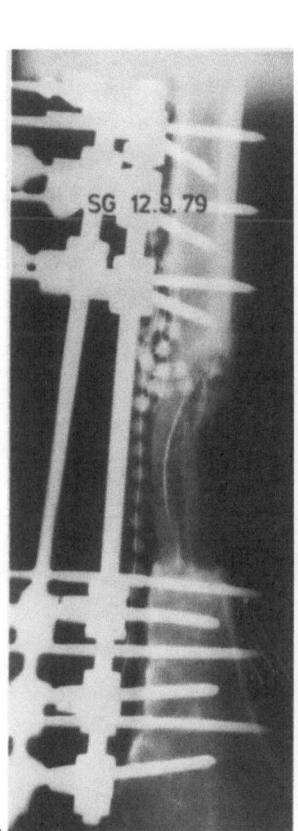

b

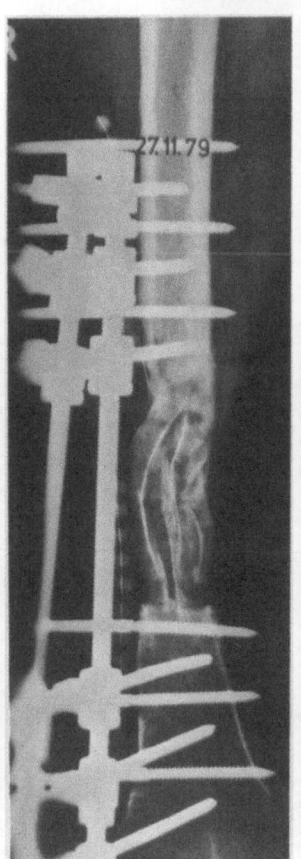

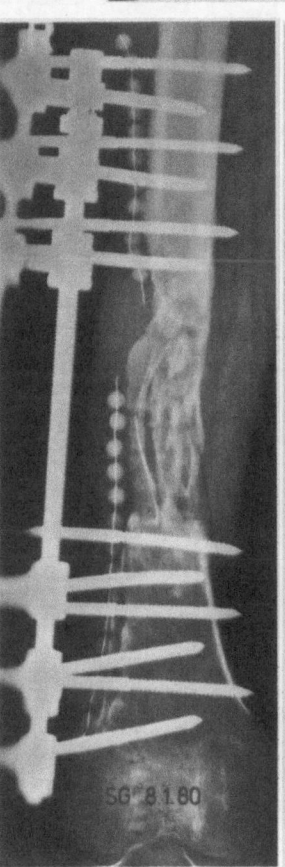

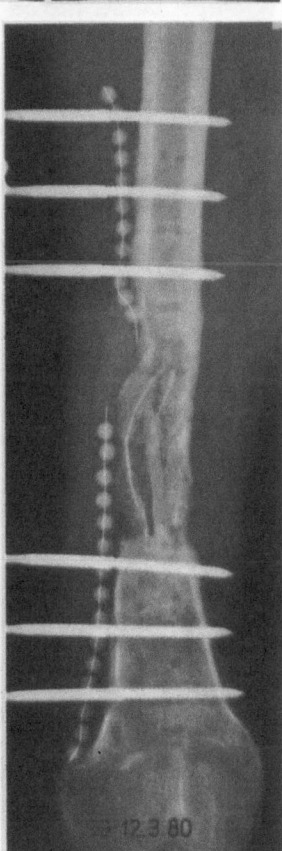

c

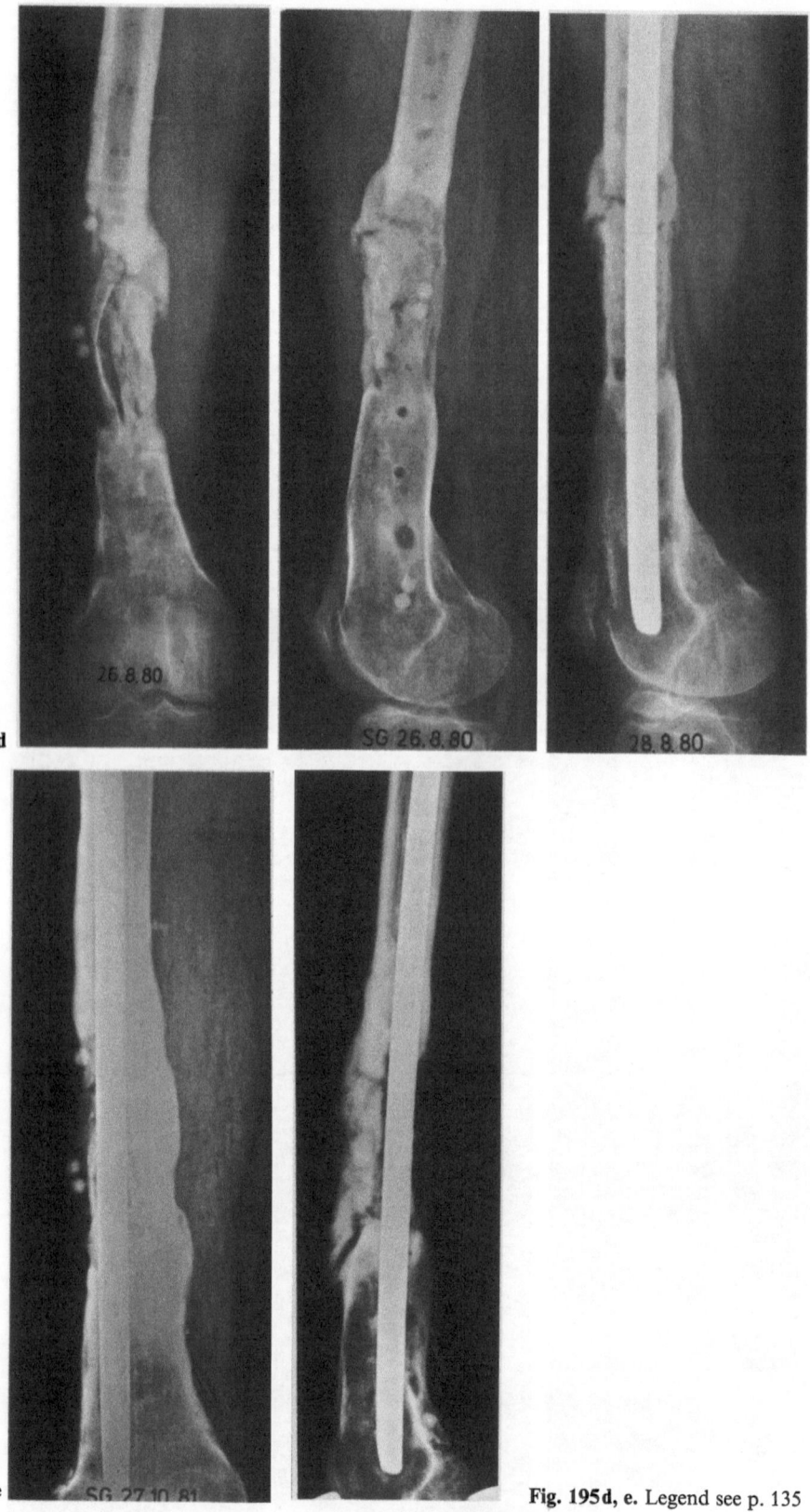

Fig. 195d, e. Legend see p. 135

**Fig. 196 a–c.** Osteitis secondary to femoral fracture. Unilateral frame. R.M., 1943, 34 years, ♀, 206687.

**a** Fourteen months previously: closed femoral fracture. Compression plating, infection, suction irrigation (abroad). At presentation: osteitis, sinus. Treatment: plate removal, debridement, cancellous bone graft, unilateral frame for 2 months. Spontaneous fracture 1 week after frame removal.

**b** Refixation with reinforced unilateral frame, regrafting. After 5 months, full weight bearing and removal of frame.

**c** Six years after start of treatment: complete recovery

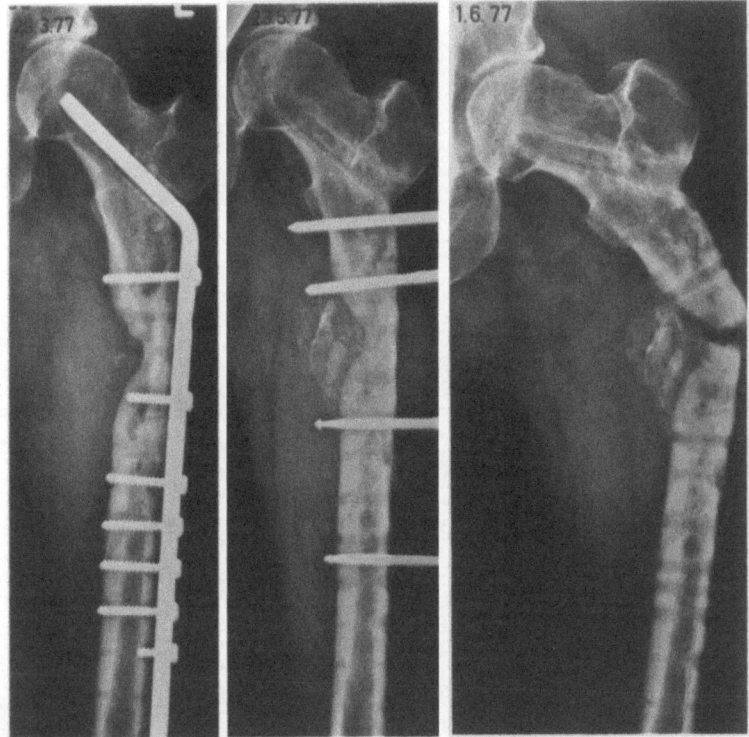

a

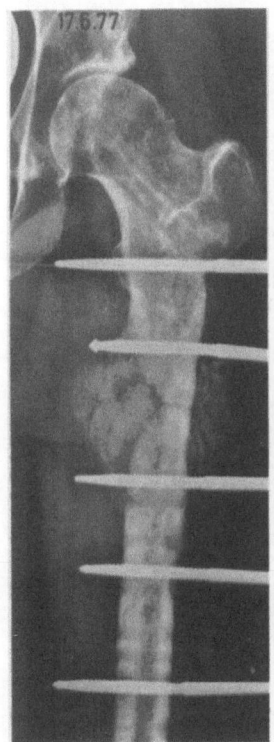

b

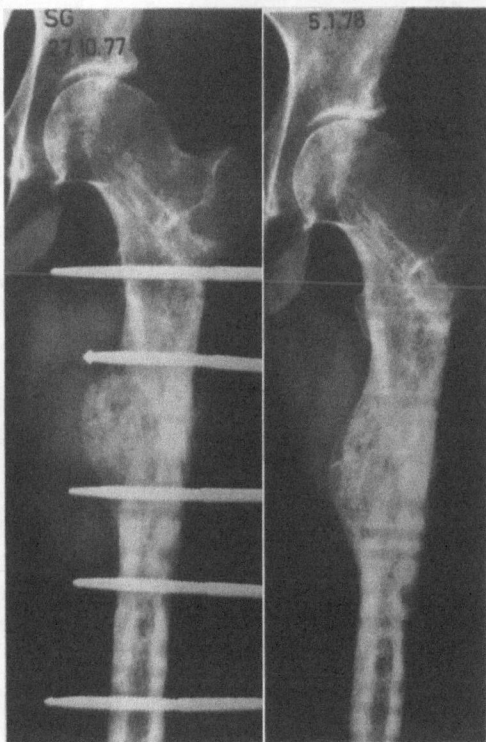

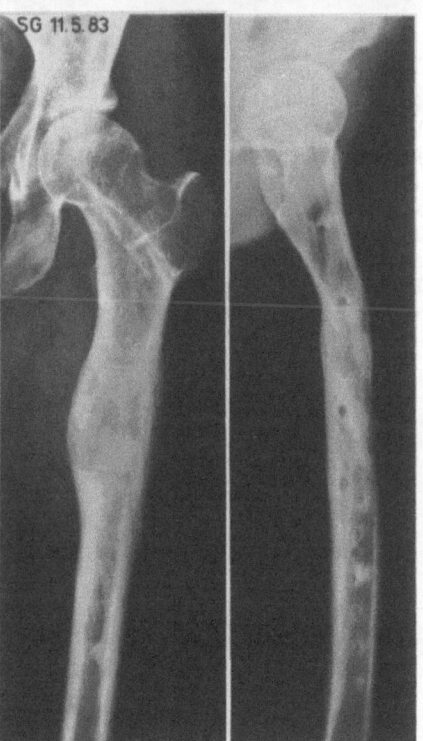

c

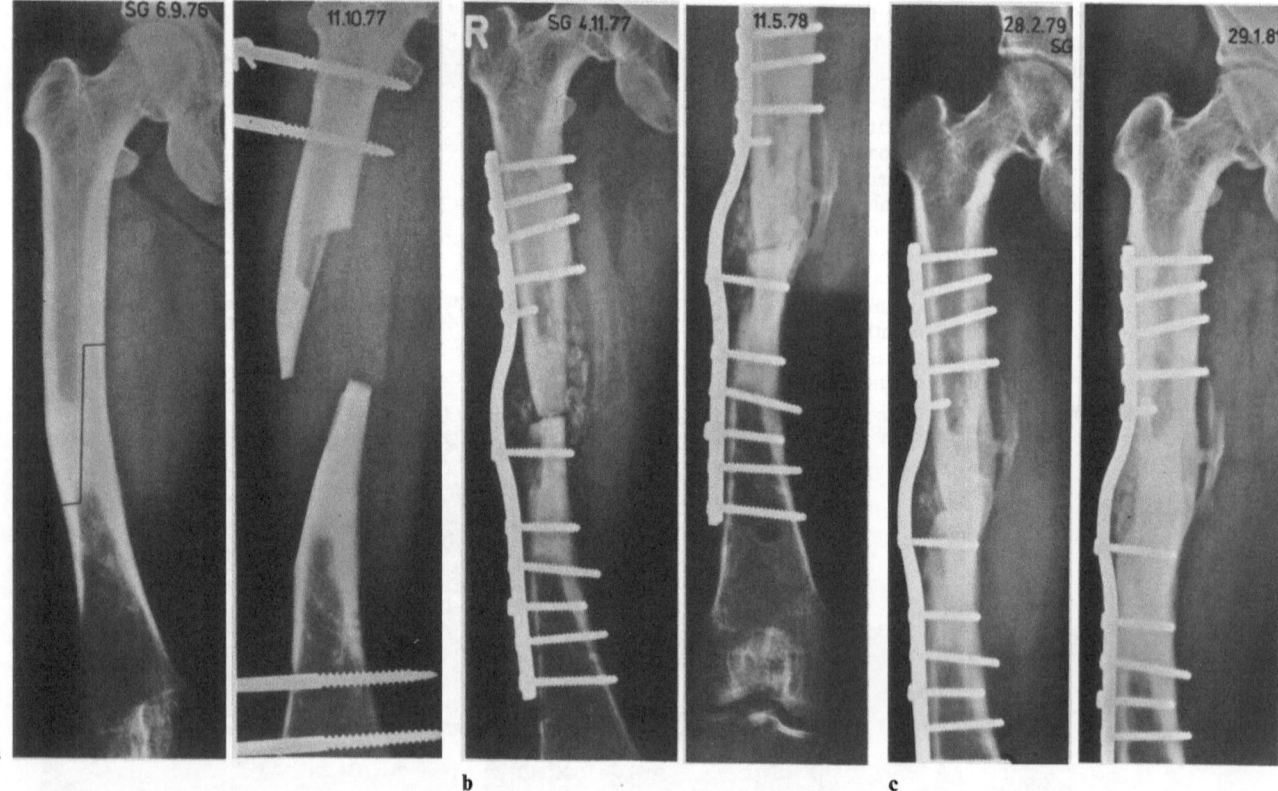

**Fig. 197 a–c.** Lengthening osteotomy of the femur. WAGNER apparatus. T.S., 1956, 21 years, ♀, 179 840.

**a** Femoral fracture in childhood. At presentation: 8-cm limb shortening, 20° varus deformity. Four weeks after distraction with Wagner lengthening frame.
**b** Two weeks and 7 months after internal fixation with wave plate and cancellous bone graft: gradual consolidation.
**c** $1^1/_4$ and $3^1/_4$ years after osteotomy: osseous remodeling is complete. Normal limb length and alignment

**Fig. 198 a–e.** Arthrodesis of the knee joint. Bilateral frame.▶ K.I., 1897, 77 years, ♀, 183 253.

**a** Osteoarthritis of the knee with marked varus deformity.
**b** Compression arthrodesis with small bilateral frame (2 pins).
**c** Four weeks postoperatively: frame removal + plaster cast for 6 weeks.
**d** $3^1/_2$ months postoperatively: arthrodesis is solid.
**e** $7^1/_2$ years postoperatively: functional bone remodeling is complete

# 7 Knee (Figs. 198–201)

**Examples:**

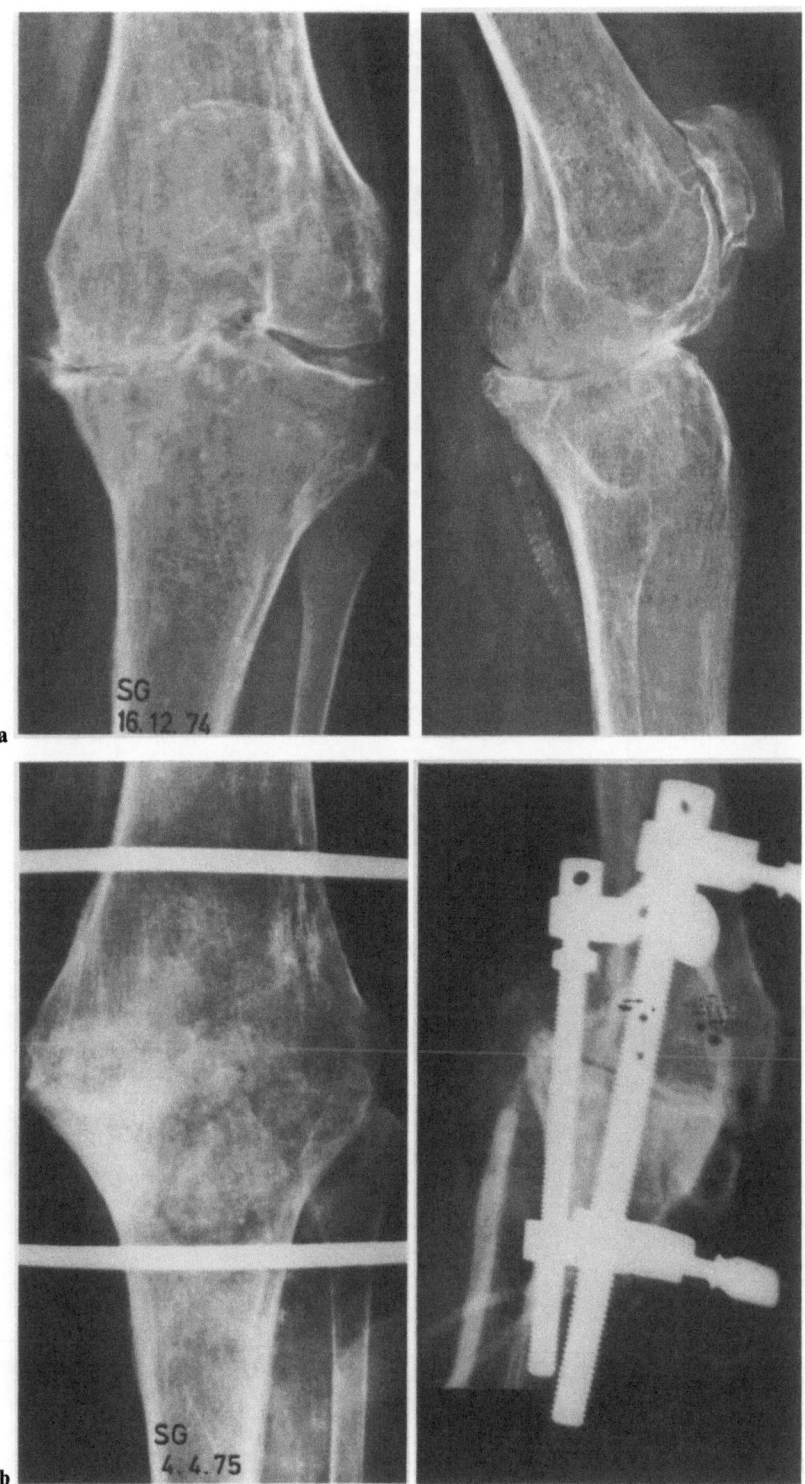

Fig. 198 a, b

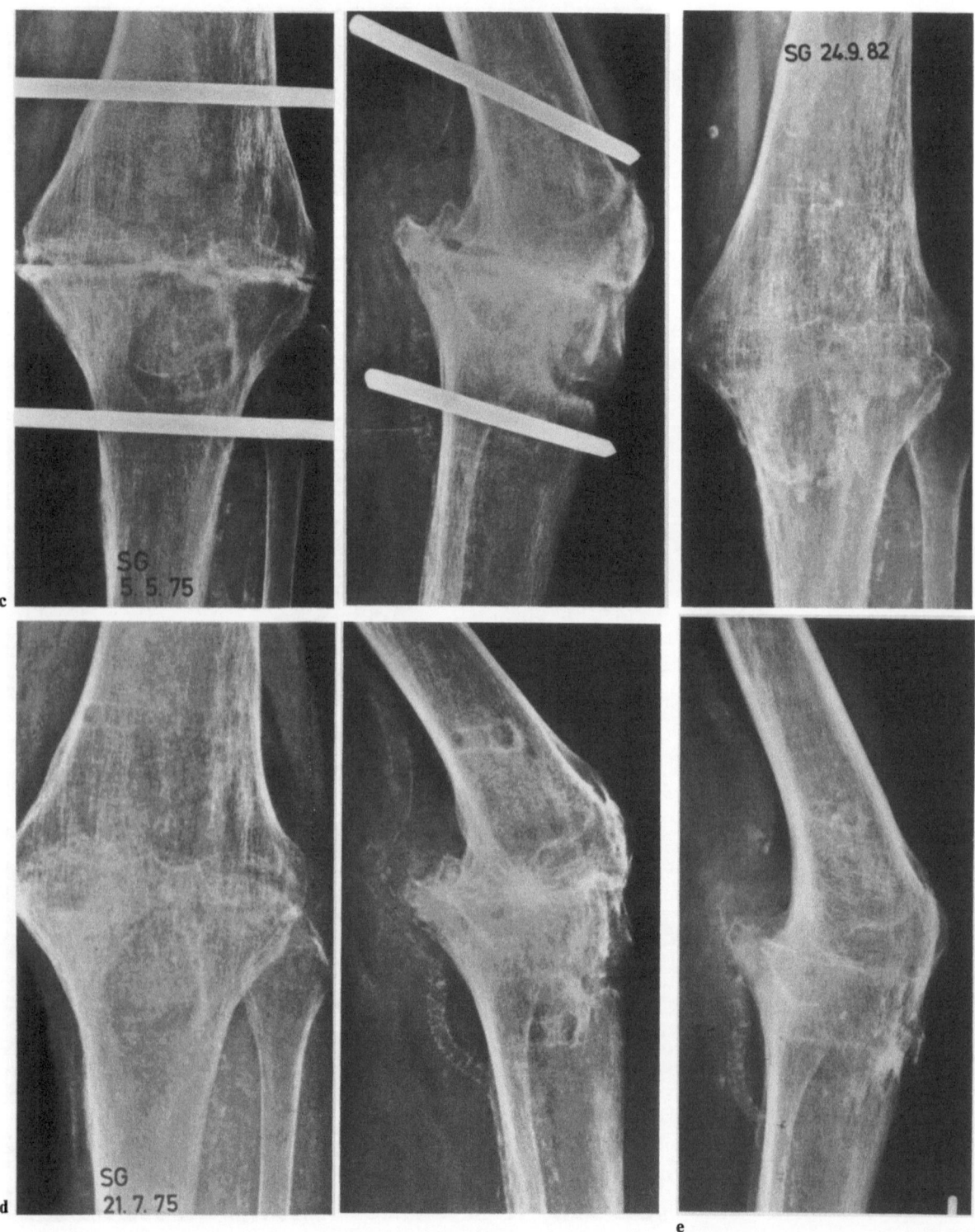

**Fig. 198c–e.** Legend see p. 138

**Fig. 199 a–c.** Arthrodesis of the knee joint. Bilateral frame. M.V., 1904, 78 years, ♀, 259833.

**a** Severe osteoarthritis of the knee with varus deformity.
**b** Compression arthrodesis with small bilateral frame for 5 weeks, double clamps (4 pins).
**c** Five months postoperatively: perfect result

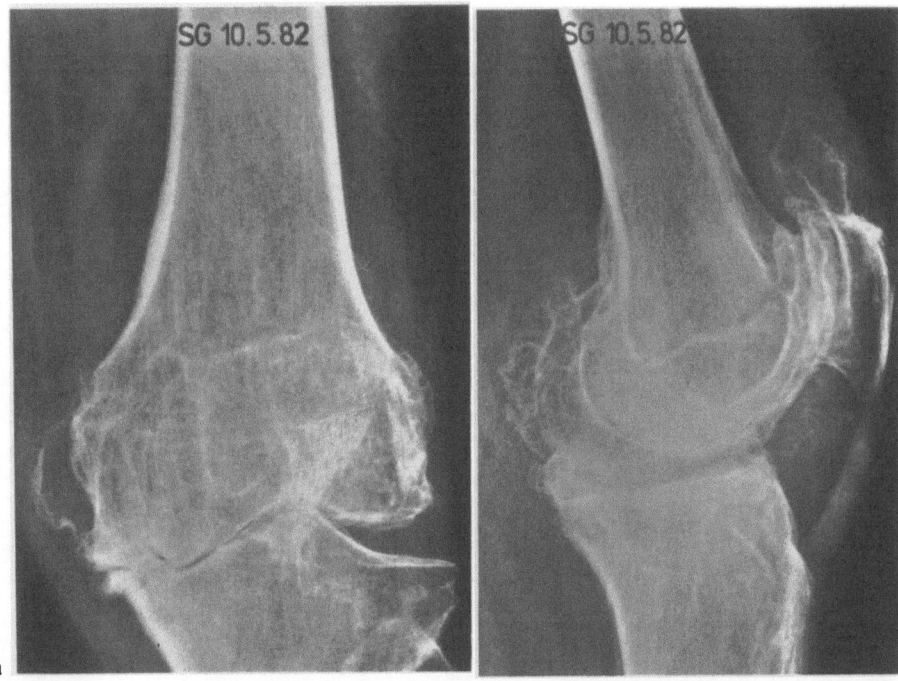

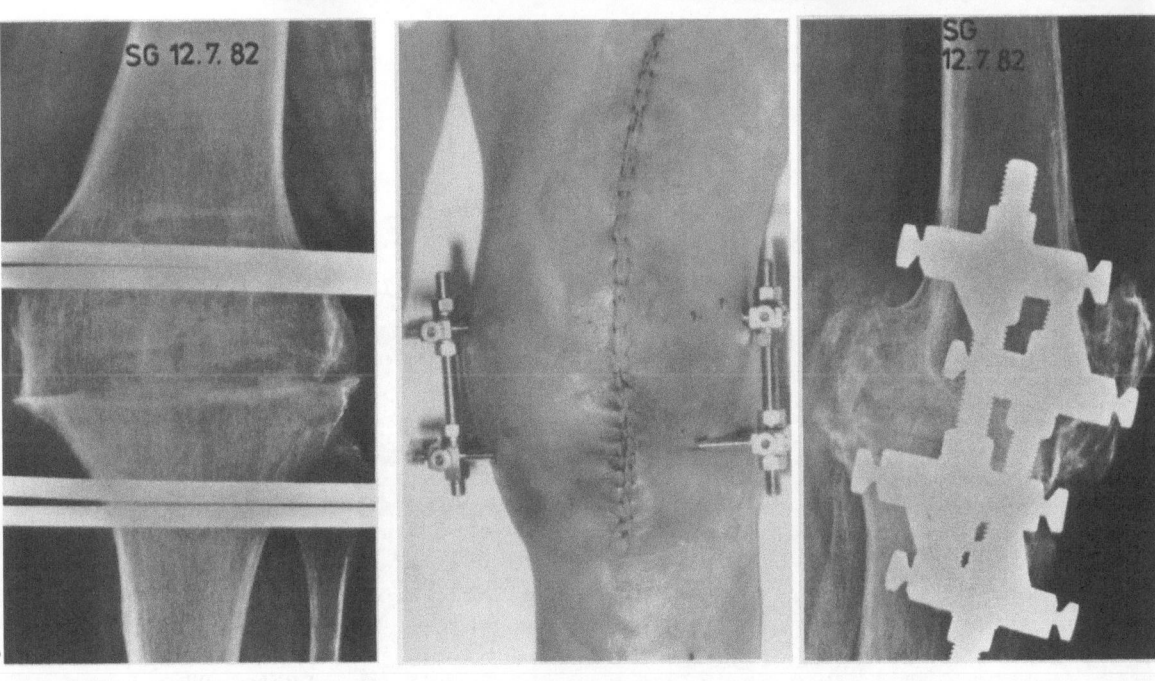

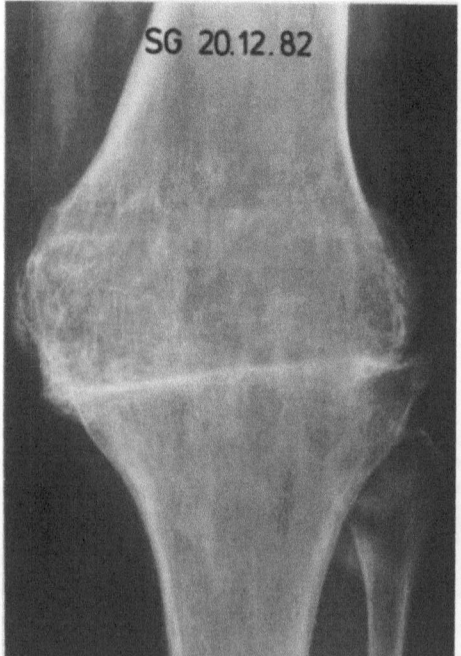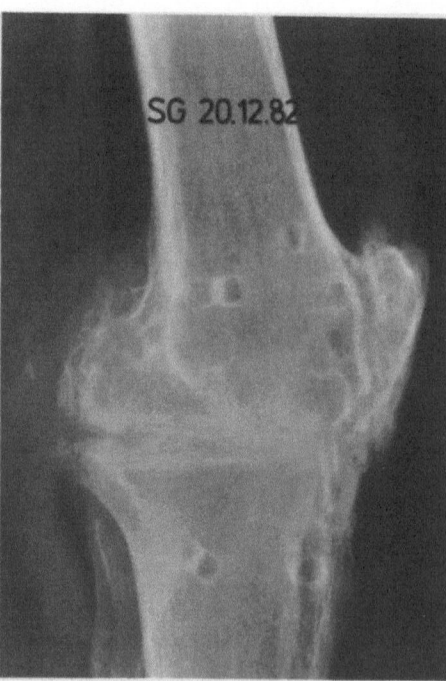

**Fig. 199c.**
Legend see p. 141

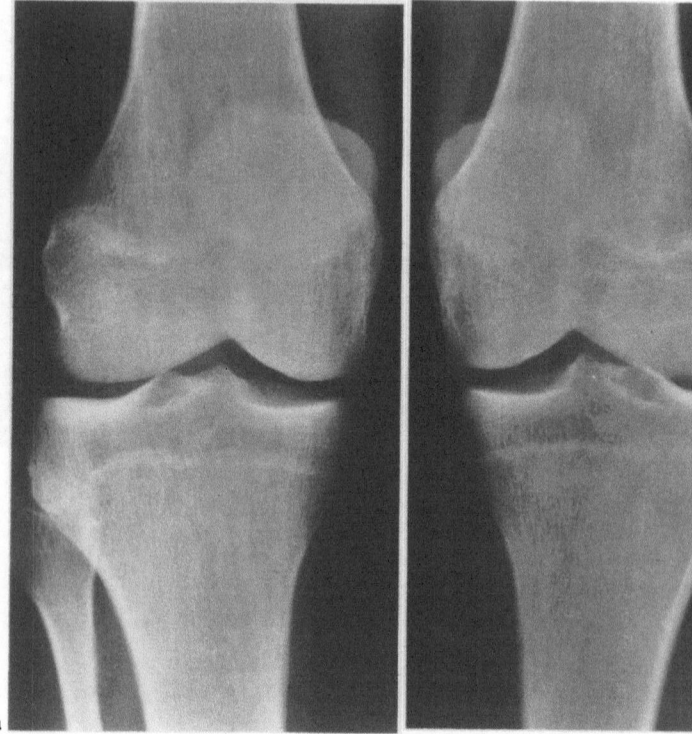

**Fig. 200 a–e.** Bilateral upper tibial osteotomy. Bilateral frame. B.W., 1942, 27 years, ♂, 127800.

**a** Genua vara.
**b** Prior to osteotomy.
**c** After osteotomy.
**d** *Right:* Bilateral compression frame applied postoperatively. *Left:* One month after osteotomy. Frame removal after 4 weeks, plaster cast for 6 weeks, full weight bearing.
**e** $4^1/_2$ months postoperatively: both osteotomies are healed. Note pin placement in anterior half of sagittal diameter to provide a tension band effect

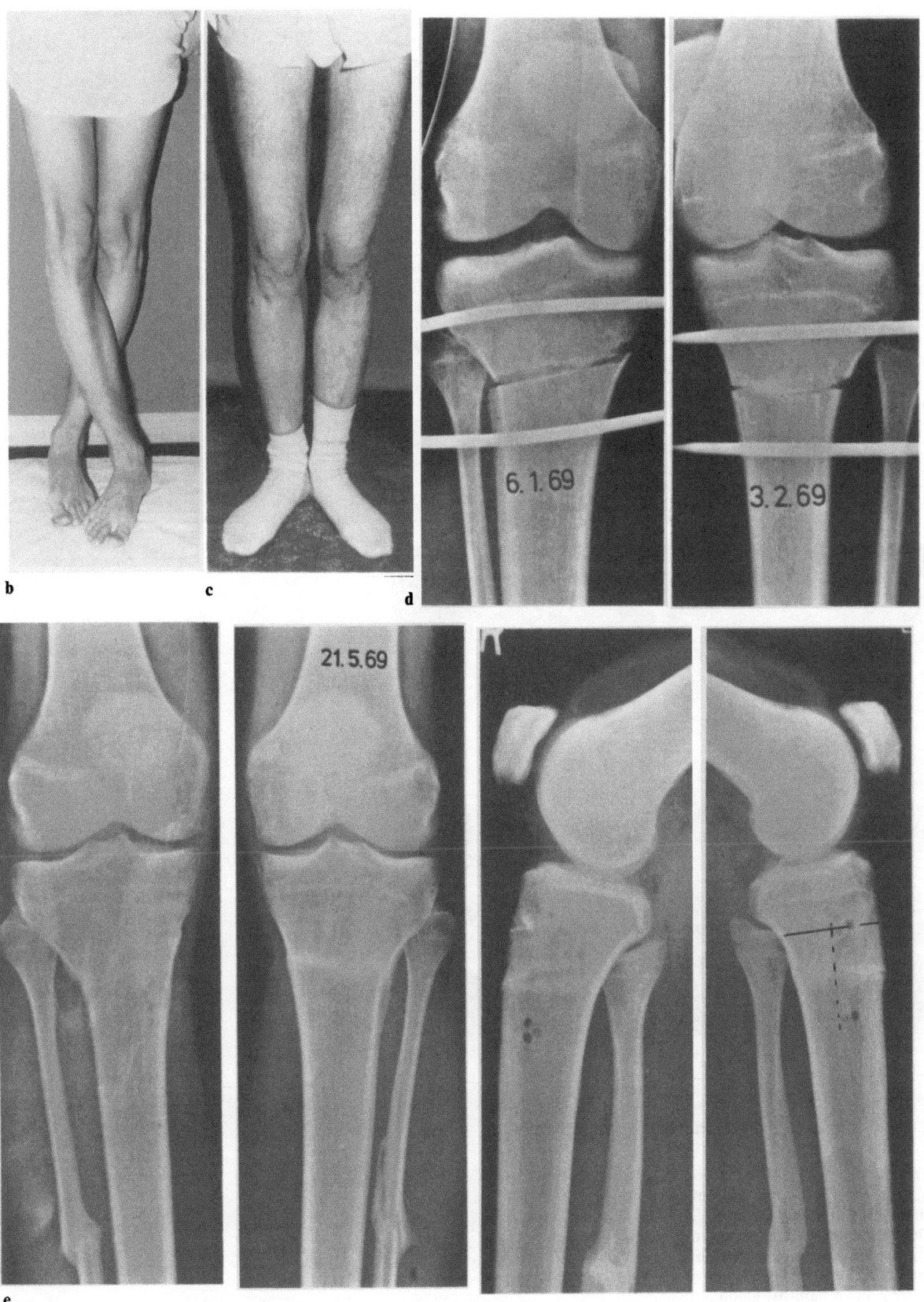

b          c          d

e

Fig. 200b–e

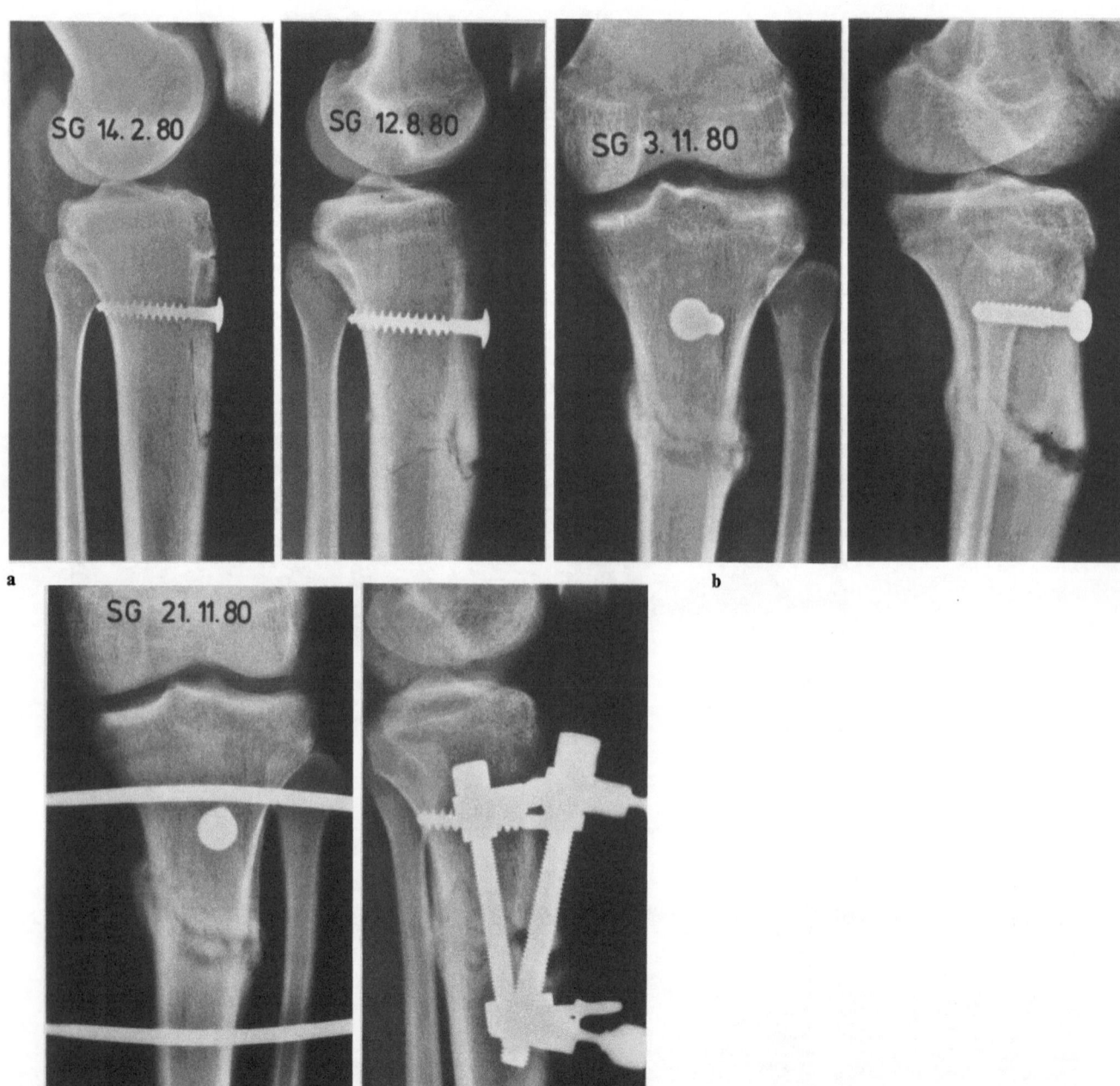

**Fig. 201 a–e.** Proximal stress fracture of the tibia with deformity. Bilateral frame. P.J., 1963, 17 years, ♂, 210476.

**a** Transposition of the tibial tuberosity for patellar subluxation. Six months later a fracture resulted from minimal trauma. Cast immobilization.
**b** Delayed union with deformity, anterior bowing.
**c** $3^1/_2$ months postinjury: tension band fixation with small bilateral frame, axial correction.
**d** After 2 and 4 months: union.
**e** Seven months after external fixation: complete recovery. Note former anterior pin location for tension band effect

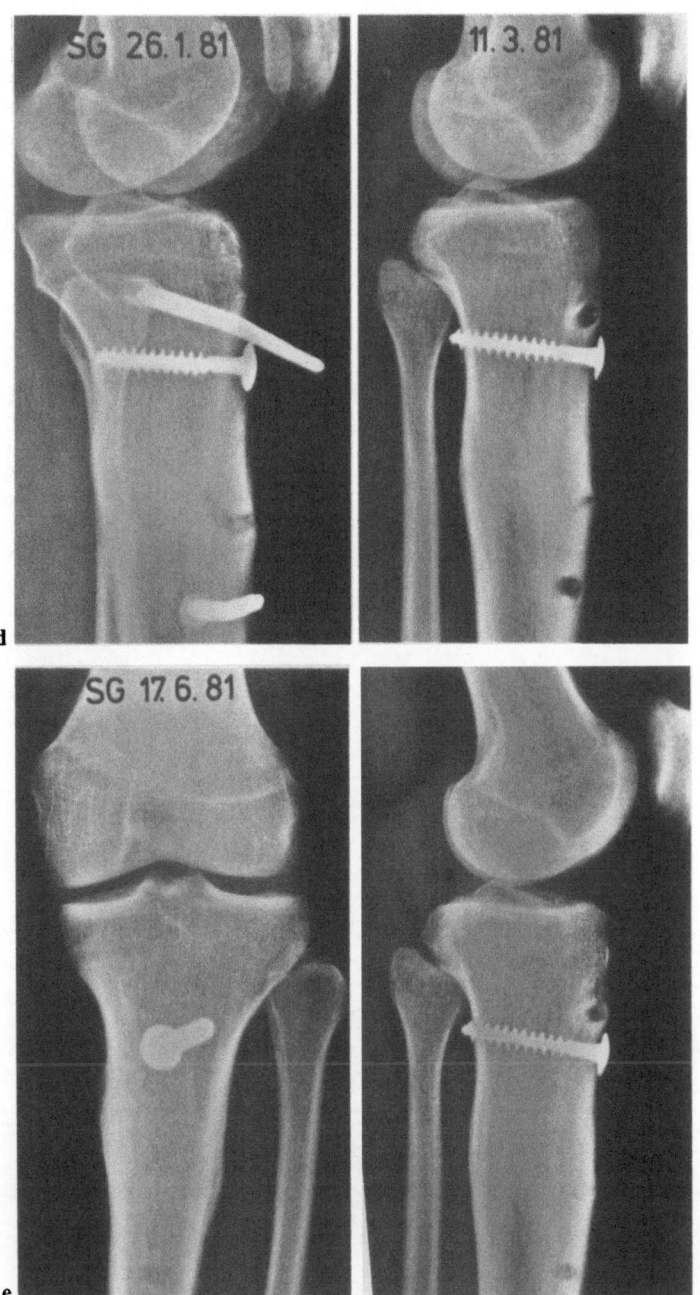

Fig. 201 d, e

## 8 Tibia (Figs. 202–240)

**Examples:**

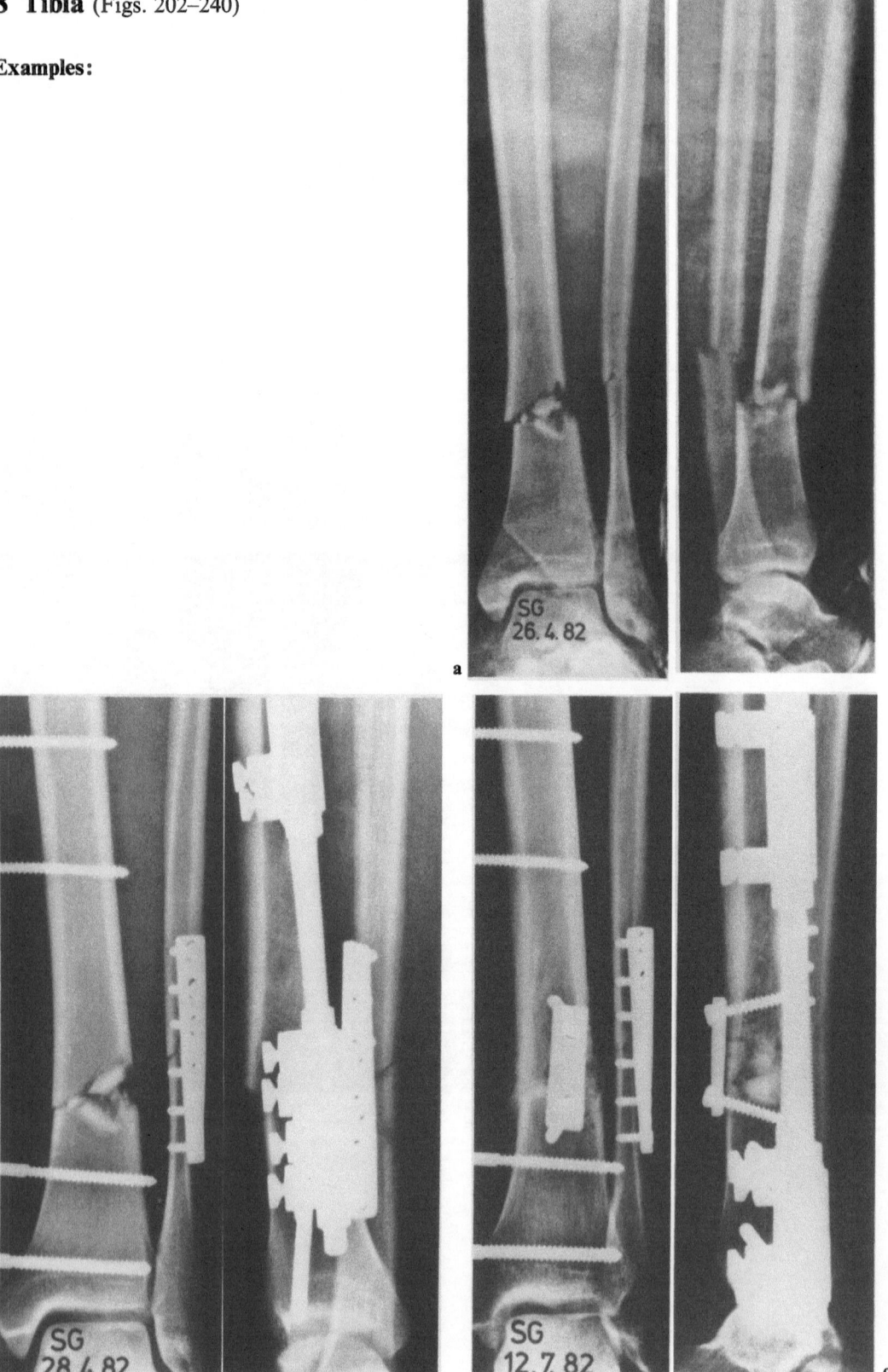

Fig. 202a–c

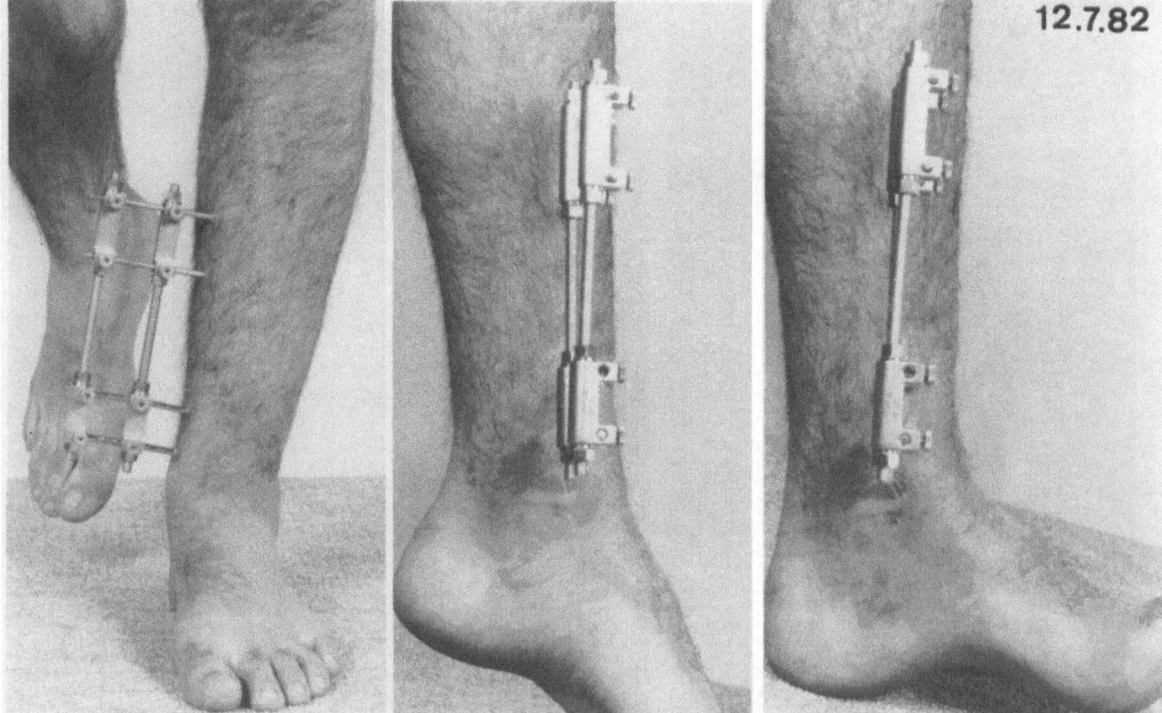

d

**Fig. 202 a–e.** Closed tibial fracture. Compartment syndrome. Unilateral frame + supplementary internal fixation of the fibula. R.W., 1962, 20 years, ♂, 259 514.

**a** Closed fracture. Dehne cast. Development of anterior compartment syndrome.

**b** Two days postinjury: fasciotomy and internal plating of the fibula. Closed unilateral frame for 10 weeks. Three weeks later: cancellous bone grafting of the tibia and internal fixation with 2-hole semitubular plate.

**c** Ten weeks after external fixation: fracture is solid, the compartment syndrome is relieved.

**d** The leg has full weight-bearing capacity. Foot mobility is normal, and the compartment syndrome has resolved. The fixator is removed.

**e** One year postinjury: complete recovery

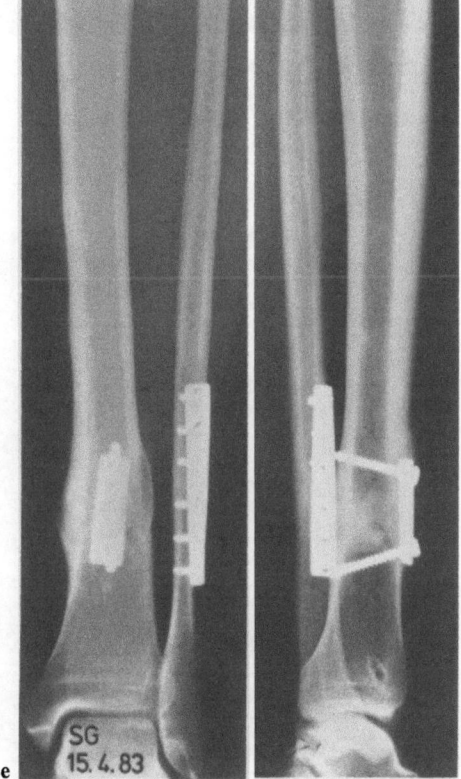

e

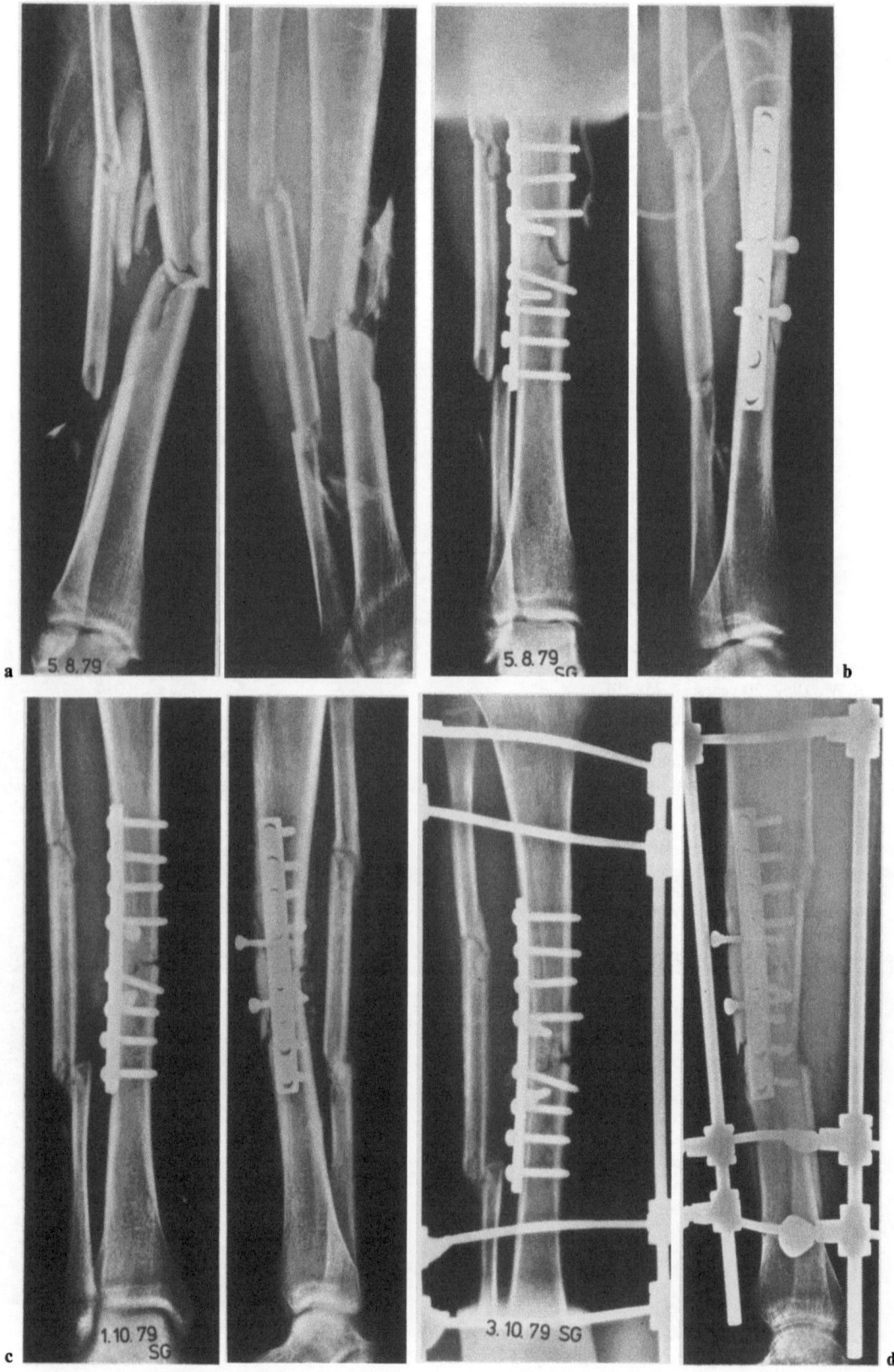

**Fig. 203a–d**

**Fig. 203 a–f.** Open fracture. Internal plating. Instability. Bilateral frame. N.J., 1962, 17 years, ♂, 231001.

**a** Grade II open tibial fracture.

**b** Internal fixation with a lateral plate.

**c** Two months postinjury: instability, fragment necrosis. Skin coverage inadequate for local secondary procedures. Hence:

**d** Stabilization with bilateral neutralization frame for 5 months.

**e** Three months postinjury: posteromedial cancellous bone grafting and removal of 2 screws (4 weeks prior). Five months postinjury: removal of plate and devitalized fragment of tibial border (4 weeks prior). Fixator is removed.

**f** Fifteen months postinjury: complete recovery

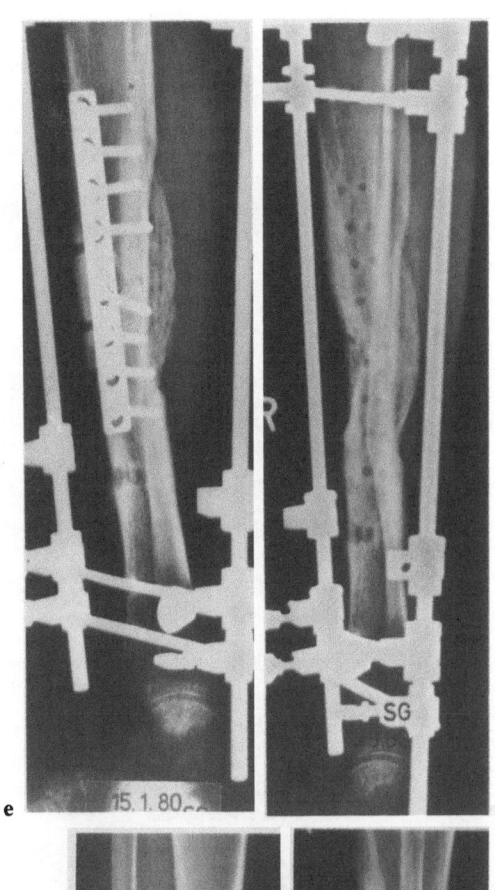

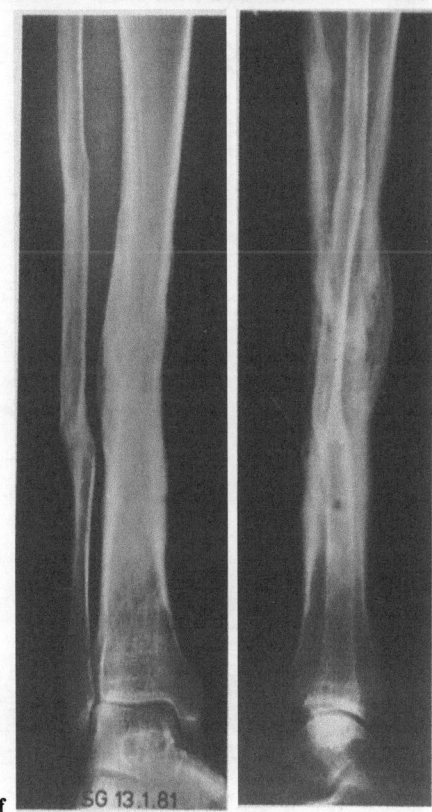

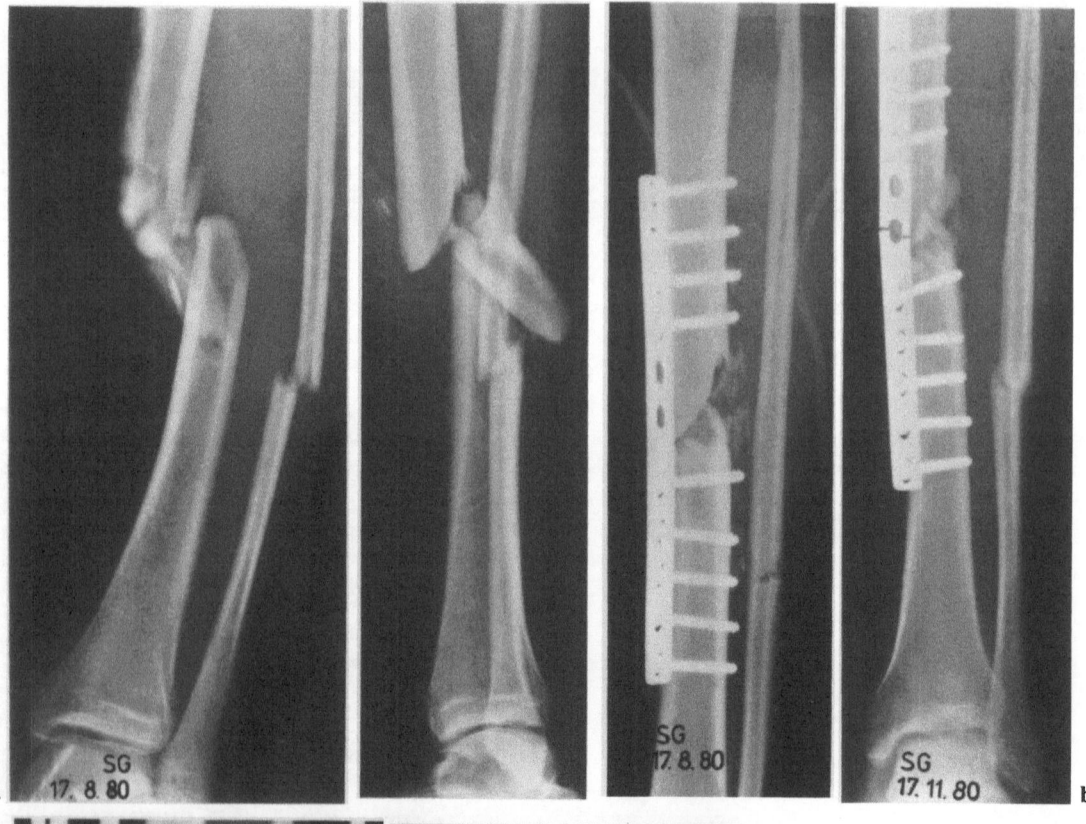

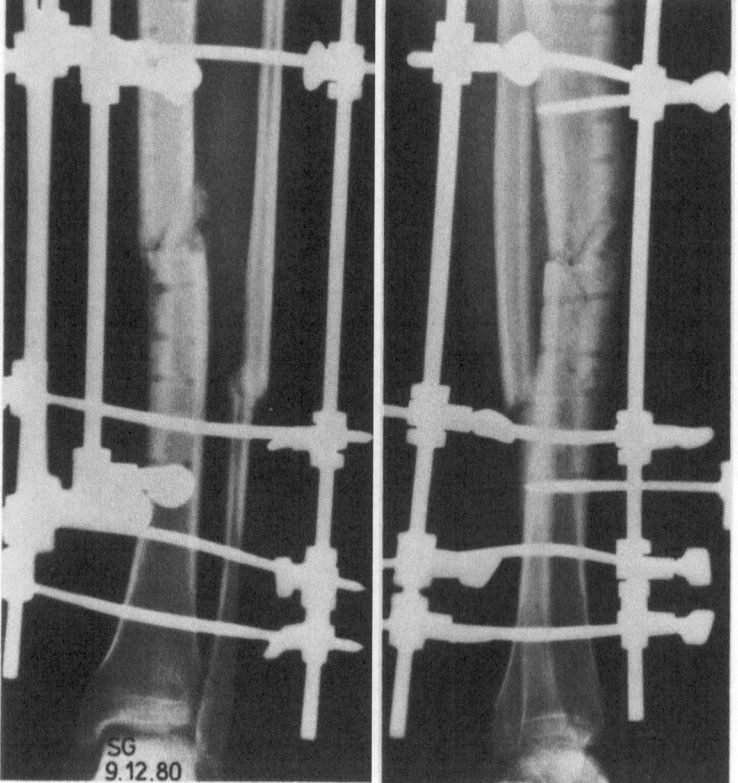

**Fig. 204 a–e.** Open fracture. Internal plating. Plate fracture. Infection. Bilateral frame. Z.N., 1960, 20 years, ♂, 241853.

**a** Grade II open fracture.
**b** Debridement. Cancellous bone graft, posteromedial plate. Persistent sinus, *Staphylococcus aureus*. After 3 months: plate fracture. Immediate sequestrectomy, removal of implants. Bilateral frame for 6 months.
**c** Three weeks after external fixation: anterolateral cancellous bone graft.
**d** Graft take after 4 and 11 months.
**e** $2^1/_2$ years postinjury: complete recovery

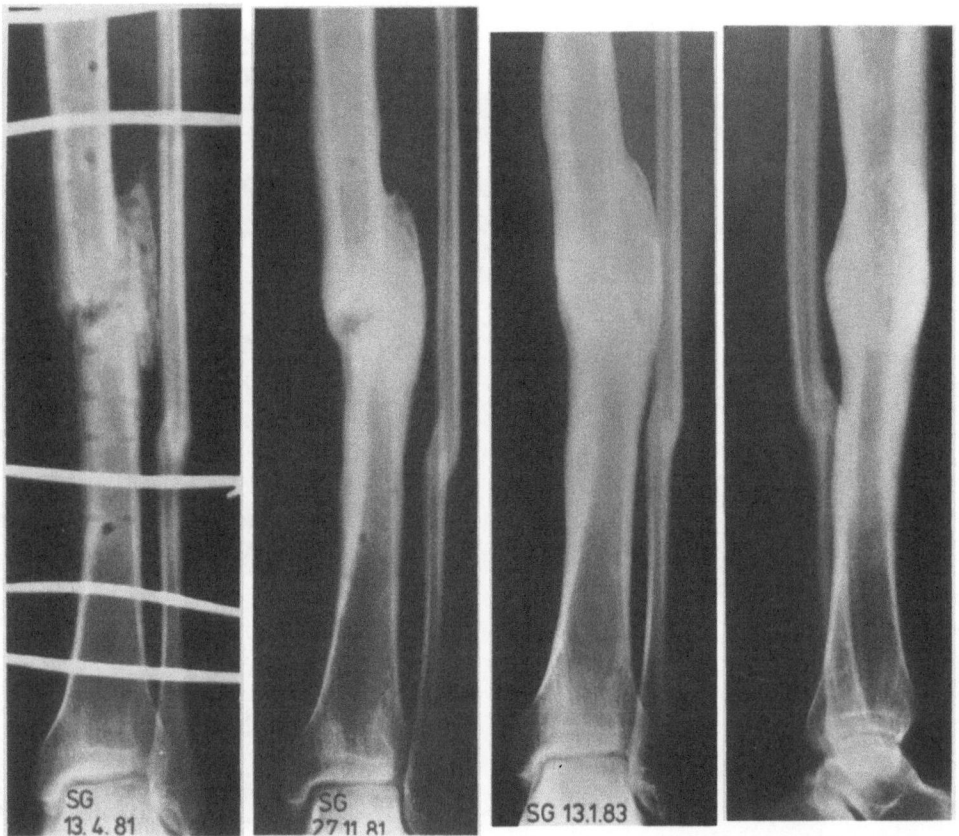

**Fig. 204 d, e**  d      SG 13.4.81      SG 27.11.81      SG 13.1.83      e

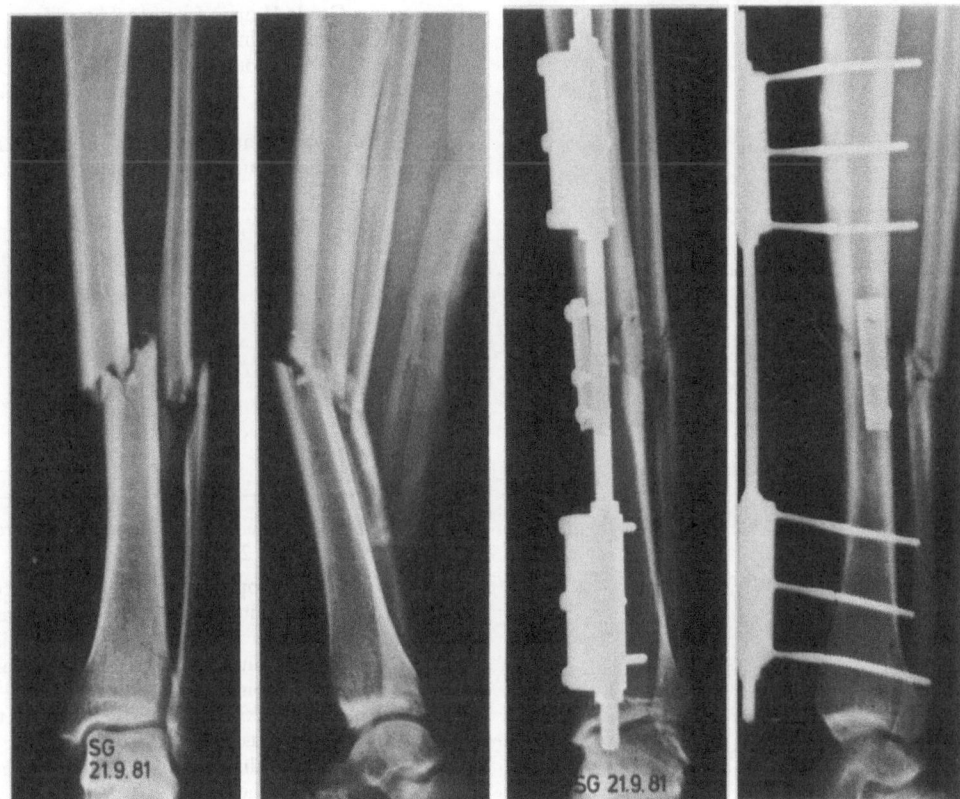

**Fig. 205 a, b.**
Legend see p. 152   a      SG 21.9.81      SG 21.9.81      b

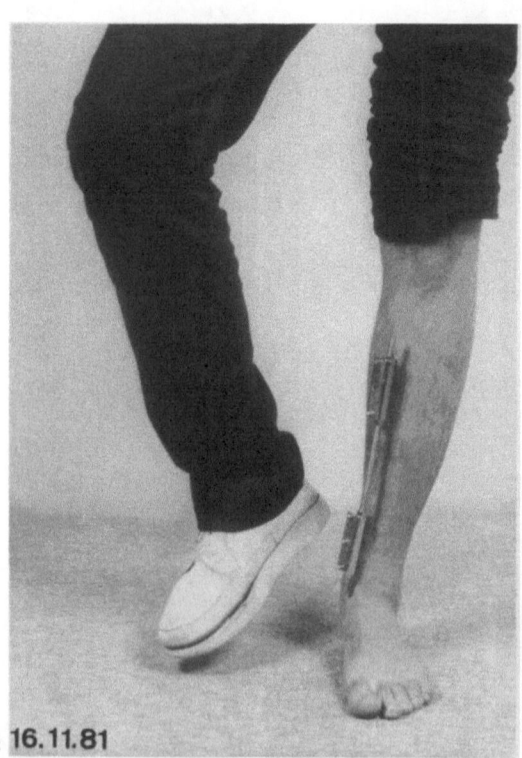

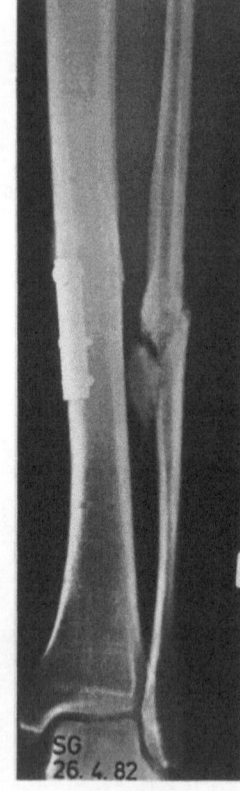

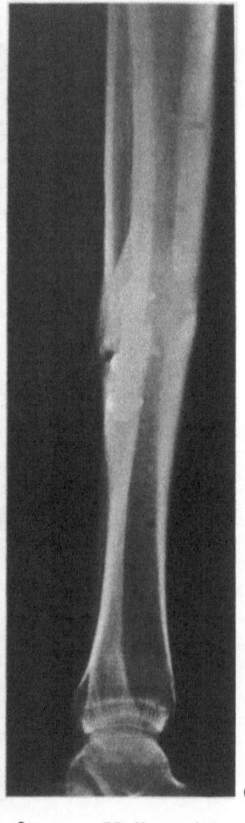

**Fig. 205 a–e.** Open fracture. Unilateral frame + minimal internal fixation. P.F., 1959, 22 years, ♂, 171 508.

**a** Grade II open fracture 24 h old.
**b** Minimal internal fixation of posterior tibial border and unilateral compression frame for 8 weeks.
**c** Clinically, full weight bearing is possible 7 weeks after fracture.
**d** Seven months postinjury: complete recovery.
**e** Fourteen months postinjury: complete recovery

**Fig. 206 a–e.** Open fracture. Unilateral frame. H.E., 1964, 18 years, ♀, 223 506.

**a** Grade II open fracture with severe contusions.
**b** Minimal internal fixation + unilateral frame for 5 months.
**c** Six weeks postinjury. Skin necrosis. Nine weeks postinjury. Granulations. Meshed skin grafts.
**d** Three months postinjury: Minimal internal fixation removed. Proximal screws replaced due to reddening. Posterior cancellous bone graft.
**e** $7^{1}/_{2}$ months postinjury: complete recovery with excellent skin coverage

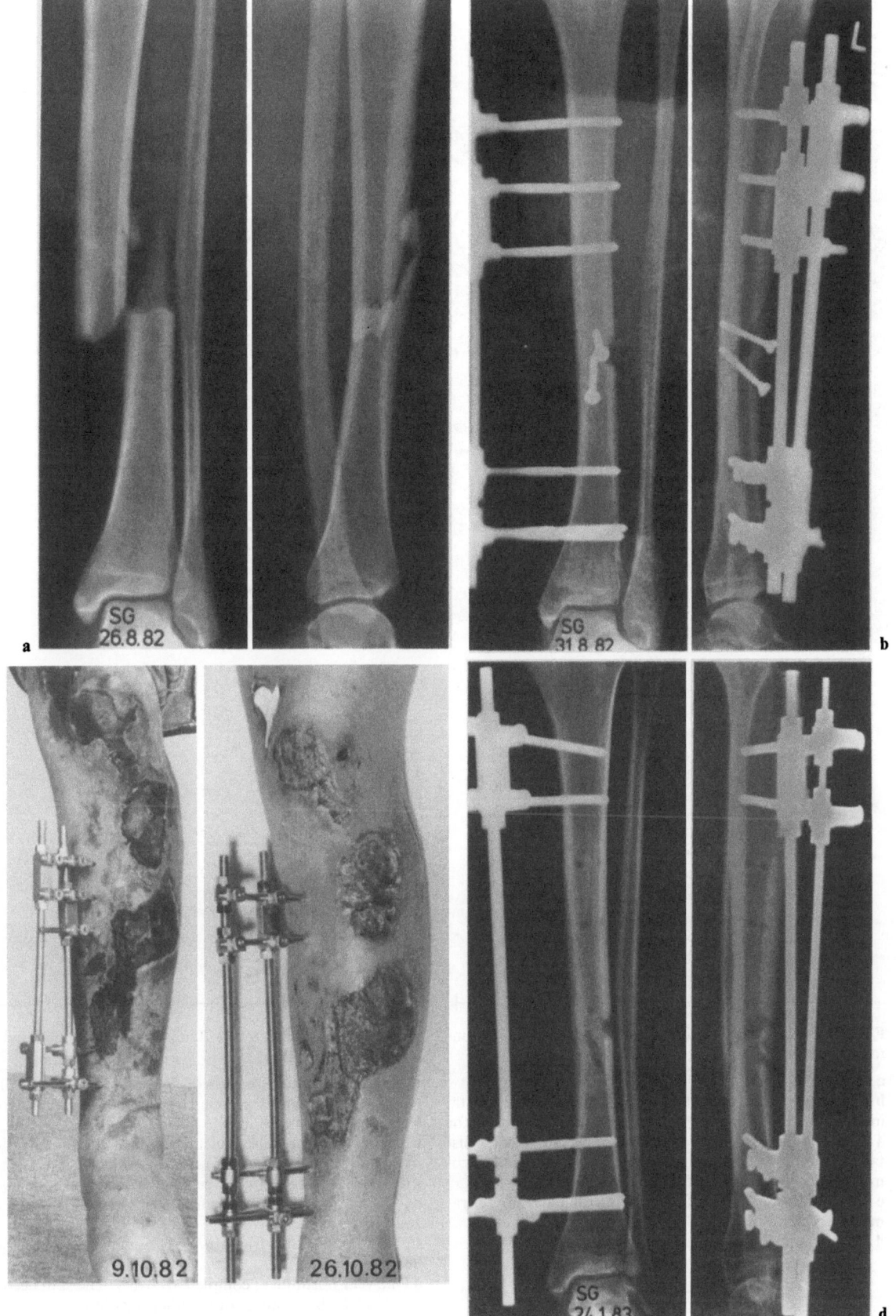

a   SG
26.8.82

b   SG
31 8 82

c   9.10.82   26.10.82

d   SG
24.1.83

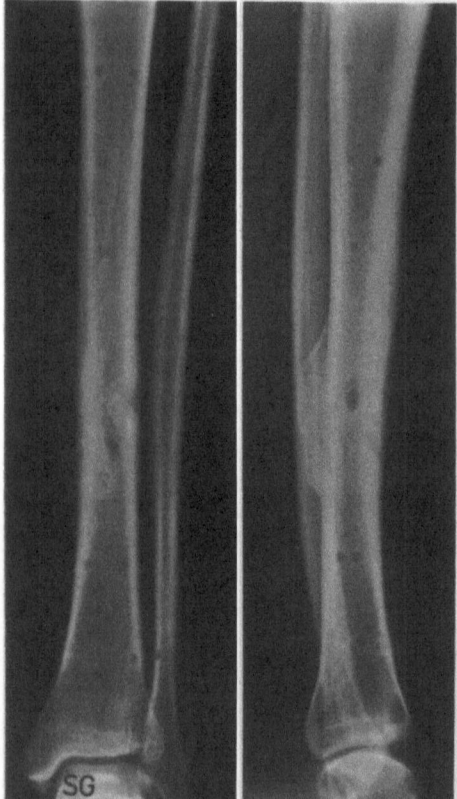 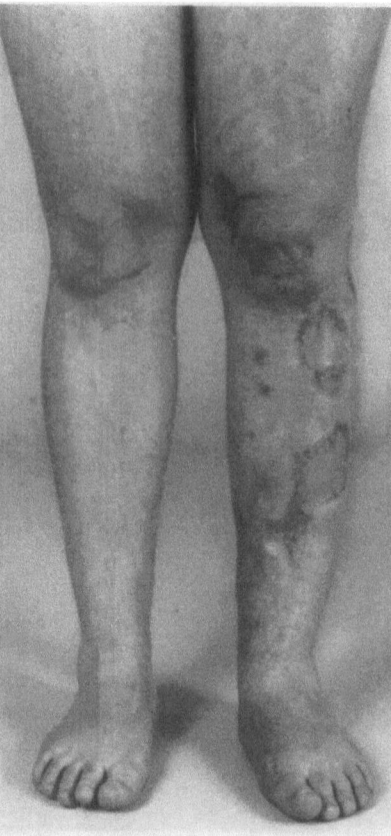

**Fig. 206e.**
Legend see p. 152

**Fig. 207 a–d.** Open fracture. Unilateral frame + minimal internal fixation. R.A., 1958, 23 years, ♂, 254447.

**a** Grade II open fracture.
**b** Three weeks after minimal internal fixation, supplemental internal fixation of fibula + unilateral compression frame for 4 months. Thirteen weeks postinjury: fracture is solid distally but not proximally due to lack of viable bone: posteromedial cancellous bone graft.
**c** Five months postinjury: failure of proximal healing; intramedullary nail is inserted.
**d** $1^1/_2$ years postinjury: complete recovery

**Fig. 208 a–g.** Open fracture. Unilateral frame + minimal internal fixation. B.B., 1965, 17 years, ♂, 261888.

**a** Multiple injuries. Progress of femoral fracture with plate fracture, intramedullary nail, cancellous bone graft, union.
**b** Grade III open fracture.
**c** Six weeks after debridement, minimal internal fixation, unilateral frame for $5^1/_2$ months. Dry skin necrosis.
**d** Ten weeks postinjury, 5 weeks since posterior bone graft.
**e** $5^1/_2$ months postinjury: cancellous bone and fracture are solid. Fixator is removed.
**f** Eight months after fracture. Only a small area of dry skin necrosis remains.
**g** One year postinjury: complete recovery. The skin necrosis has resolved by spontaneous epithelialization

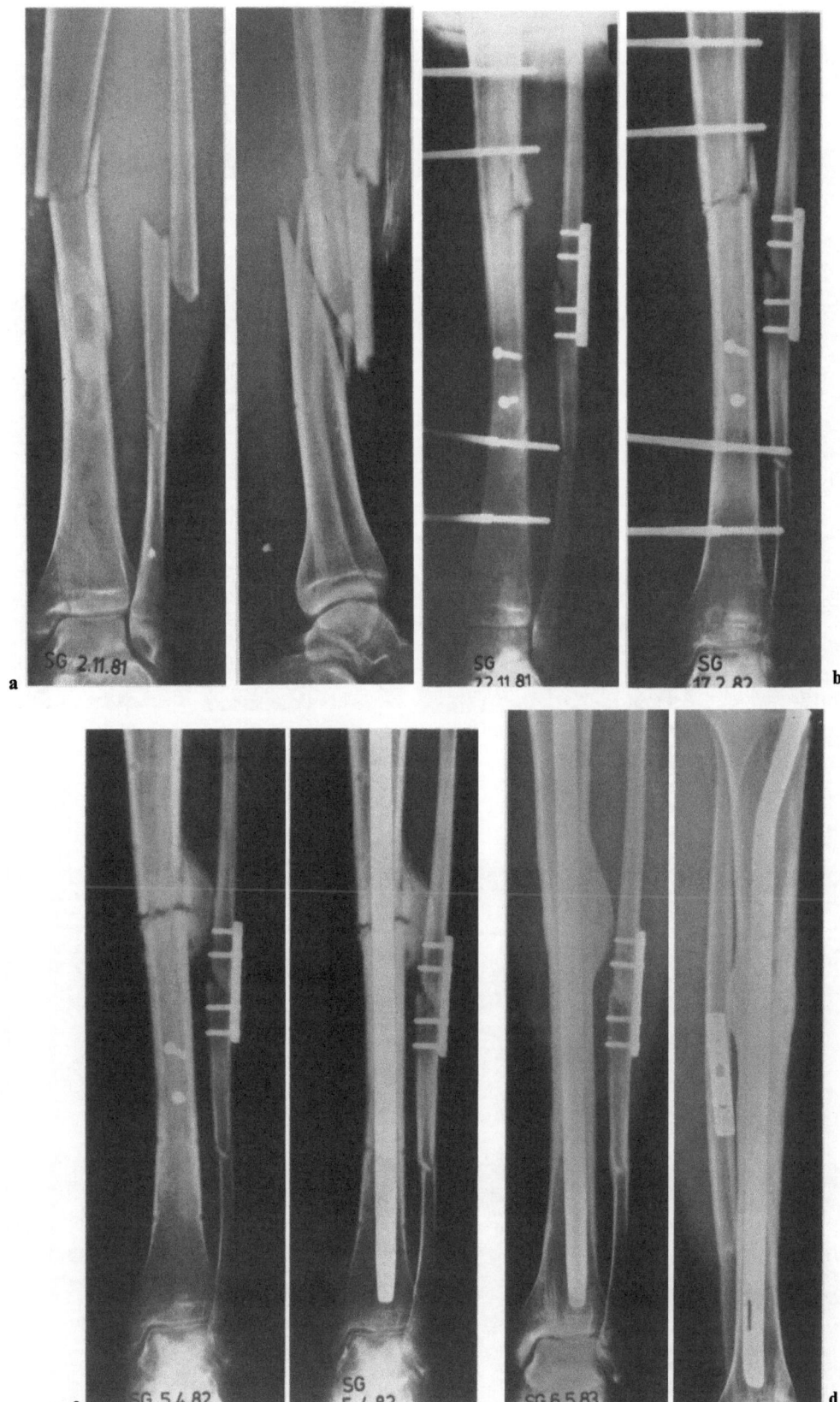

**Fig. 207 a–d**

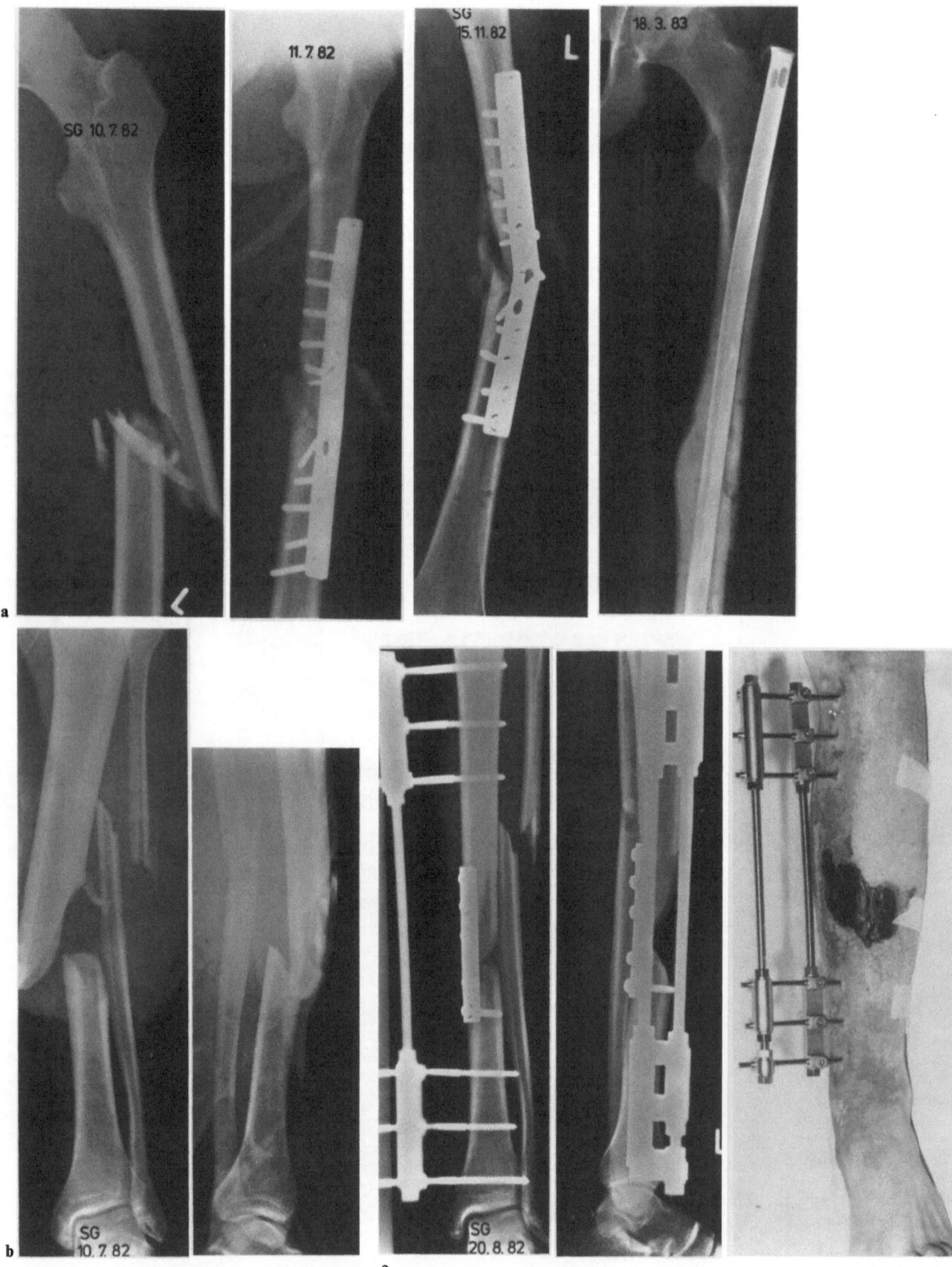

**Fig. 208a–g.**
Legend see p. 154

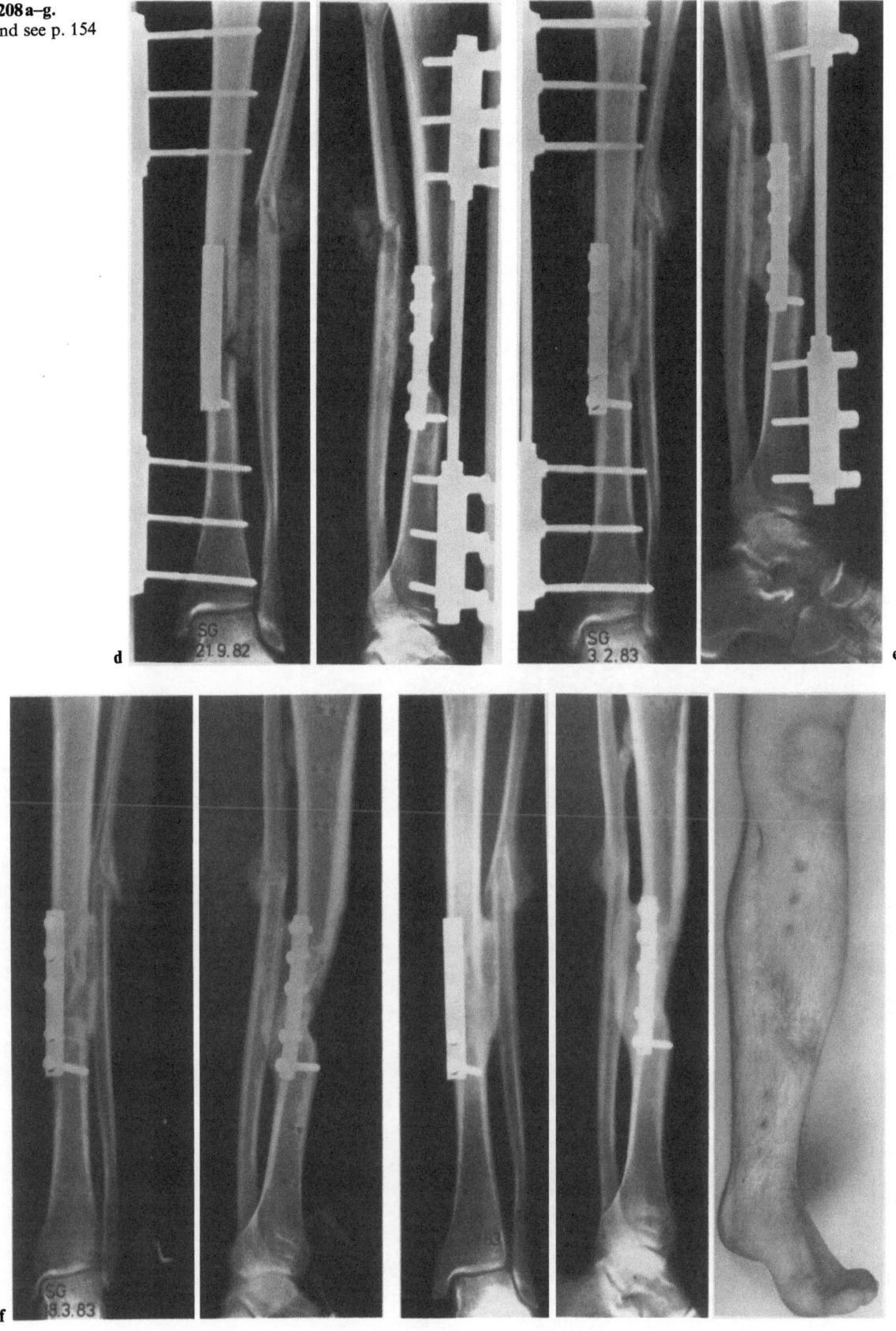

d

e

f

g

SG
21. 9. 82

SG
3. 2. 83

SG
8.3.83

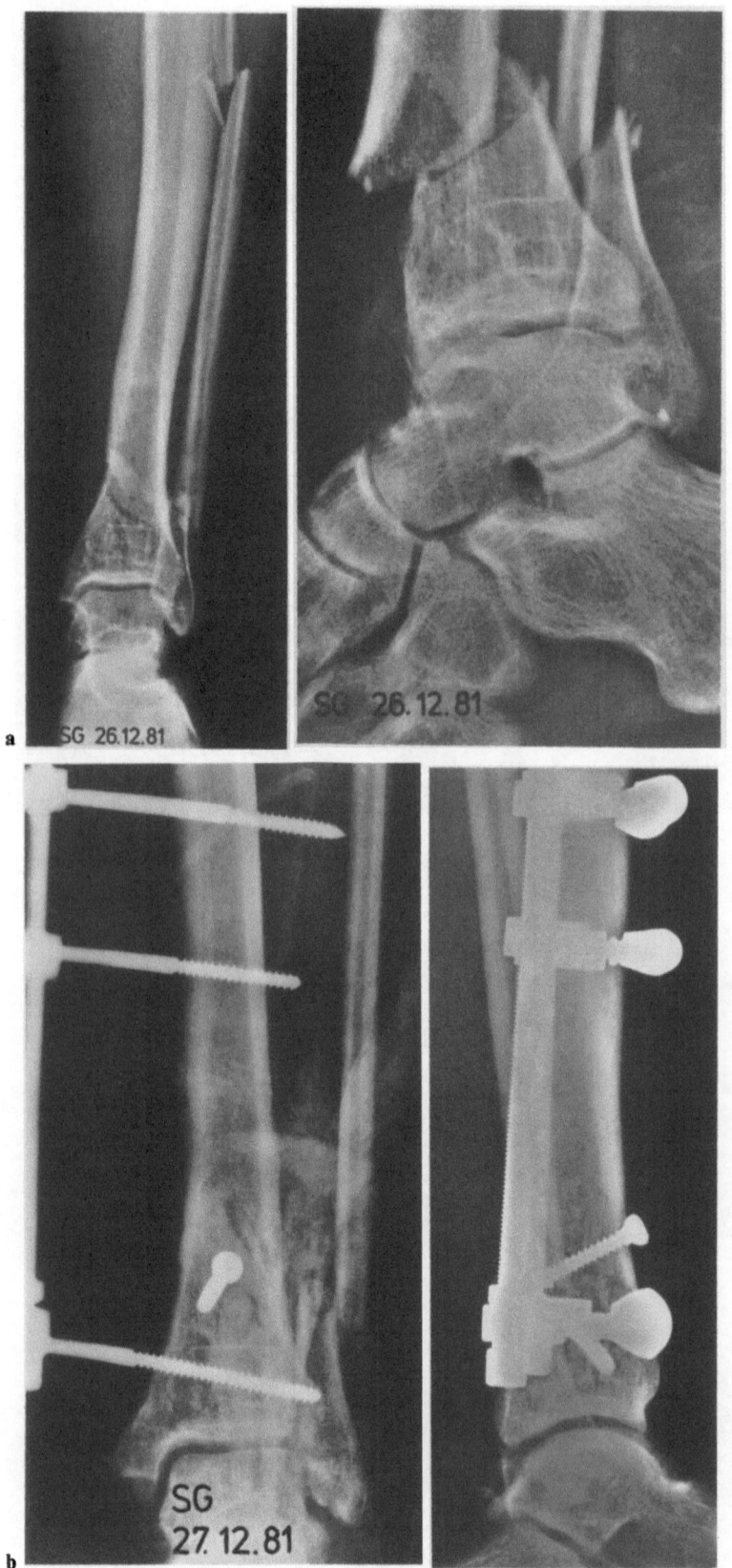

Fig. 209a, b

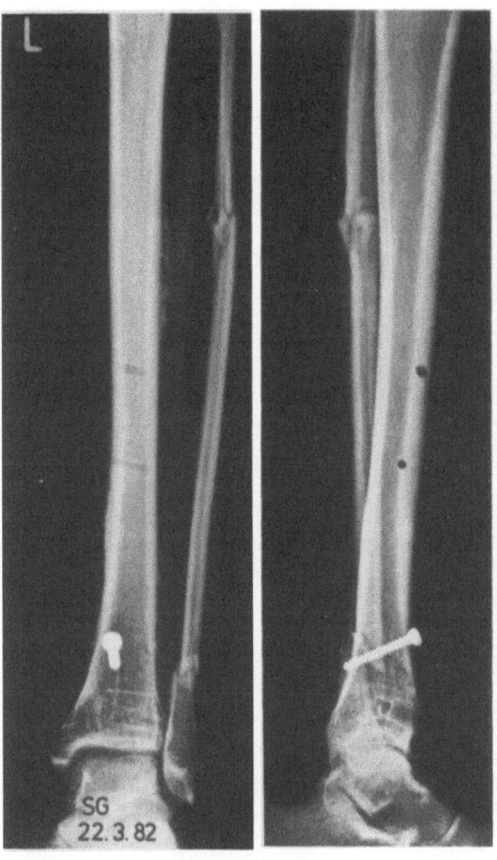

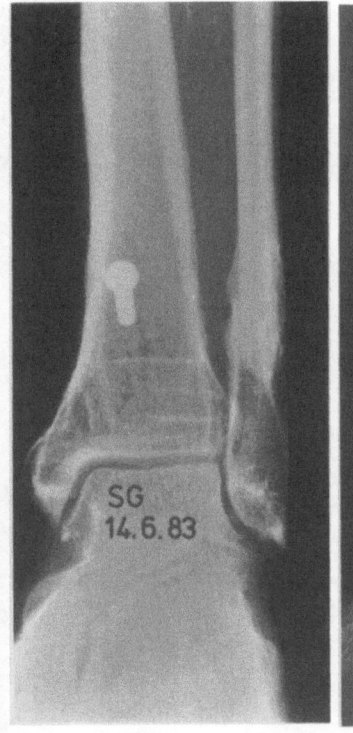

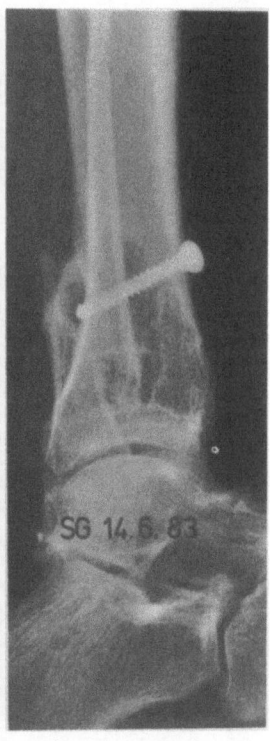

**Fig. 209 a–d.** Open fracture. Unilateral frame + minimal internal fixation. G.R., 1956, 25 years, ♂, 255967.

**a** Grade II open fracture with short distal fragment.
**b** Minimal internal fixation with 1 lag screw + unilateral neutralization frame for 3 months.
**c** Three months postinjury: tibial fracture is united, but the fibular fracture is not yet solid.
**d** Eighteen months postinjury: complete recovery

**Fig. 210 a–i.** Open fracture, unilateral frame, shortening. B.E., 1917, 66 years, ♂, 269614.

**a** Multiple injuries. Pertrochanteric fracture, internal fixation. Full weight bearing after 2 months.
**b** Fracture of femoral shaft. Internal fixation. Full weight bearing after 2 months.
**c** Humeral fracture, internal fixation. Arm could be used for cane-assisted gait! Normal use after 2 months.
**d** Grade II open tibial fracture.
**e** Debridement, external fixation for 9 weeks. Extraction of devitalized fragment 1 week later.
**f** Gradual shortening by 4 cm over 3-week period.
**g** $2^1/_2$ months postinjury, immediately before removal of fixator.
**h** $2^1/_2$ months postinjury: Sarmiento brace.
**i** Five months postinjury: fracture is solid and bears weight normally; 4 cm shortening

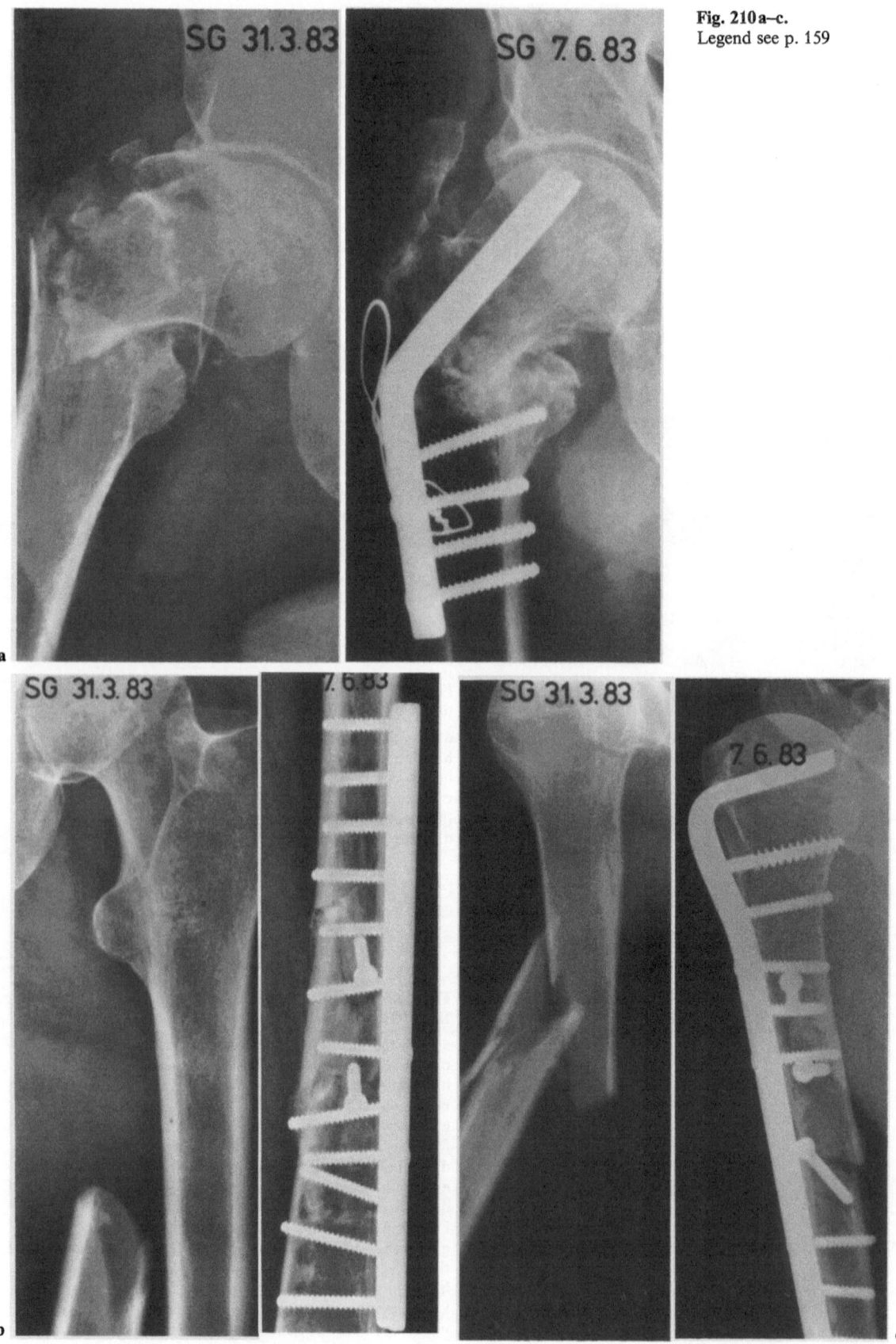

Fig. 210 a–c.
Legend see p. 159

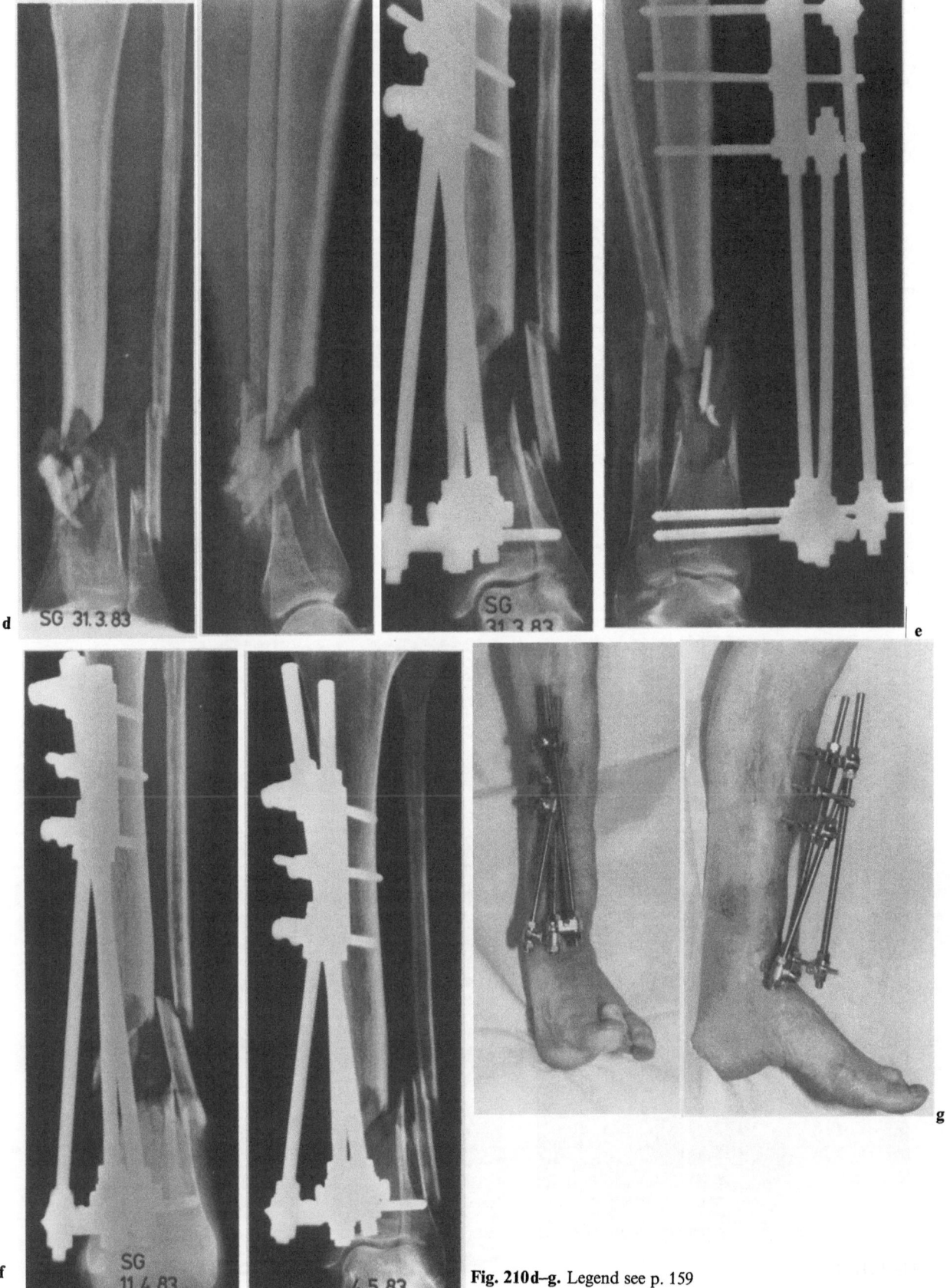

d   SG 31.3.83

SG
31.3.83                                                          e

f   SG
    11.4.83                    4.5.83

**Fig. 210d–g.** Legend see p. 159

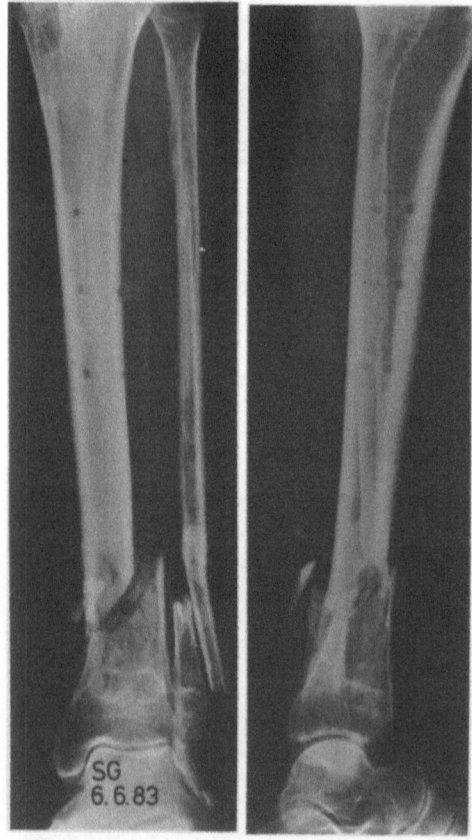
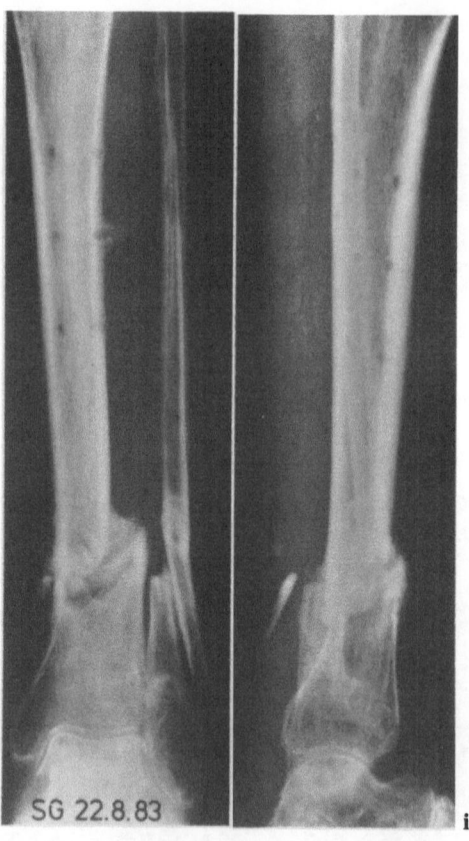

Fig. 210h, i
Legend see p. 159

SG
6. 6. 83

h

SG 22.8.83

i

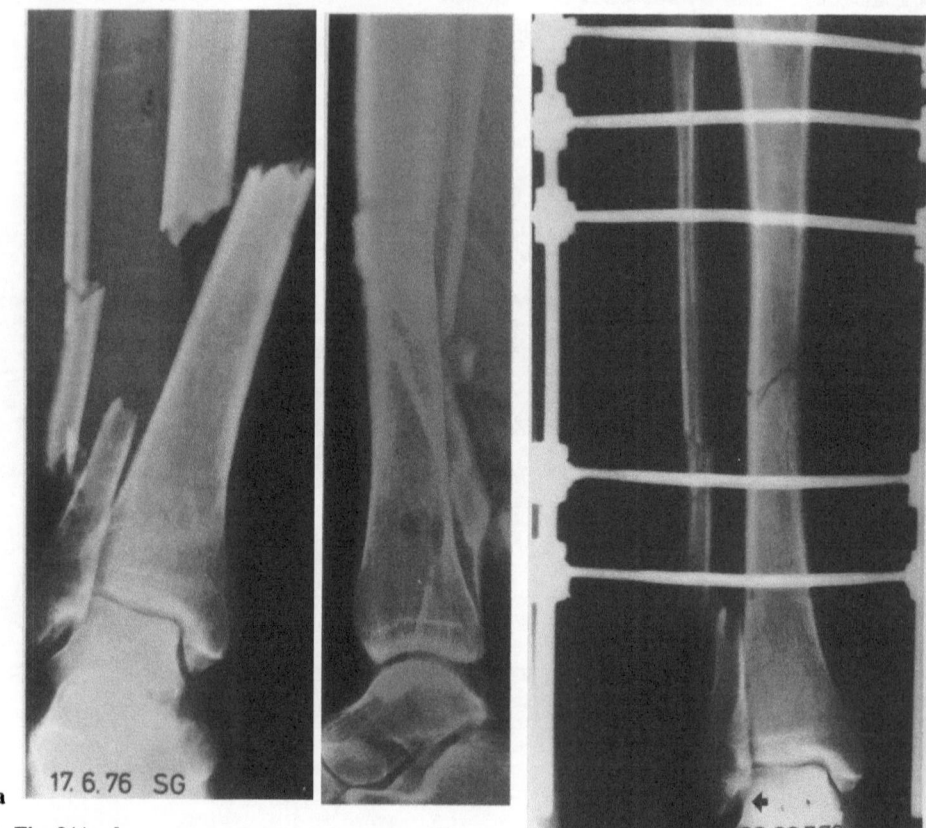

17. 6. 76  SG

a

Fig. 211 a, b

SG 23.7.76

b

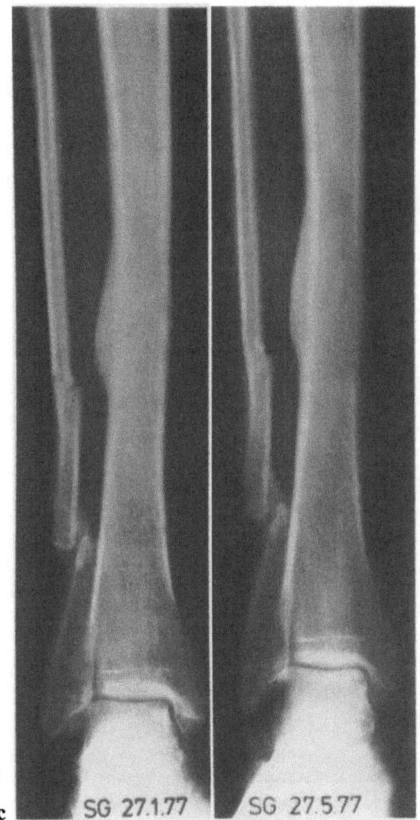

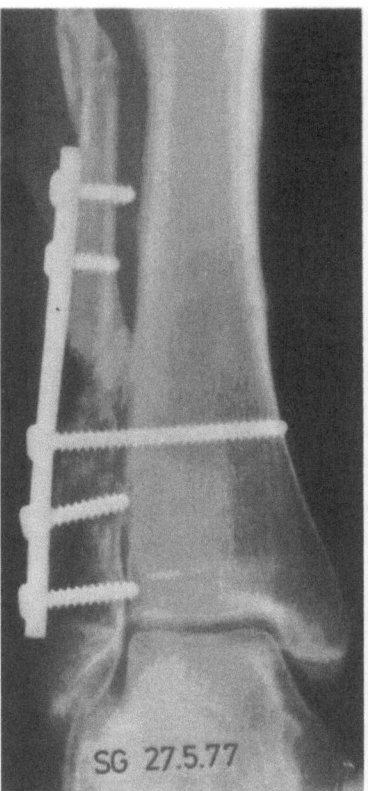

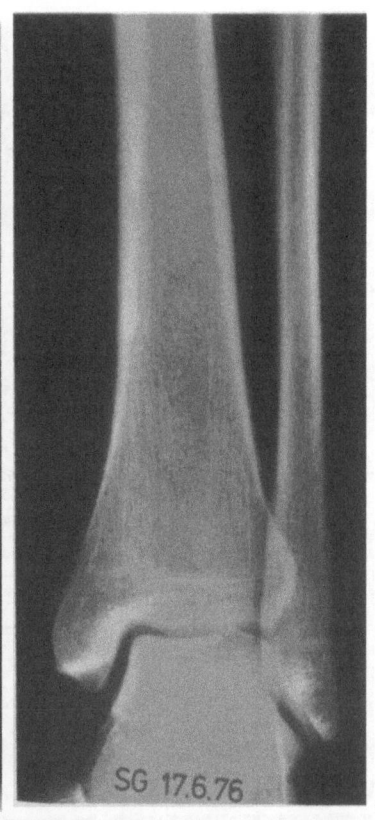

c    SG 27.1.77    SG 27.5.77

SG 27.5.77

SG 17.6.76                                    d

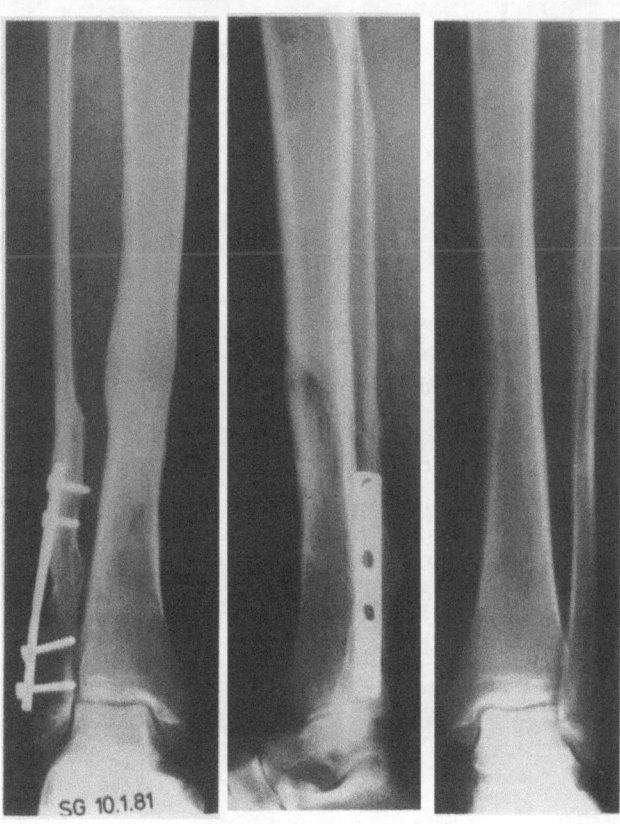

**Fig. 211 a–e.** Open fracture with disruption of ankle mortice. Bilateral frame. H.H., 1930, 46 years, ♀, 80456.

**a** Grade III open segmental fracture of the fibula.
**b** Five weeks after application of bilateral compression frame. Fibula is too short ( → ).
**c** Six and 10 months postinjury: excellent remodeling of tibial fixation callus, deformity of distal fibula with incongruity of tibiofibular articulation.
**d** Status following distal fibular osteotomy and matching of tibiofibular joint to opposite side.
**e** 4$^1/_2$ years postinjury: complete recovery with equality of injured and uninjured extremities

SG 10.1.81                                    e

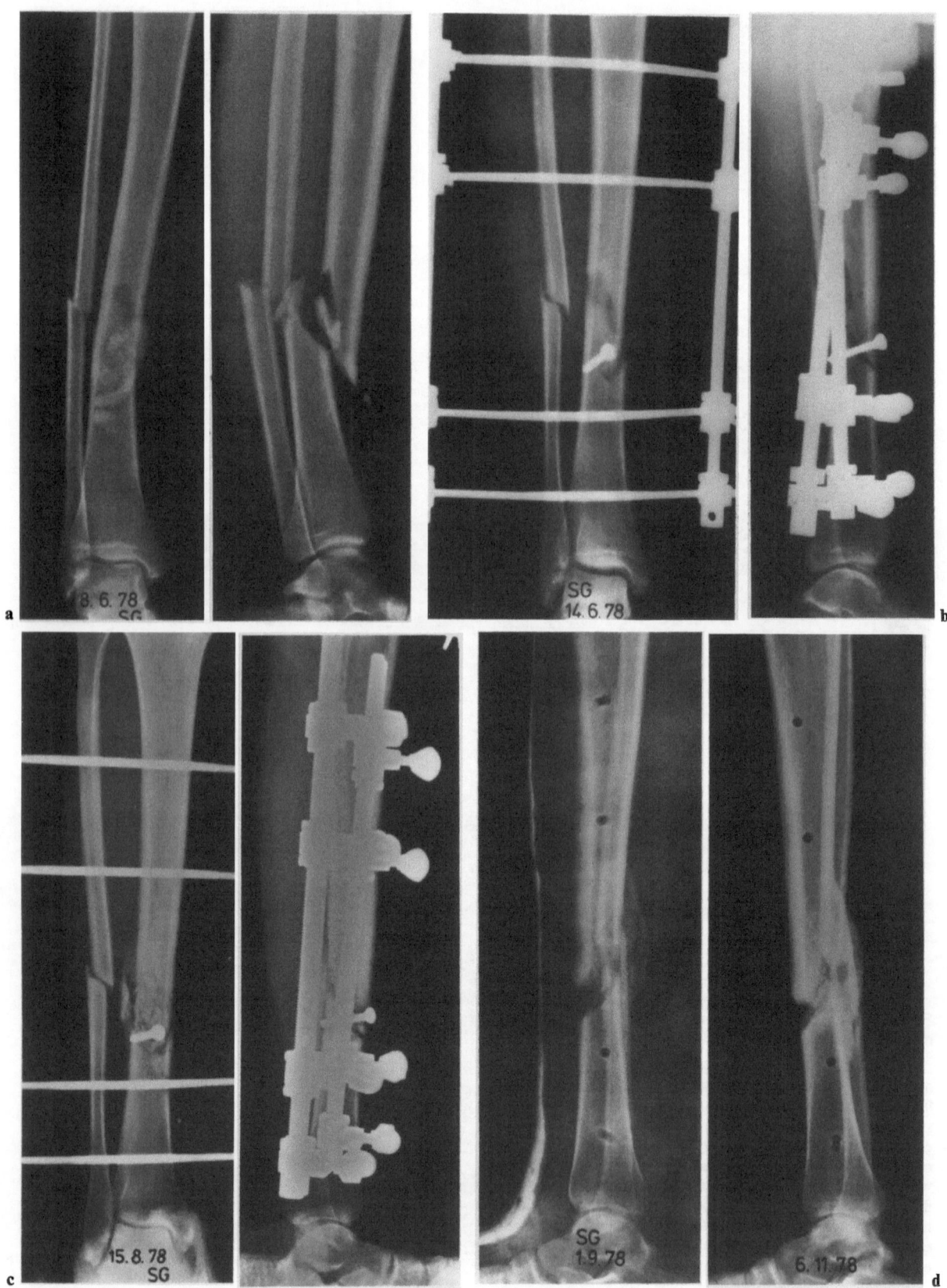

Fig. 212a–d

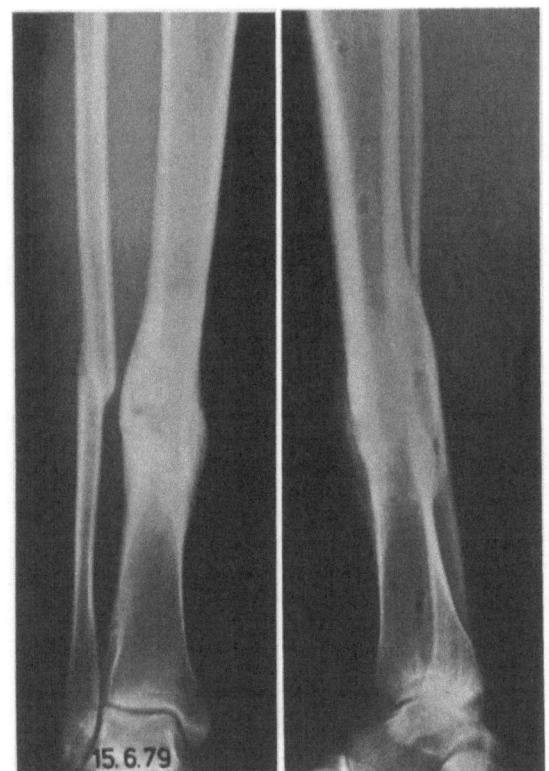

**Fig. 212 a–e.** Open fracture. Bilateral frame + minimal internal fixation. Z.J., 1958, 20 years, ♀, 185950.

**a** Grade II open fracture.
**b** Minimal internal fixation + bilateral neutralization and compression frame for 12 weeks.
**c** Ten weeks postinjury. Six weeks after autogenous, posteromedial cancellous bone graft.
**d** Two weeks after removal of frame and screw. Sarmiento brace. Five months postinjury: cancellous graft take.
**e** One year postinjury: complete recovery

**Fig. 213 a–e.** Open fracture. Bilateral frame. Nonunion. Internal plating. G.O., 1921, 56 years, ♂, 208360.

**a** Grade II open fracture.
**b** Three weeks after bilateral neutralization frame. Soft tissues are healed.
**c** Five months postinjury, after 10 weeks' external fixation and walking cast: nonunion.
**d** Compression plating, no bone graft.
**e** End result at 1¹⁄₂ years: complete recovery

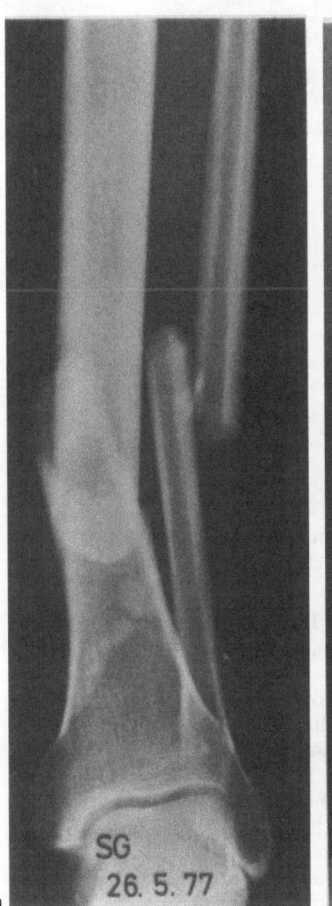
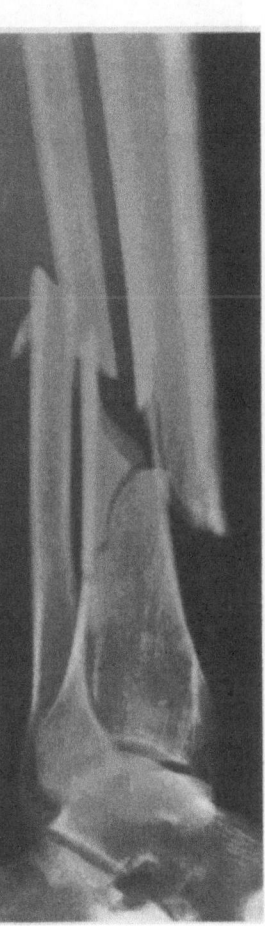
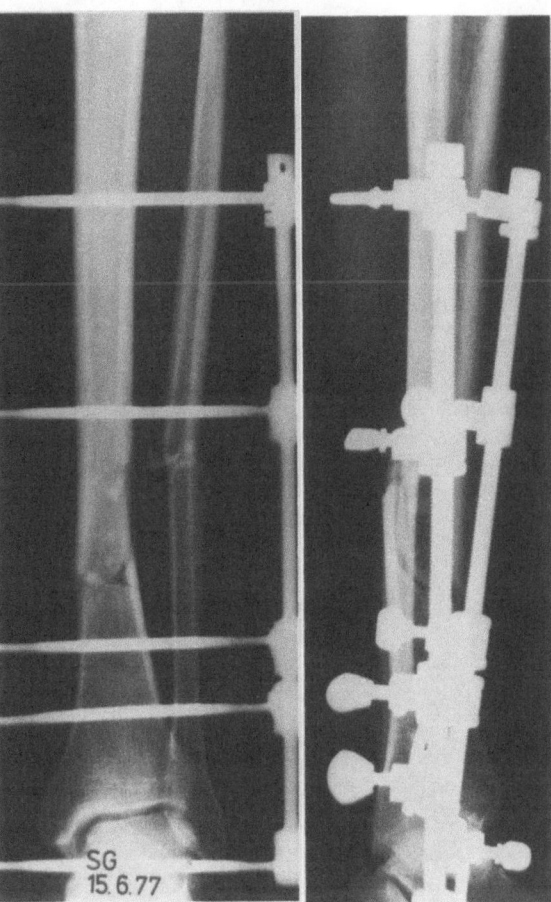

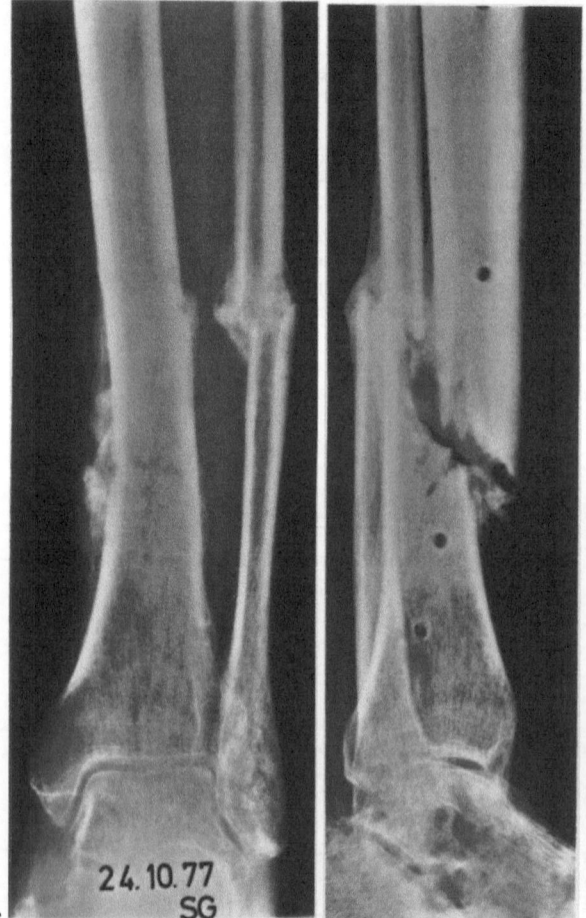

24.10.77
SG

c

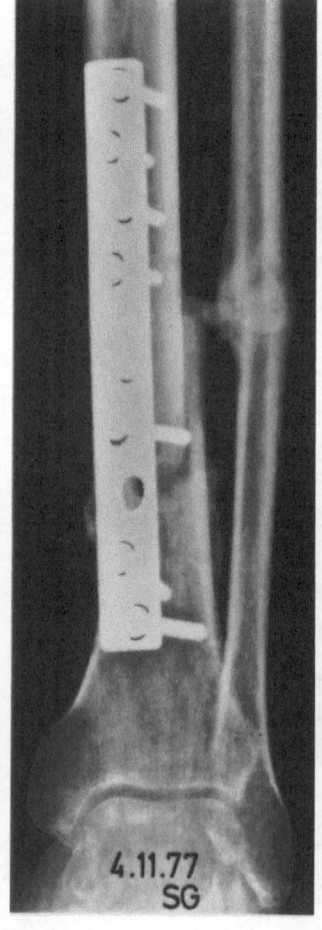

4.11.77
SG

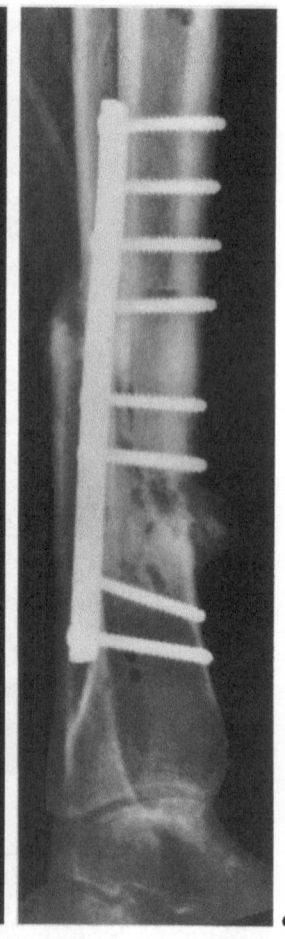

d

**Fig. 213c–e.** Legend see p. 165

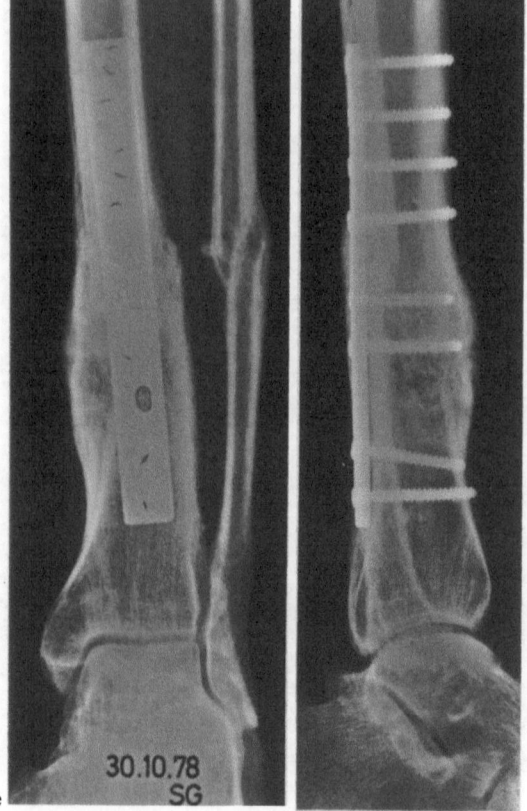

30.10.78
SG

e

**Fig. 214 a–h.** Bilateral open fracture. Bilateral frame + minimal internal fixation on left side. G.E., 1940, 42 years, ♀, 260290.

**a** Multiple injuries. Grade II open fracture on right side.
**b** Seven weeks after neutralization frame: cancellous bone graft.
**c** Grade III open fracture on left side.
**d** Ten weeks after neutralization frame + minimal internal fixation, 2 weeks after cancellous bone graft.
**e** Two months postinjury, 1 week after bilateral cancellous bone graft. Active exercise of feet and knee.
**f** Equinus prophylaxis with molded plastic sole and elastic tension.
**g, h** Result at 1 year: Fractures are solid. Good walking ability, almost normal joint motion on both sides

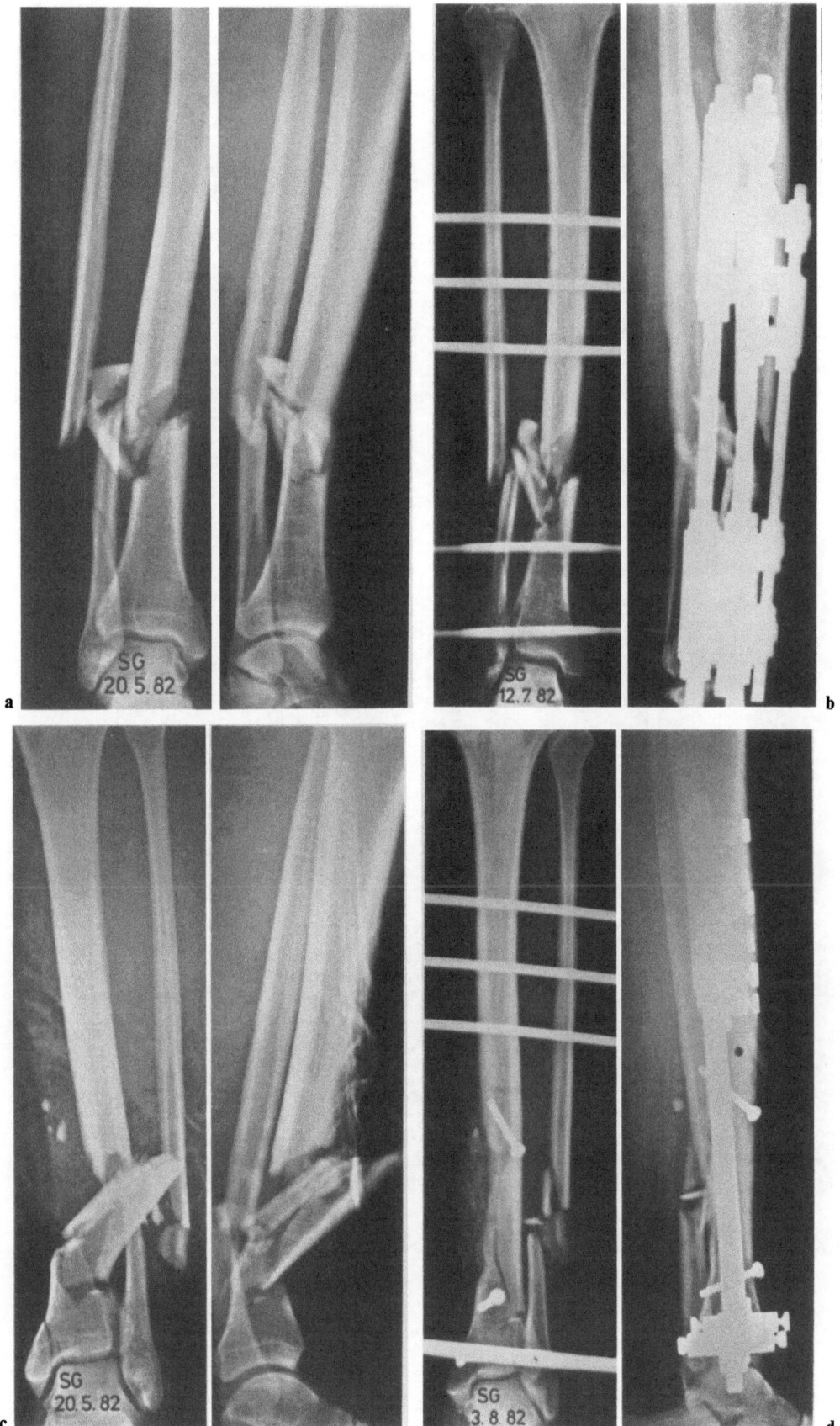

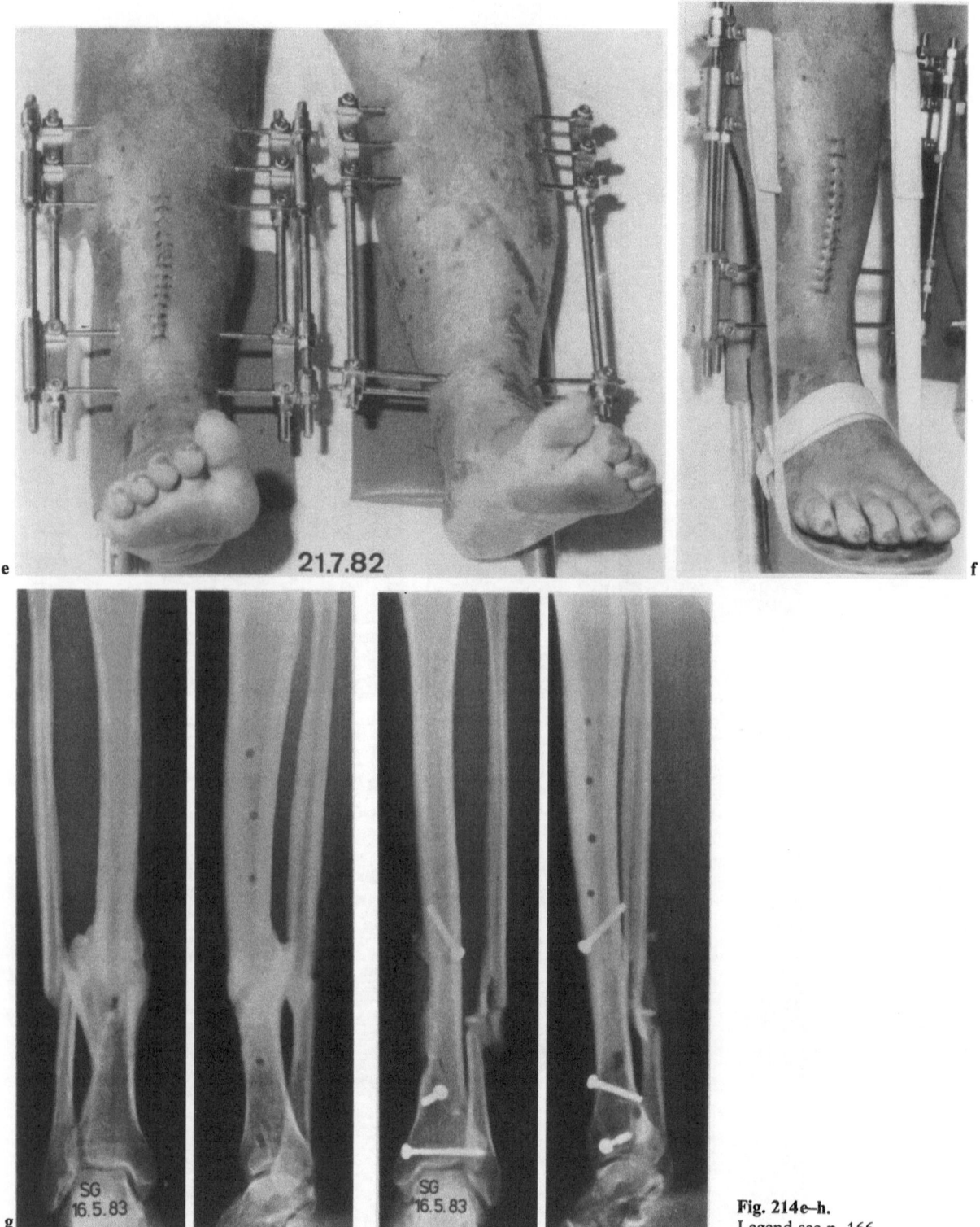

21.7.82

e

f

g

SG
16.5.83

h

SG
16.5.83

**Fig. 214e–h.**
Legend see p. 166

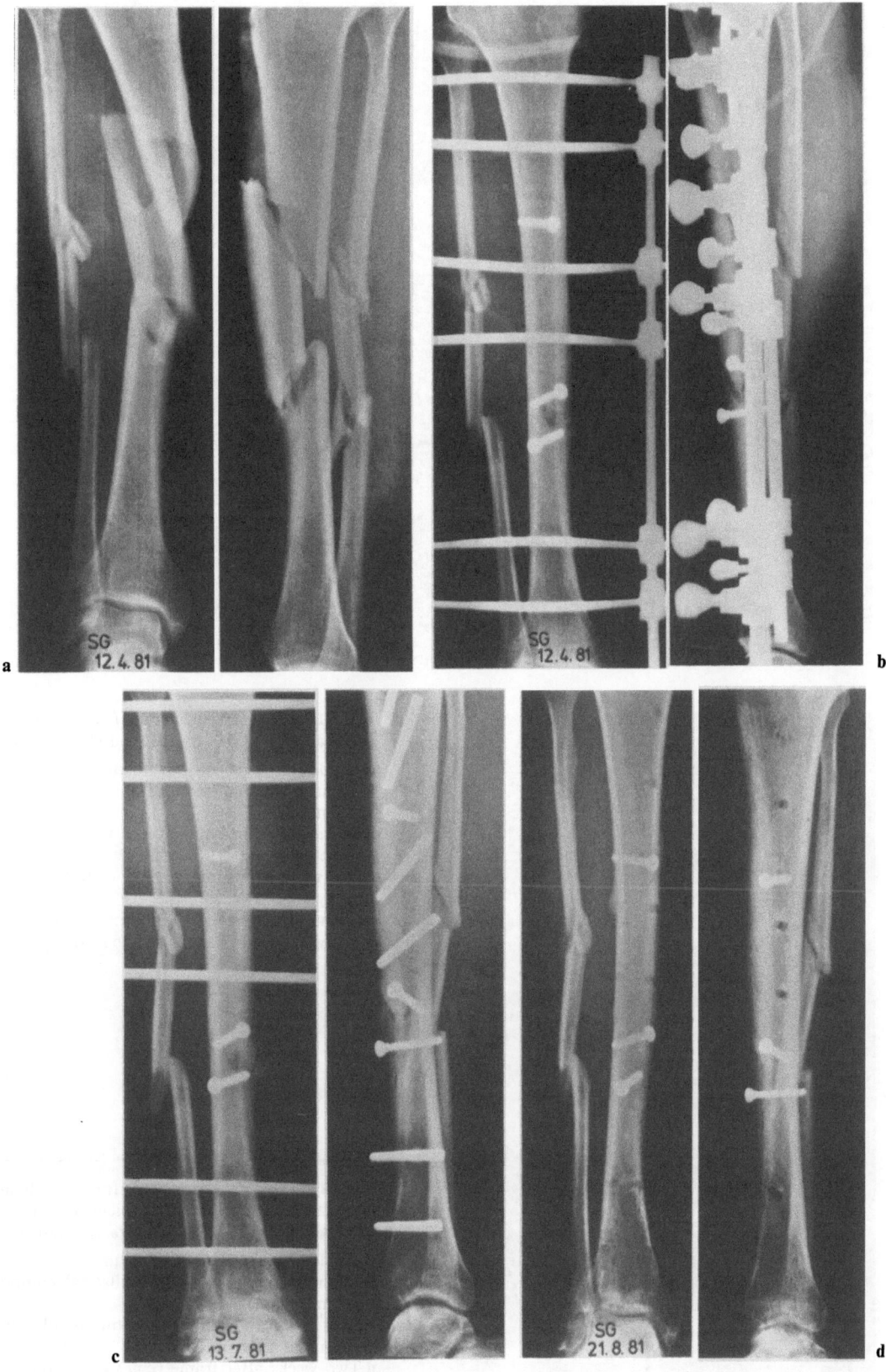

**Fig. 215a–d.** Legend see p. 170

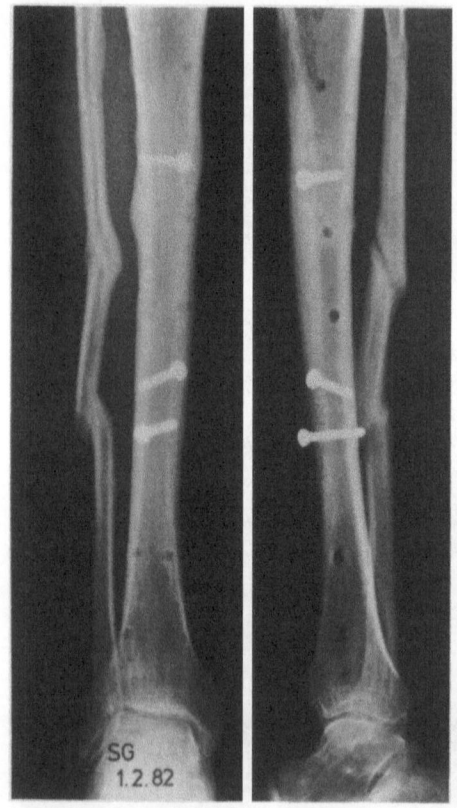

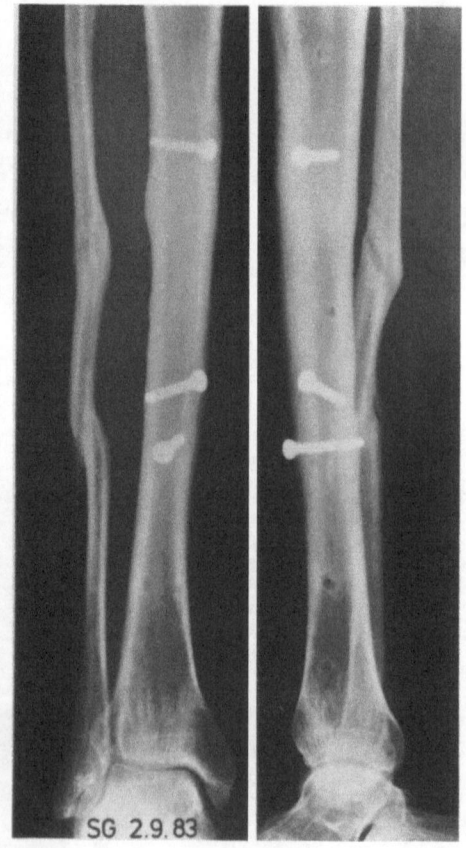

Fig. 215 a–f. Open segmental fracture. Bilateral frame + minimal internal fixation. E.A., 1928, 53 years, ♂, 248 755.

a Grade II open segmental fracture.

b Minimal internal fixation + bilateral neutralization frame for 3 months.

c Three months postinjury the fracture is clinically solid. Sarmiento brace for 6 weeks.

d 4$^1/_2$ months postinjury: start of full, unprotected weight bearing.

e Ten months postinjury: union.

f 2$^1/_2$ years postinjury: complete recovery

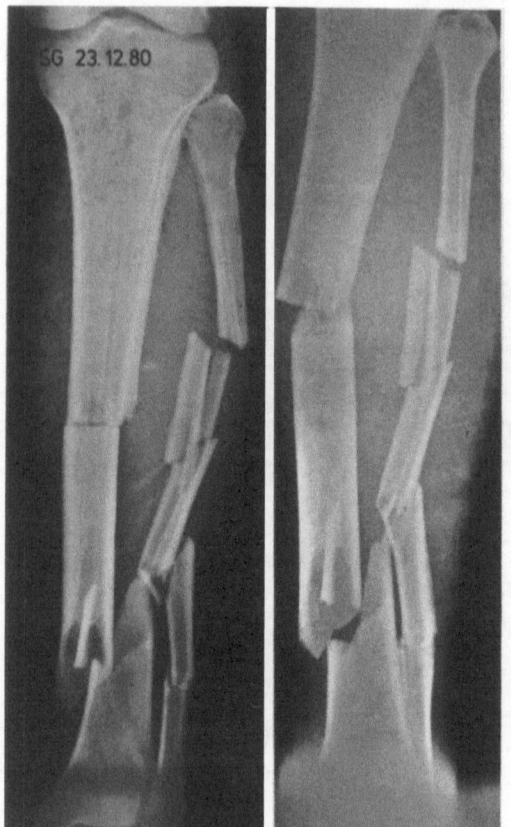

Fig. 216 a–e. Open segmental fracture. Bilateral frame + minimal internal fixation. Incipient nonunion. Intramedullary nailing. G.A., 1928, 52 years, ♂, 245 686.

a Grade II open segmental fracture.

b Minimal internal fixation + bilateral compression frame for 4 months.

c Four months postinjury: fracture is solid distally; incipient nonunion proximally.

d Two weeks after frame removal: intermedullary nailing, no bone grafting.

e One year postinjury: complete recovery

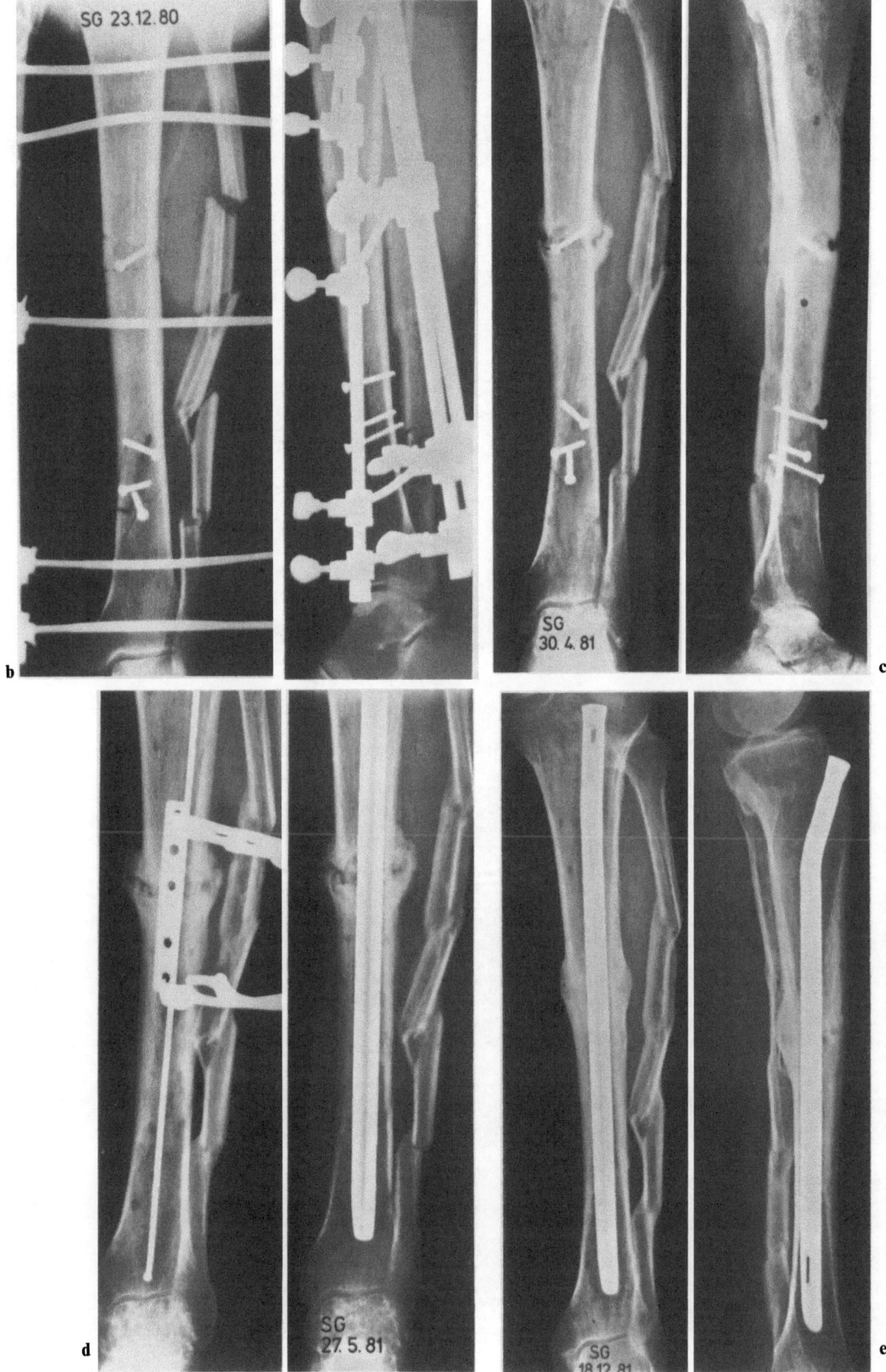

SG 23.12.80

b

SG
30. 4. 81

c

d

SG
27. 5. 81

SG
18.12.81

e

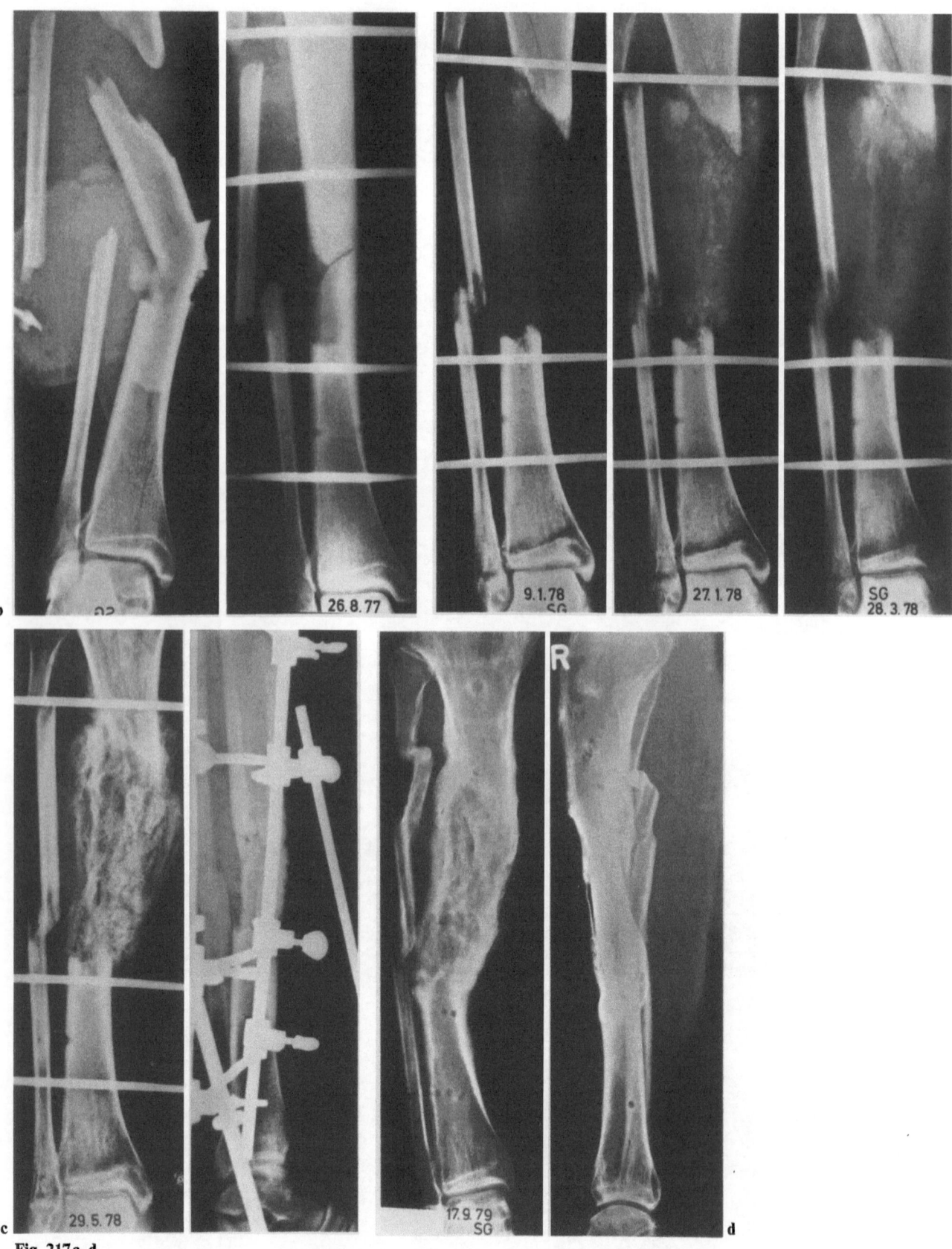

a, b

c

Fig. 217a–d

d

**Fig. 217 a–g.** Open segmental fracture. Bilateral frame. Infection. Bone loss. Reconstruction. H.W., 1950, 27 years, ♂, 210 749.

**a** Grade III open fracture. Debridement, bilateral frame for 9 months. Infection. Sequestrectomy.
**b** Thiersch graft. Posterolateral cancellous bone grafts and weight bearing.
**c** Nine months postinjury: removal of fixator, weight-relieving caliper.
**d** Two years postinjury: full weight bearing and resumption of work as truck driver. Varus deformity of ankle joint.
**e** 4$^1/_2$ years postinjury: Normal function. Fracture united with 1 cm shortening. Varus is corrected by osteotomy.
**f, g** 4$^1/_2$ years postinjury: The foot shows good trophism, the joints have good mobility, and the patient is free of complaints

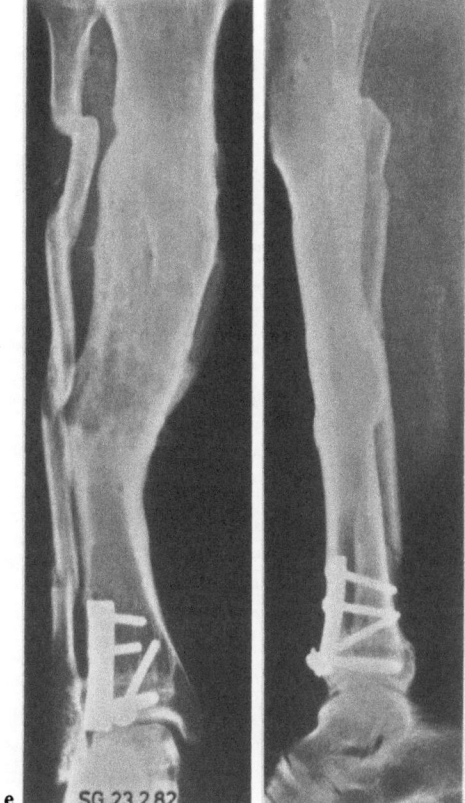

e    SG 23.2.82

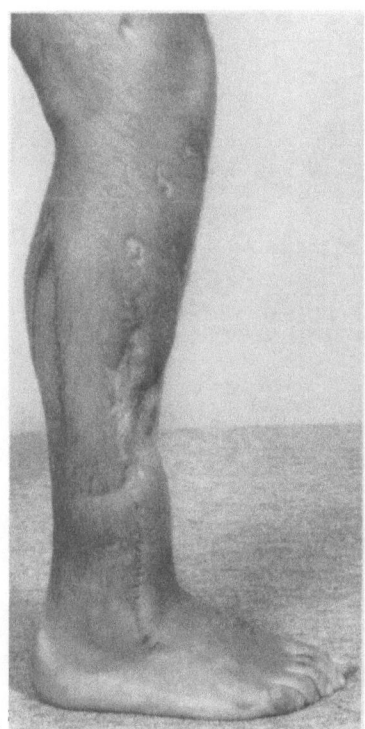
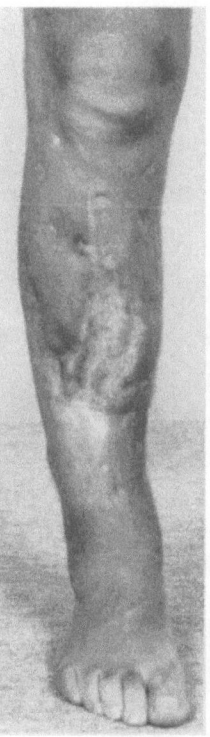
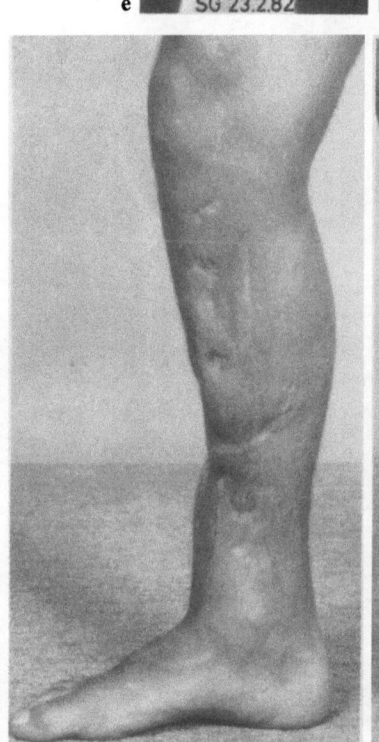
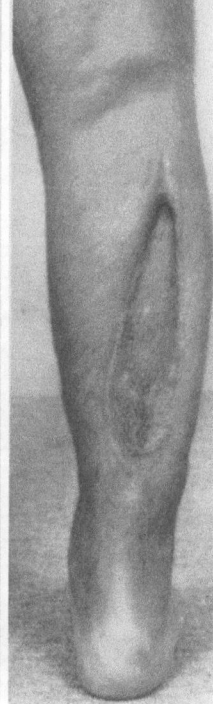

f

g

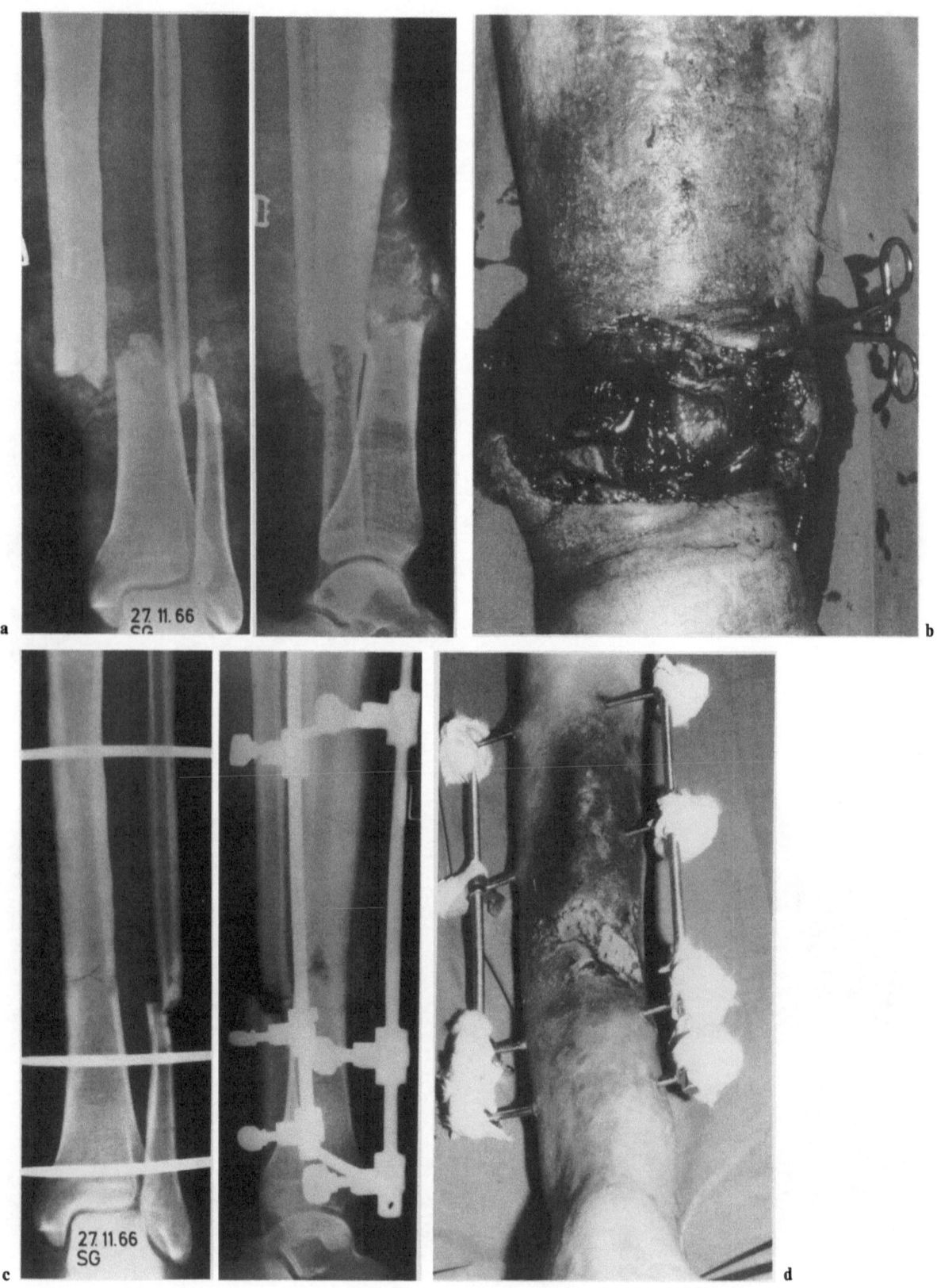

**Fig. 218a–d**

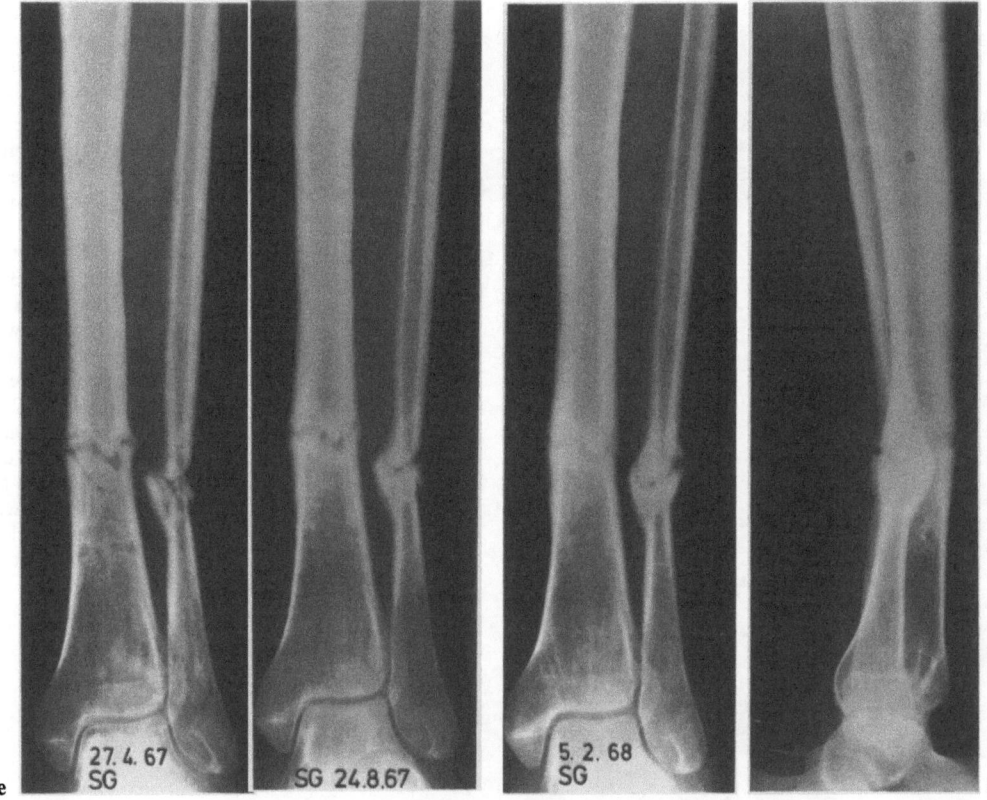

27. 4. 67
SG

SG 24.8.67

5. 2. 68
SG

e                                                                                                                    f

**Fig. 218 a–f.** Open fracture in the presence of a chronic crural ulcer. Infected fracture. Bilateral frame. W.W., 1934, 32 years, ♂, 109 116.

**a** Grade III open fracture with crural ulcer.
**b** Local findings: tibial fracture at the center of the crural ulcer with a mixed infection.
**c** Bilateral compression frame for 4 months.
**d** Three weeks postinjury: split-thickness skin graft.
**e** Gradual consolidation at 5 and 9 months postinjury.
**f** Fifteen months postinjury: tibia is united but fibular non-union persists. The ulcer is healed, and there is no infection

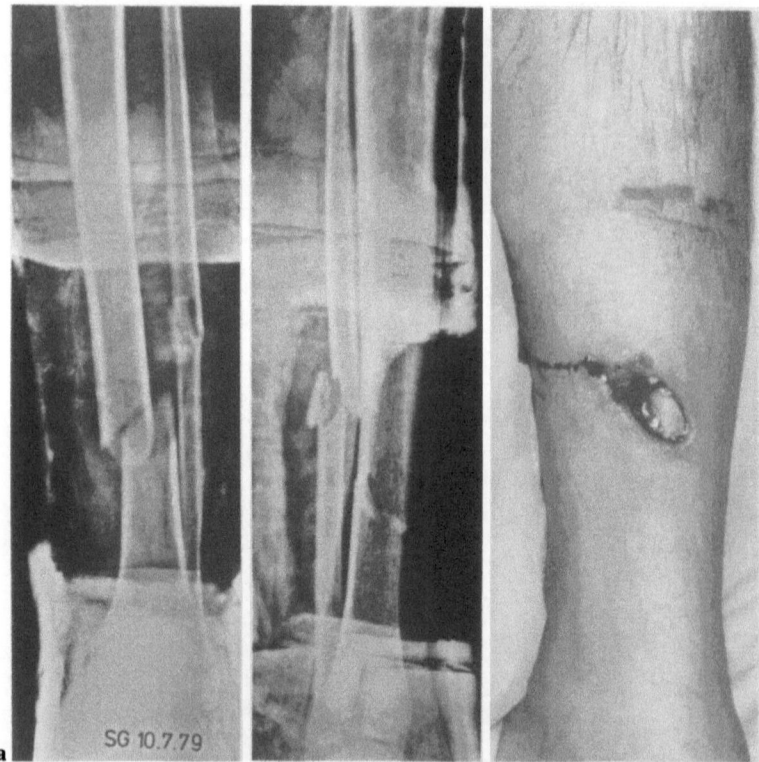

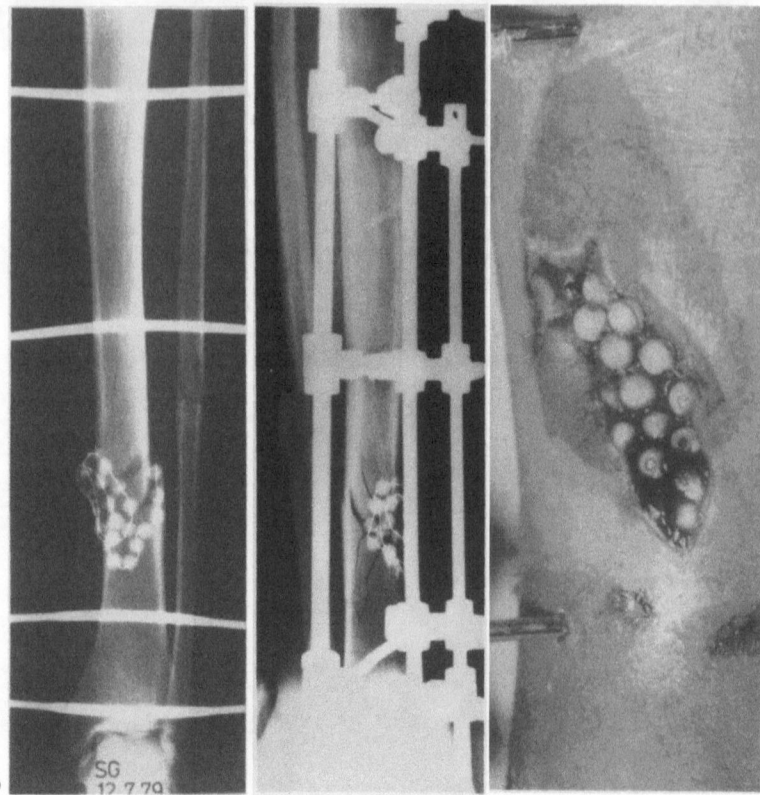

**Fig. 219 a–f.** Infected fracture following open fracture and primary cast immobilization. Bilateral frame. N.G., 1944, 35 years, ♂, 230325.

**a** Four weeks previously: open tibial fracture immobilized in plaster (abroad). At presentation: infected fracture, ulcer, visible fragments in ulcer.

**b** Stabilization with bilateral neutralization frame for 3 months. Gentamycin-PMMA beads under plastic film for 10 days, followed by open cancellous bone graft.

**c** Cancellous bone graft. Split-thickness skin applied 2 weeks later.

**d** Three months after start of treatment: provisional union. Fixator is removed. Sarmiento brace for 2 months.

**e** Four months after external fixation: fracture is solid, ulcer is healed.

**f** $3^1/_2$ years after initial treatment: complete recovery

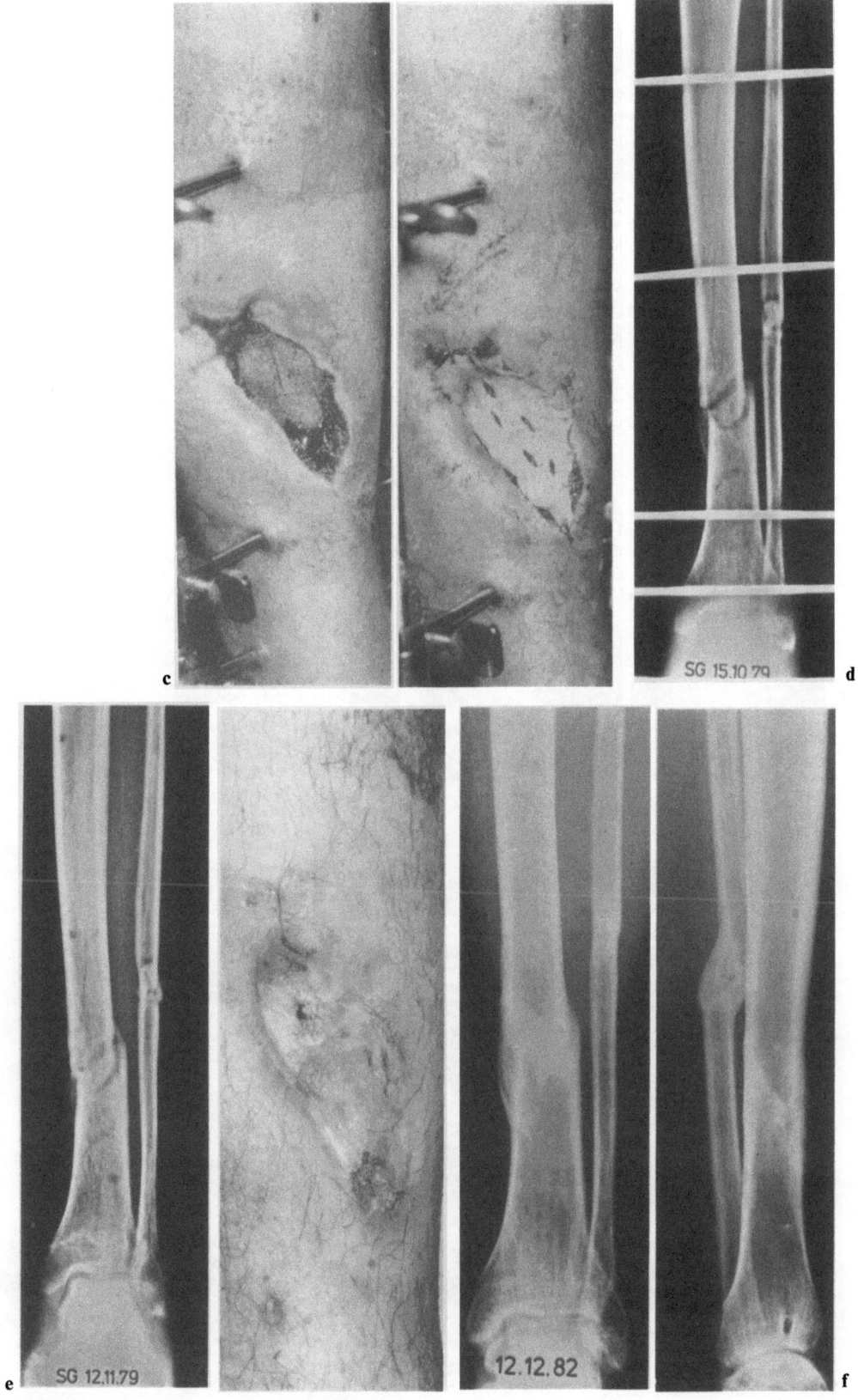

c

d

SG 15.10.79

e   SG 12.11.79

12.12.82

f

**Fig. 219c–f**

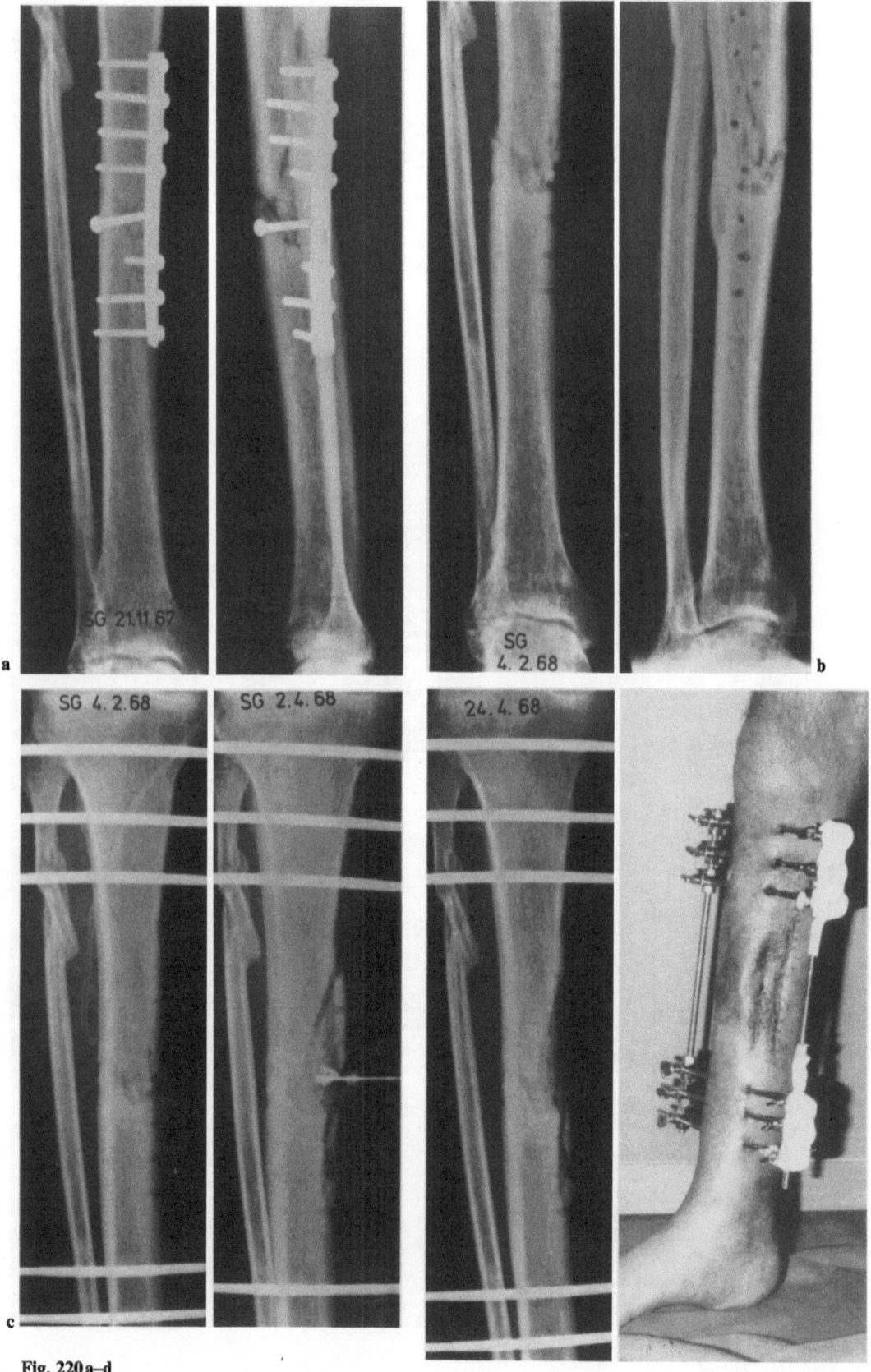

**Fig. 220 a–d**

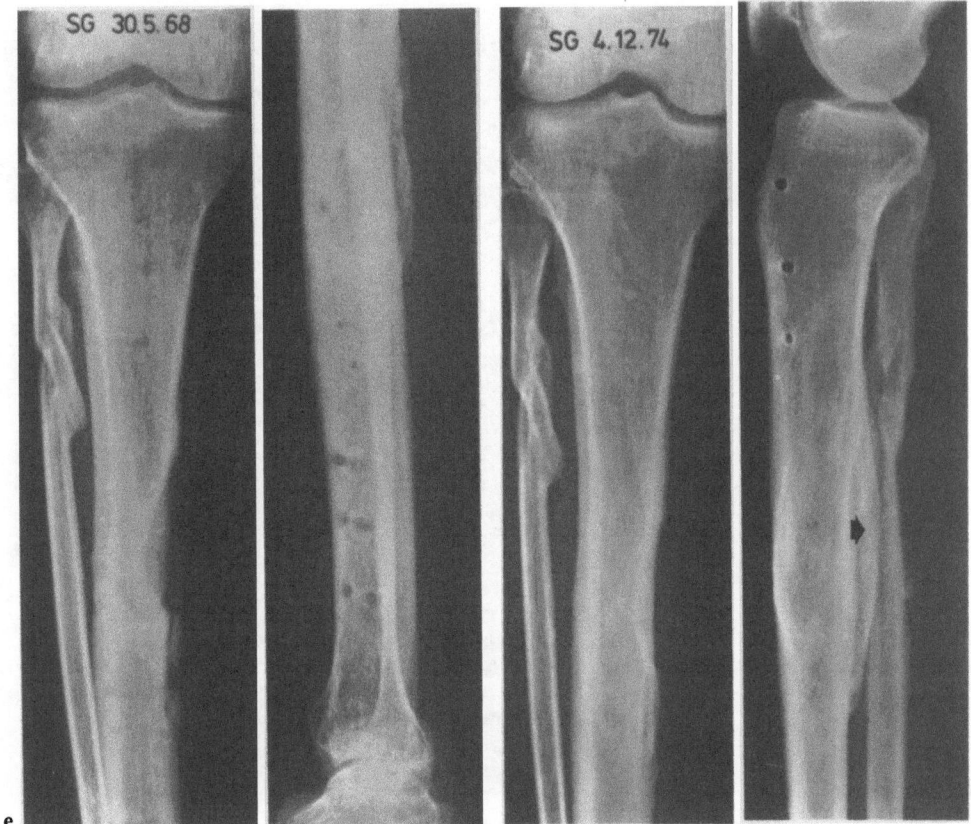

**Fig. 220 a–f.** Infected fracture following open fracture and internal fixation. Bilateral frame. K.W., 1910, 57 years, ♂, 117976.

**a** Five months after open fracture, internal fixation, infection. Removal of plate. Plaster.

**b** At presentation: Patient had slipped, sustaining a refracture; osteitis, sinus.

**c** Bilateral frame for 3 months and posteromedial bone graft. Sinography, sequestrectomy, bone graft.

**d** Ten weeks after external fixation: fracture and infection are healed. Fixator is removed.

**e** Six months after start of treatment.

**f** Seven years after treatment: complete recovery. Note posterior cancellous bone graft (→)

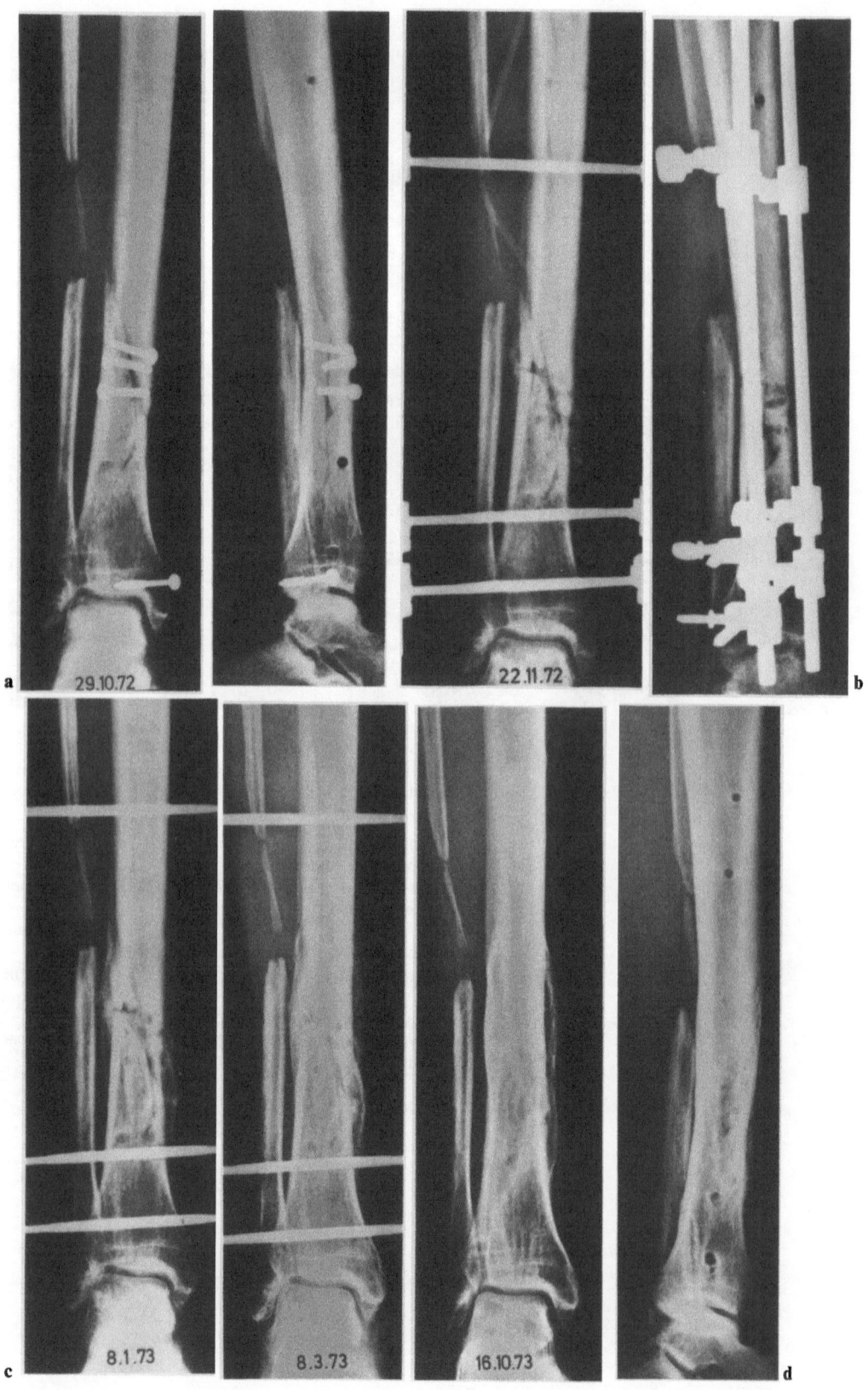

**Fig. 221a–d**

**Fig. 221 a–d.** Infected fracture following open fracture and internal fixation. Bilateral frame. G.St., 1935, 37 years, ♂, 163 532.

**a** Status 3 months after open fracture, internal fixation, infection, extraction of septic fibular fragment and attempted external fixation (abroad). At presentation: infected fracture, sinuses, sequestrum.
**b** One month after debridement the loose screws are removed. Bilateral neutralization frame for 4 months. Posteromedial cancellous bone graft.
**c** Progress 2 and 4 months after external fixation.
**d** One year after start of treatment: complete recovery

◀————————————————————

**Fig. 222 a–d.** Infected fracture following open fracture and internal fixation. Unilateral and bilateral frame. I.M., 1947, 33 years, ♂, 239 674.

**a** Three months previously: Grade II open fracture. Intramedullary nailing, infection (abroad). At presentation: infected fracture, medullary phlegmon, sinus.
**b** One month after nail removal and 7 months of unilateral-bilateral frame applied distant from septic focus. Sequestrum on anterior tibial border: posterior cancellous bone graft, sequestrectomy, Thiersch graft.
**c** Seven months after external fixation: infection and fracture are healed. Fixator is removed.
**d** 1 $^1/_2$ years after start of treatment: fracture and infection are healed

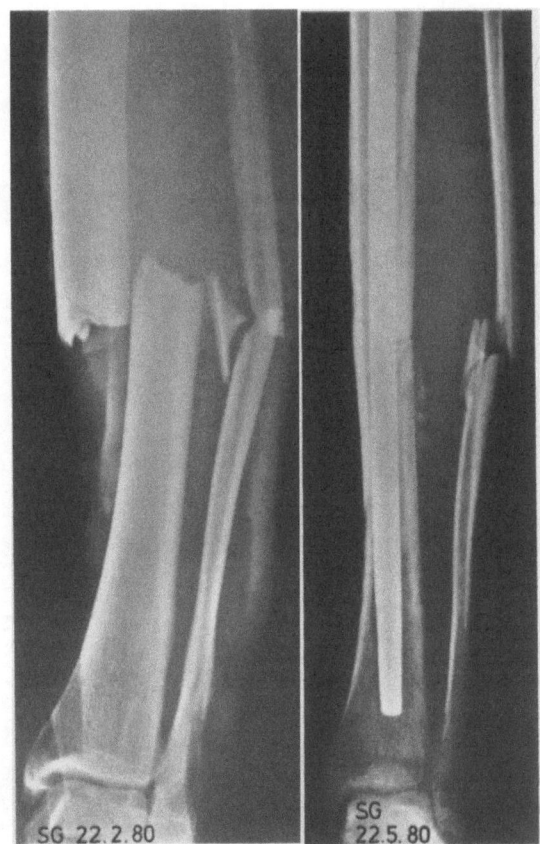

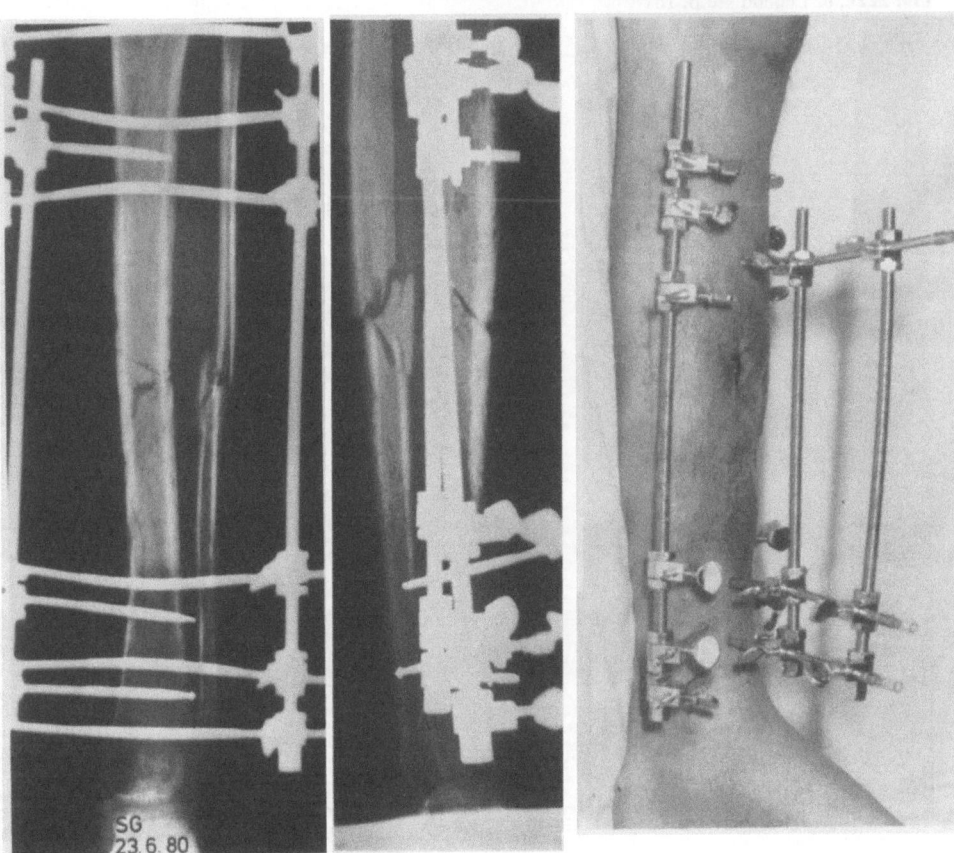

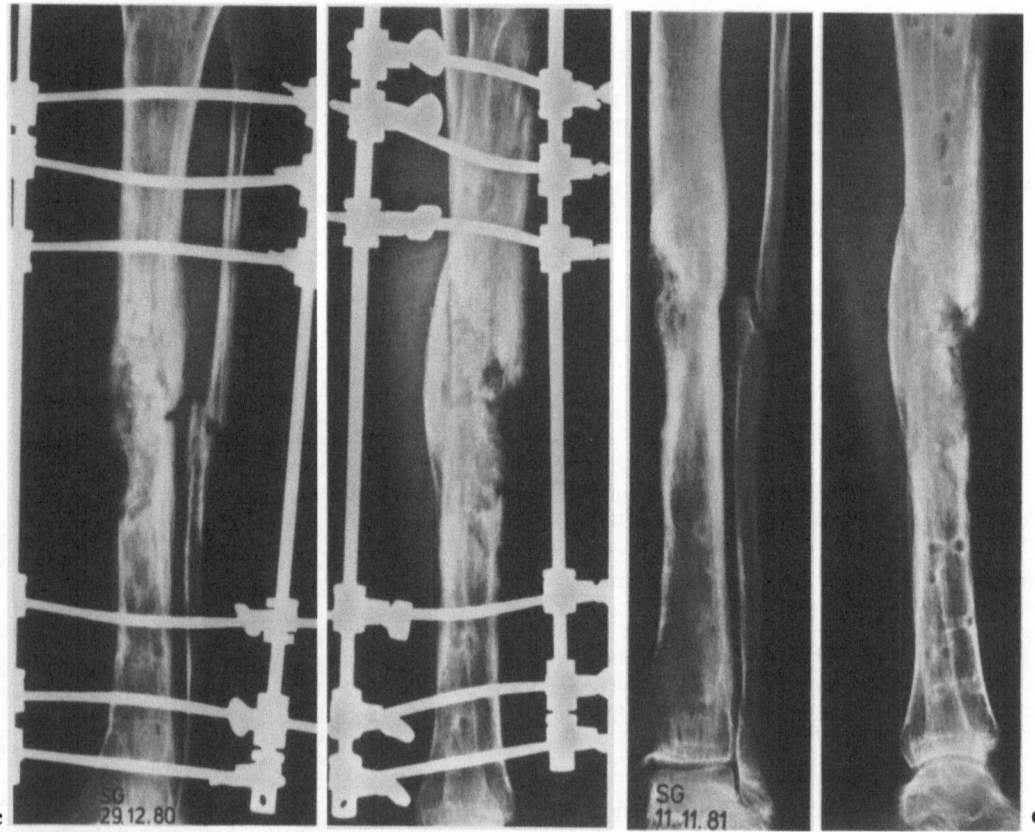

**Fig. 222c, d.** Legend see p. 181

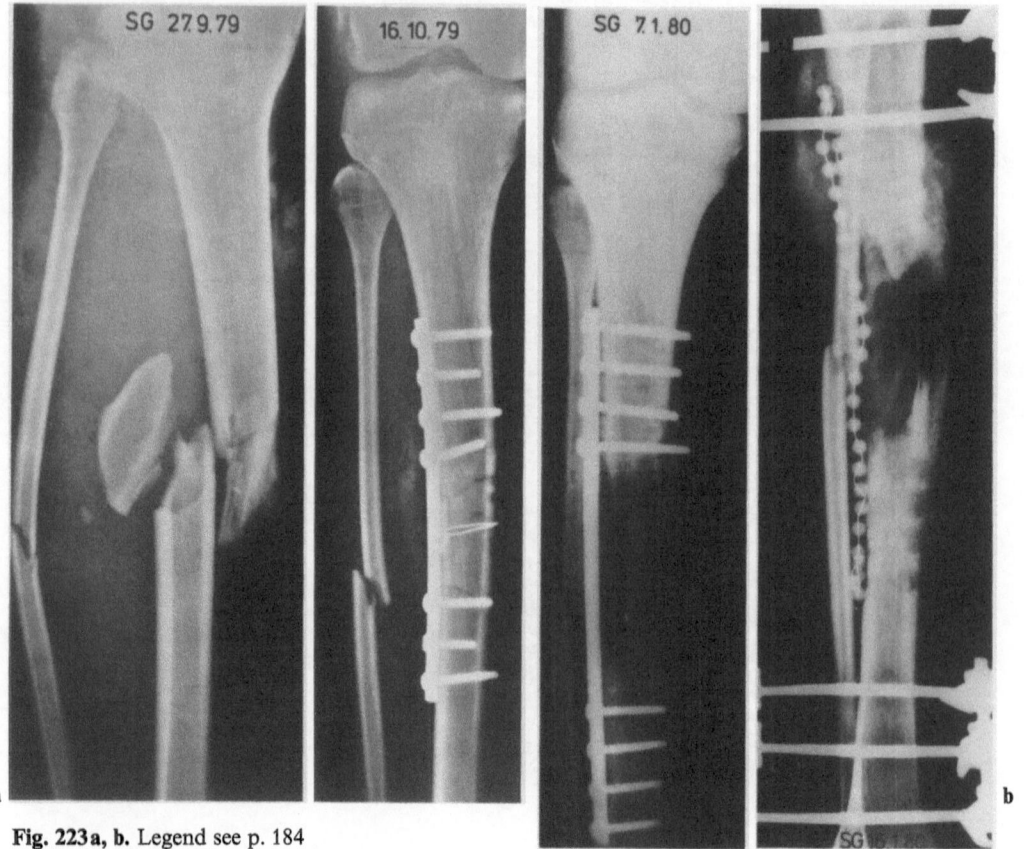

**Fig. 223a, b.** Legend see p. 184

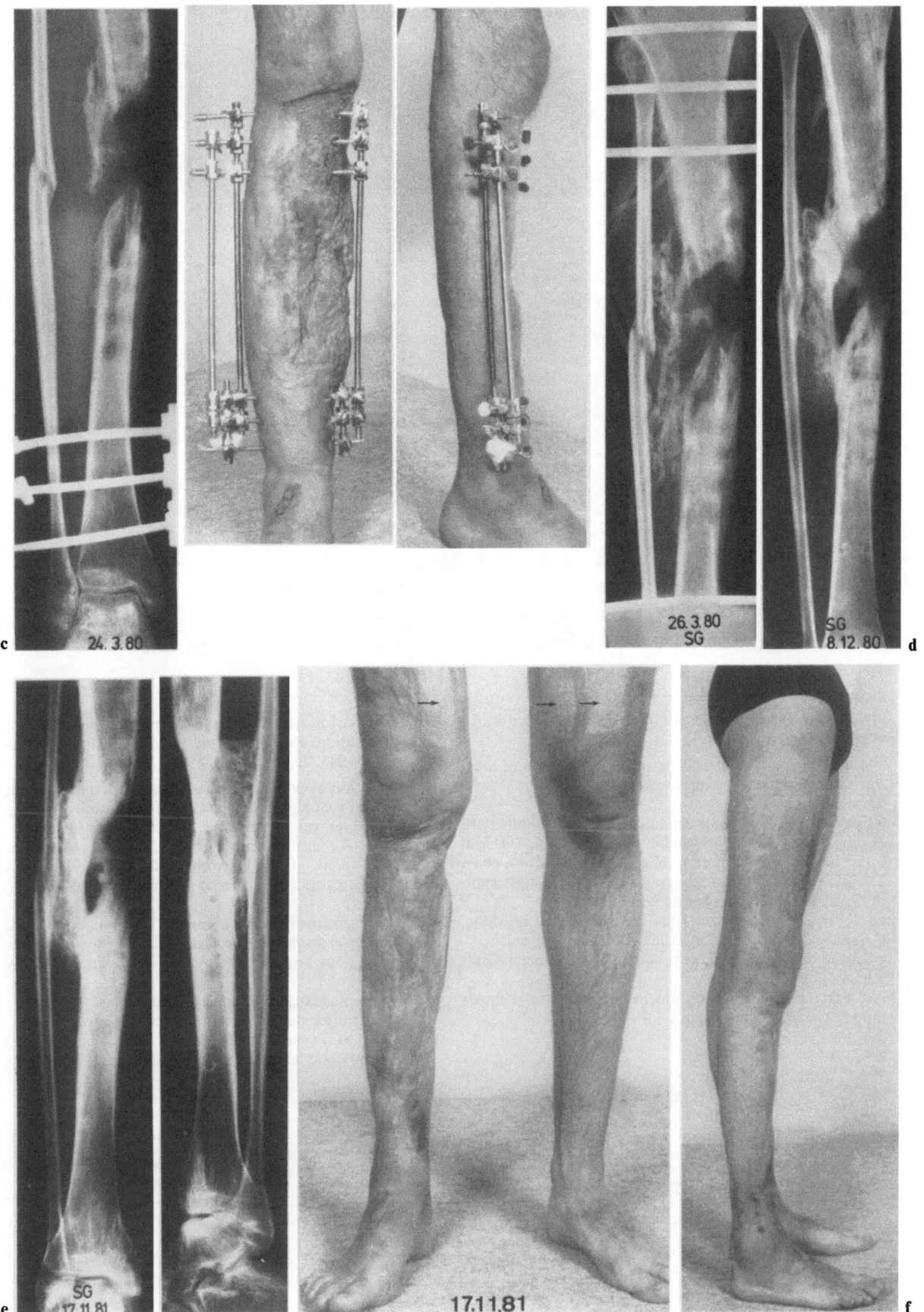

**Fig. 223c–f.** Legend see p. 184

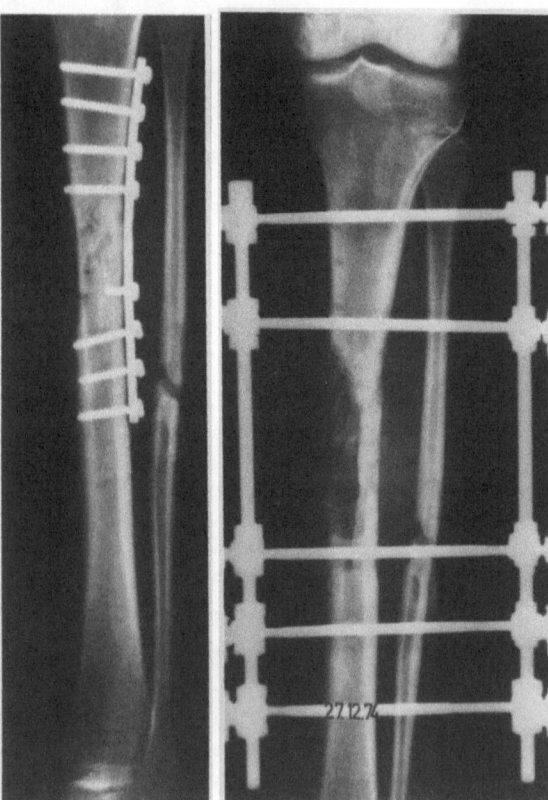 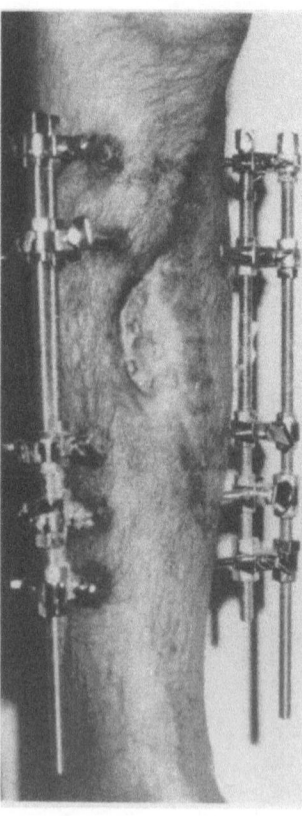

Fig. 224a

**Fig. 223a–f.** Infected open fracture. Bilateral frame. R.R., 1960, 20 years, ♂, 222696.

**a** Grade III open fracture. Plate fixation. Infection of tibial fracture: debridement, sequestrectomy, replacement of plate (abroad).
**b** Infected fracture with defect, large ulcer over middle third of tibia. Extensive debridement. Plate removal, bilateral frame for 4 months. Insertion of gentamycin-PMMA chain into plate bed. First cancellous bone graft. Multiple split-thickness skin grafts applied at 3-week intervals.
**c** $2^1/_2$ months after external fixation: healing of infection, restoration of cutaneous coverage. Tibial defect persists.
**d** Second bone graft through posterolateral approach. Graft take $8^1/_2$ months later.
**e, f** Fracture and infection are healed, function is nearly normal [Thiersch donor sites ($\rightarrow$)]

**Fig. 224 a–e.** Infected fracture following open fracture and internal fixation. Bilateral frame. Secondary internal fixation. F.R., 1945, 29 years, ♂, 178947.

**a** Five months previously: open fracture, internal fixation, infection (abroad). At presentation: infected, poorly healing fracture. Removal of implants, debridement, sequestrectomy, bilateral neutralization frame for 4 months. Open cancellous bone graft. Thiersch graft. Local findings 4 months postoperatively. Frame removal, weight-relieving caliper.
**b** One year postoperatively: nonunion is no longer infected. Application of contoured posterior plate. Two weeks later cancellous bone grafting of concavity and skin closure by suture.
**c** Three months later: nonunion is consolidated.
**d** $7^1/_2$ years after start of treatment: complete recovery.
**e** Function at 2 years after treatment: Patient has resumed work as professional alpine ski racer

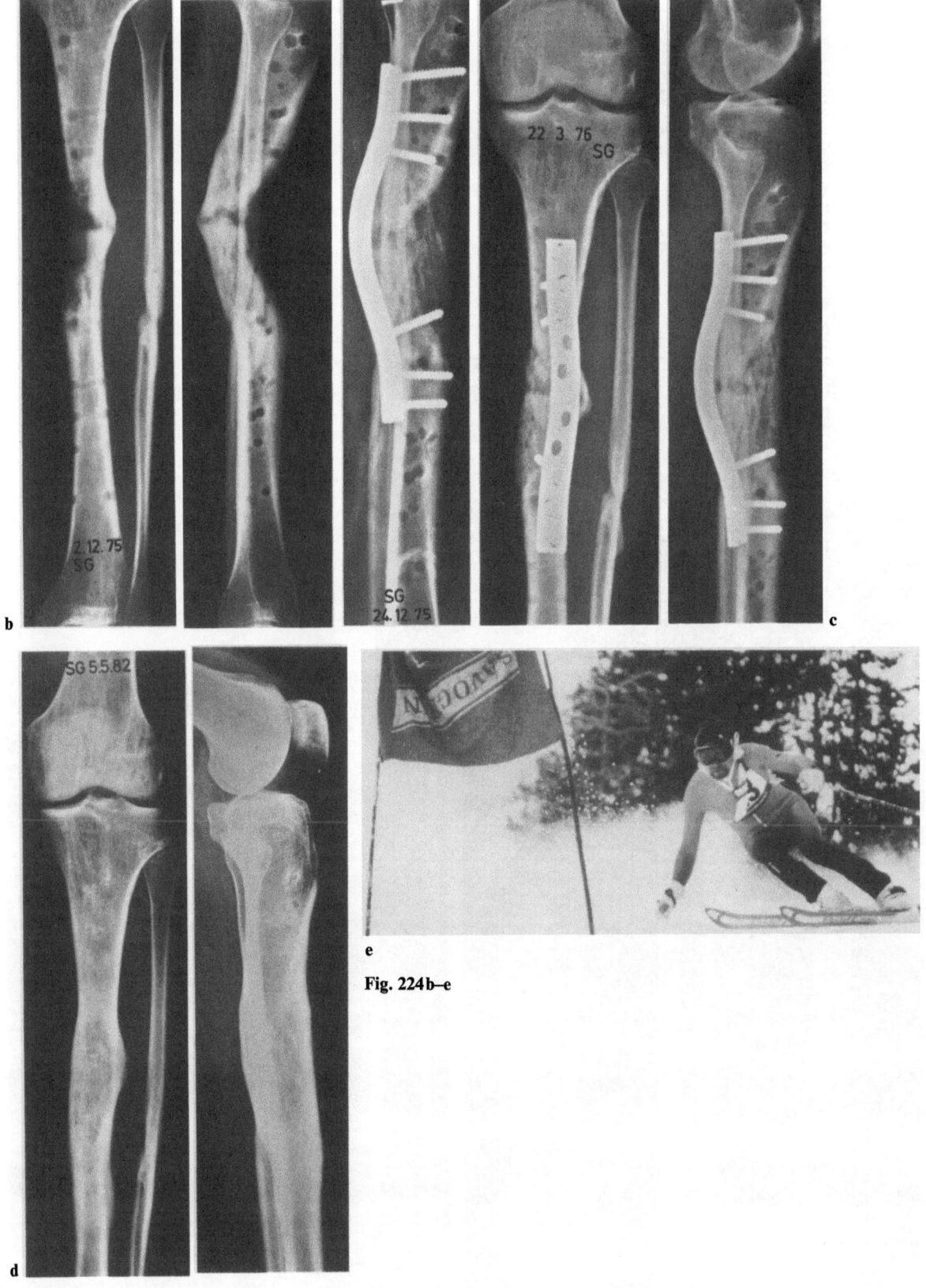

b

2.12.75
SG

SG
24.12.75

22  3  76
SG

c

SG 5.5.82

d

e

**Fig. 224b–e**

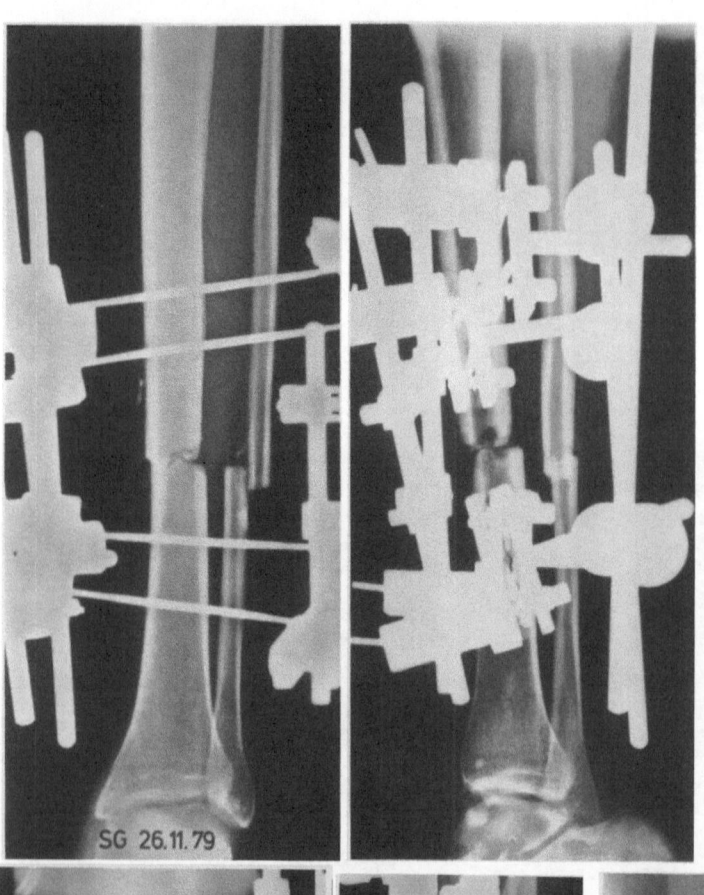

Fig. 225a–c

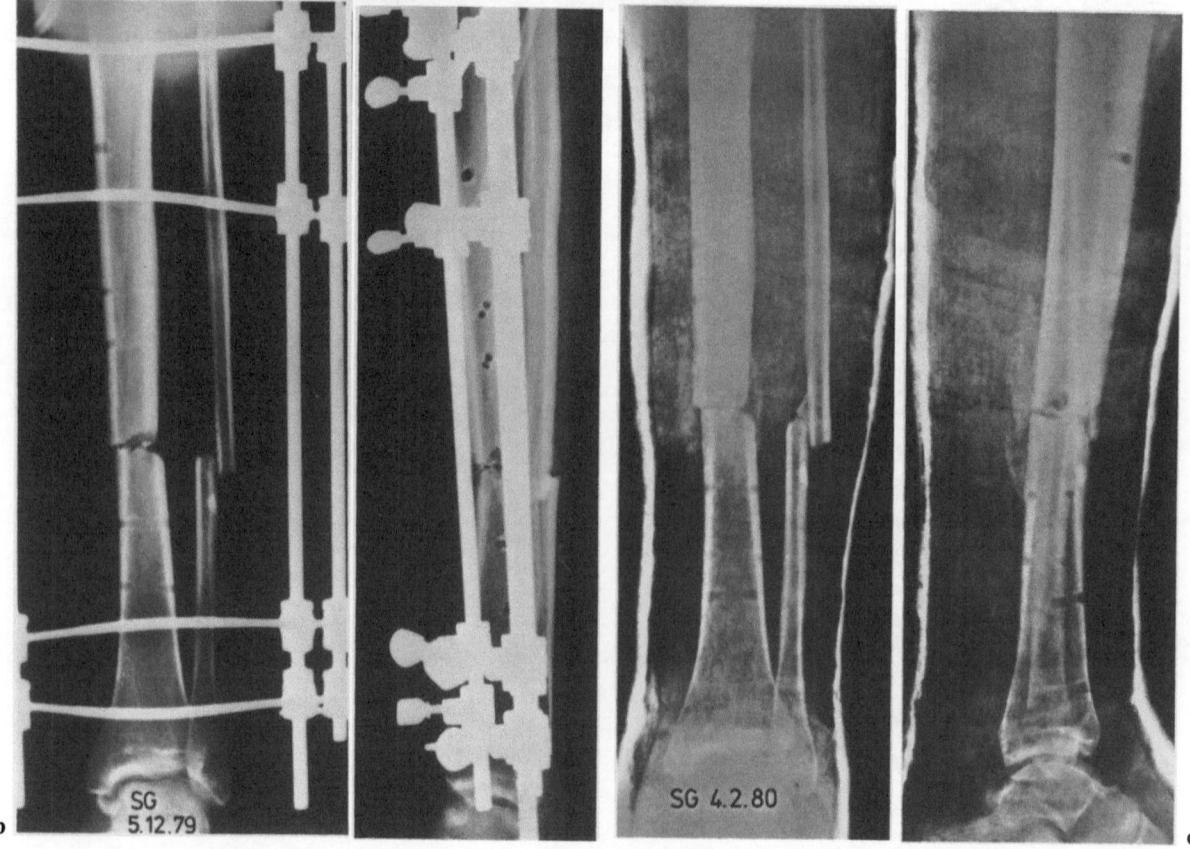

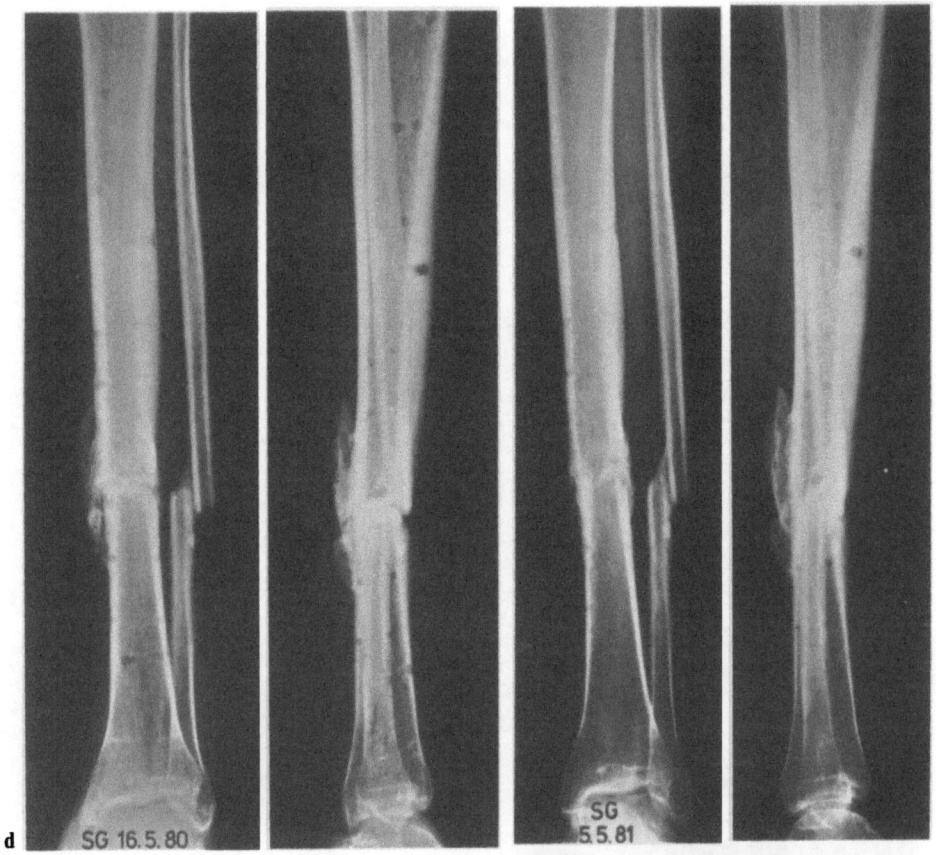

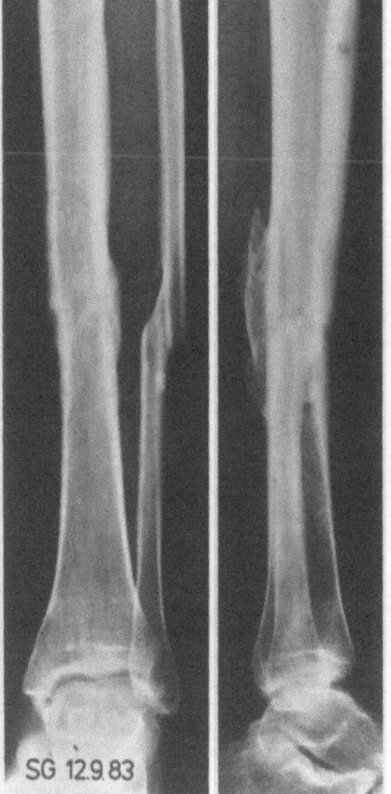

**Fig. 225 a–f.** Infected fracture following open fracture and external fixation. Bilateral frame. A.G., 1954, 25 years, ♂, 232152.

**a** Two months earlier: multiple injuries with open fracture, external fixation (abroad). At presentation: infected fracture, unstable external fixator. All pin tracks are infected.
**b** Treatment: removal of unstable fixator. Bilateral compression frame for 8 weeks. Posterior cancellous bone graft 3 weeks later.
**c** Two months after start of treatment: Sarmiento brace.
**d** Five months after start of treatment: fracture is solid.
**e** After 17 months: complete recovery.
**f** Four years postinjury: complete recovery

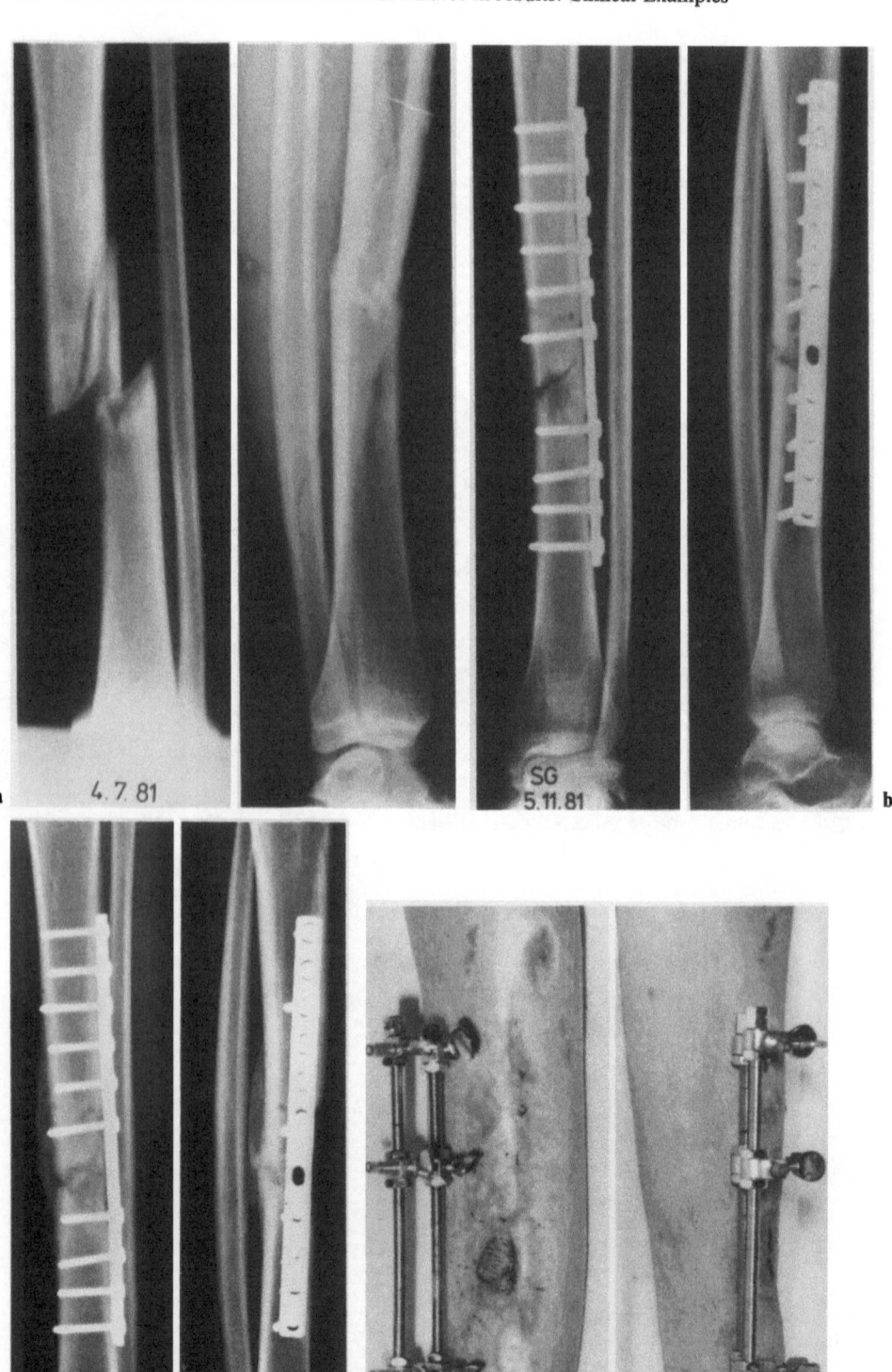

**Fig. 226a–d**

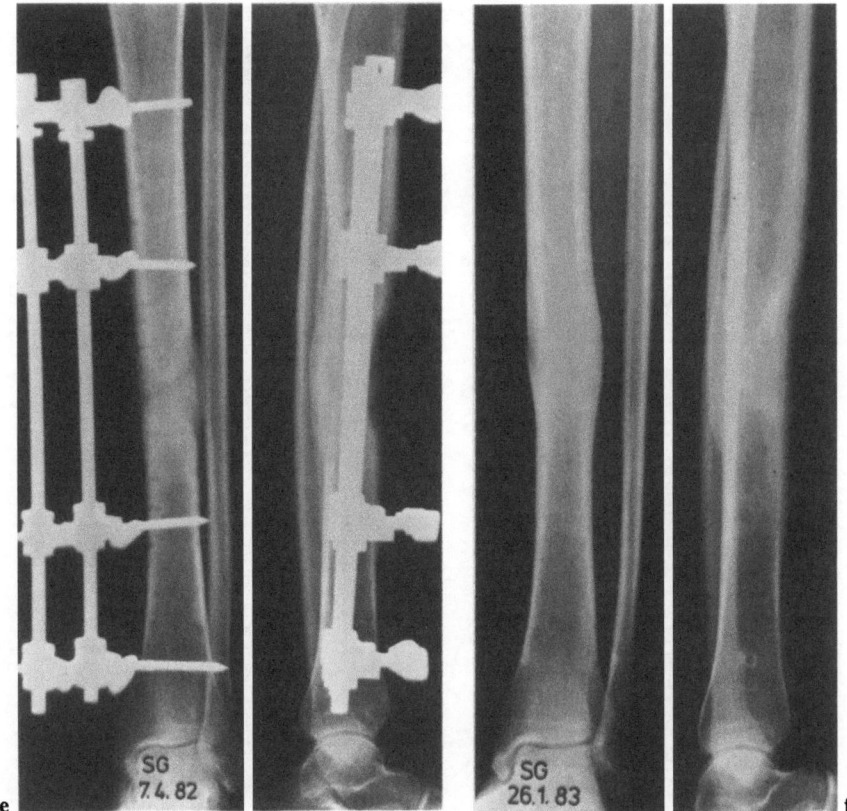

**Fig. 226 a–f.** Infected fracture following open fracture and internal fixation. Unilateral frame. St.M., 1967, 14 years, ♀, 254 500.

**a** Grade II open tibial fracture. Internal fixation. Infection (abroad).
**b** At presentation 4 months after internal fixation: infected fracture, ulcer, sinus.
**c** One month after posteromedial cancellous bone graft. Removal of plate + unilateral frame for 4 months. Thiersch graft.
**d** Six weeks after unilateral compression frame.
**e** Four months after external fixation: fracture is solid.
**f** One year, 2 months after initial treatment: complete recovery

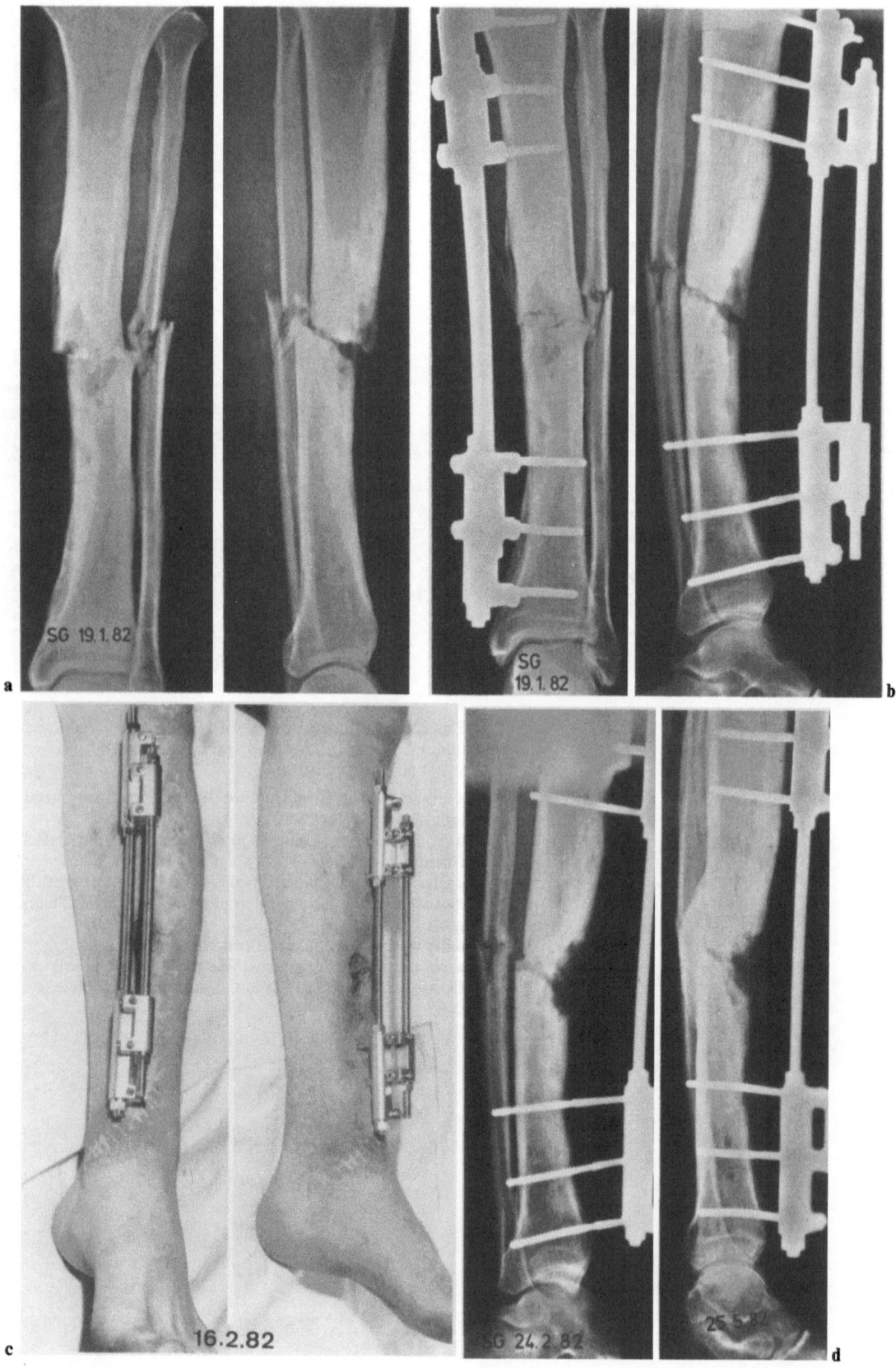

**Fig. 227 a–d**

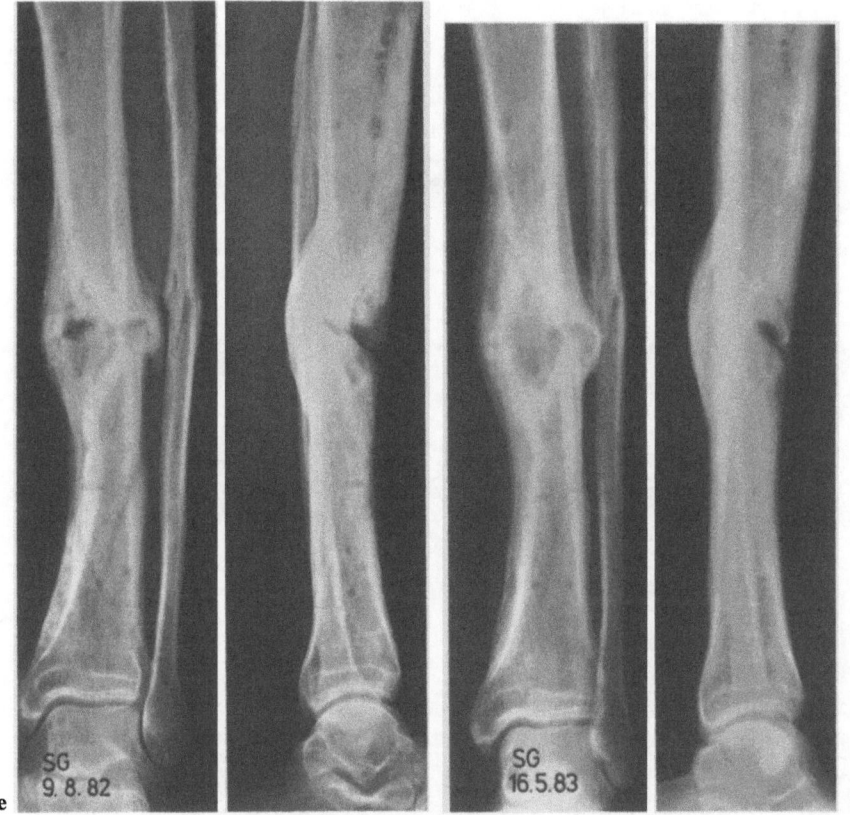

**Fig. 227 a–f.** Infected fracture following open fracture and internal fixation with osteitis. Unilateral frame. I.A., 1947, 35 years, ♂, 256644.

**a** 1½ years previously: open fracture. Internal fixation with plate, infection, plate removal, sinus (abroad). At presentation: open fracture through saucerization with sinus.
**b** Unilateral compression frame for 4 months.
**c** One month after external fixation: sinus.
**d** One month postinjury: posterior cancellous bone graft. Three months later: posterior bridging of fracture.
**e** Seven months postinjury: fracture is solid.
**f** One year, 4 months postinjury: full weight bearing, no residual sinus

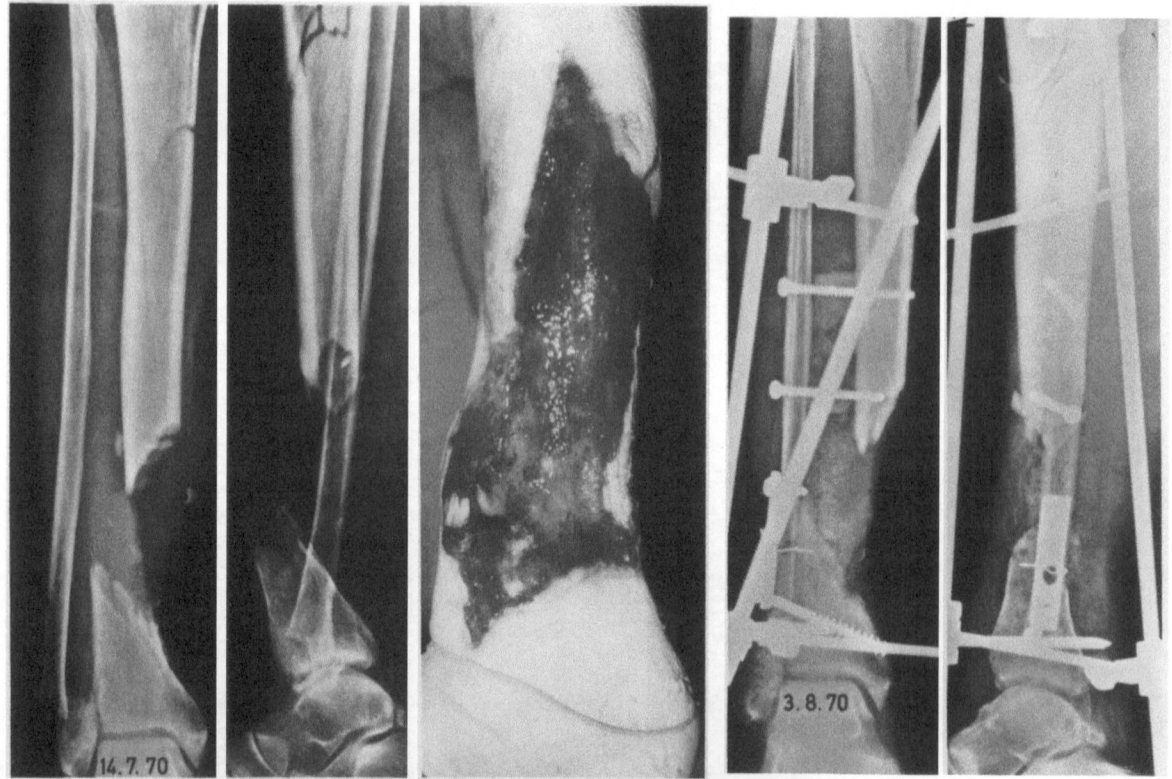

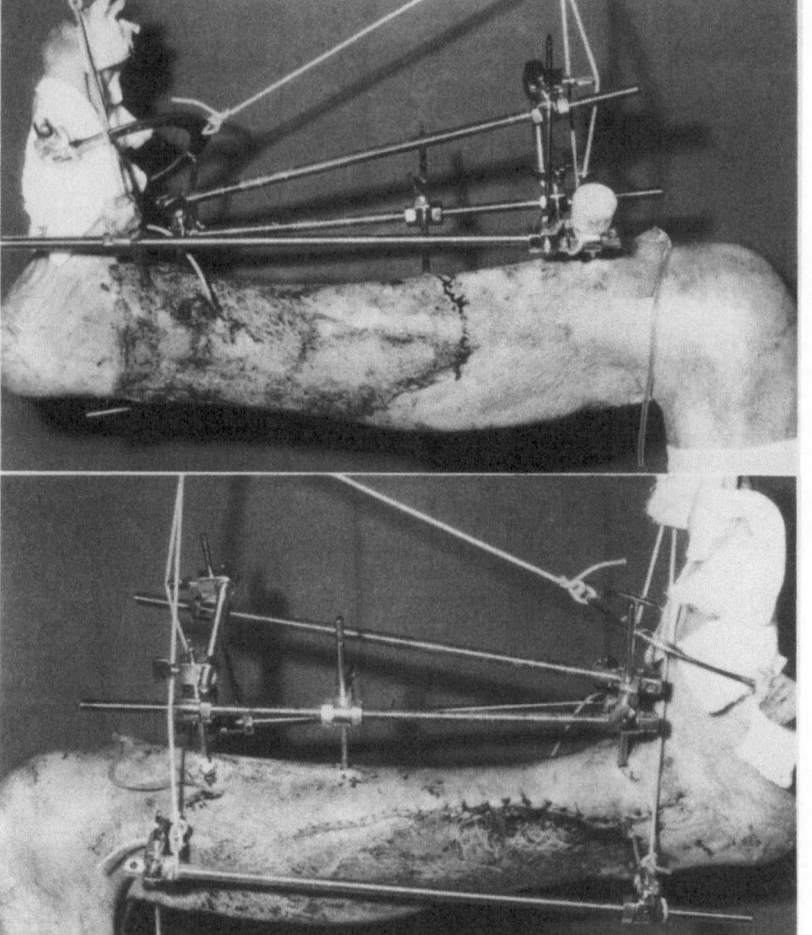

Fig. 228 a–e. Infected fracture with osseous defect following open fracture and amputation injury of opposite side. Unilateral and bilateral frame + minimal internal fixation. K.J., 1922, 48 years, ♂, 141979.

**a** Six weeks prior: open fracture with defect on right side, amputation injury of left tibia (abroad). At presentation: infected fracture with defect, lack of medial skin coverage.

**b** Three weeks after debridement, tibiofibular grafting, minimal internal fixation of fibula, external fixation for 4 months. Meshed Thiersch graft.

**c** Two weeks after Thiersch graft: cutaneous coverage is restored. Local care with tibia suspended. Equinus prevention with stirrup and Steinmann pins.

**d** Two years postinjury: Full weight bearing protected by below-knee caliper. Skin "unstable" medially and distally. Opposite side: below-knee prosthesis.

**e** Five years postinjury: stress-competent distal tibia, orthosis. No infection. Removal of implants

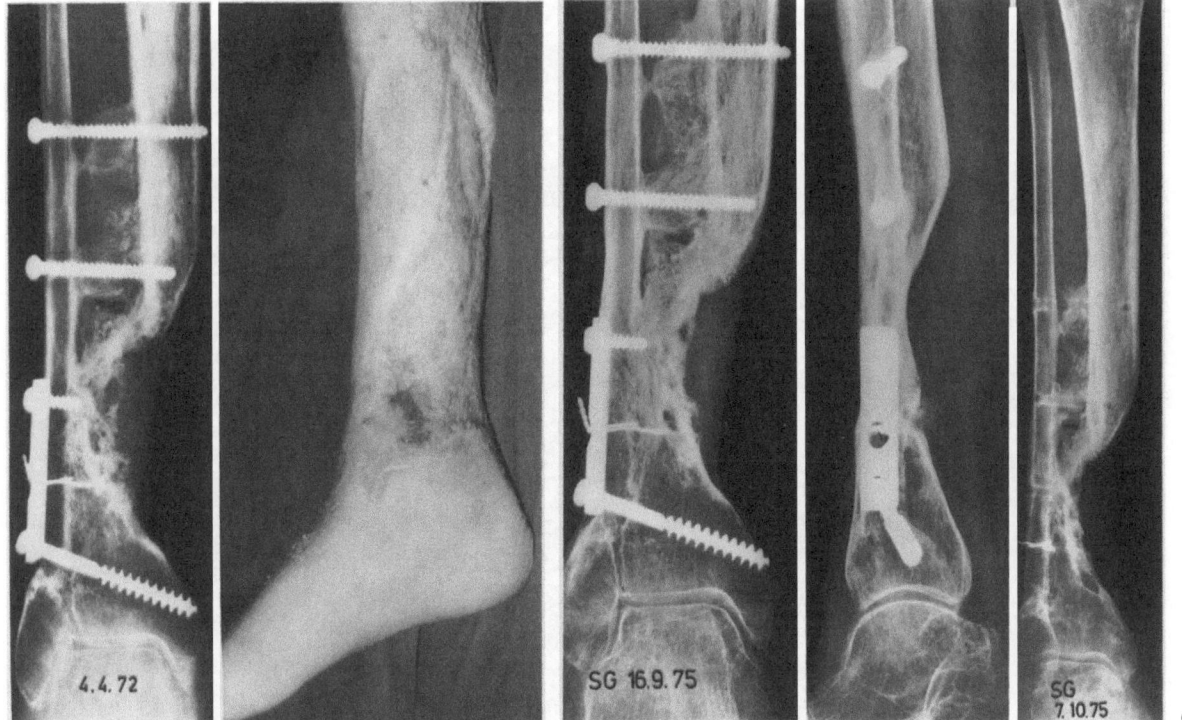

d    4.4.72                                    SG 16.9.75                                    SG
                                                                                             7.10.75    e

**Fig. 228d, e**

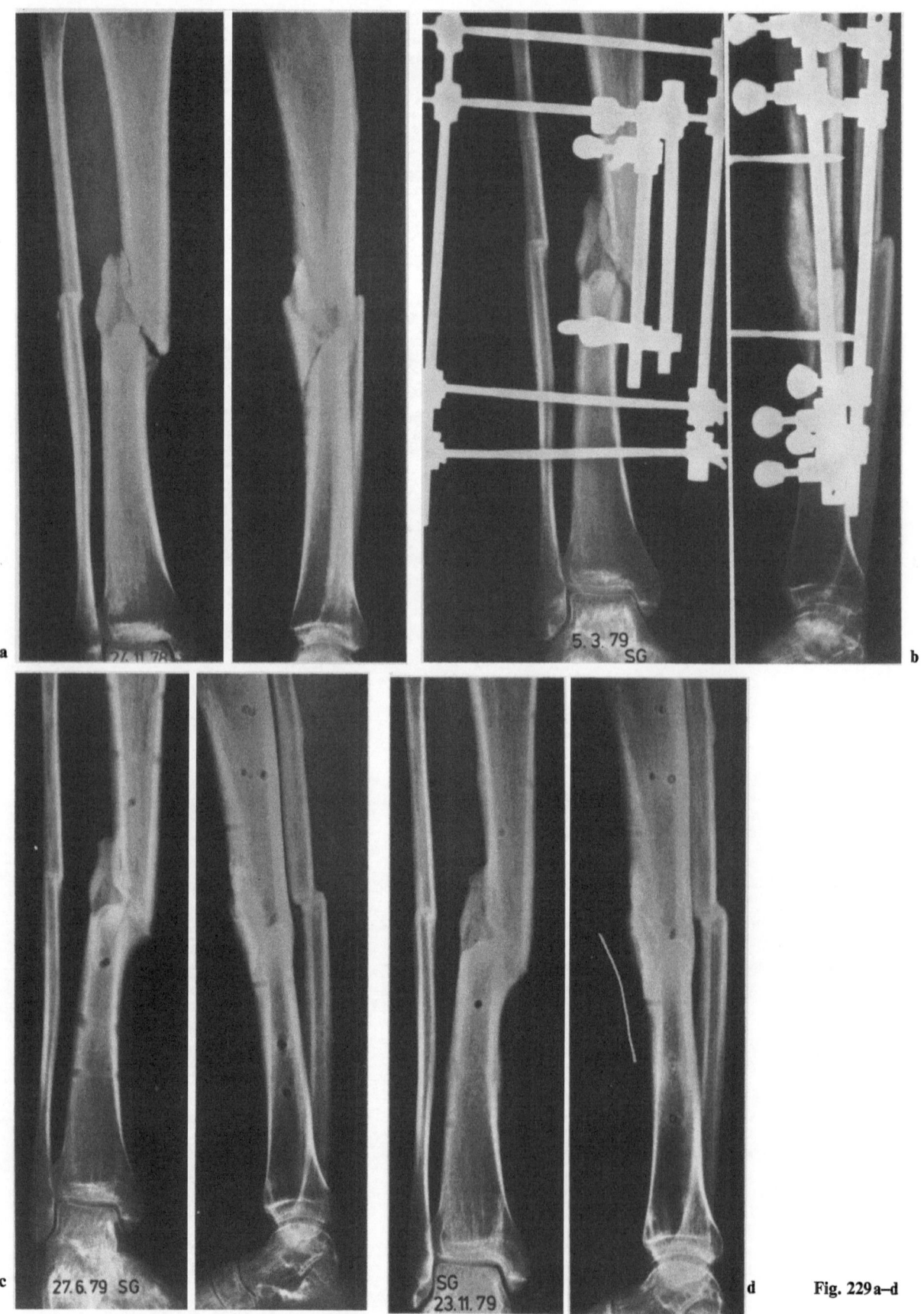

Fig. 229a–d

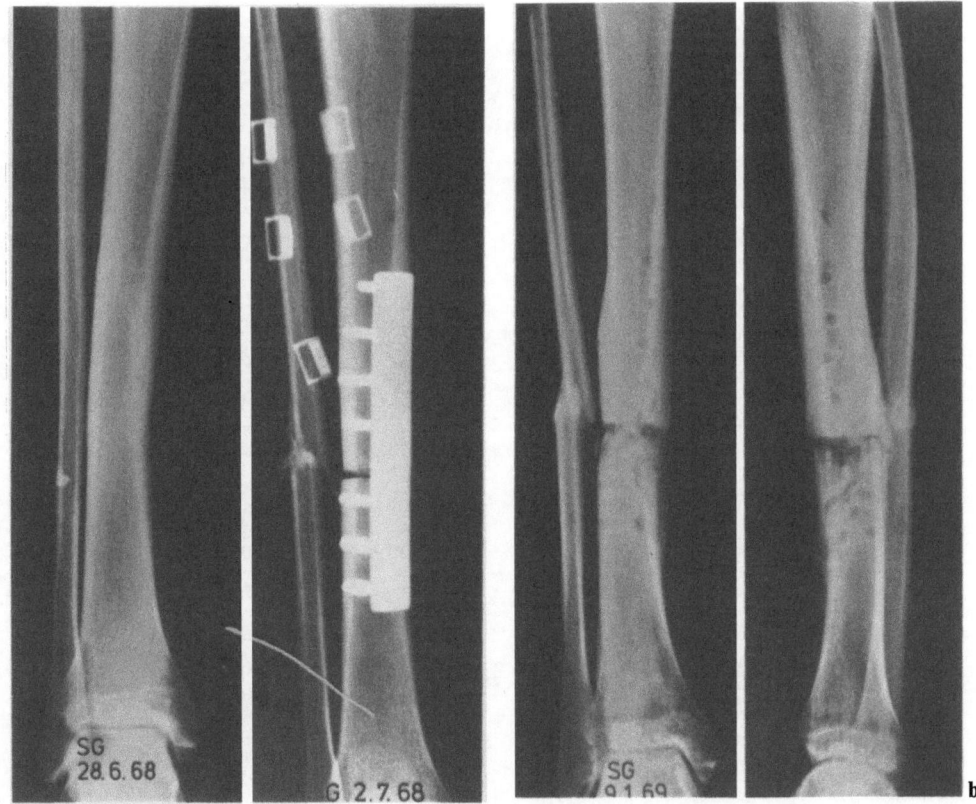

**Fig. 229 a–d.** Infected nonunion following open fracture and primary cast immobilization. Bilateral frame. G.E., 1955, 23 years, ♂, 224645.

**a** Ten months previously: open fracture. Plaster. Infection (abroad).
**b** At presentation: infected nonunion, sinus. Without local measures, unilateral and bilateral neutralization frame for 3 months, then Sarmiento brace for 2 months.
**c** Six months after initial treatment: nonunion is solid, sinus has closed spontaneously.
**d** Eleven months after external fixation: complete recovery

**Fig. 230 a–f.** Infected nonunion following corrective osteotomy. Bilateral frame. C.F., 1940, 29 years, ♂, 127884.

**a** Malrotation following healed tibial fracture, osteotomy, infection, plate removal (abroad).
**b** At presentation 6 months after osteotomy: infected nonunion, sinus.
**c** Two weeks after bilateral compression frame for 3 months, decortication + cancellous bone graft.
**d** After 10 weeks external fixation, 2 weeks before removal and Sarmiento brace for 6 weeks. Eight months after external fixation: nonunion and sinus are healed.
**e, f** Fourteen years after initial treatment: complete recovery

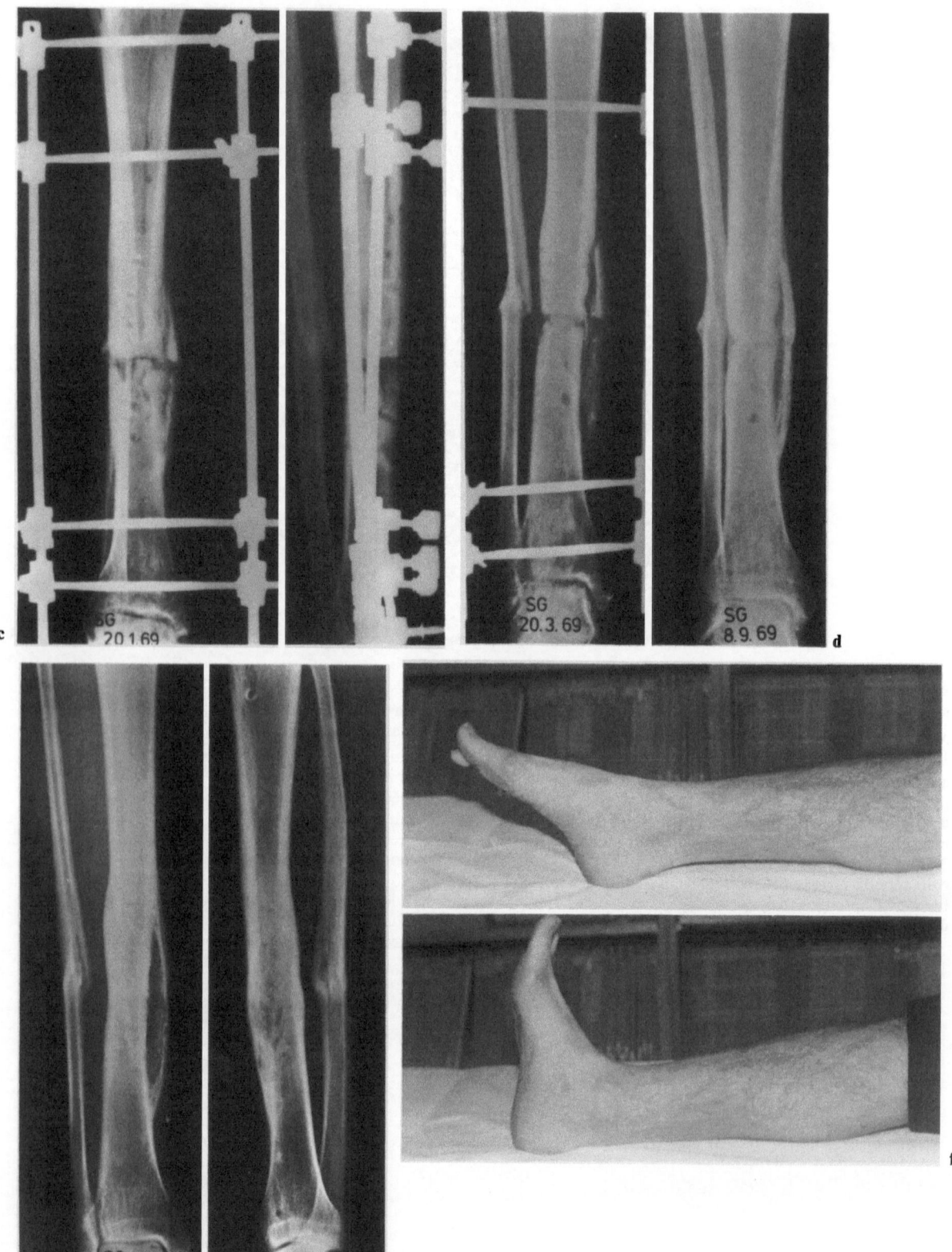

**Fig. 230c–f.** Legend see p. 195

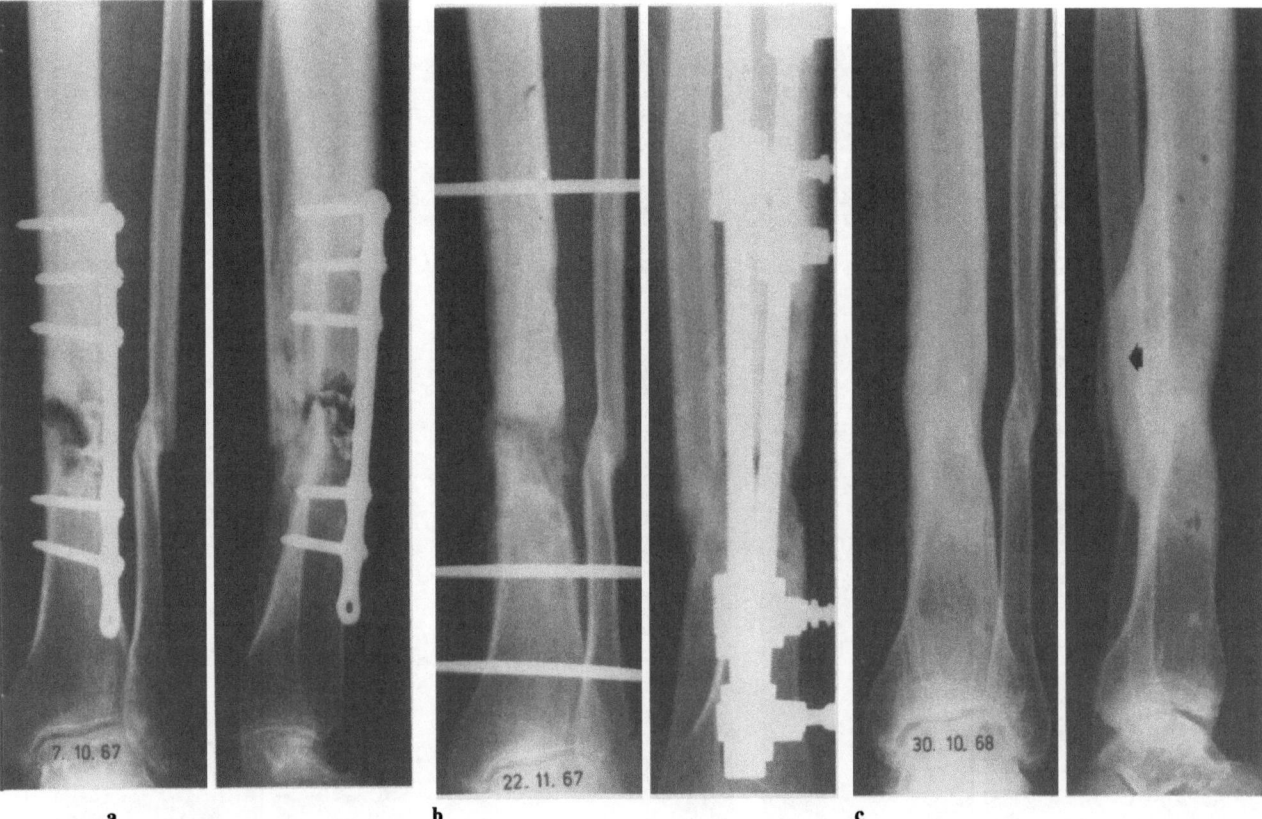

a    b    c

**Fig. 231 a–c.** Infected nonunion following closed fracture and internal fixation. Bilateral frame. K.K., 1944, 23 years, ♂, 116905.

**a** Six months prior: closed fracture, internal fixation, infection (abroad). At presentation: infected nonunion, sinus. Plate removal, suction irritation.
**b** Six weeks after start of treatment: bilateral neutralization frame for 3 months, posteromedial cancellous bone graft. After removal of fixator 2 months in walking cast.
**c** One year after start of treatment: complete recovery. Note posteromedial bridge of cancellous bone ( → )

**Fig. 232 a–d.** Infected nonunion following open fracture and cast immobilization. H.H., 1946, 22 years, ♀, 96491.

**a** Two years previously: open fracture, conservative treatment in plaster. Infection. Sinus (abroad). At presentation: infected nonunion, sinus.
**b** One month after medial decortication + sequestrectomy + cancellous bone graft. Varus deformity corrected with bilateral compression frame for 10 weeks + fibular osteotomy.
**c** Ten weeks after external fixation: nonunion is solid, sinus is closed.
**d** Twenty-six months after external fixation: complete recovery

**Fig. 233 a–d.** Infected nonunion following closed fracture and internal fixation. Bilateral frame. W.H., 1934, 42 years, ♀, 191781.

**a** Eight months previously: closed tibial fracture, plate fixation, infection, plate removal (abroad). At presentation: infected nonunion with medial sinus and valgus angulation.
**b** One month prior: sequestrectomy, cancellous bone graft, bilateral compression frame for 4 months with transverse compression. Then Sarmiento brace for 2 months. Six months after initial treatment: consolidation.
**c** At 1¹/₂ years the nonunion has healed in correct axial alignment.
**d** At 5 years recovery is complete

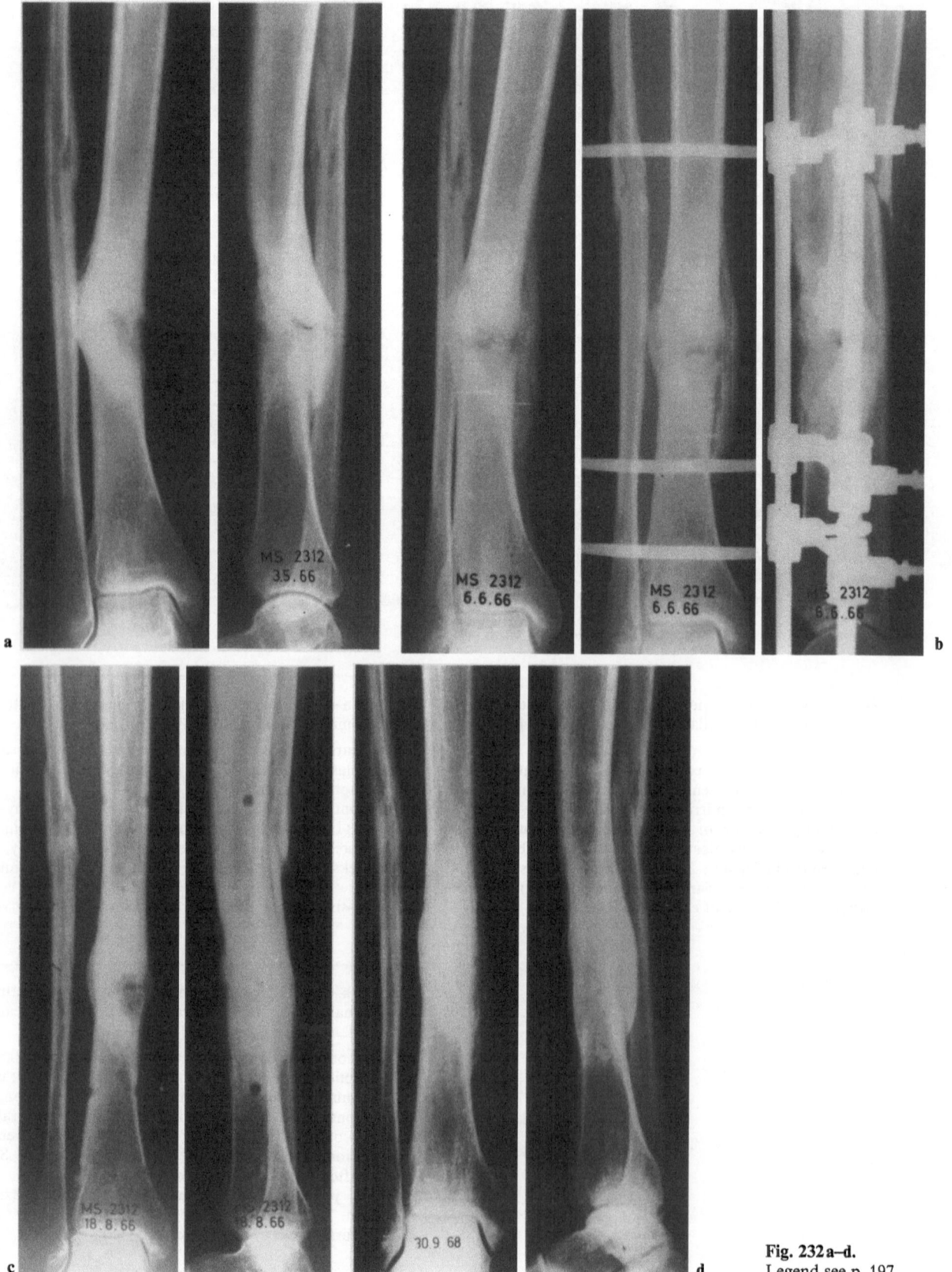

Fig. 232a–d.
Legend see p. 197

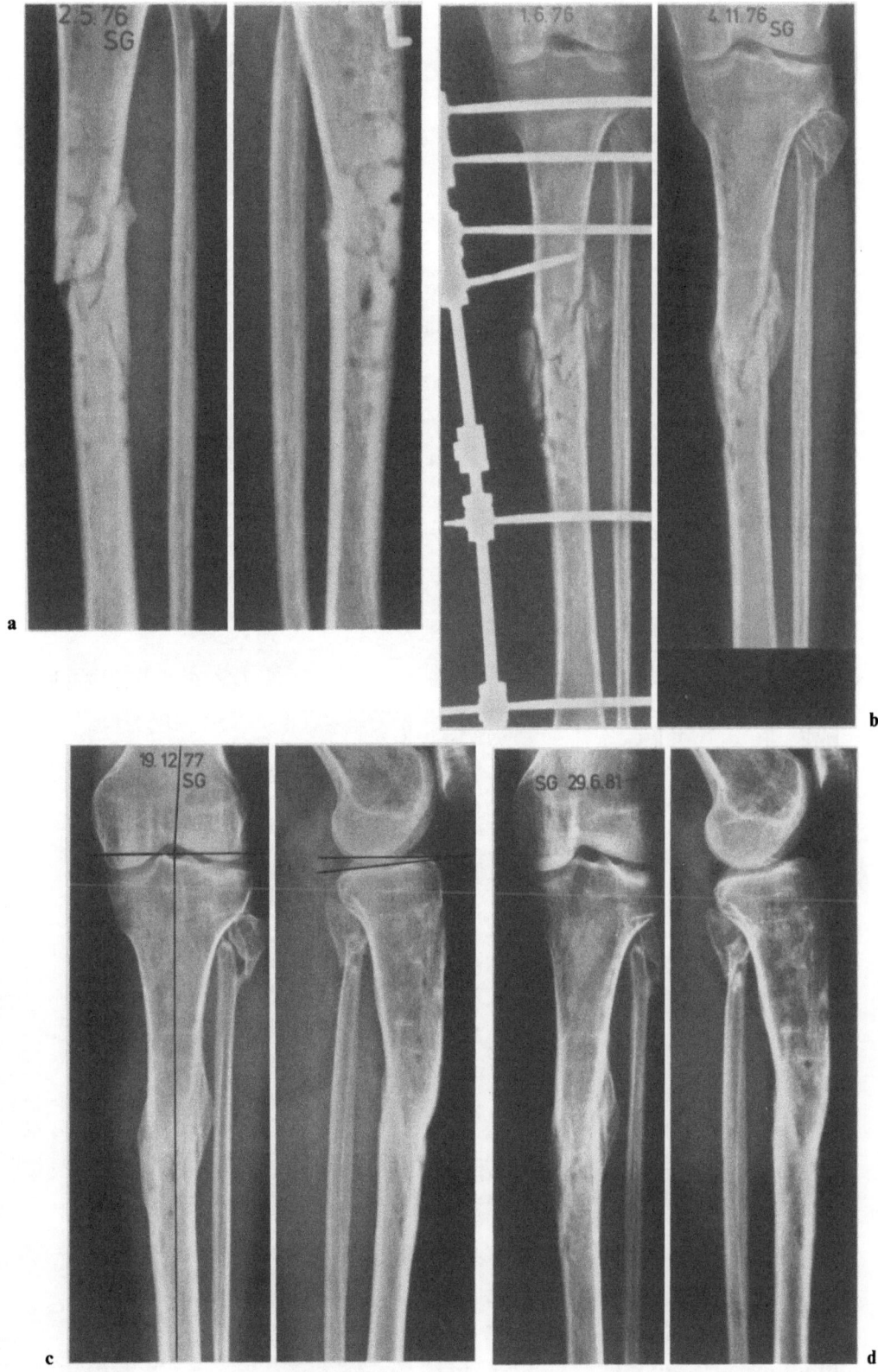

**Fig. 233a–d.** Legend see p. 197

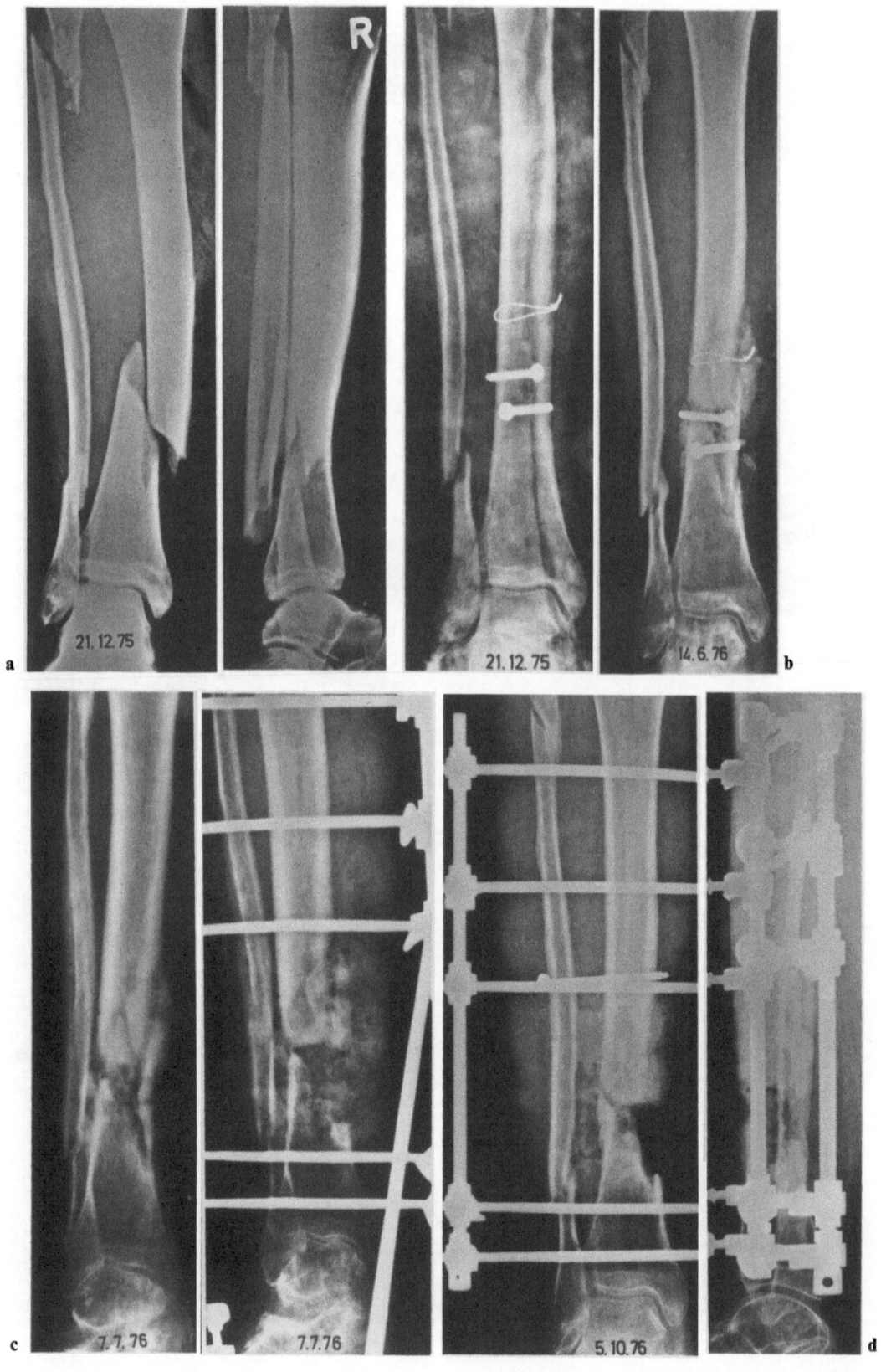

Fig. 234a–d

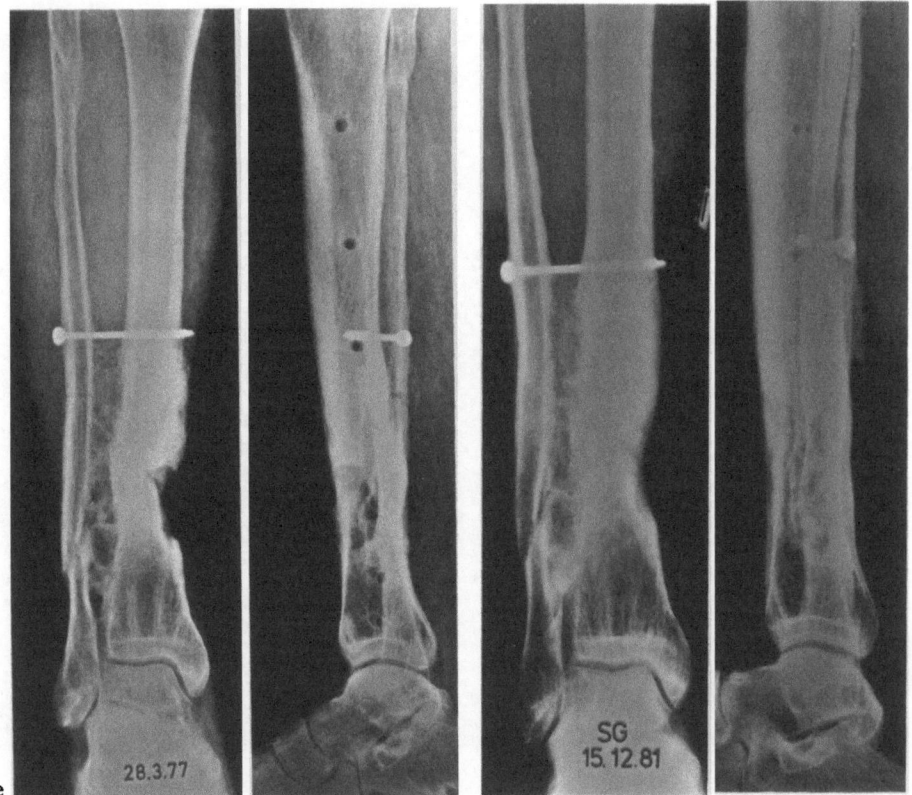

e 28.3.77    SG 15.12.81    f

**Fig. 234 a–f.** Infected nonunion following open fracture and internal fixation. Bilateral frame. B.A., 1943, 33 years, ♂, 144509.

**a, b** Open fracture, internal fixation, infection (abroad).
**c** At presentation $6^1/_2$ months after injury: infected nonunion with sinus, ulcer. Debridement, sequestrectomy, bilateral neutralization frame with anti-equinus frame for $3^1/_2$ months. Two weeks later Thiersch graft.
**d** Fibulotibial synostosis 5 weeks prior.
**e** Eight months after initial treatment: the nonunion is solid. Residual osteitis.
**f** $5^1/_2$ years after initial treatment, three additional bone debridements and Thiersch grafts: nonunion and infection are resolved. Function is normal

**Fig. 235 a–e.** Infected nonunion following open fracture and internal fixation. Bilateral frame. G.G., 1939, 23 years, ♂, 79548.

**a** Open tibial fracture, intramedullary nailing, infection. Removal of nail (abroad).
**b** At presentation 17 months postinjury: infected nonunion with osseous defect. Sinogram.
**c** Debridement, compression-resistant corticocancellous bone grafts, bilateral compression frame for 4 months. Graft take after $3^1/_2$ months.
**d** Five months after initial treatment: healing of nonunion and infection.
**e** Two years after treatment: complete recovery

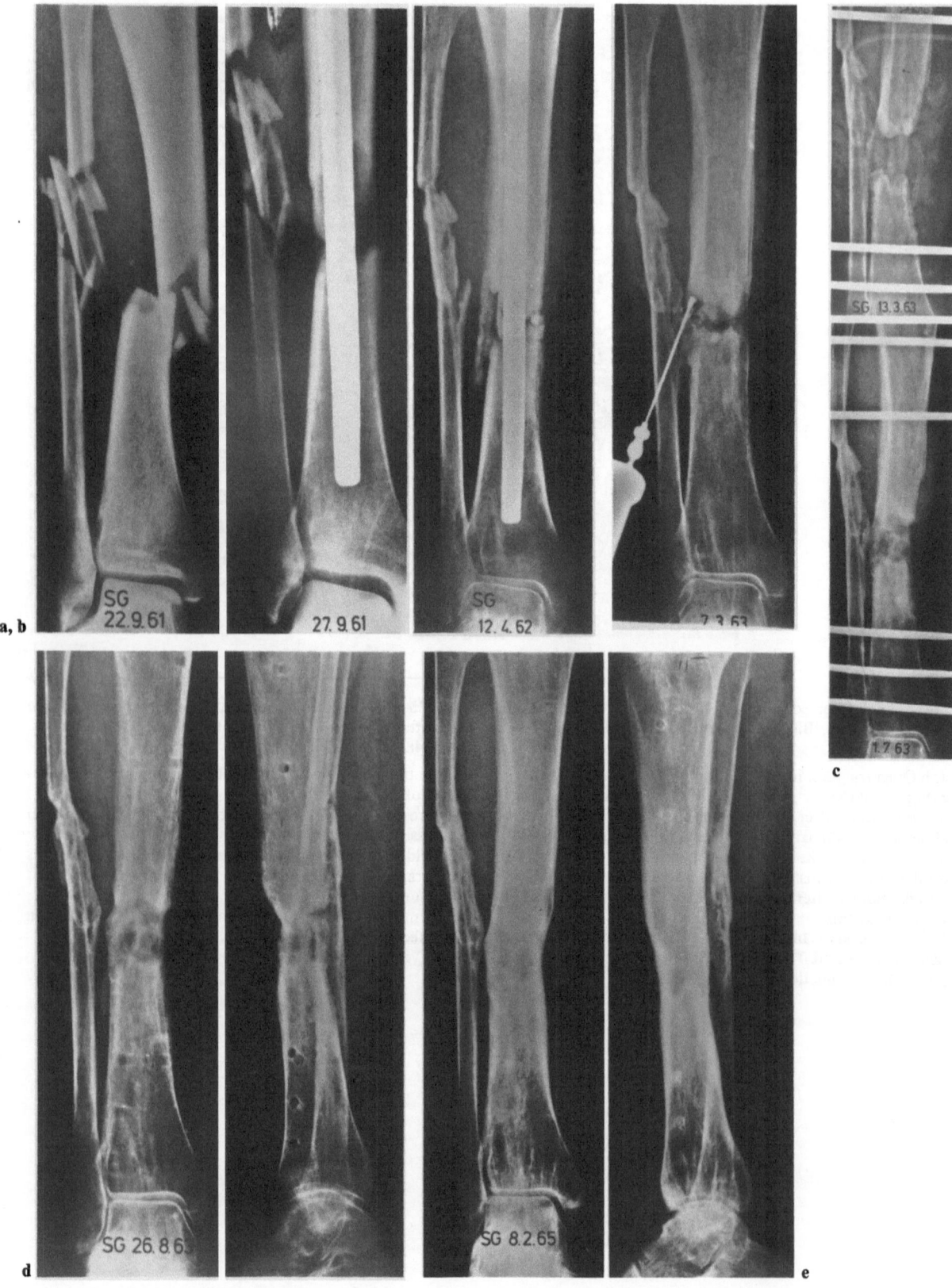

**Fig. 235a–e.** Legend see p. 201

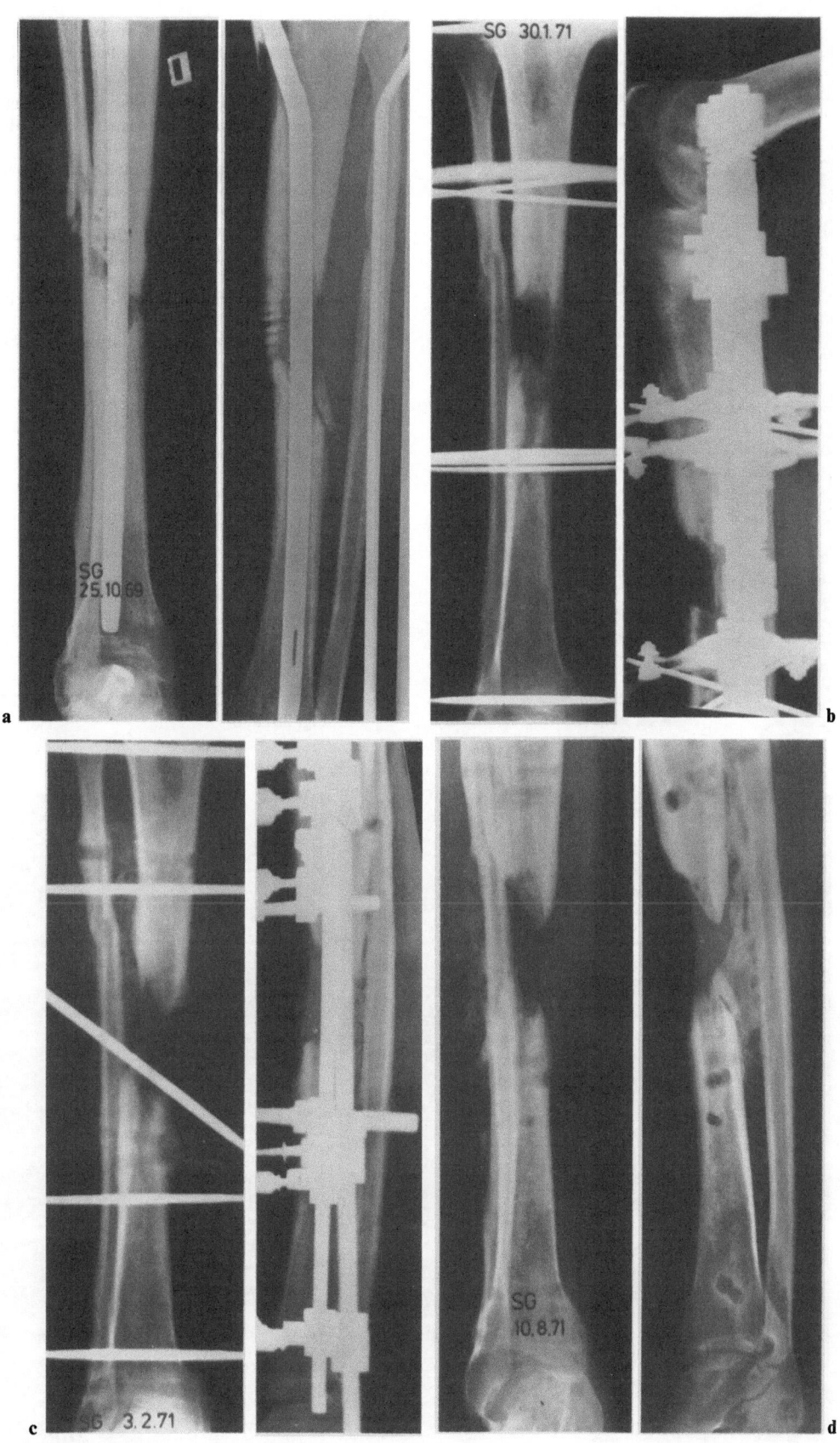

**Fig. 236a–d.**
Legend see p. 204

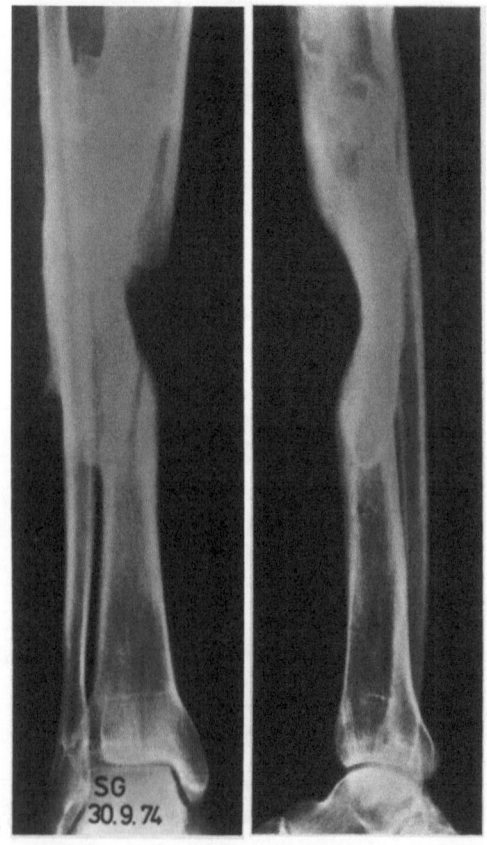

e

**Fig. 236 a–e.** Infected nonunion following closed fracture and internal fixation. Bilateral frame. S.W., 1927, 44 years, ♂, 146678.

**a** Six months previously: closed fracture, intramedullary nailing, infection. Sequestrectomy, drilling, nail extraction, external fixation (abroad).
**b** At presentation: infected nonunion with osseous defect. Loose Ilizarov frame in place.
**c** Removal of loose frame. Bilateral neutralization frame for 6 months. Open, anterolateral cancellous bone graft. Reverdin graft 1 month later.
**d** One month after removal of fixator. Infection has cleared but bone lacks adequate weight-bearing capacity. Below-knee orthosis for 1 year.
**e** Three years, 8 months after start of treatment: complete recovery

**Fig. 237a, b**

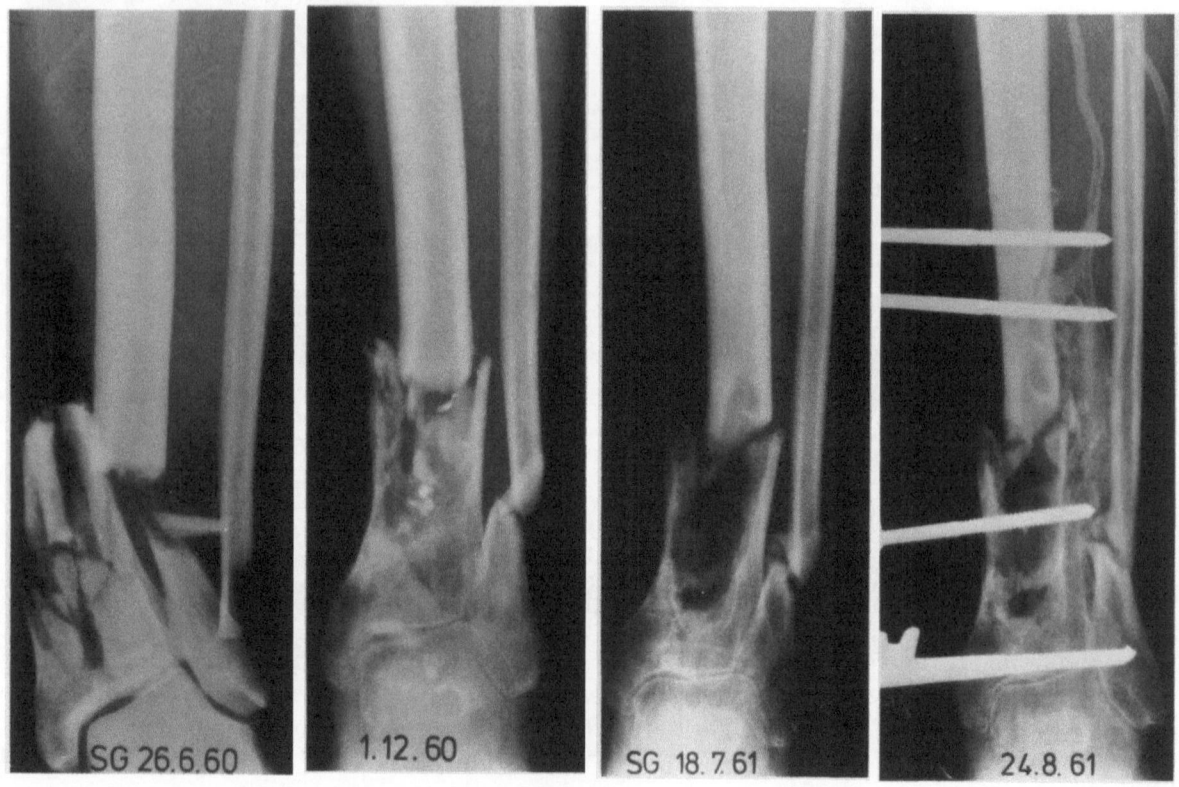

a

b

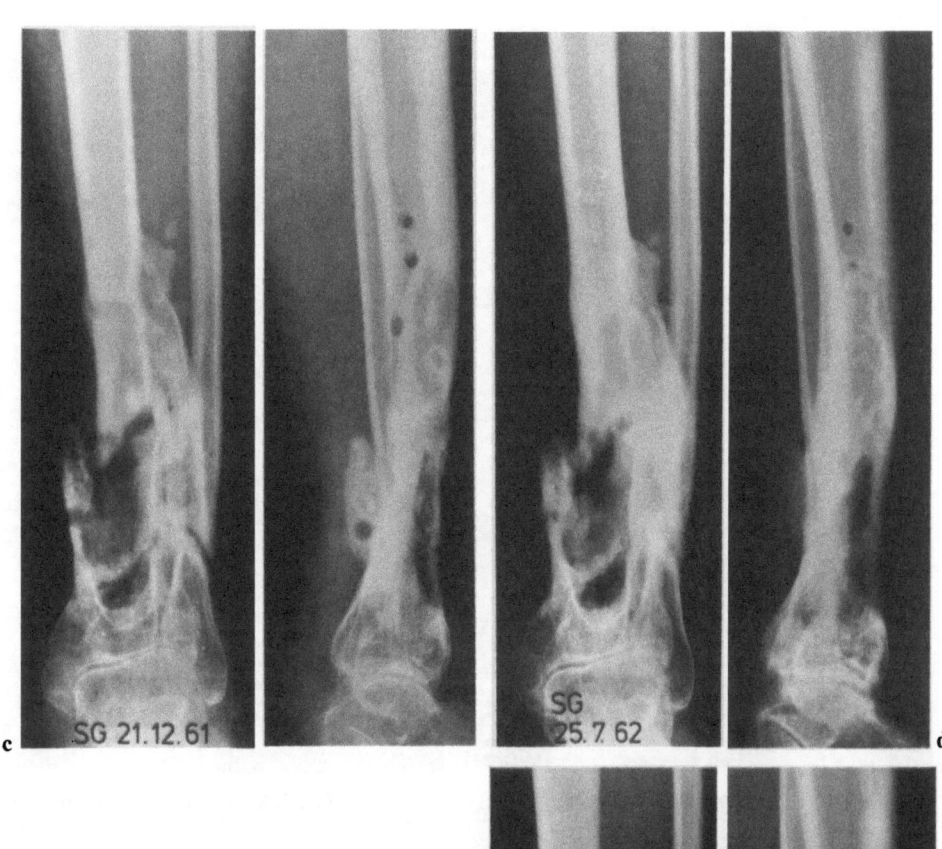

**Fig. 237 a–e.** Infected nonunion following open fracture and conservative treatment. Unilateral frame. B.B., 1938, ♂, 63325.

**a** Five months previously: open fracture, infection (abroad).
**b** At presentation 13 months postinjury: infected nonunion. Valgus unilateral frame for 4 months. Tibiofibular autogenous cancellous bone graft through lateral approach.
**c** Four months postoperatively: nonunion is reasonably solid. Saucerization + Thiersch graft.
**d** One year postoperatively: nonunion and infection are healed.
**e** Three years postoperatively: Healing is complete. Ankle joint is stiff and free of pain

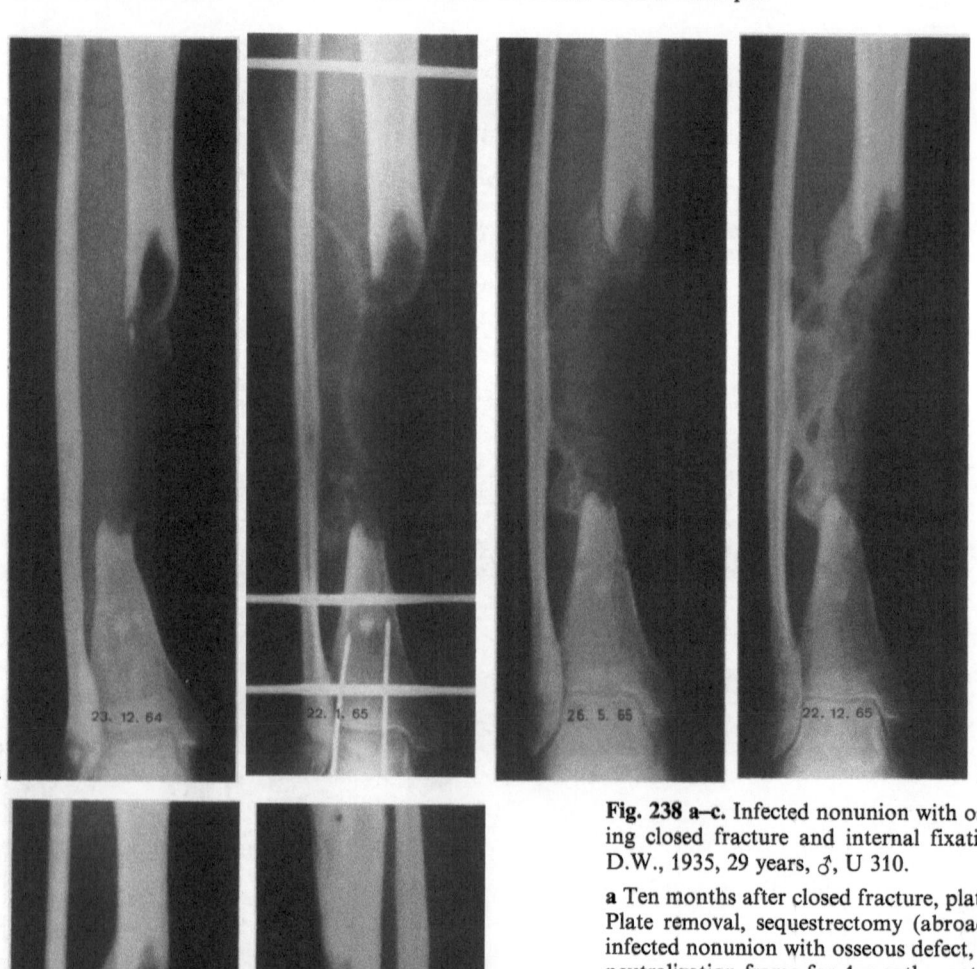

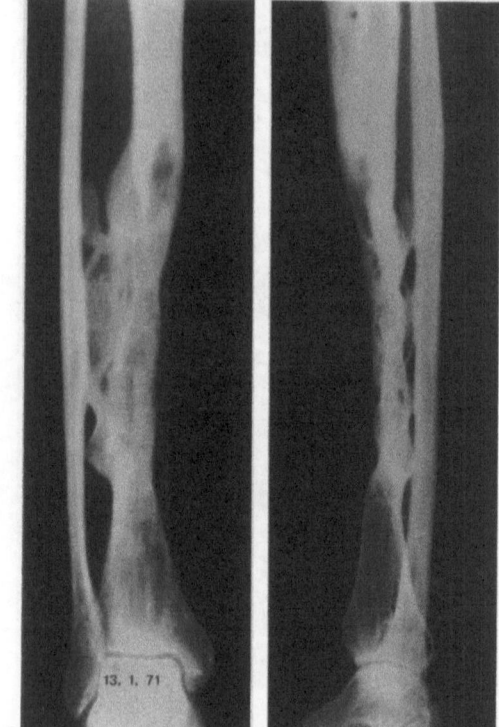

**Fig. 238 a–c.** Infected nonunion with osseous defect following closed fracture and internal fixation. Bilateral frame. D.W., 1935, 29 years, ♂, U 310.

**a** Ten months after closed fracture, plate fixation, infection. Plate removal, sequestrectomy (abroad). At presentation: infected nonunion with osseous defect, large ulcer. Bilateral neutralization frame for 4 months, anterolateral cancellous bone graft. Thiersch graft. Equinus control with axial Kirschner wire fixation of ankle joints.
**b** After removal of fixator, walking cast applied. Six months after initial treatment, 2nd bone graft is applied. Eleven months after initial treatment: limb can bear weight.
**c** Complete recovery at 6 years

**Fig. 239 a–d.** Infected nonunion following open fracture and external fixation. Osseous defect. Sagittal unilateral frame with shortening. G.P., 1945, 24 years, ♂, 127414.

**a** Three years previously: open fracture treated conservatively. Infection, external fixation (abroad).
**b** At presentation: infected nonunion, removal of loose fixator, application of a sagittal unilateral compression frame for 6 months with shortening, decortication.
**c** Six months after initial treatment: nonunion is healed.
**d** At 2 years the nonunion is healed and free of infection

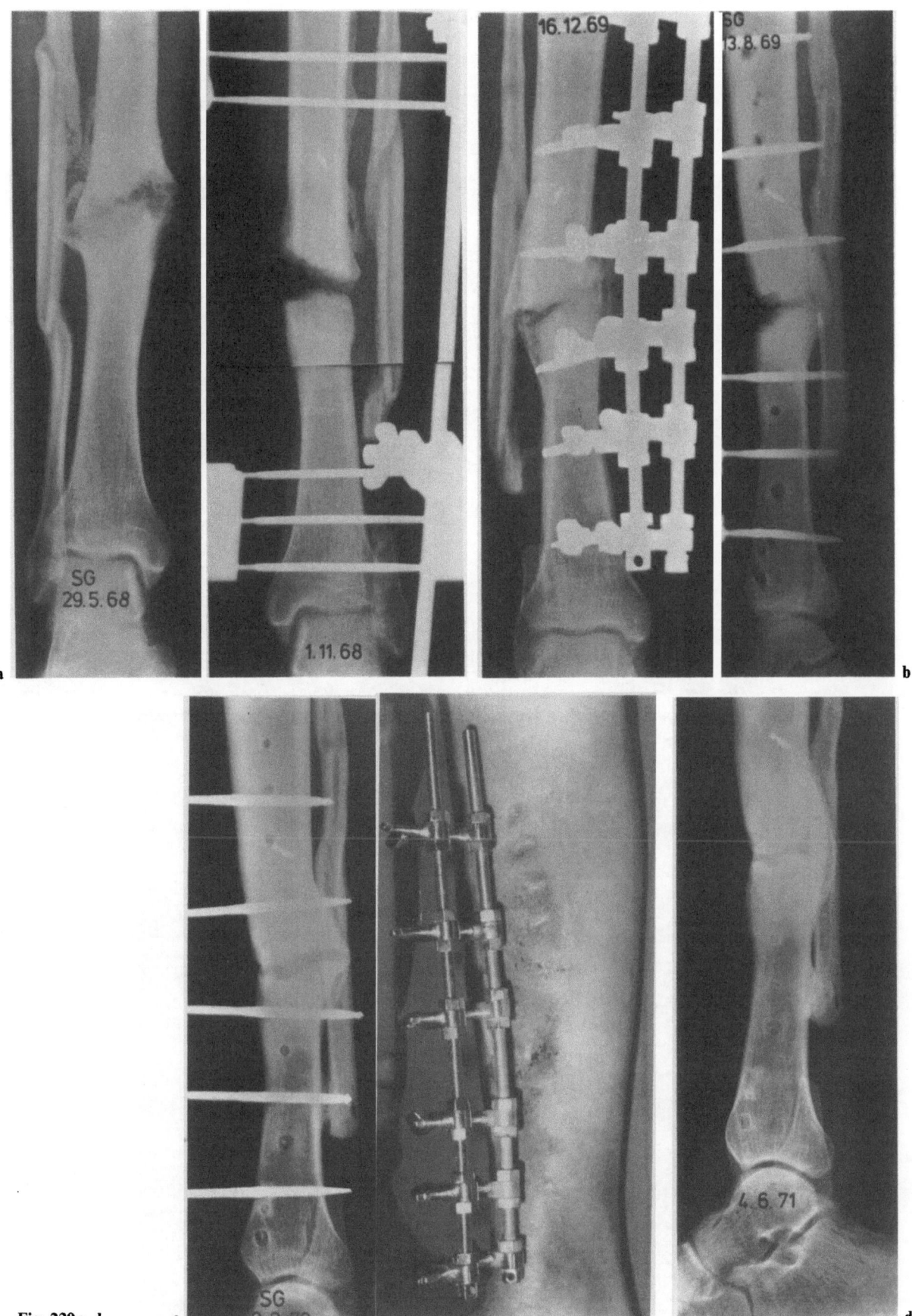

SG
29.5.68

1.11.68

16.12.69

SG
13.8.69

a

b

SG
9.2.70

4.6.71

Fig. 239a–d

c

d

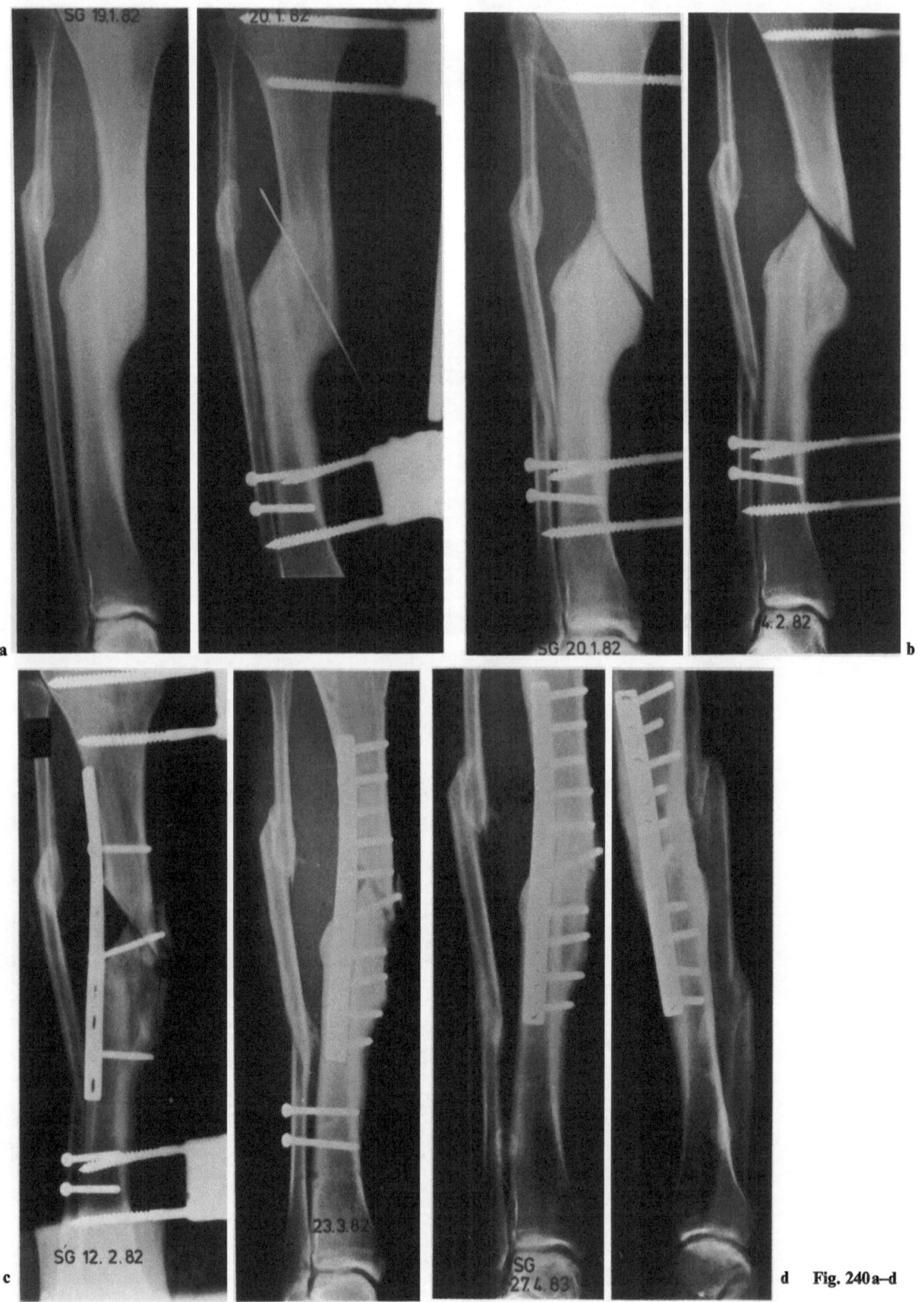

a   b   c   d   Fig. 240a–d

# 9 Ankle (Figs. 241–252)

**Examples:**

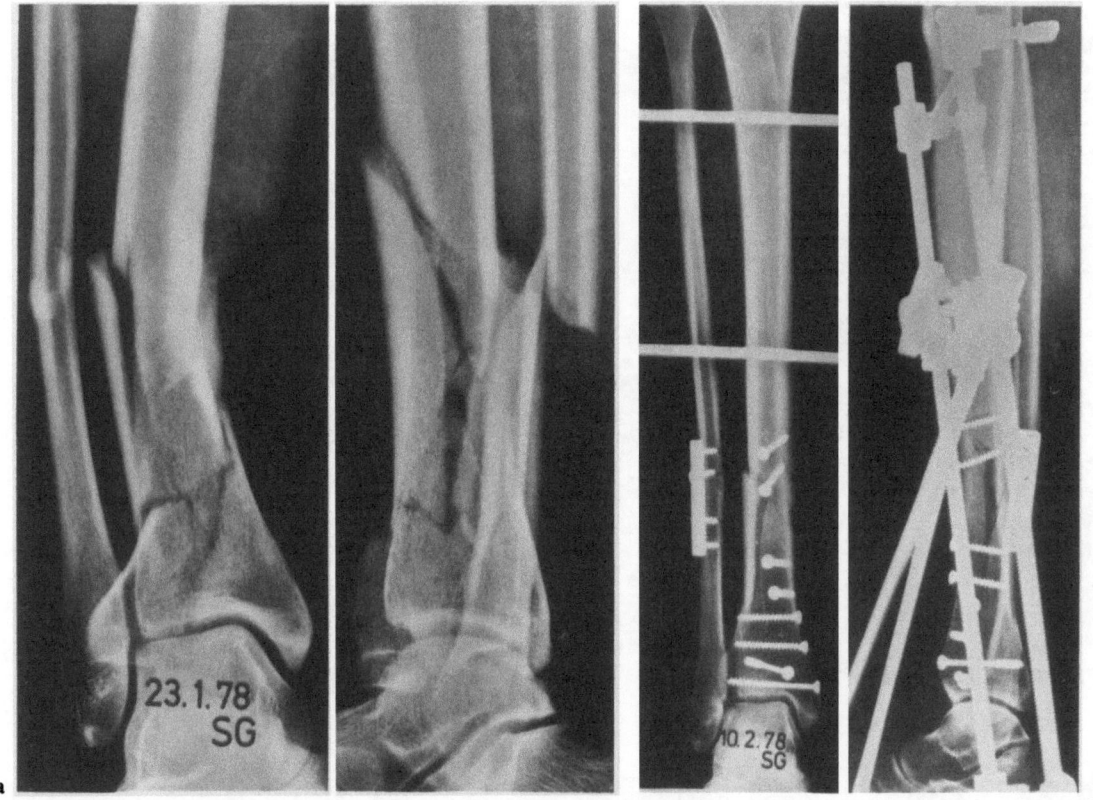

**Fig. 240 a–d.** Lengthening osteotomy. H.S., 1962, 20 years, ♀, 252480.

**a** Three years previously: tibial fracture managed conservatively (abroad). *1*: At presentation: 2.5-cm shortening, varus deformity. *2*: Intraoperative photo with Wagner frame in place: Schanz screws are inserted at desired angle of correction.
**b** Postoperatively and 1 month later: gradual lengthening and correction of axial deformity.
**c** Intraoperative photo and 6 weeks later: plating and cancellous bone graft.
**d** 1¼ years after correction: limb axis and length are normal, osteotomy is healed. Plate removal is planned

**Fig. 241 a–d.** Open tibial fracture with involvement of the ankle joint. Internal fixation + bilateral frame. S.T., 1935, 43 years, ♀, 215057.

**a** Grade II open impacted fracture of the distal tibia. Internal fixation + bilateral frame with anti-equinus frame for 8 weeks. Walking cast for 6 weeks.
**b** 2½ weeks postinjury: first-intention healing of soft tissues.
**c** Six months postinjury: fracture is consolidated. Initiation of normal weight bearing.
**d** Five years postinjury: normal walking ability. Incipient osteoarthritis of the ankle joint

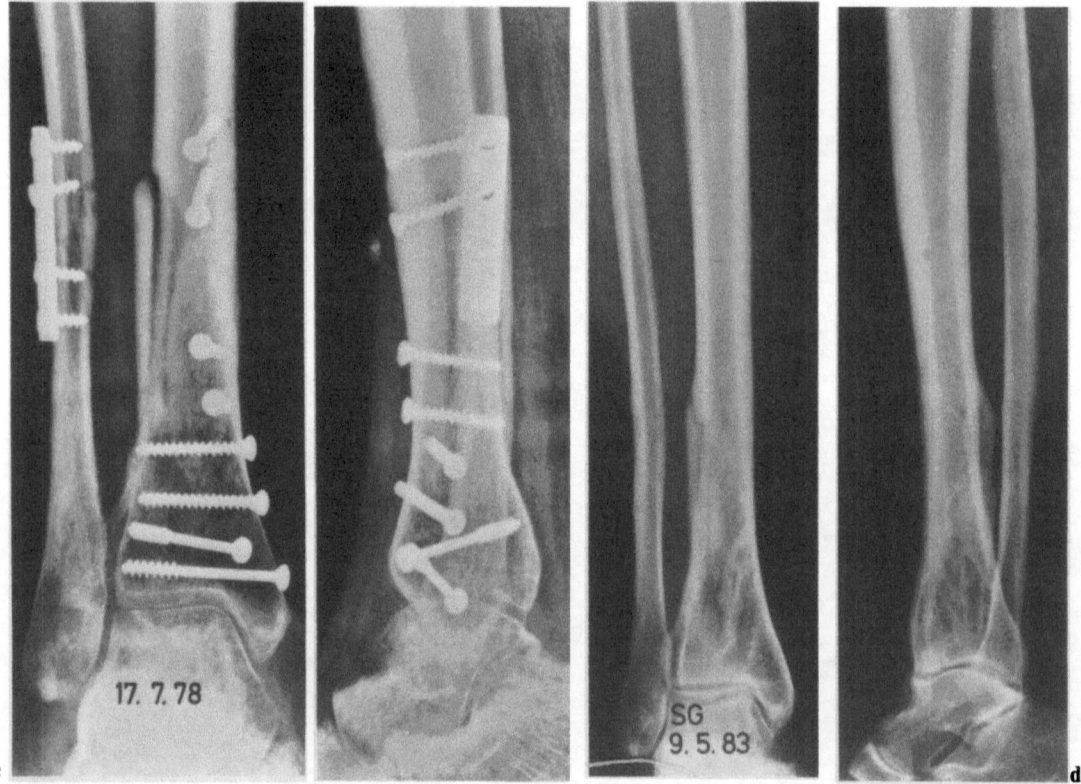

**Fig. 241c, d.** Legend see p. 209

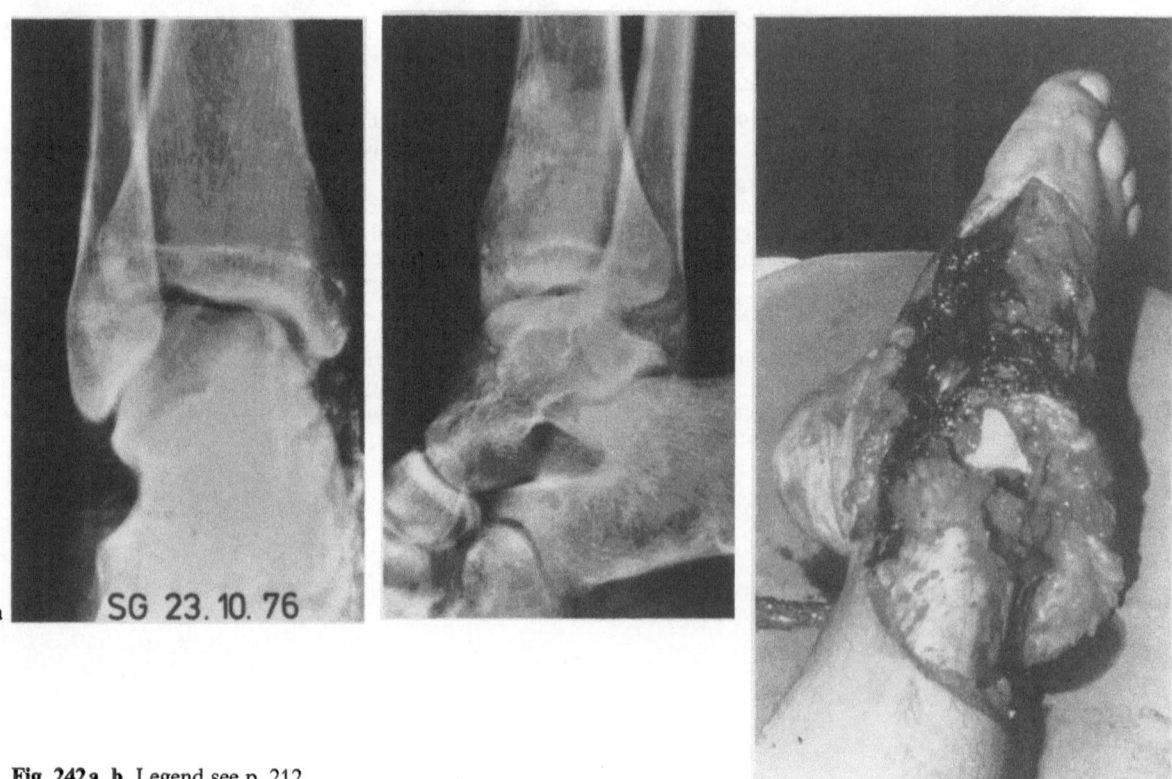

**Fig. 242a, b.** Legend see p. 212

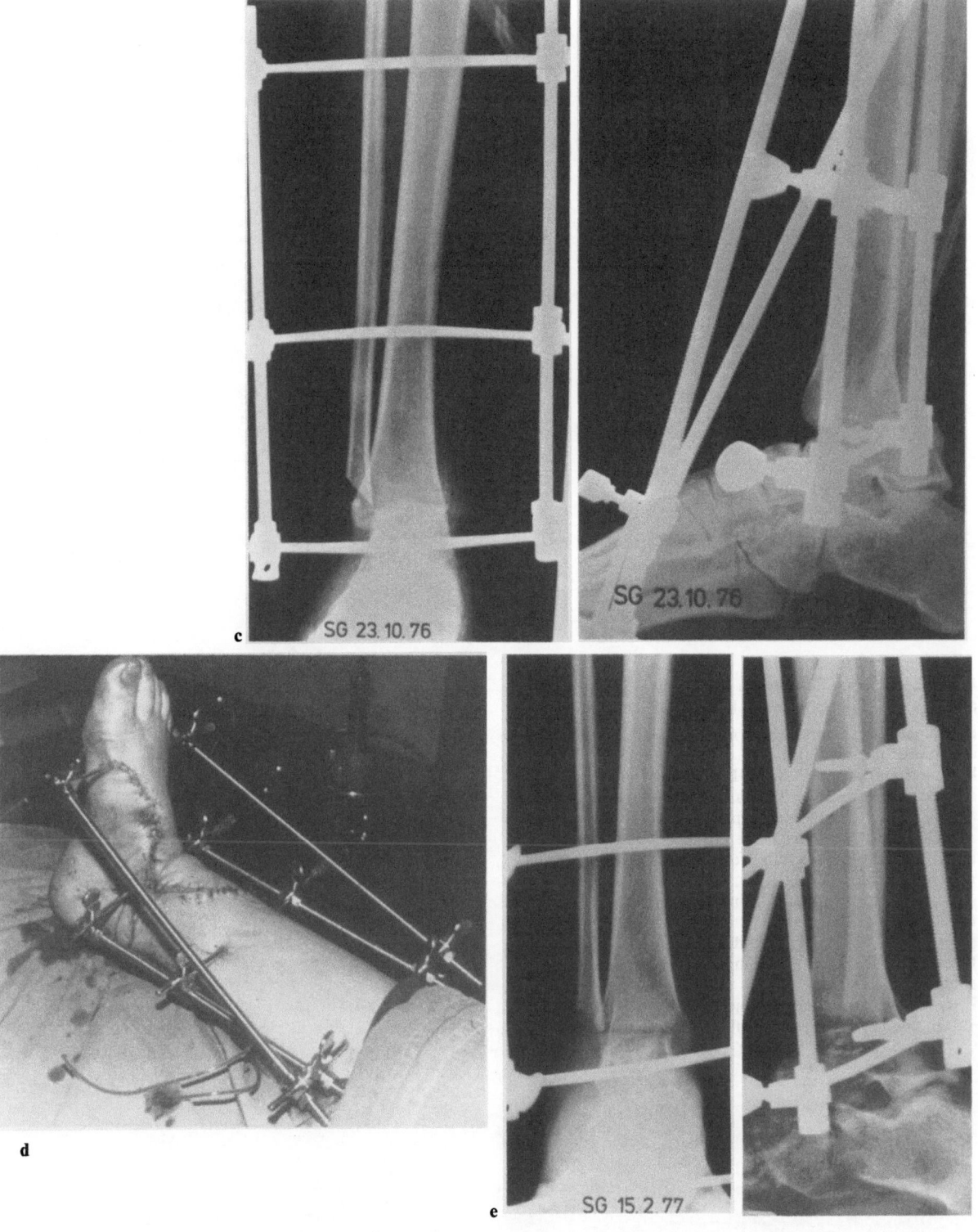

c

SG 23.10.76

SG 23.10.76

d

e

SG 15.2.77

**Fig. 242c–e.** Legend see p. 212

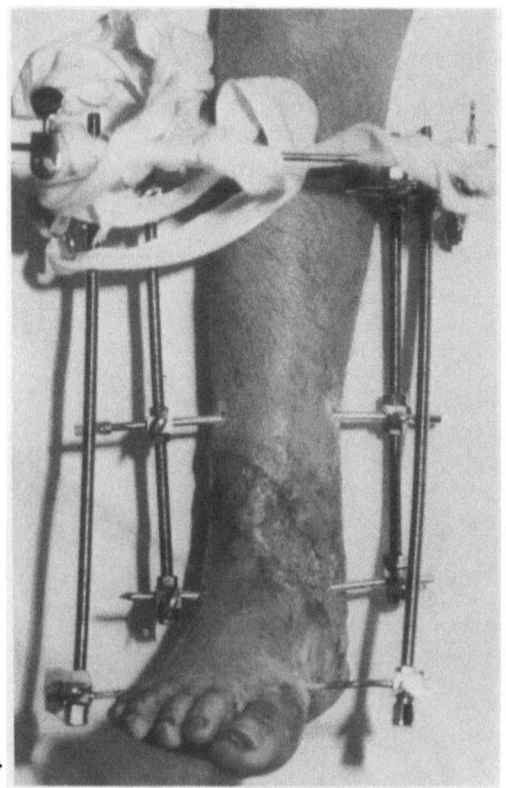

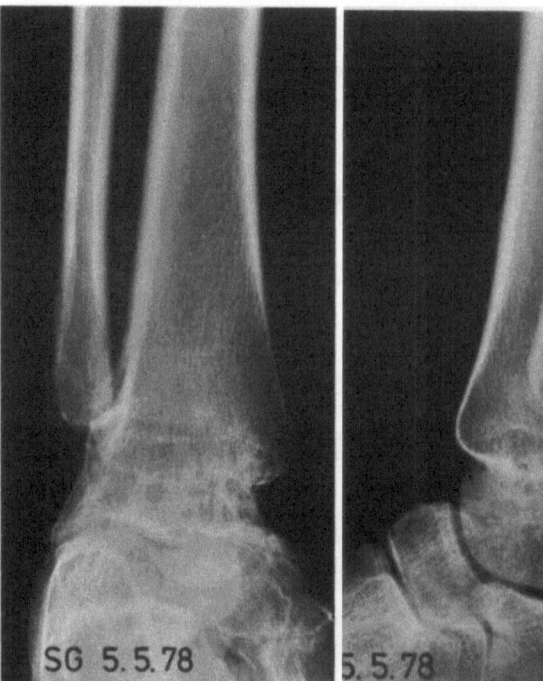

f

**Fig. 242f, g**

**Fig. 242 a–i.** Open dislocation of the ankle joint. Primary arthrodesis. Bilateral frame. R.I., 1960, 16 years, ♀, 202166.

**a** "Innocent" radiograph does not demonstrate severe damage to articular cartilage.

**b** Clinical appearance: Grade II soft tissue injury.

**c** Primary arthrodesis with bilateral compression frame for 4 months. Soft tissue care, repair of anterior tibial artery and all extensor tendons, nerve suture.

**d** Stable conditions favorable for soft tissue healing. Equinus prophylaxis.

**e** Four months postinjury: arthrodesis is solid.

**f** Soft tissues are healed

**g** Sixteen months postinjury: ideal arthrodesis.

**h** Seven years postinjury: compensatory hypermobility of subtalar joint.

**i** No subjective complaints, objective shortening of tibia by 1.5 cm, mild residua from pedal compartment syndrome

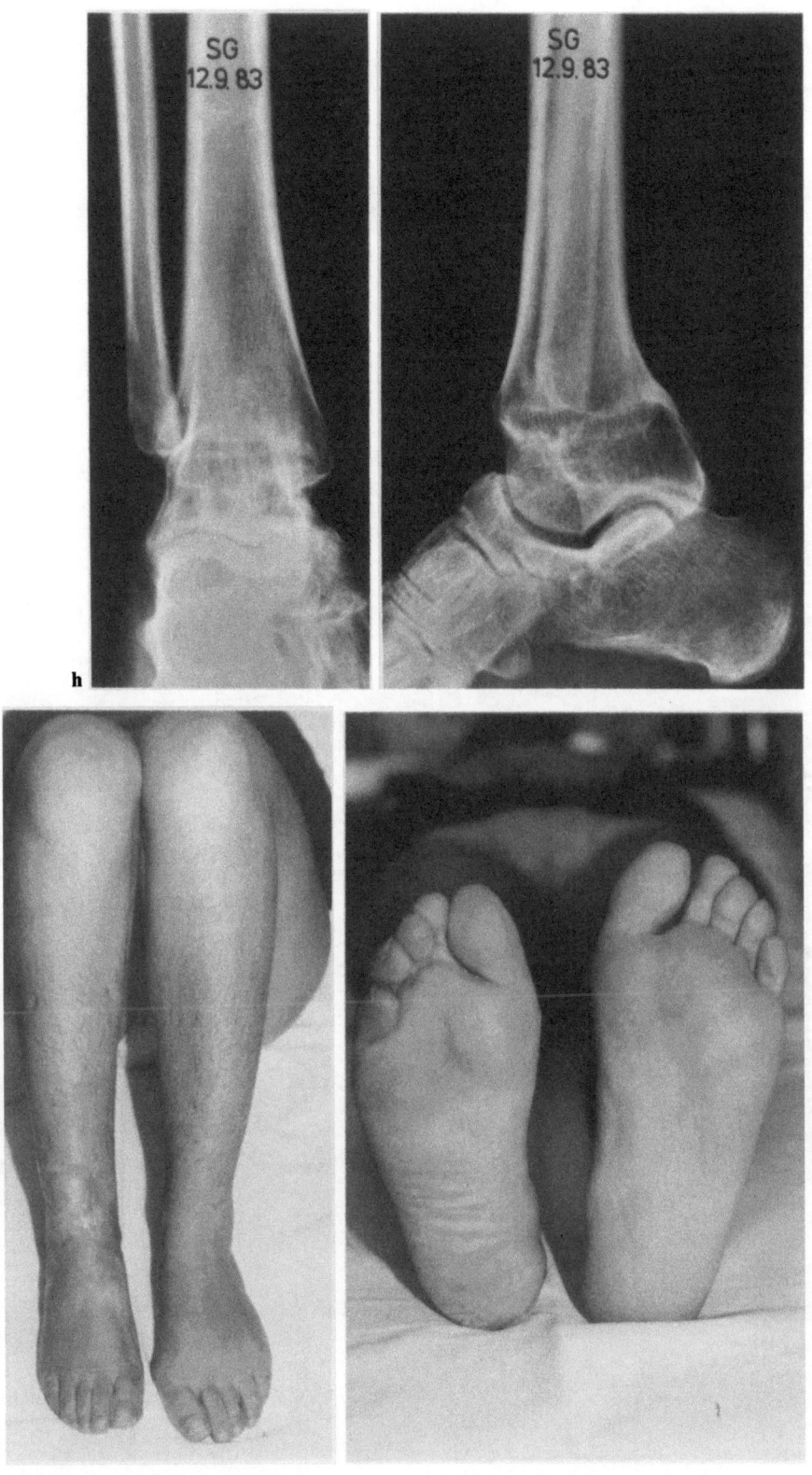

Fig. 242h, i

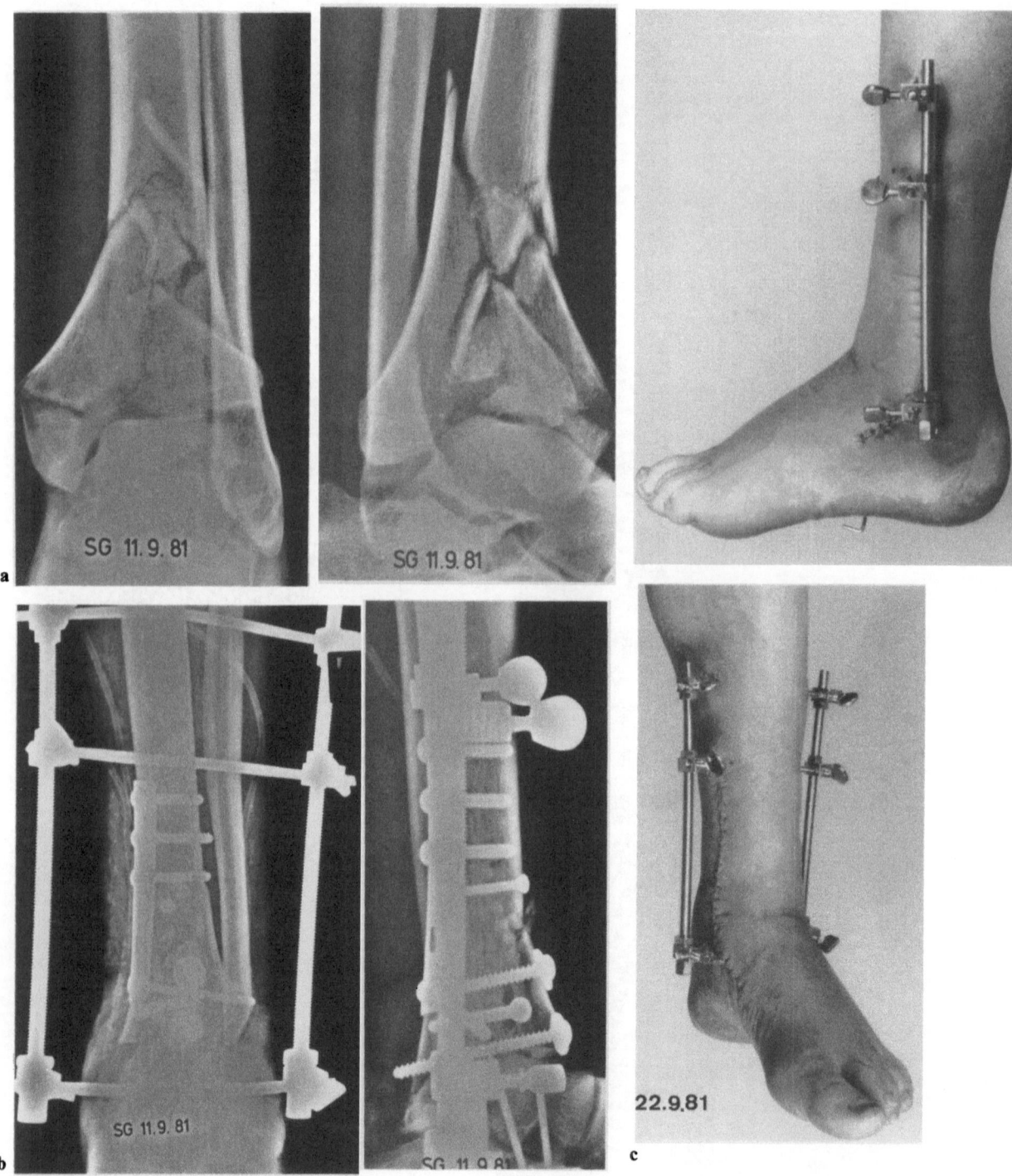

Fig. 243a–c

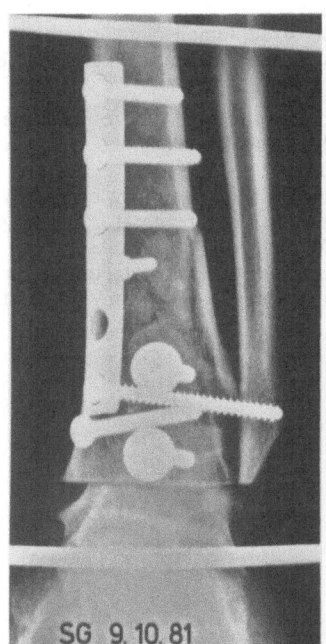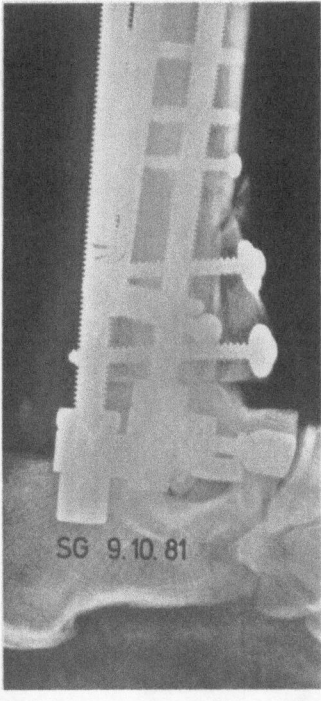

**Fig. 243 a–f.** Closed impacted fracture. Primary arthrodesis. Bilateral frame. C.G., 1937, 44 years, ♂, 187 584.

**a** Impacted fracture; shattered distal tibia.
**b** Primary compression arthrodesis with bilateral frame for 6 weeks + cancellous bone graft.
**c** Eleven days postinjury: normal trophism.
**d** One month postinjury, 2 weeks before frame removal and walking cast for 10 weeks.
**e** Eleven months postinjury: painful, distal tibiofibular nonunion. Synostosis of distal fibula.
**f** 1 3/4 years postinjury: normal walking ability

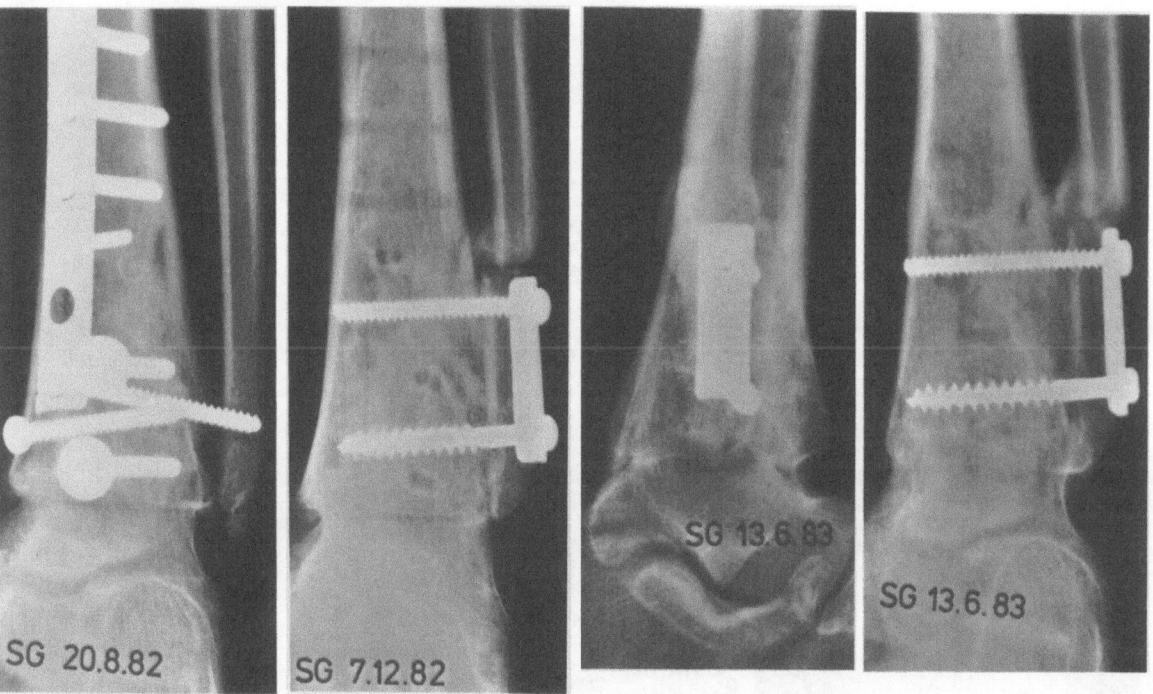

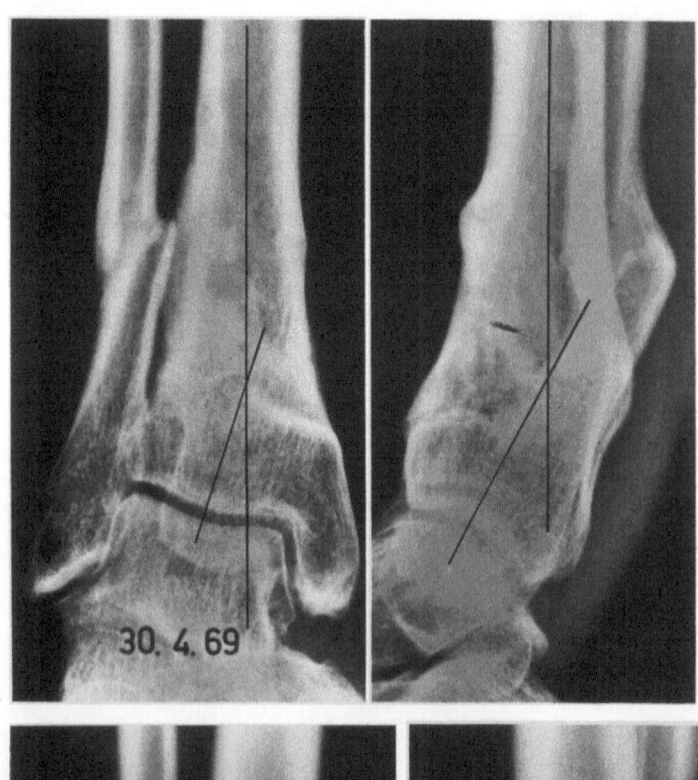

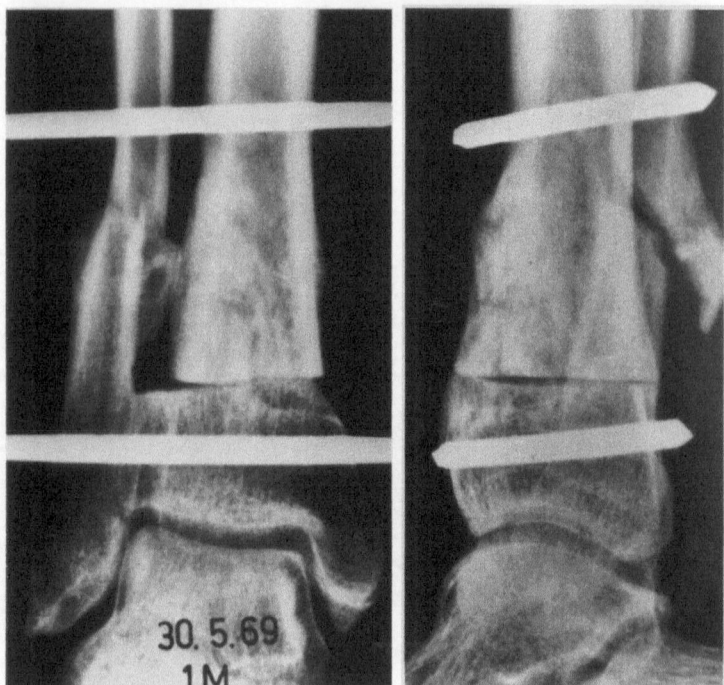

**Fig. 244 a–c.** Supramalleolar corrective osteotomy. Bilateral frame. B.E., 1941, 28 years, ♀, 131022.

**a** Axial deformity secondary to tibial fracture (abroad): 18° valgus, 22° posterior angulation.
**b** One month after corrective osteotomy. Fixation with small bilateral frame for 4 weeks. Walking cast for 6 weeks.
**c** Eighteen months after osteotomy: normal limb alignment. Osteotomy is remodeled

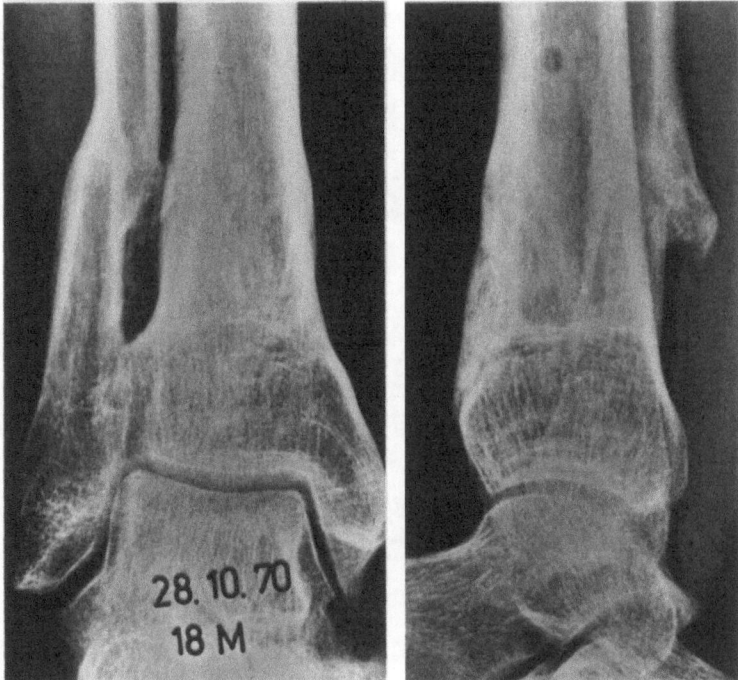

Fig. 244c

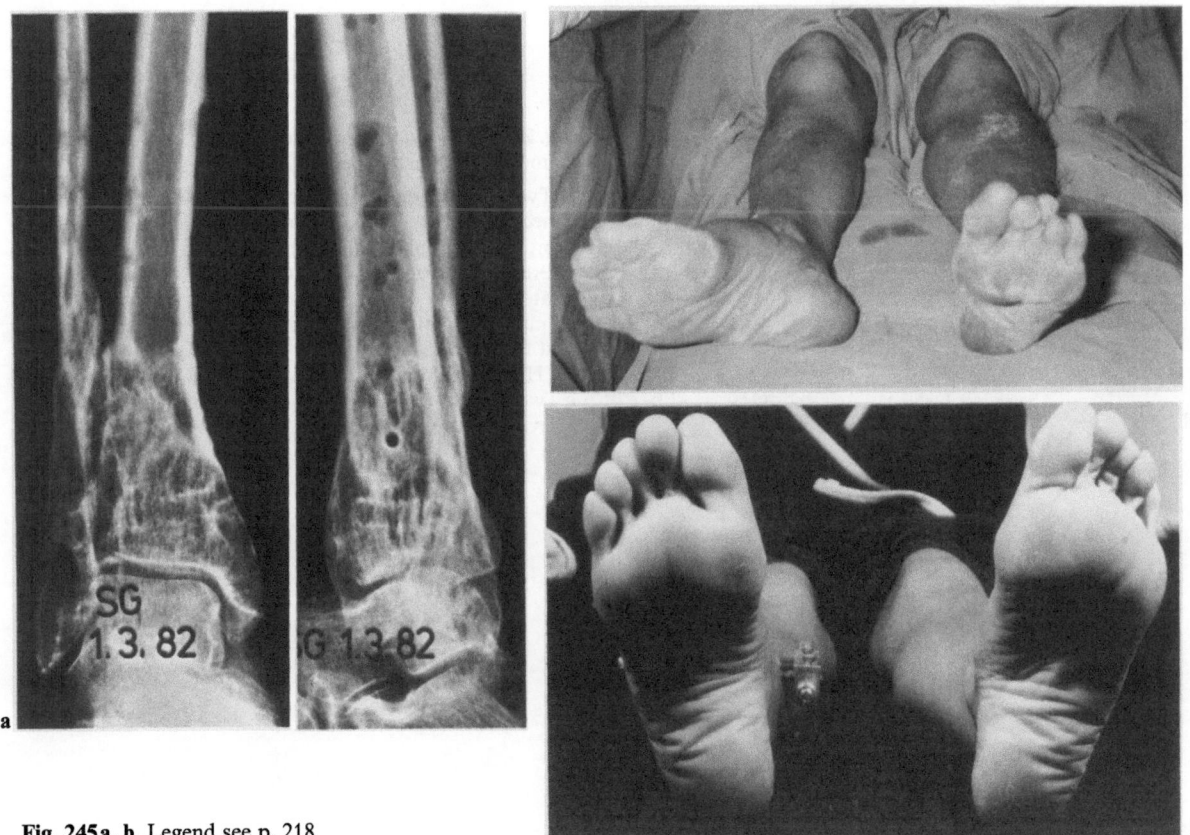

Fig. 245a, b. Legend see p. 218

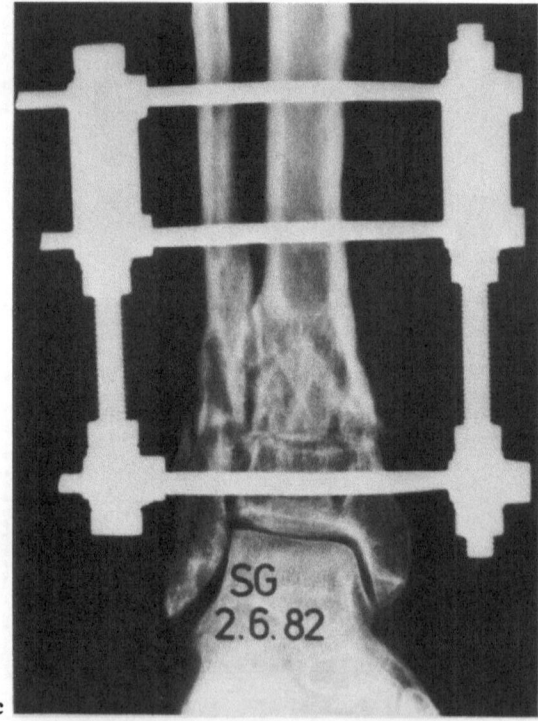
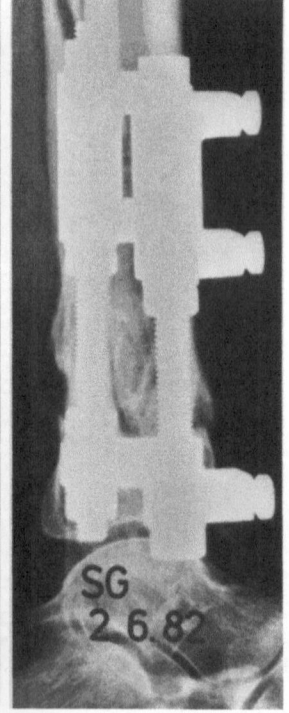

c

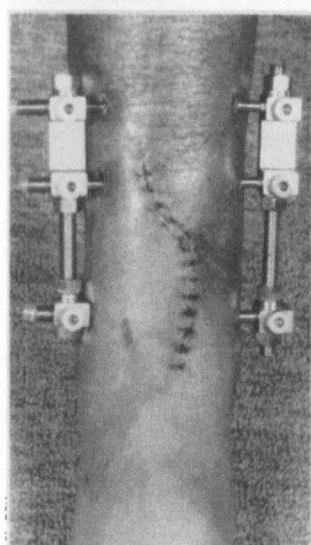
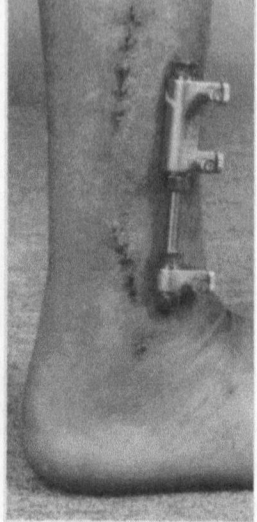

d

**Fig. 245 a–f.** Supramalleolar derotation osteotomy. Bilateral frame. M.H., 1930, 52 years, ♀, 257 554.

**a** Two years previously: open fracture, internal fixation, cancellous bone, implant removal (abroad). At presentation: gross rotational malalignment of 35°.
**b** Preoperative malrotation. Corrected malrotation, small bilateral frame.
**c** Small bilateral compression frame for 4 weeks, walking cast for 4 weeks.
**d** "Humane" frame. Partial weight bearing.
**e** Two months postoperatively, osteotomy is solid.
**f** Seven months after osteotomy: complete recovery

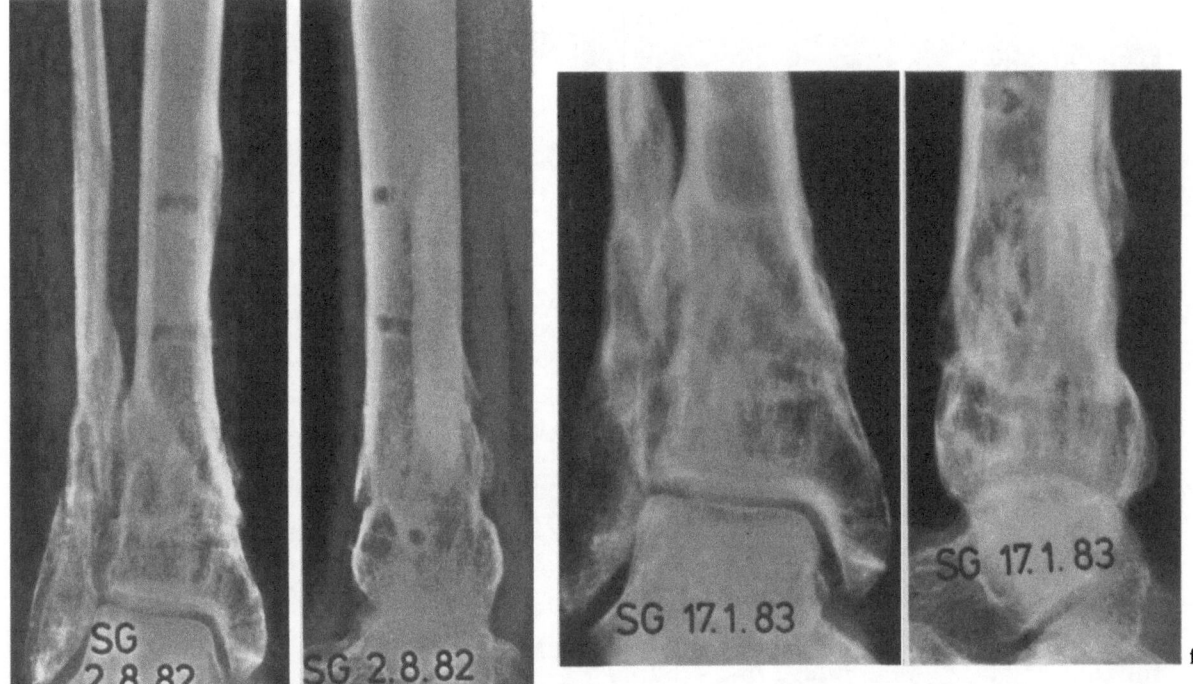

Fig. 245e, f

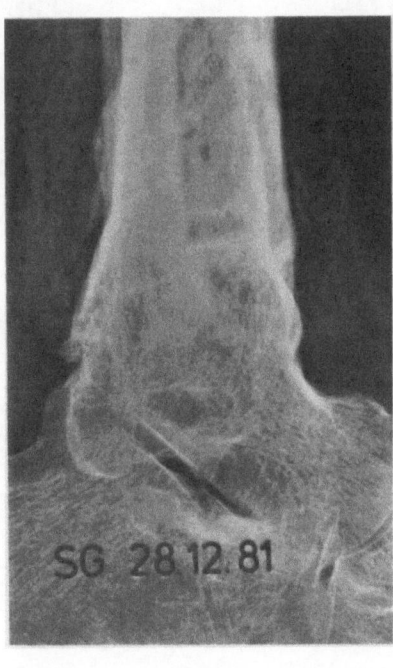
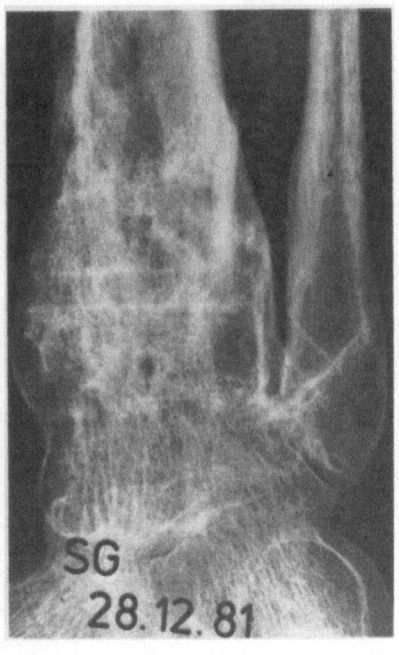

Fig. 246 a–c. Correction of deformity secondary to arthrodesis. Bilateral frame. K.M.-L., 1945, 36 years, ♀, 230809.

a Two years previously: impacted fracture, internal fixation, arthrodesis 7 months prior (abroad). At presentation 2¹/₂ years postinjury: foot deformity with 25° equinus, 20° varus, 20° medial torsion.
b Corrective osteotomy. Bilateral compression frame for 5 weeks, walking cast for 5 weeks.
c Six months postoperatively: osteotomy is solid, function is good owing to correction of deformity

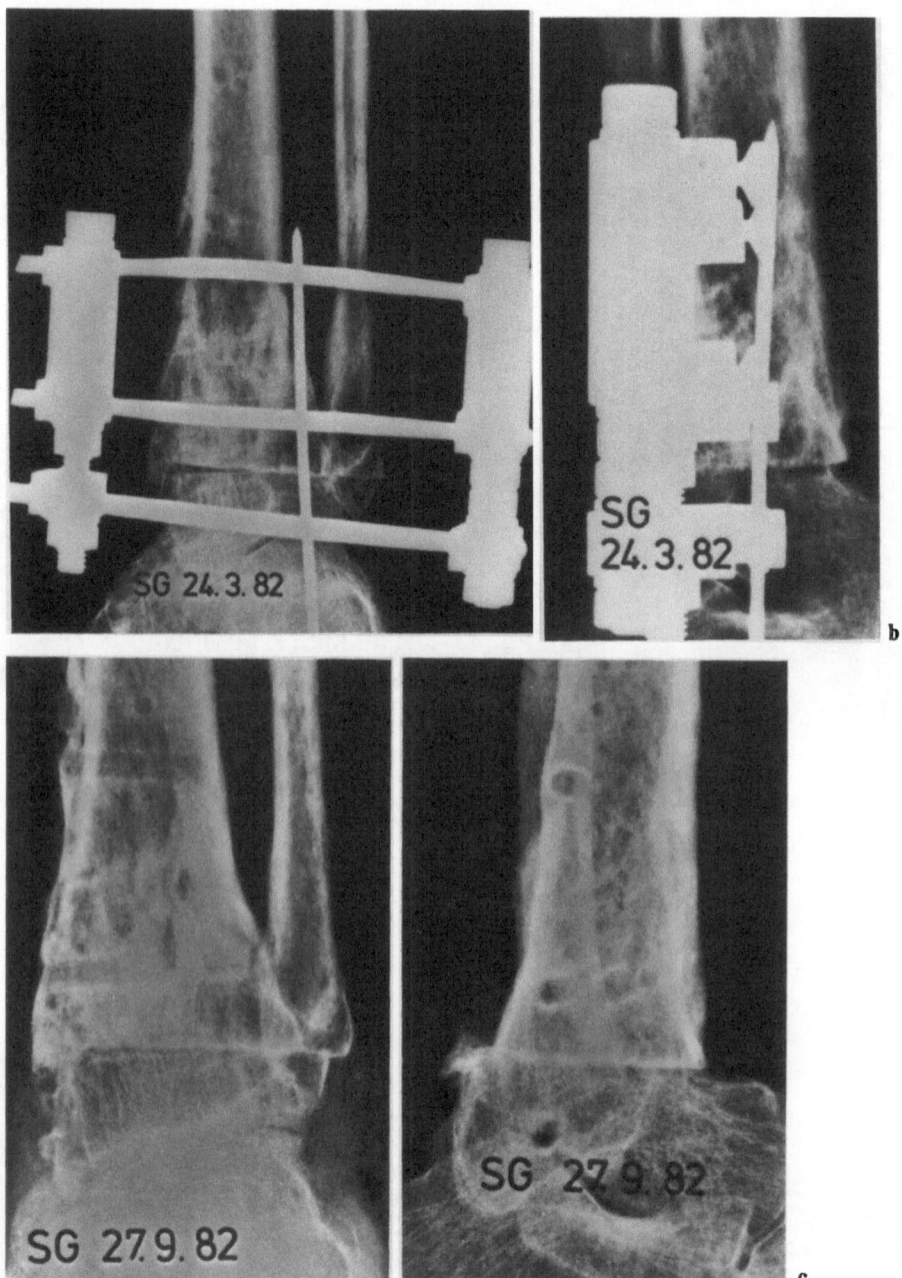

**Fig. 246b, c.** Legend see p. 219

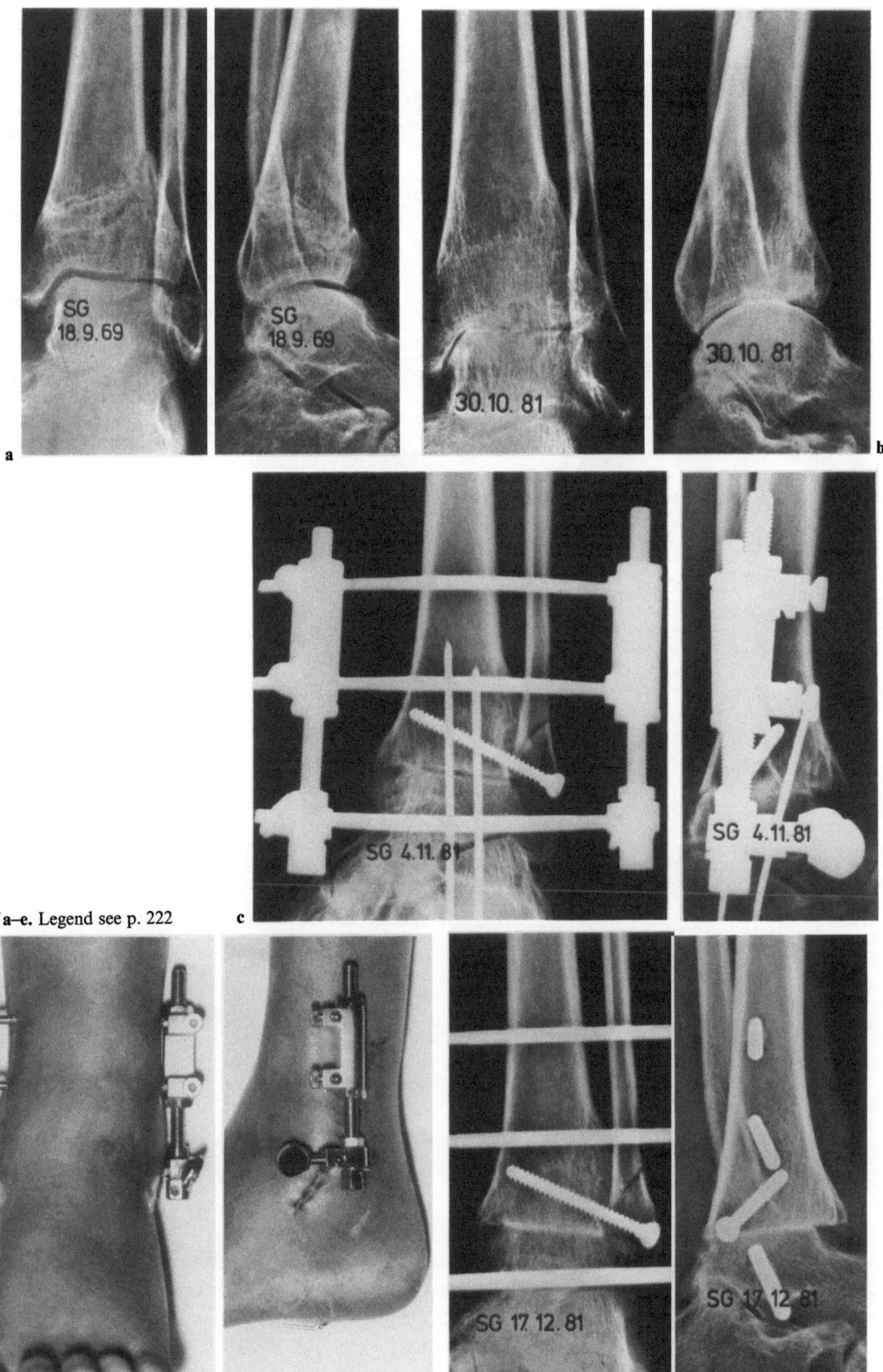

**Fig. 247 a–e.** Legend see p. 222

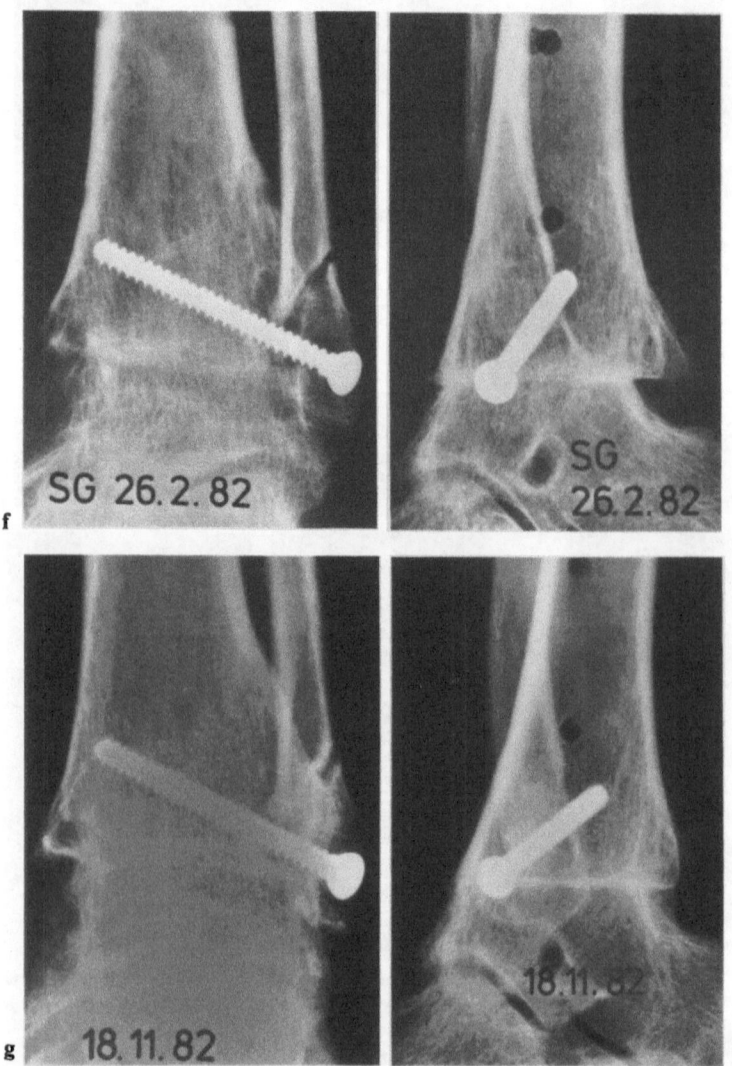

**Fig. 247 a–g.** Secondary arthrodesis for post-traumatic osteoarthritis. Bilateral frame. P.H., 1945, 36 years, ♂, 134512.

**a** Twelve years previously: impacted supramalleolar fracture of the tibia (abroad).

**b** At presentation: painful osteoarthritis.

**c** Arthrodesis with small bilateral compression frame for 6 weeks, Kirschner wire fixation of hindfoot, walking cast for 4 weeks.

**d** Clinical appearance at 12 days postoperatively.

**e** Six weeks postoperatively: removal of external fixator.

**f** Four months postoperatively: excellent healing.

**g** One year postoperatively: anatomically and functionally perfect arthrodesis

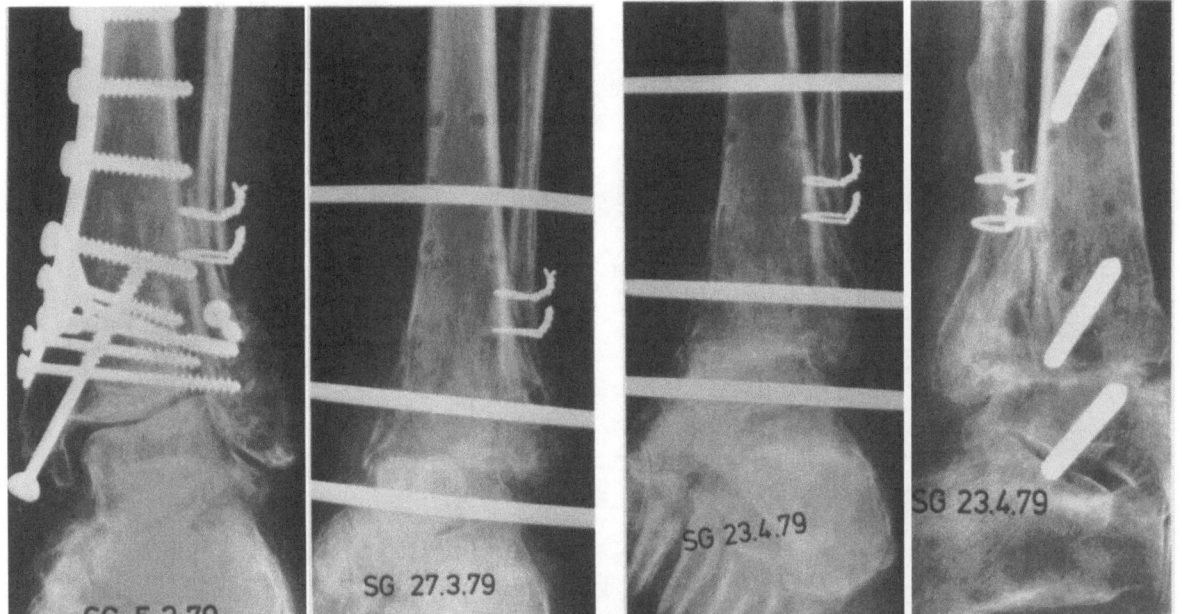

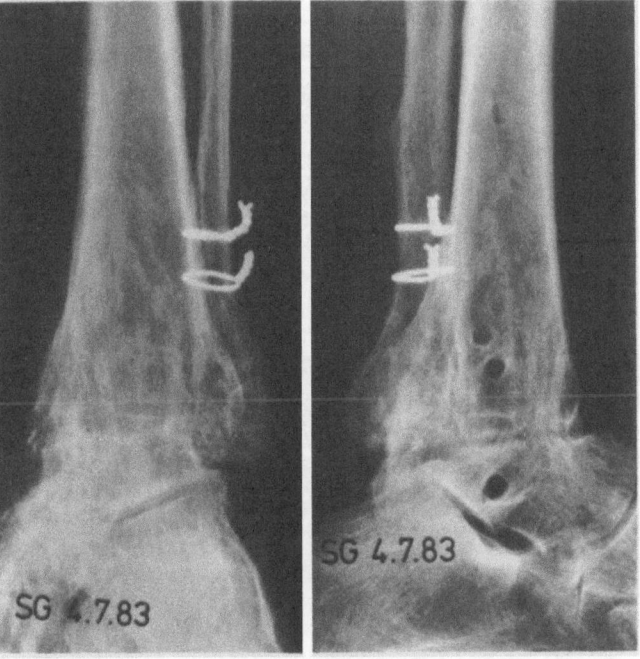

**Fig. 248 a–c.** Secondary arthrodesis following impacted fracture and internal fixation. Bilateral frame. P.A., 1916, 63 years, ♀, 225777.

**a** Eight months previously: impacted fracture, internal fixation without bone grafting (abroad). At presentation: pain, deformity, joint incongruity. Arthrodesis with bilateral compression frame for 4 weeks, walking cast for 6 weeks.

**b** Four weeks after arthrodesis, immediately before removal of frame: consolidation.

**c** 4$^{1}/_{2}$ years after arthrodesis: no complaints, normal walking ability

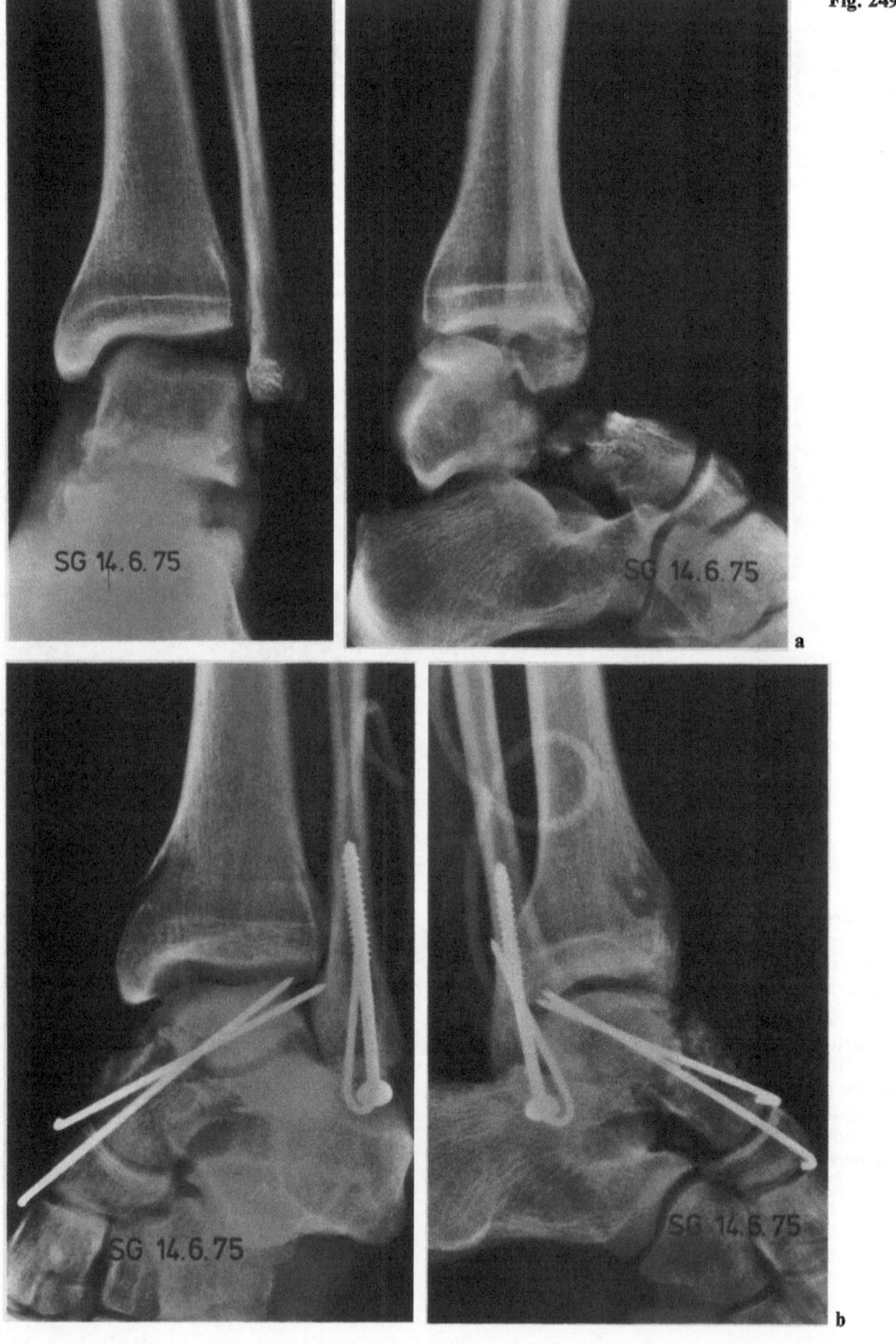

Fig. 249 a, b

**Fig. 249 a–g.**
Secondary arthrodesis following talus fracture. Bilateral frame. H.J., 1950, 25 years, ♂, 188362.

**a** Fracture-dislocation of talus + avulsion of lateral malleolus.
**b** Internal fixation.
**c** Four months postinjury: fracture is united.
**d** Seventeen months postinjury: necrosis of body of talus.
**e** Twenty-one months postinjury: arthrodesis with bilateral compression frame.
**f** Five months after arthrodesis: union.
**g** Six years after arthrodesis: arthrodesis is perfect, walking ability is virtually normal

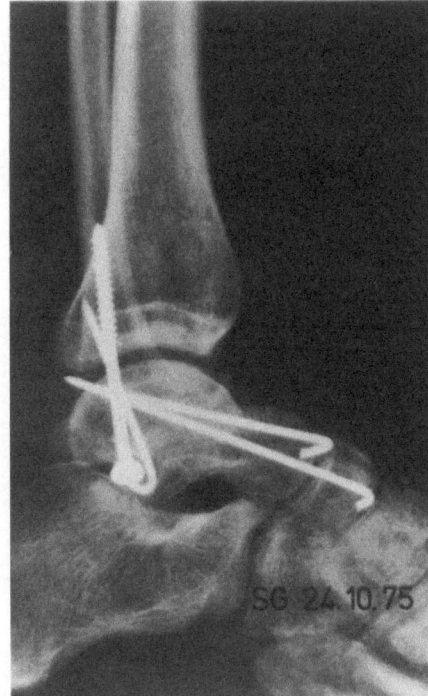
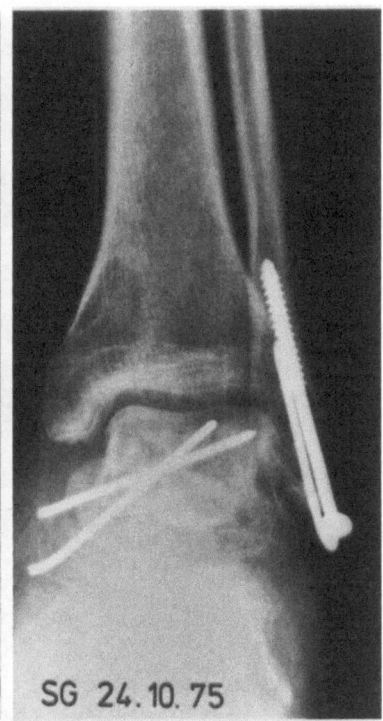

c

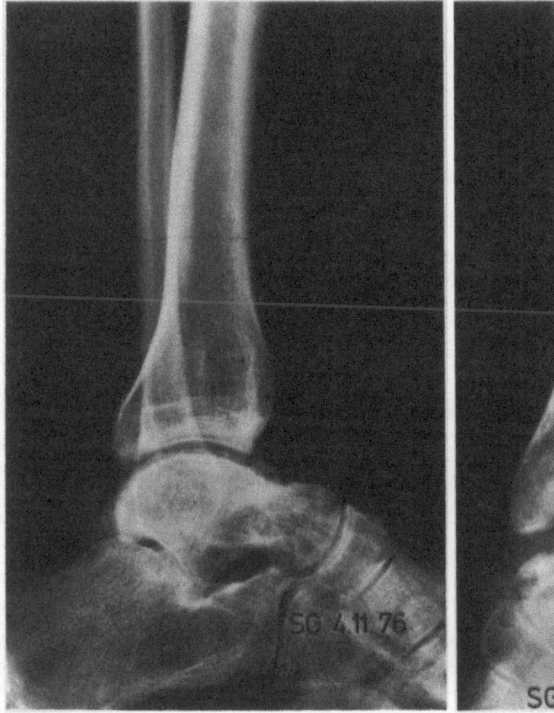
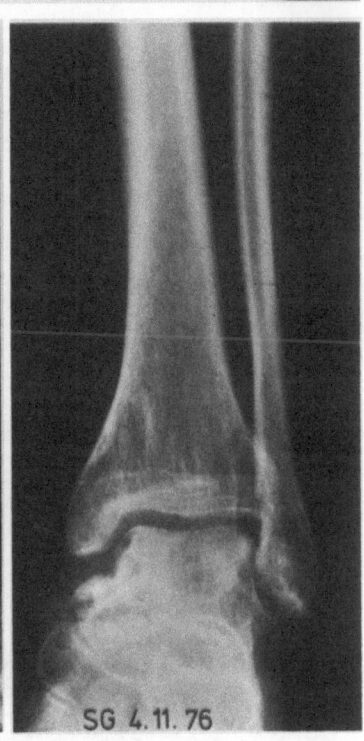

d

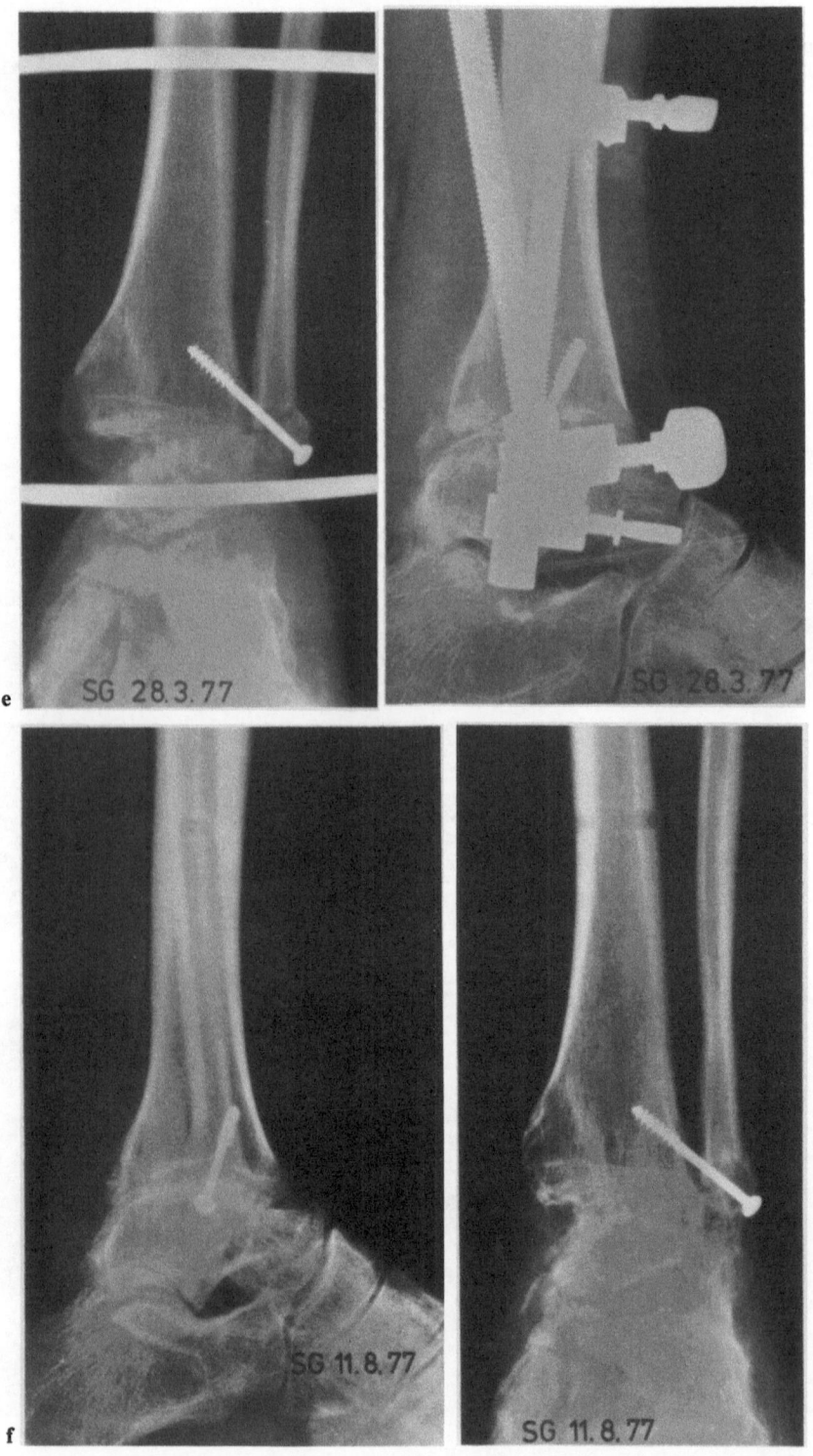

Fig. 249e, f. Legend see p. 225

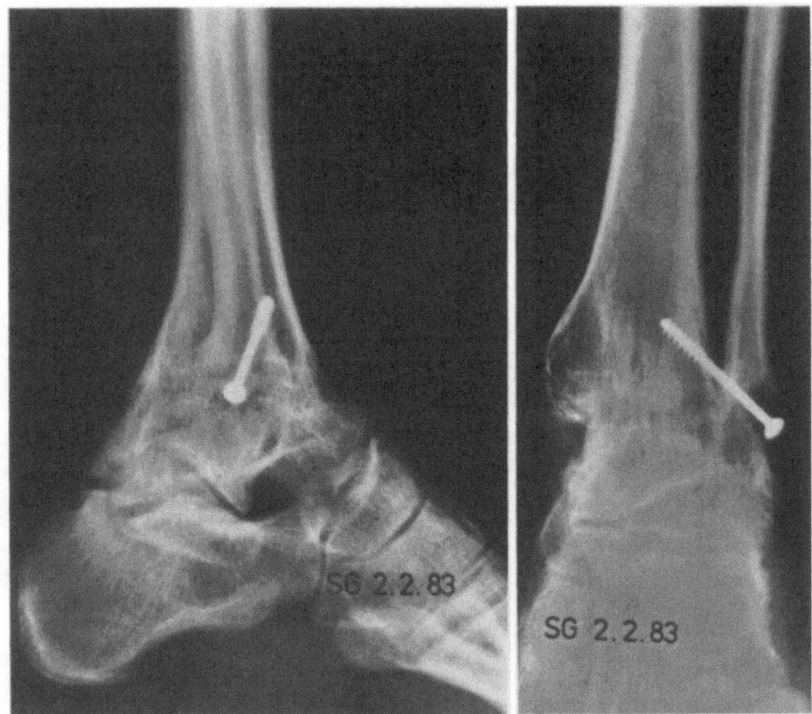

**Fig. 249g.** Legend see p. 225

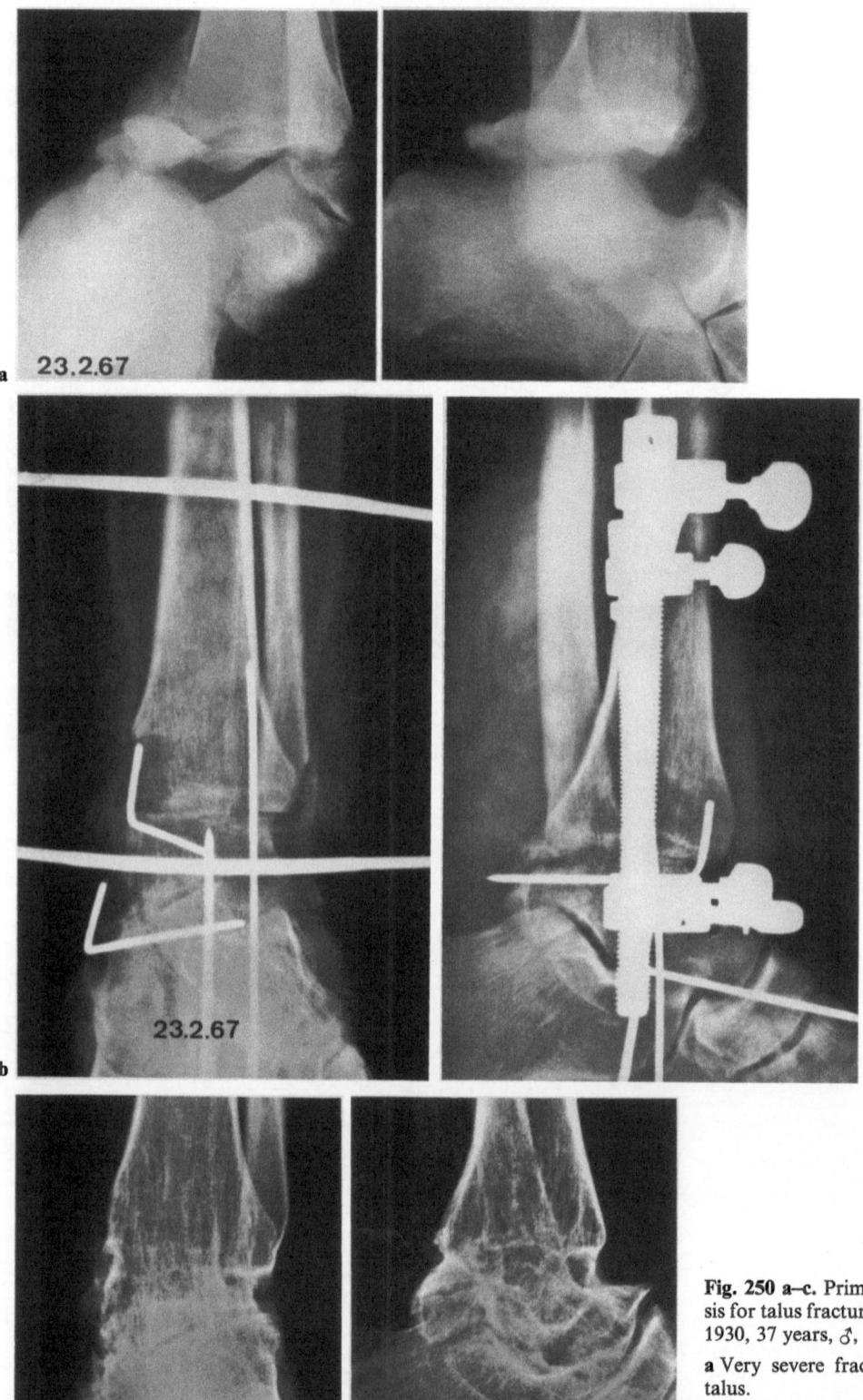

**Fig. 250 a–c.** Primary tibiotalar arthrodesis for talus fracture. Bilateral frame. H.E., 1930, 37 years, ♂, 111 282.

**a** Very severe fracture-dislocation of the talus.
**b** Primary tibiotalar arthrodesis following open reduction and internal fixation of talar fracture. Bilateral compression frame.
**c** Eight years postinjury: Patient has minimal complaints and is able to engage in sports (tennis, skiing)

**Fig. 251 a–c.** Arthrodesis for infected fracture. Bilateral frame. H.A., 1920, 54 years, ♀, 180239.

**a** Eight months previously: fracture-dislocation, internal fixation, infection (abroad). At presentation: septic arthritis of ankle joint.
**b** Resection-compression arthrodesis. Bilateral frame for 6 weeks + axial Kirschner wire fixation of hindfoot for 2 weeks + walking cast for 6 weeks.
**c** Three years after arthrodesis: Patient is free of complaints, requires 1.5 cm heel elevation

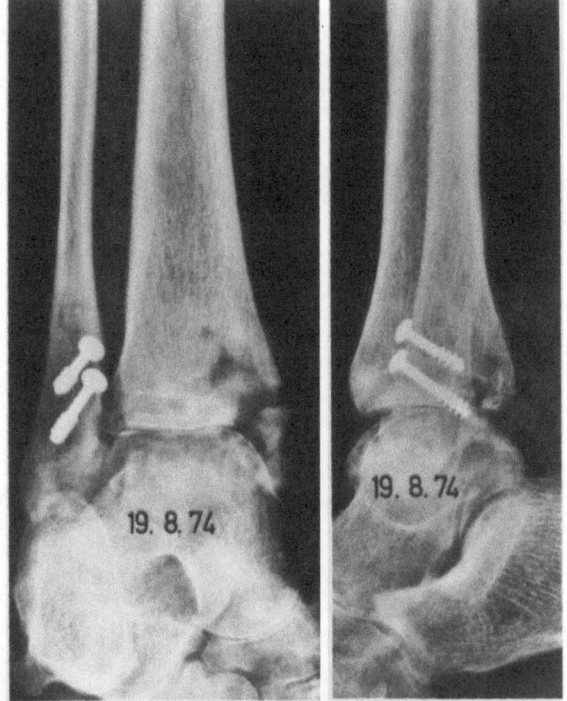

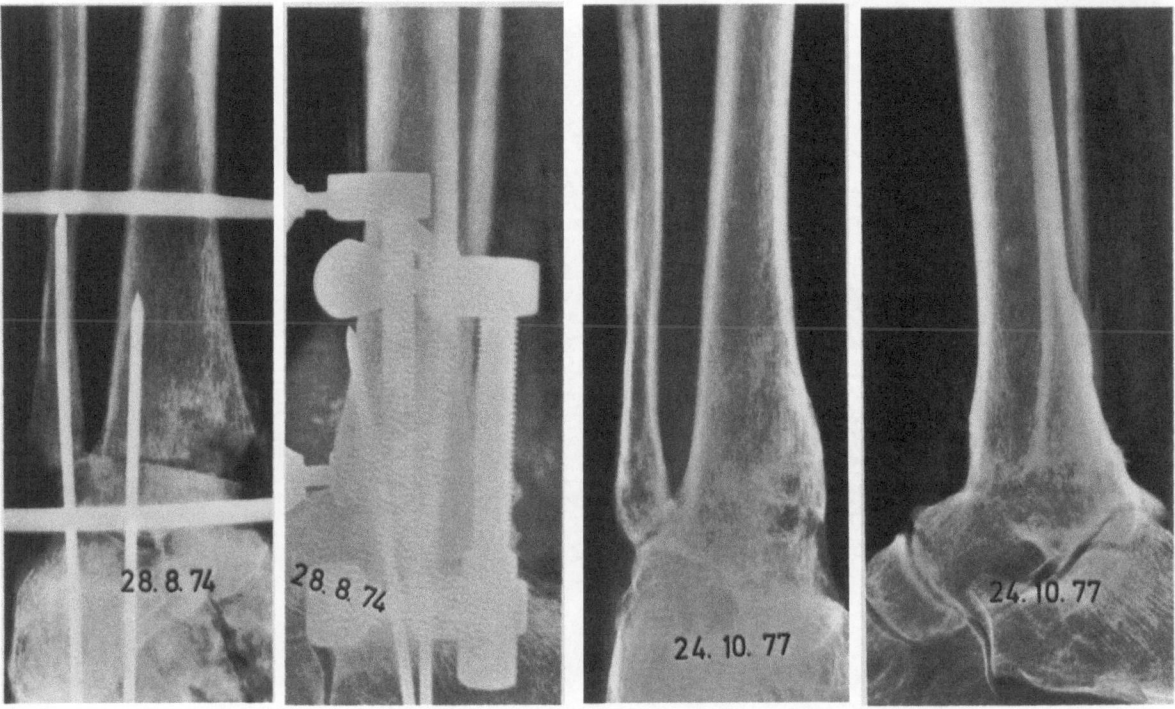

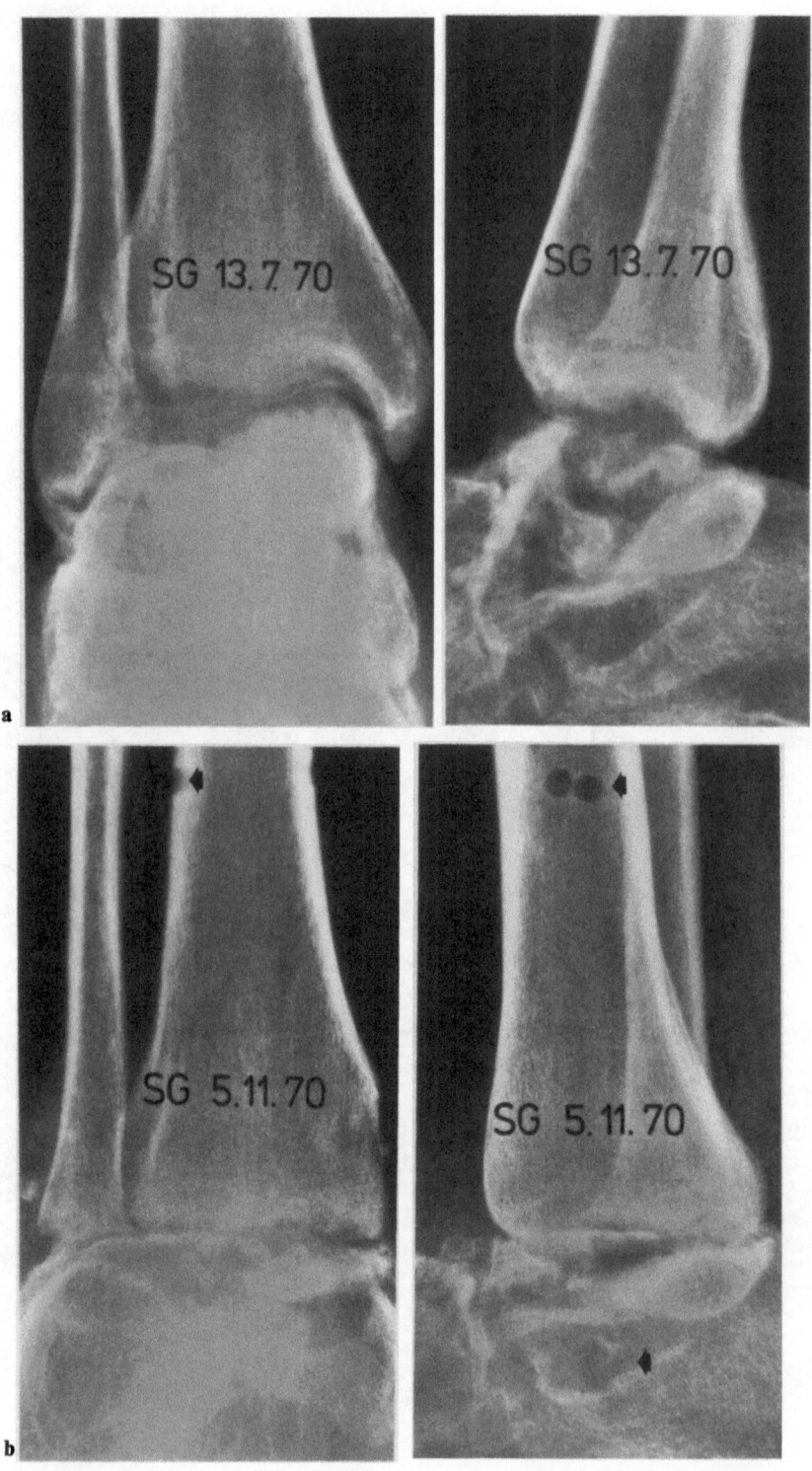

Fig. 252a, b

**Fig. 252 a–c.**
Tibiotalar arthrodesis for osteitis of the talus secondary to fracture. Bilateral frame. S.F., 1947, 23 years, ♂, 141986.

**a** Two years previously: open talus fracture (abroad). At presentation: septic arthritis of ankle and subtalar joints, sinus.
**b** Three months after operation, resection arthrodesis and talectomy. Bilateral compression frame for 6 weeks, walking cast for 6 weeks (→ former site of the 2 pins). Arthrodesis undergoing consolidation. Weight-relieving caliper for 6 months.
**c** $10^{1}/_{2}$ years after talectomy and arthrodesis between tibia and calcaneus: Patient is free of complaints, trabecular remodeling is complete

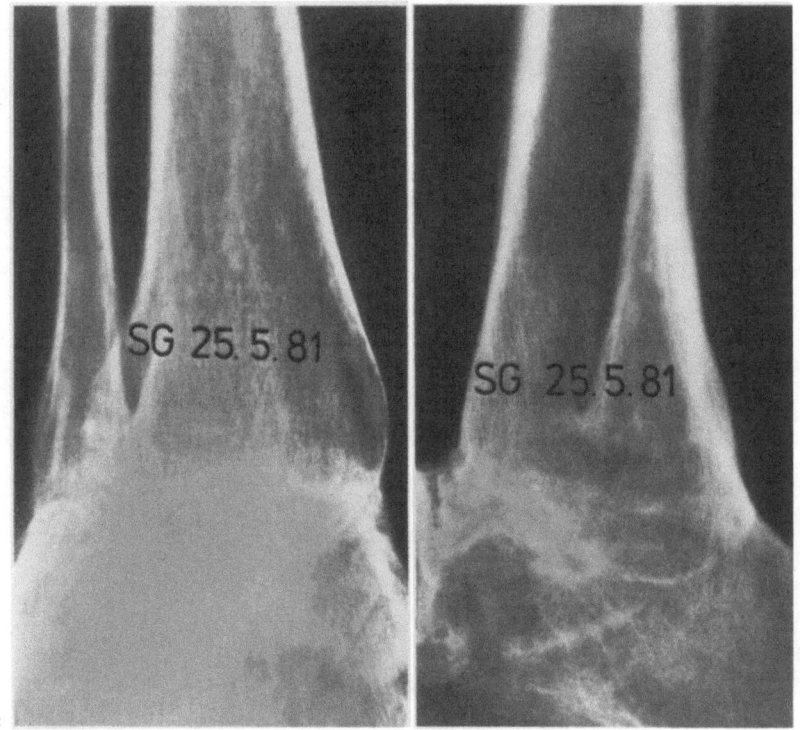

# 10  Soft Tissues (Figs. 253–260)

**Examples:**

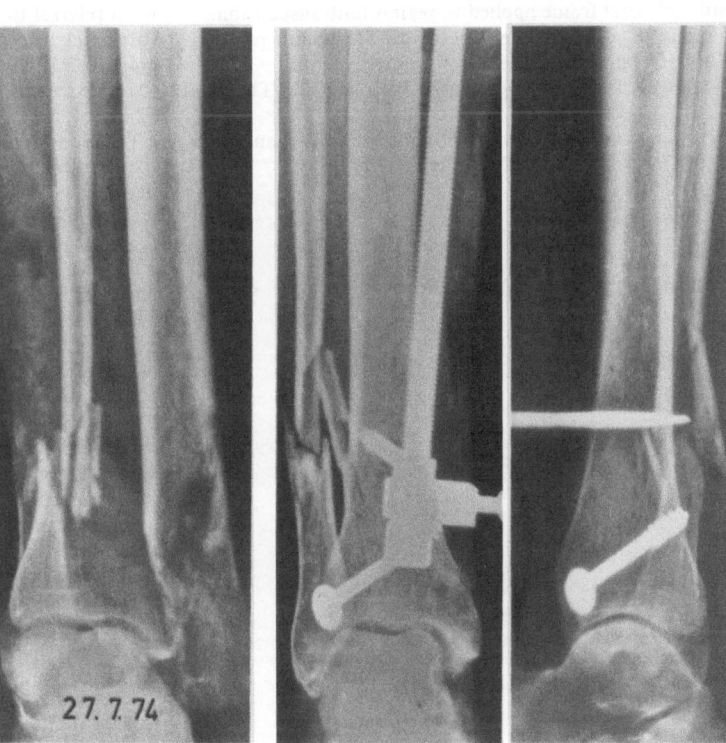

**Fig. 253a, b.** Legend see p. 232

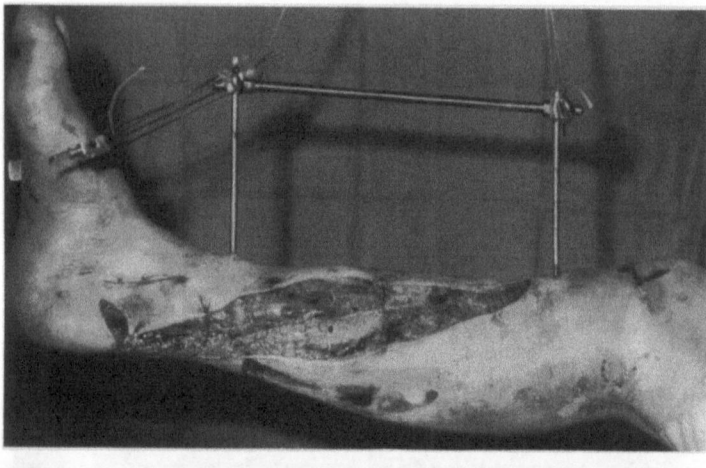

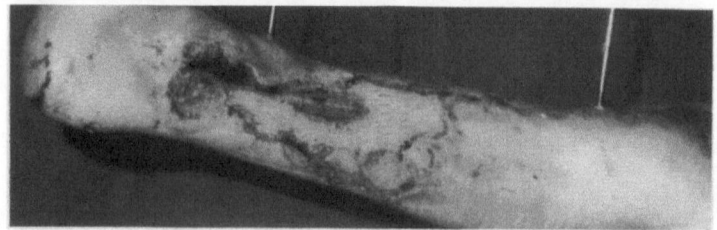

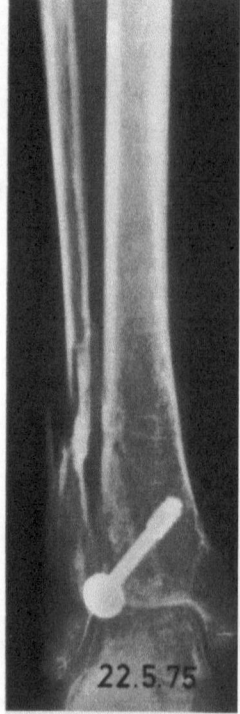

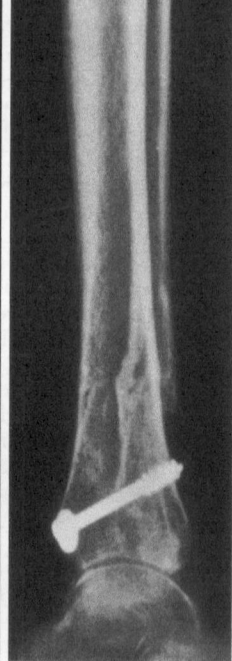

22.5.75

**Fig. 253 a–e.** Skin coverage following a fracture. Unilateral frame. B.K., 1918, 56 years, ♀, 179491.

**a** Grade III open fracture of the distal tibia.
**b** Minimal internal fixation with 1 cancellous lag screw. Small unilateral frame applied to permit limb suspension.
**c** Suspension, equinus prevention with Steinmann pin and traction. Open wound care.
**d** Coverage of granulating surface with meshed Thiersch graft at 2 weeks postinjury.
**e** Ten months postinjury: fracture and soft tissues are healed. Good walking and standing ability

**Fig. 254 a–n.** Skin coverage following a fracture. Unilateral frame + skin traction. T.P., 1961, 22 years, ♂, 273092.

**a** Grade III open fracture. Internal fixation. Skin closure not obtainable. Infection (abroad).
**b** On referral to our clinic 1 day after injury: broadly open soft-tissue defect on anterior side of lower leg. Epigard coverage for 3 days. Wound cleansed. Tibia ( → ) and plate (o) exposed to the air; gap between skin margins (* *) about 12 cm.
**c** Three days postinjury: removal of plate, minimal internal fixation, sagittal unilateral frame with anti-equinus component.
**d** Gradual skin closure over 3 weeks using techniques e, f, g.
**e** Longitudinal posterior relaxing incision of skin and crural fascia. Skin traction.
**f** Daily augmentation of traction with shot weights.
**g** Gradual closure of skin over exposed tibia. Thiersch graft of posterior relaxing incision. Curettage of tibial surface parallel to cutaneous fronts.
**h** Six months postinjury: Radiograph shows posteromedial cancellous bone graft ( → ) applied 4 months after fracture. The anterior tibial border is necrotic. Planned: resection of necrotic tibial border and direct replacement with autogenous cancellous bone; orthosis.
**i** Six months postinjury: 80% weight bearing (1 cane). The skin is closed. Cicatrix of cancellous bone graft ( → ).
**k** Functional brace for 6 months.
**l** 1 year postinjury: skin closed.
**m** Relaxing incision closed.
**n** 1 year postinjury: fracture is healed

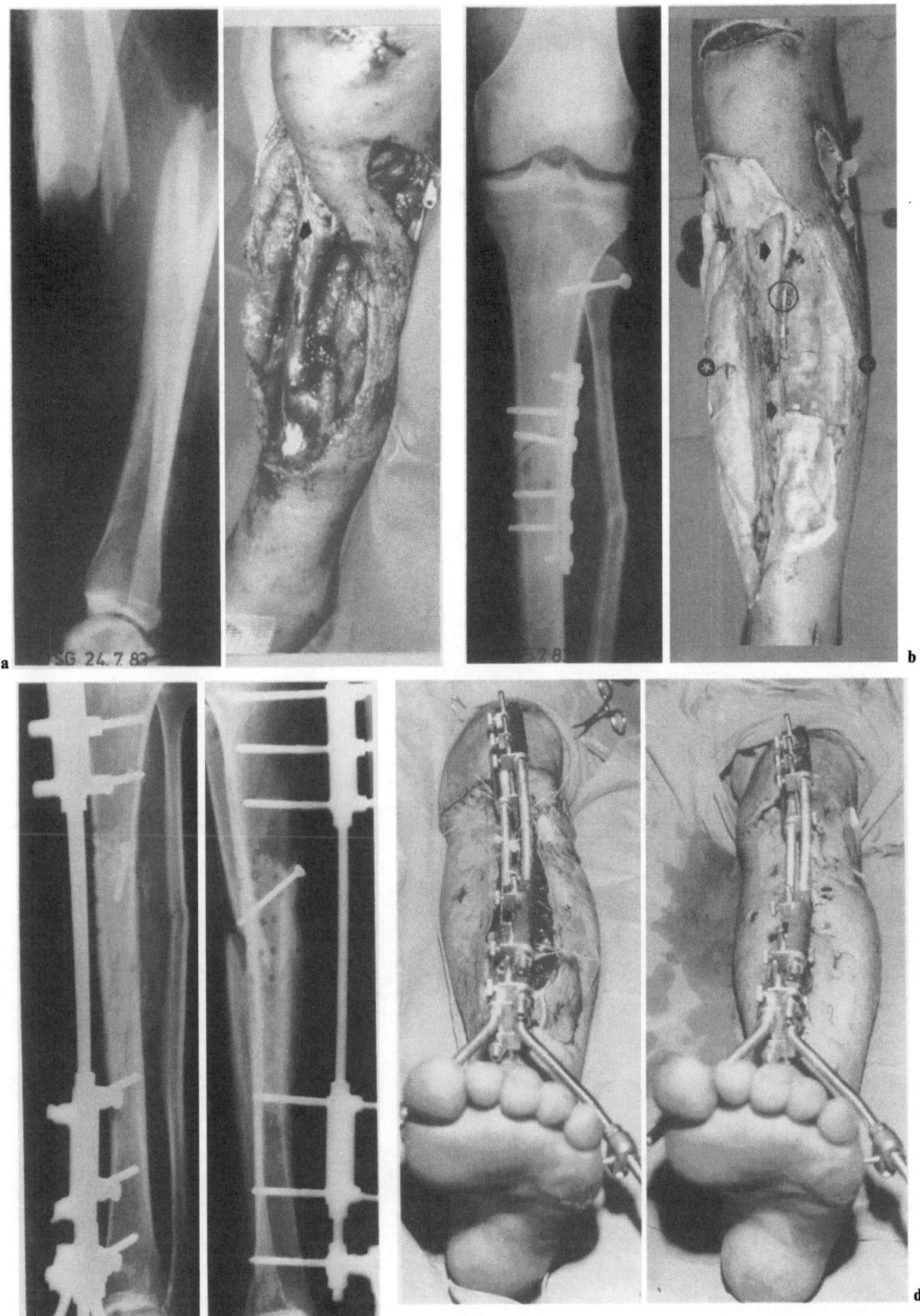

a

b

c

Fig. 254a–d

d

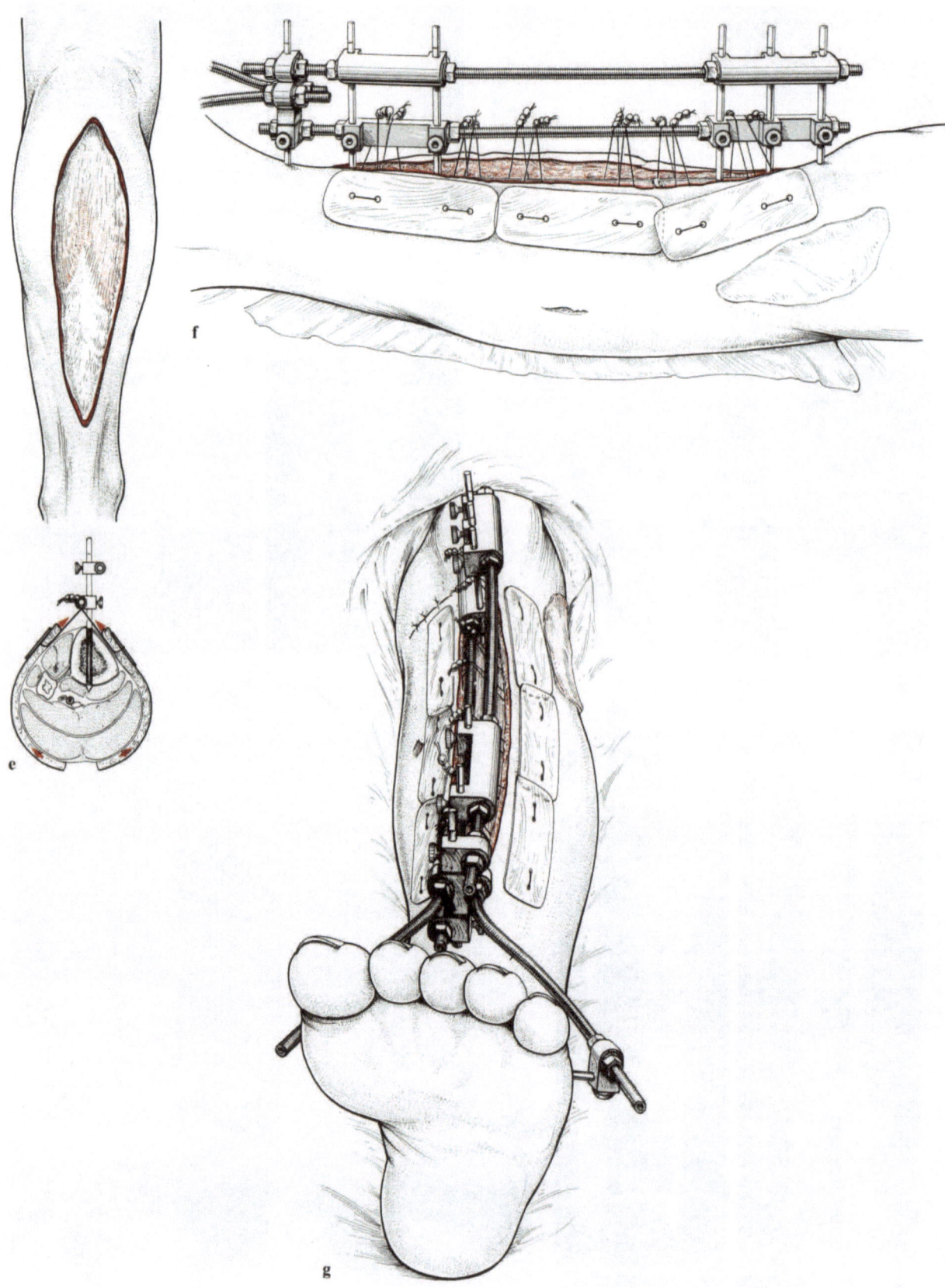

**Fig. 254e–g.** Legend see p. 232

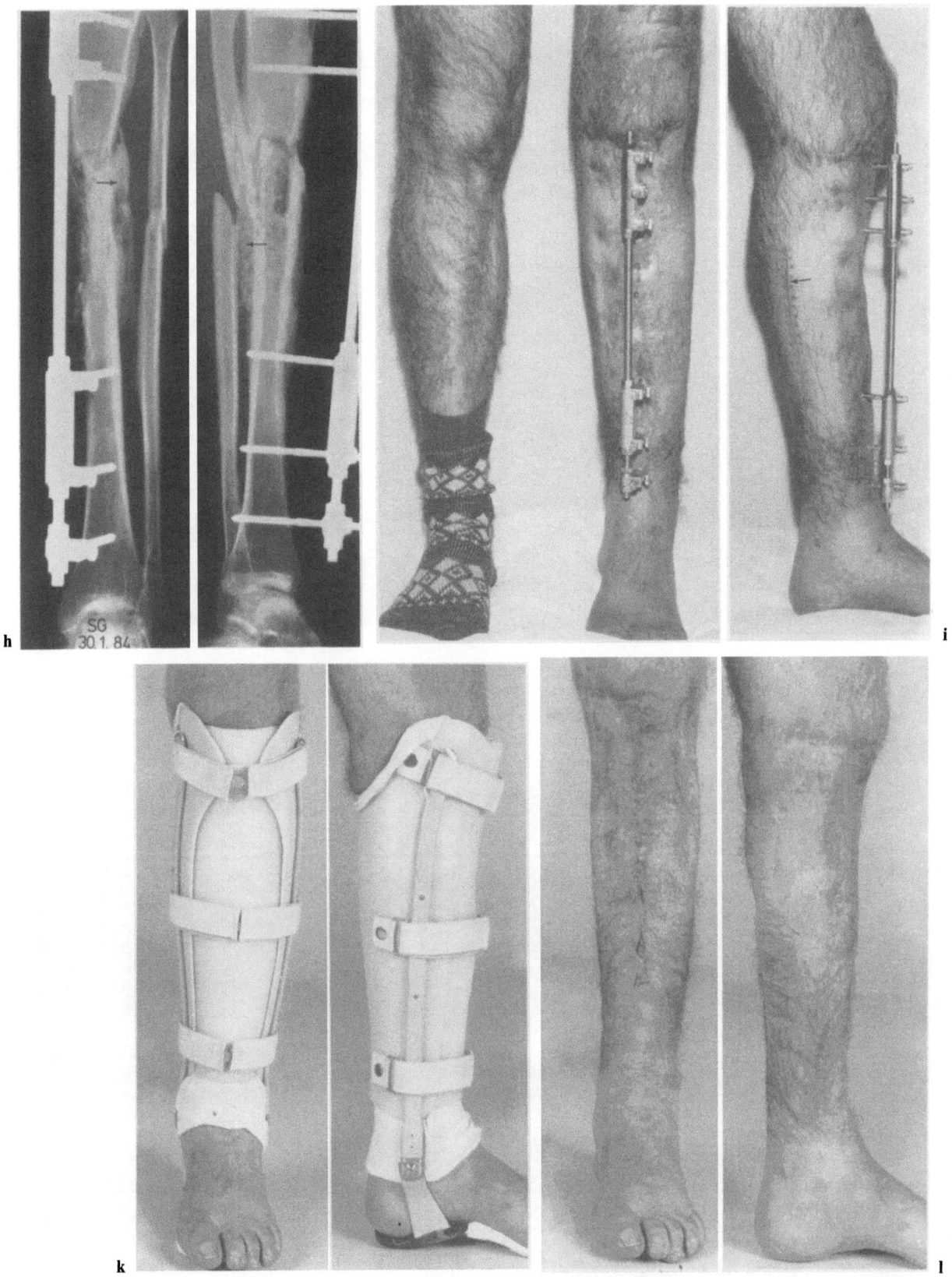

**Fig. 254h–l.** Legend see p. 232

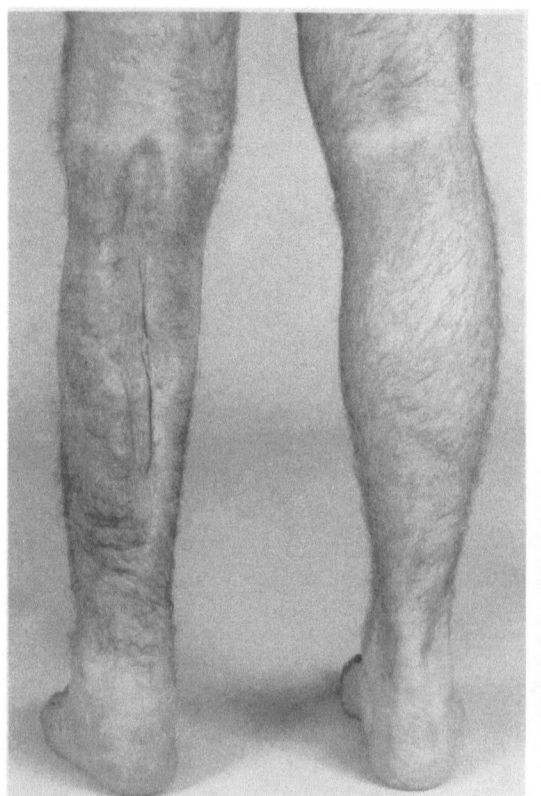

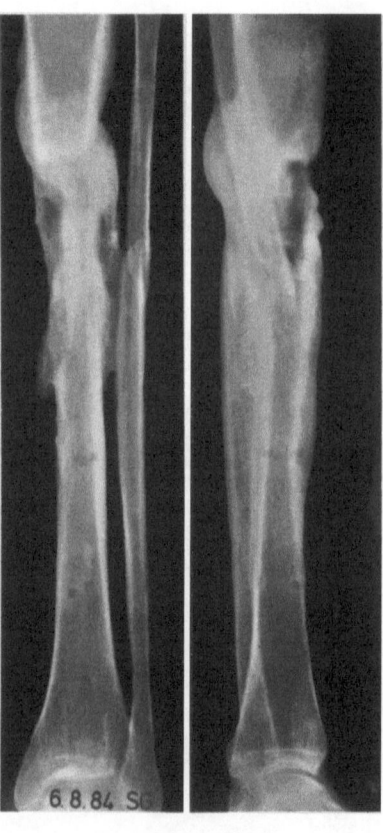

**Fig. 254m, n.**
Legend see p. 232

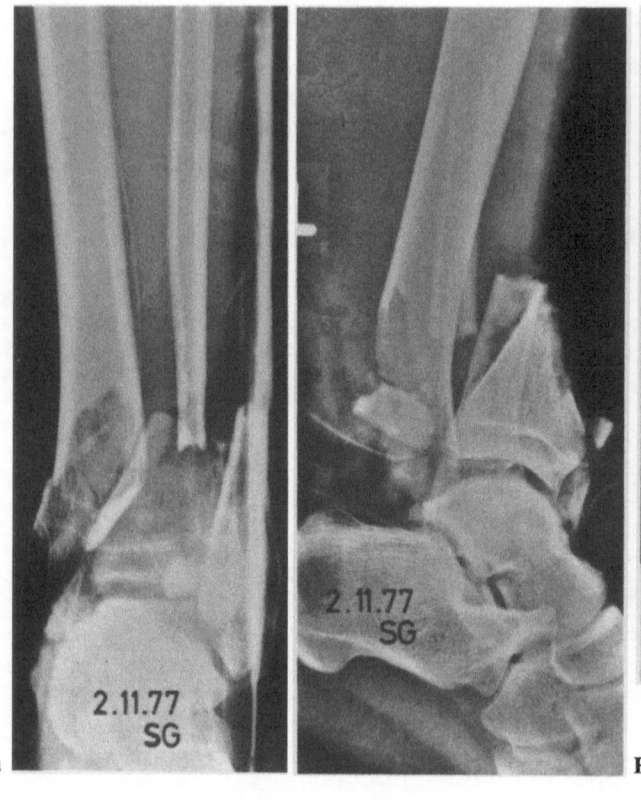

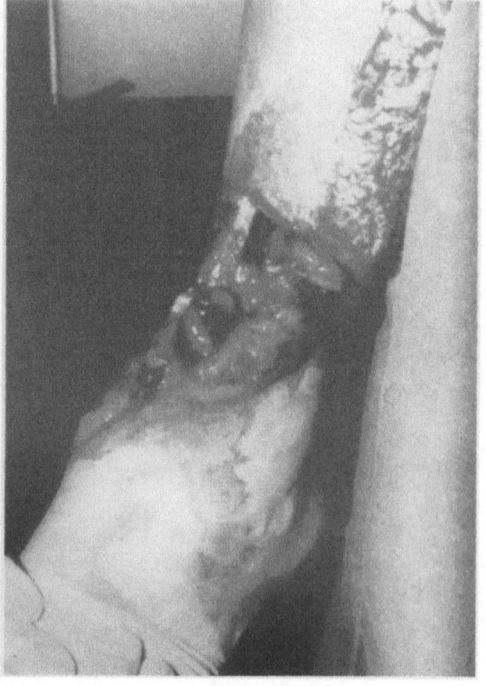

Fig. 255a

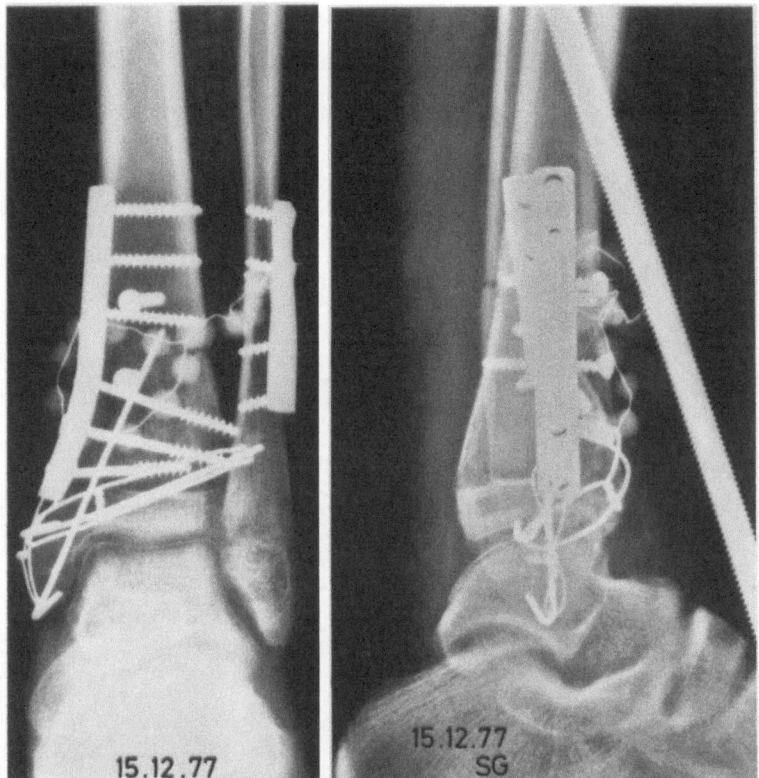

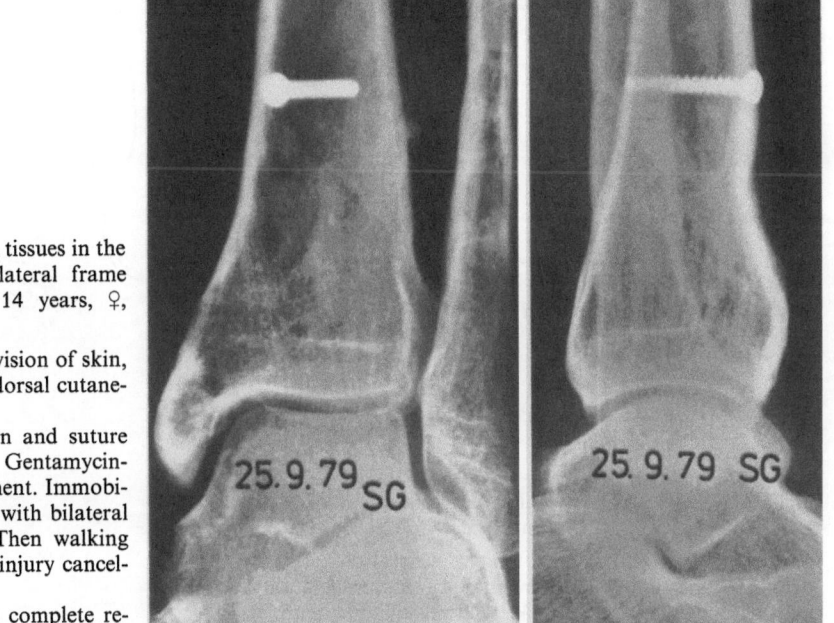

**Fig. 255 a–c.** Immobilization of soft tissues in the presence of an open fracture. Bilateral frame spanning the joint. Z.A., 1963, 14 years, ♀, 212870.

**a** *1*: Grade III open fracture. *2*: Division of skin, tendons, dorsalis pedis artery and dorsal cutaneous nerves.

**b** Two weeks after internal fixation and suture of artery, tendons and nerves. Gentamycin-PMMA beads. Open wound treatment. Immobilization of soft tissues for 5 weeks with bilateral frame from tibia to metatarsus. Then walking cast for 5 weeks. Three weeks postinjury cancellous bone graft + Thiersch graft.

**c** One year, 10 months postinjury: complete recovery

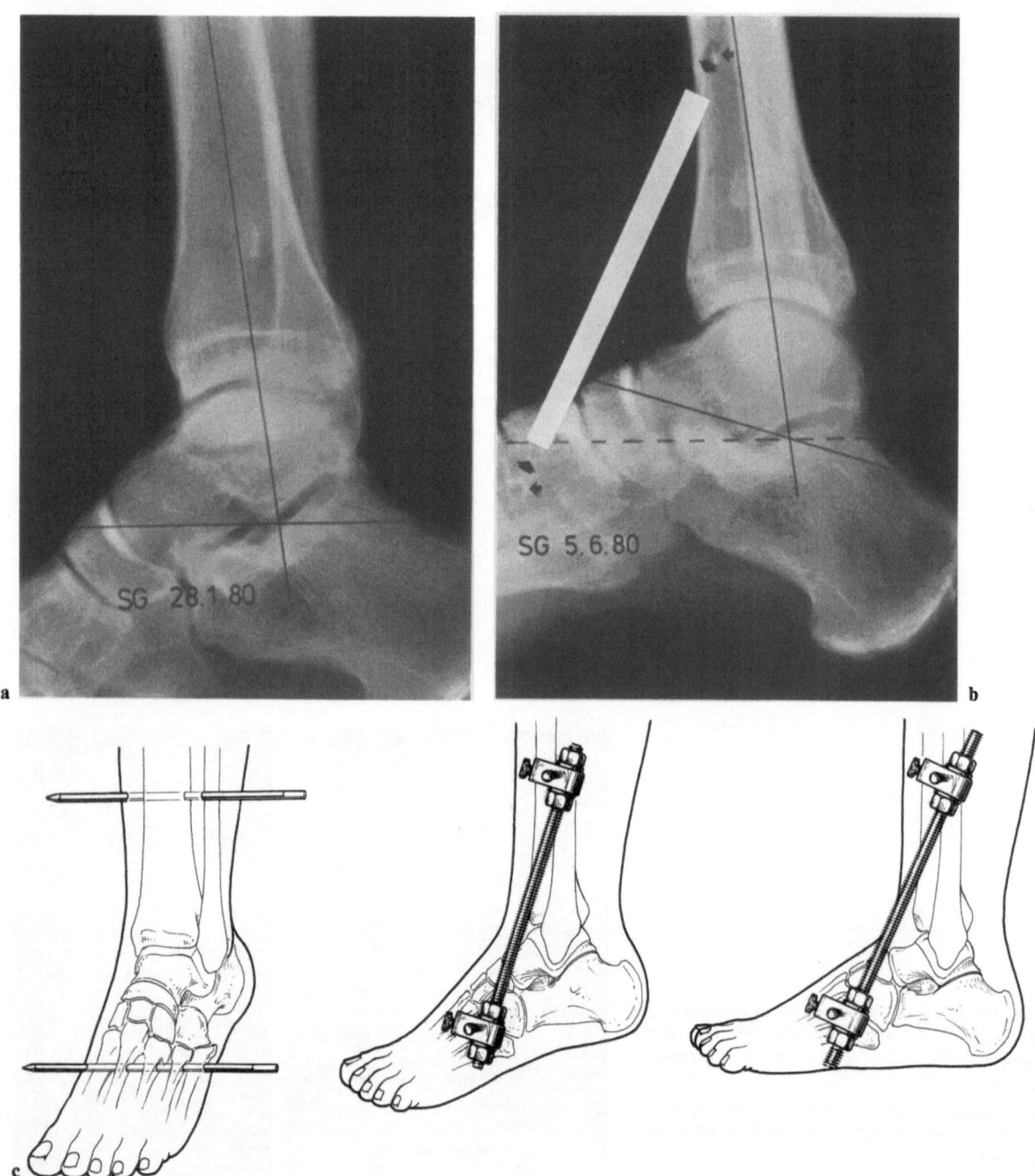

**Fig. 256 a–c.** Correction of equinus deformity. Bilateral tension frame. K.R., 1954, 26 years, ♂, 235763.

**a** $1^1/_2$ years previously: type C fracture-dislocation, internal fixation, removal of implants (abroad). At presentation: maximum dorsiflexion of ankle −10°. Bilateral tension frame for 2 weeks with staged, daily correction; no further operative intervention. Then walking cast for 3 weeks.
**b** Four months after correction: permanent gain of 20° dorsiflexion. Indicated are the angular gain of dorsiflexion, the drill holes for the Steinmann pins (→), and the tension frame (*bars*). Disadvantage: cartilage compression.
**c** Technique for assembling the small bilateral frame

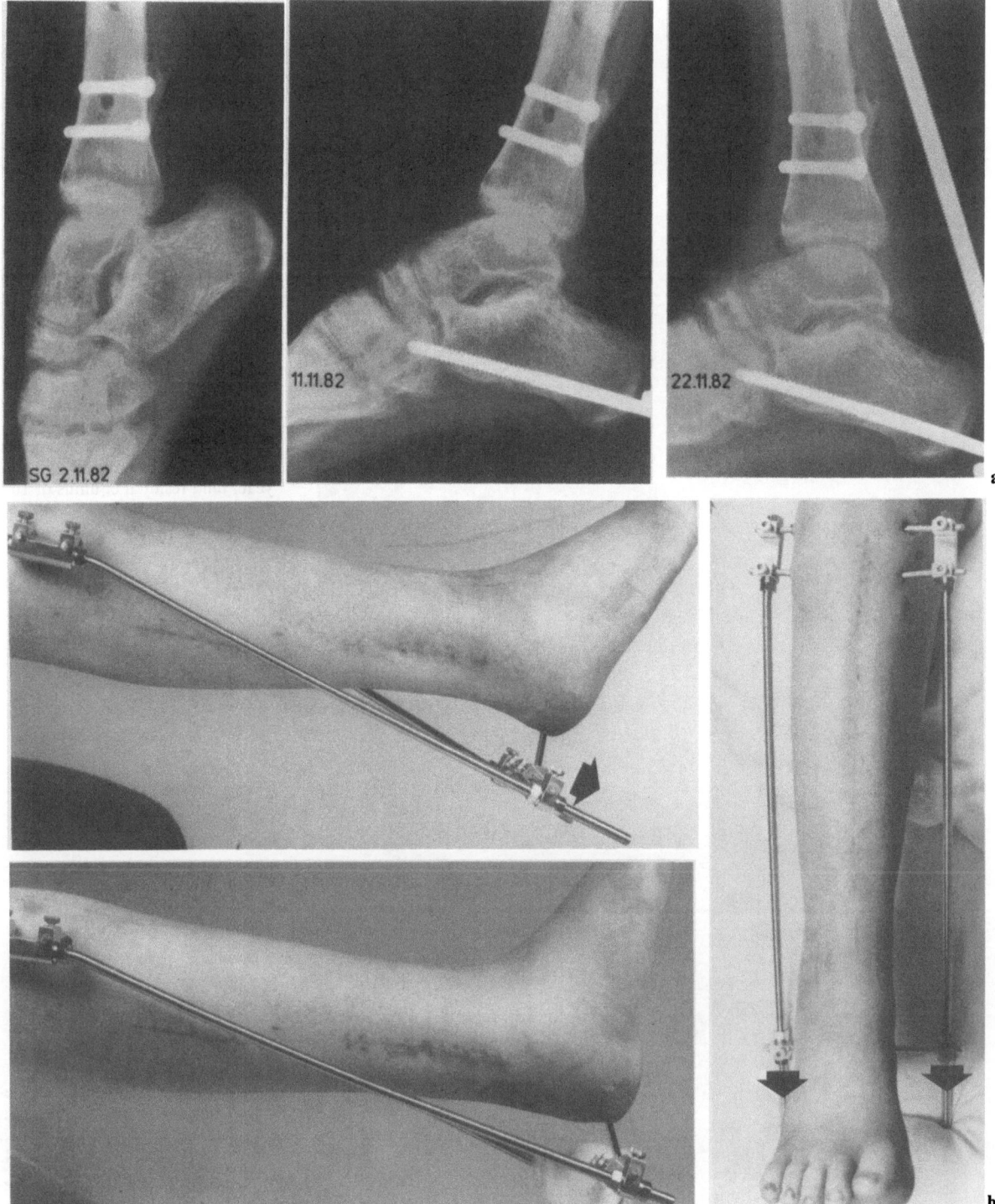

**Fig. 257a, b.** Legend see p. 240

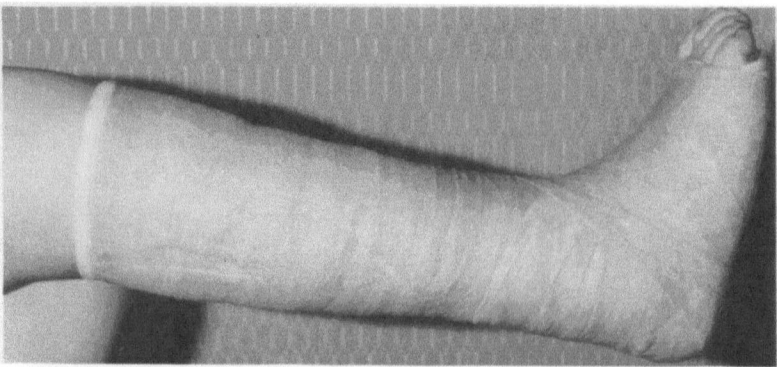

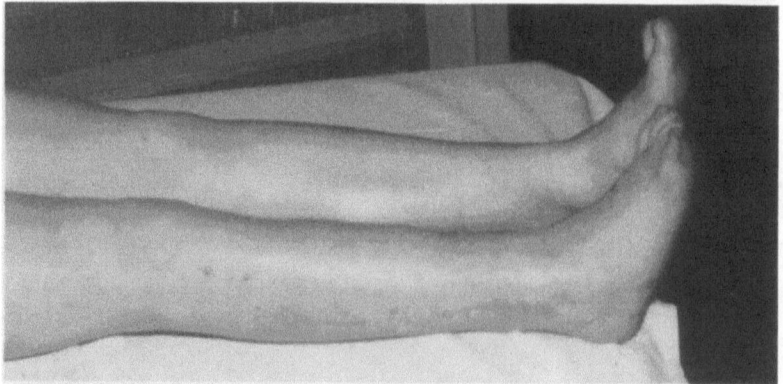

**Fig. 257 a–c.**
Correction of equinus deformity.
Bilateral thrust frame. A.B., 1965,
17 years, ♀, 261092.

**a** Extreme equinus deformity of the
foot secondary to tibial lengthening
osteotomy for congenital hypoplasia. Correction by tenomyotomy of
all pedal flexors and staged correction for 3 weeks with a soft-tissue
thrust frame.
**b** The thrust frame is a bilateral
frame anchored in the upper tibia.
A transverse Steinmann pin engages against a 5-mm Schanz screw
embedded in the calcaneus. Correction is effected by moving the lower
clamps distally ( → ) by a small
amount each day. Advantage: no
cartilage compression.
**c** After 6 weeks: molded tibial
orthosis for 6 months. Result at 1
year: mild residual equinus of 10°

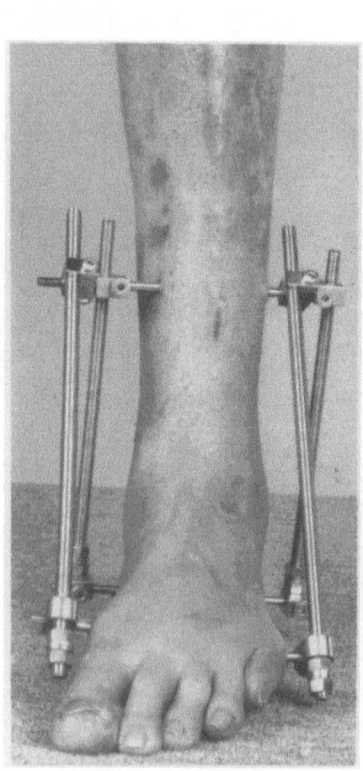

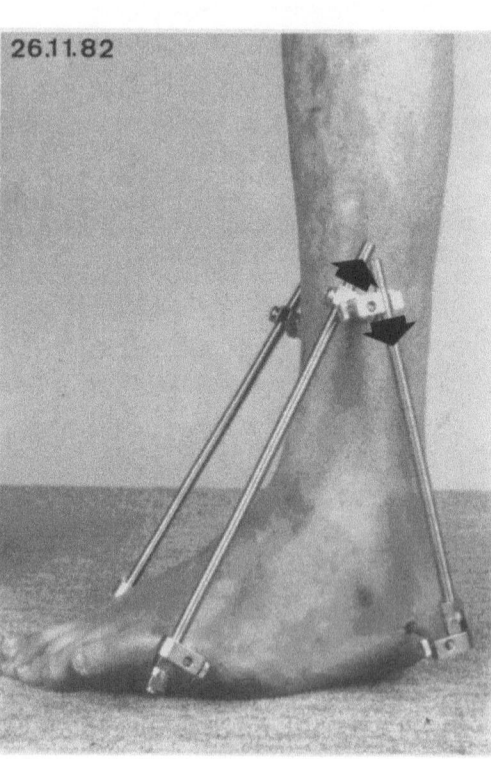

26.11.82

**Fig. 258.**
Correction of equinus deformity. Combined tension
and thrust frame. R.M.,
1958, 24 years, ♂, K 5966-4.

Post-traumatic equinus deformity with trophic disturbances secondary to compartment syndrome (abroad). → Combined tension
and thrust system, appropriate for unusually "hard"
equinus deformities and for
feet with impaired circulation and trophic disturbances

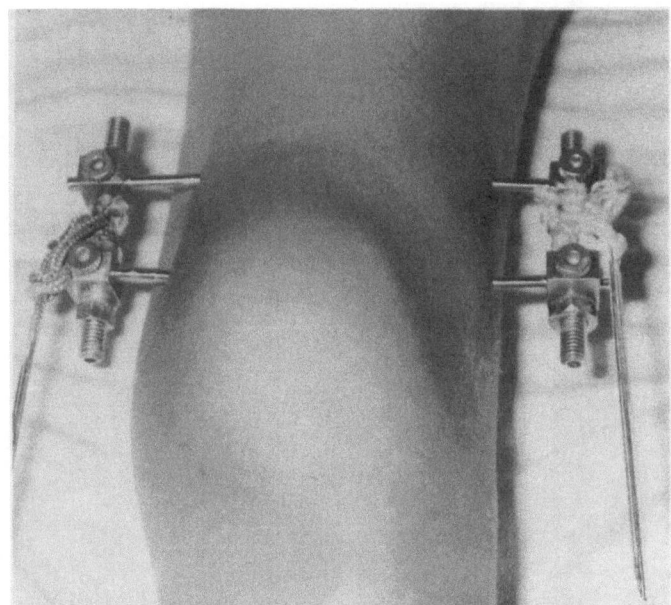

a

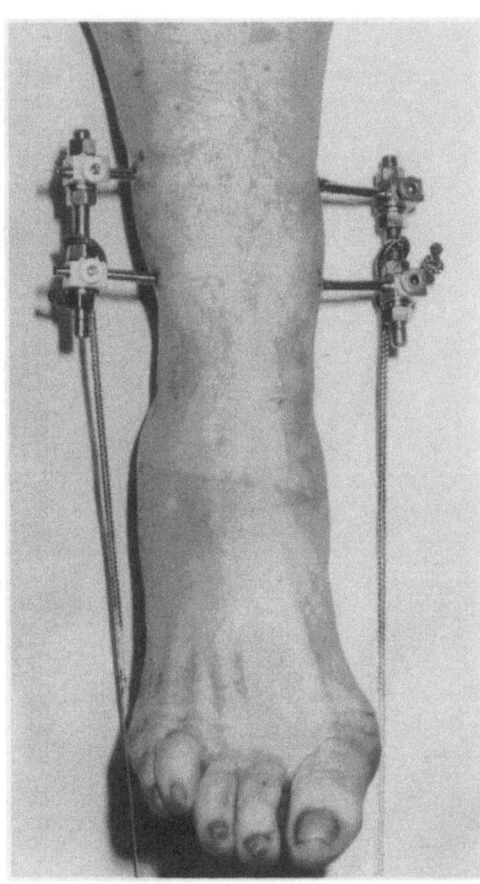

b

**Fig. 259 a, b.** Prolonged skeletal traction of the femur and tibia. Small bilateral frame.

**a** Femoral traction for prolonged period. M.G., 1960, 22 years, ♀, 246898. Bilateral compression frame + supracondylar traction of femur for pathologic fracture associated with Ewing's sarcoma. The prestressed frame remains stable.

**b** Tibial traction for prolonged period. F.I., 1921, 61 years, ♀, 179635. Bilateral compression frame + supramalleolar traction of tibia for distal femoral fracture in presence of total knee prosthesis. The prestressed frame remains stable

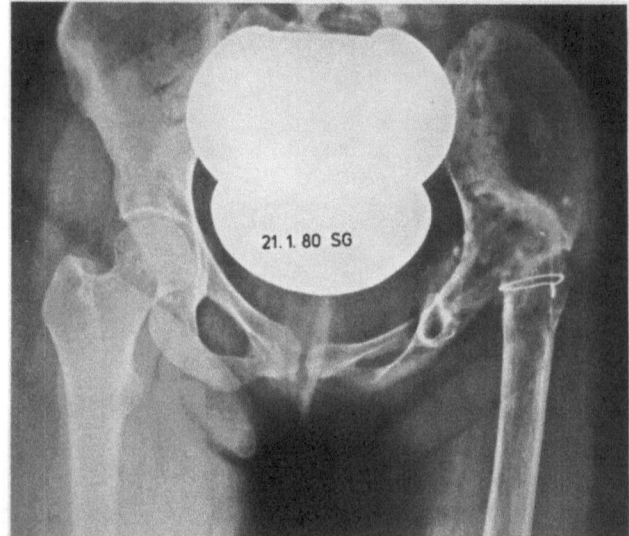

a

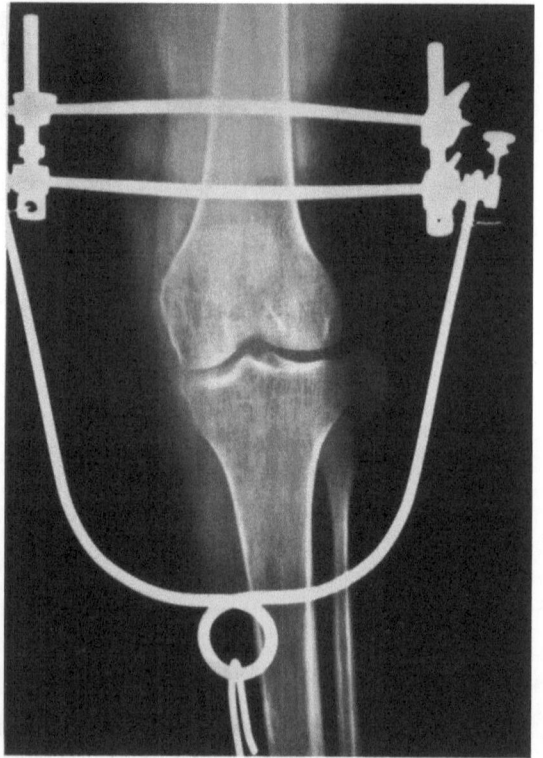

b

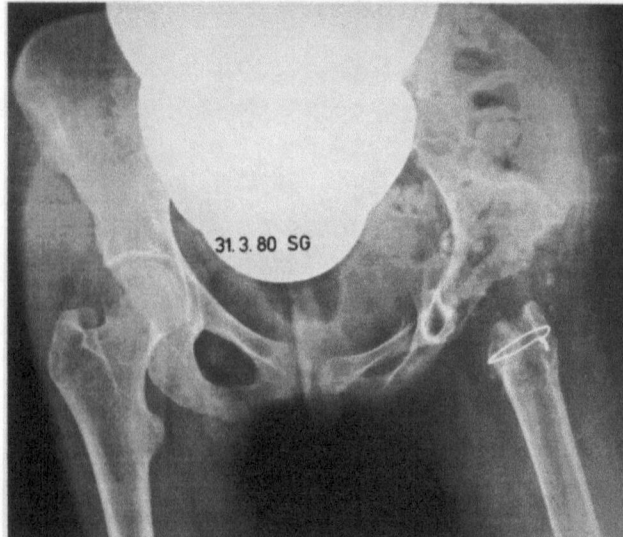

c

**Fig. 260 a–c.** Heavy skeletal traction of the femur. Small bilateral frame. B.S., 1956, 23 years, ♀, 232163.

**a** Defect following infection of a total hip prosthesis (abroad). At presentation: shortening. Insertion of a new total hip is proposed.
**b** 20 kg of supracondylar traction applied through pre-stressed bilateral frame for 10 days.
**c** Ten days after start of traction a 6–8 cm length gain was obtained (note wire loop), whereupon a new total hip was implanted

# M The Threaded External Fixator in Children and Adolescents. Technique. Clinical Examples

CH. BRUNNER

## 1 Introduction

The majority of fixations in pediatric orthopedics are accomplished by means of a plaster cast or Kirschner wires. Internal fixations with cerclage wire, lag screws, plates, etc. are rarely indicated. In certain cases, however, pediatric osteotomies and fractures have been managed with the aid of external skeletal fixation, as in adults. We, too, employ both unilateral and bilateral external frames in certain of our pediatric patients as a means of effecting compression, neutralization or distraction. We find external fixation particularly useful for the conduct of staged corrective procedures. With the threaded external fixator, staged corrections can be carried out easily and conveniently over a period of several days. A gradual approach of this type is indicated in all cases where the proposed correction carries a significant risk of neurovascular injury. It will give the neurovascular bundles an opportunity to adapt, while exerting a gradual yet effective stretching action on the shortened muscles.

In the management of *pediatric fractures,* it is best to adopt a conservative strategy whenever possible. As stated in the book *Fracture Treatment in Children and Adolescents* (WEBER, BRUNNER, FREULER), only 12% of all pediatric fractures require operative treatment. The main indications for internal fixation in such cases (plates, screws, Kirschner wires) are intraarticular fractures, fractures involving a growth zone, and open fractures. For grade III open fractures, however, external fixation is being employed with increasing frequency.

In the area of *pediatric orthopedics,* external fixation is most commonly used for corrective osteotomies of the proximal femur. The second most common use is for limb lengthenings, and the third is for axial corrections that involve an open-wedge type osteotomy.

Below we shall examine cases from our files which illustrate the applications of the external fixator in the following areas:

- open fractures
- corrections of the proximal femur
- limb lengthenings
- axial corrections
- special situations.

## 2 The External Fixator for Severe Open Fractures in Children, Infected Fractures and Infected Nonunions

Grade I open fractures in children do not carry a high risk of infection owing to the rapid fracture repair and excellent blood flow which characterize the pediatric age group. However, grade II and grade III open fractures require stable, primary operative fixation, just as in adults, in order to encourage soft-tissue healing. We tend to favor external fixation over internal fixation methods (plates and screws), depending on the nature of the soft-tissue injury. When external fixation is employed, it is important to secure primary closure of the medullary canal, as this will promote a rapid recovery of the endosteal blood flow. This can sometimes be achieved with one or two small lag screws. If the bone has satisfactory compressive strength at this stage, a unilateral external frame may be applied. Otherwise a bilateral frame is required.

*Example 1* (Fig. 261)

Grade III open fracture of the proximal tibia with severe soft-tissue injury.

*The problem:* A 12-year-old girl was run over by an automobile, sustaining an open grade III fracture of the proximal tibia with massive degloving of the skin, in addition to other serious injuries. The degloving contraindicates ordinary internal fixation. Traction would not immobilize the limb sufficiently for soft-tissue healing, and an ordinary external frame would have to be applied through the soft-tissue lesions.

*The solution:* First the medullary canal is closed with cortex lag screws. The unilateral frame now provides optimum stability. The two proximal screws are driven into the epiphysis and connected by a double clamp such that the threaded rod runs between the screws. This arrangement is optimum for soft-tissue healing. After six weeks the fixator is removed, at which time the limb is functionally sound. Coexisting injuries also healed completely during the course of the fixation.

→

**Fig. 261 a–d.** Grade III open fracture of the proximal tibia with severe soft-tissue disruption. G.F., 1970, 12 years, ♀, 262860.

**a** Grade III open tibial fracture with soft-tissue lesion extending to the tibial tuberosity.
**b** Operation: fixation with unilateral frame + 2 cortex lag screws (to close medullary canal), debridement of soft tissues.
**c** Three weeks postinjury: soft tissues are healed, course is uneventful.
**d** Two small screws are still in place

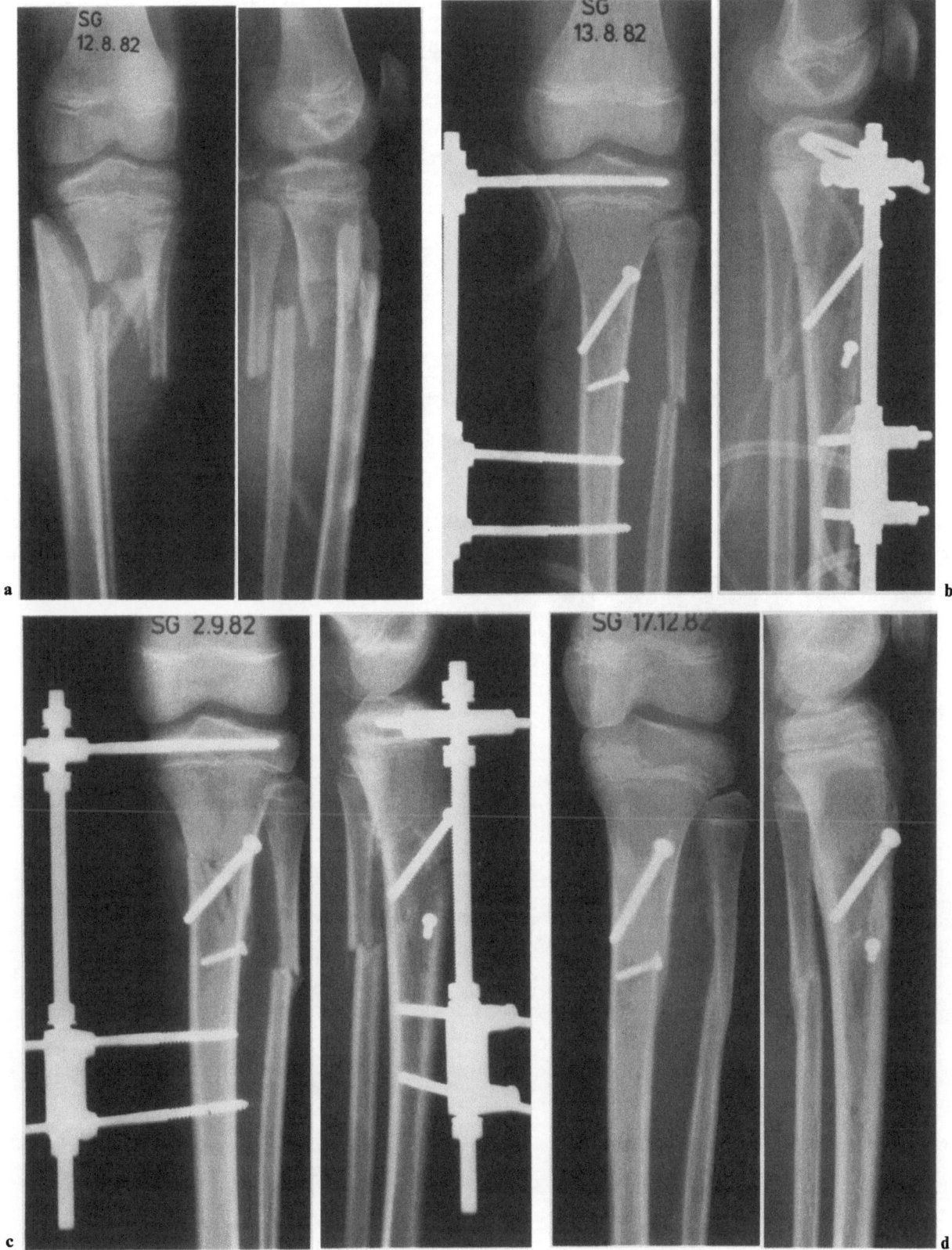

**Fig. 261a–d**

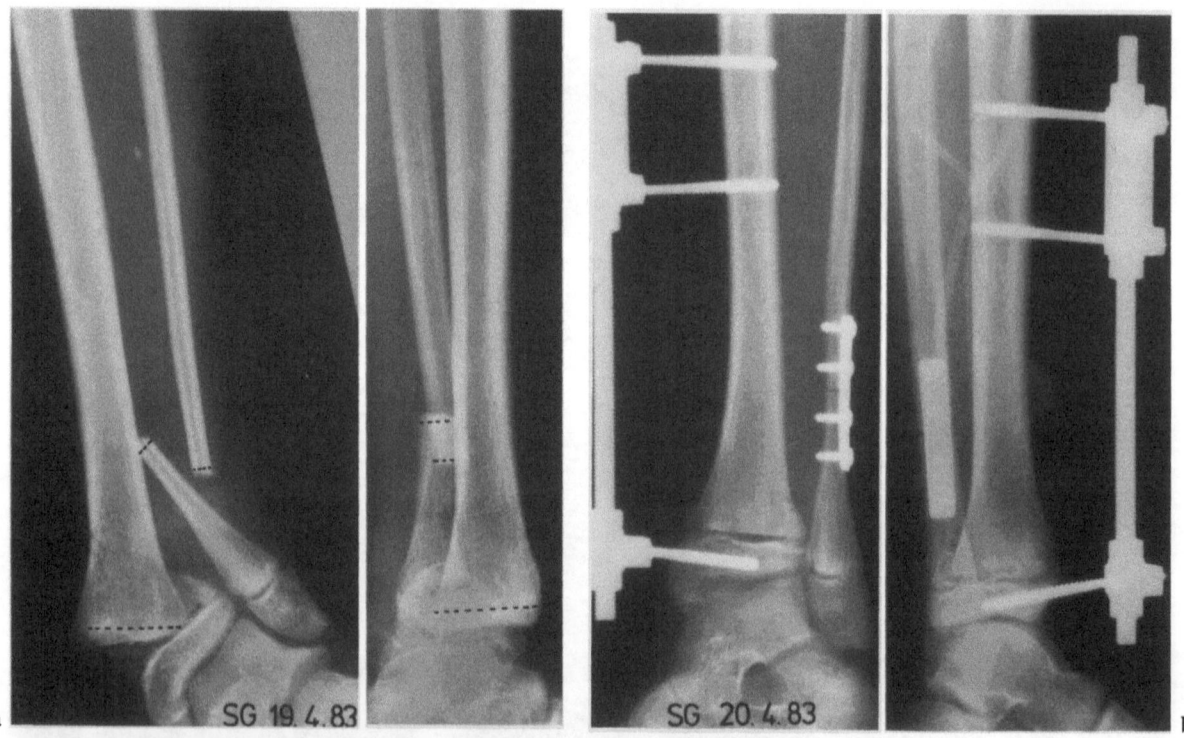

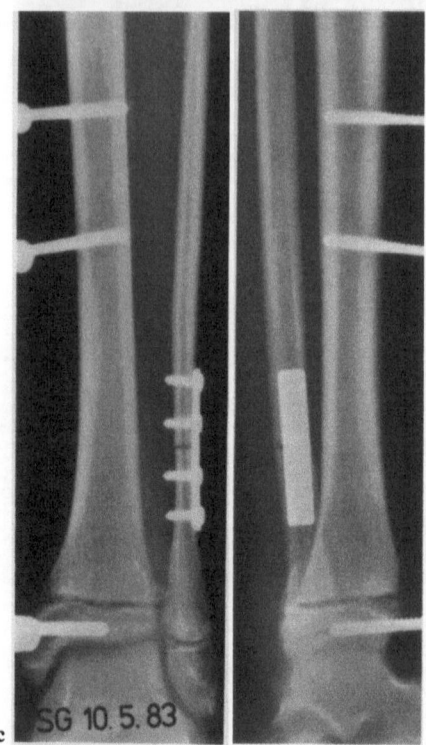

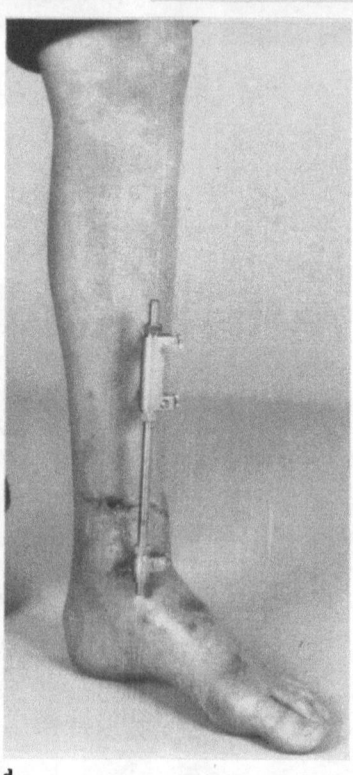

**Fig. 262 a–e.**
Heavy bone contamination in a grade II open tibial fracture. R.D., 1971, 12 years, ♂, 269 542.

**a** Preoperative status: grade II open tibial fracture, tibial metaphysis heavily contaminated with road dirt. A 1-cm bone resection is planned.
**b** Postoperative status: after debridement, 1 cm resected from distal tibia and from fibula. Small 4-hole plate applied to fibula, unilateral compression frame applied to tibia.
**c** Three weeks postinjury: soft tissues are healing well, no problems with fixation materials.
**d** Clinical status 3 weeks postinjury: soft tissues are healing, external fixator is in place and permits partial weight bearing; after frame removal, walking cast applied for additional 3 weeks.
**e** Four months postinjury: complete recovery, normal epiphyseal plate growth

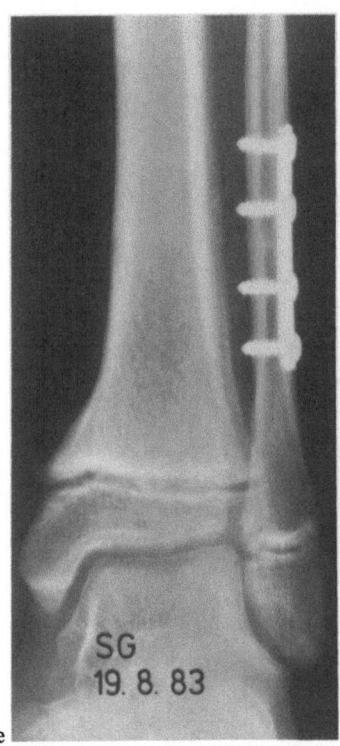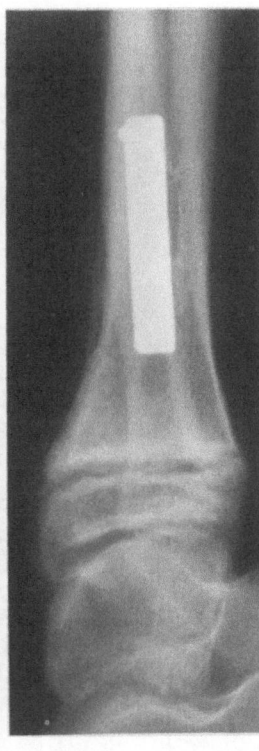

**Fig. 262e**

*Example 2* (Fig. 262)

Grade II open tibial fracture with gross contamination of the bone.

*The problem:* When a 12-year-old boy fell from his bicycle, the distal tibia was fractured and dragged against the asphalt, causing road dirt to be driven deep into the bone. The epiphyseal plate is exposed.

*The solution:* Following meticulous cleansing of the wound, the tibia is shortened by 1 cm in its metaphyseal portion. An equal amount of bone is resected from the fibula, and a unilateral frame is applied with one cortex screw in the epiphysis and two proximal screws in the midshaft. This assembly is stable enough to permit undisturbed soft-tissue healing. At eight weeks postinjury the fracture and soft tissues are healed, and the frame is removed. Follow-up radiographs at five months show normal growth in the distal epiphyseal plate.

*Example 3* (Fig. 263)

Infected fracture following conservative treatment.

*The problem:* A femoral shaft fracture in a 14-year-old boy was treated by traction on a supracondylar Kirschner wire. An infection developed along the wire tract. Because extensive distal stripping of the periosteum occurred at the time of injury, the Kirschner wire lay within the fracture hematoma, permitting the infection to spread to the fracture site. The infection and relative instability are an impediment to fracture healing.

*The solution:* Two unilateral frames are erected at right angles to each other. The resulting stability is sufficient to permit complete healing of the infection and fracture following debridement, suction irrigation and secondary cancellous bone grafting (Fig. 263). At 16 months postoperatively, recovery is complete.

*Example 4* (Fig. 264)

Infected nonunion of the tibia with bone loss, and arthritis of the ankle joint.

*The problem:* A 14-year-old boy was involved in a farm vehicular accident, sustaining an open tibial fracture contaminated with manure, in addition to a contused and lacerated wound on the lateral side of the ankle. Primary treatment consisted of calcaneus traction. A severe coli infection of the tibia and infectional arthritis of the ankle joint ensued.

*The solution:* A bilateral external frame is applied, at which time the tibiotalar joint is denuded of cartilage. The distal Steinmann pin fixes the talus against the tibia to secure the arthrodesis. The tibial infection is controlled by sequestrectomy and suction irrigation. The initial result is a nonunion with an osseous defect. After resolution of the infection, and while the original external fixator is still in place, two different cancellous bone grafts are performed to restore the tibial stock. At seven months postinjury the leg is again able to bear weight. Two years later the tibia is normal, with a good arthrodesis of the ankle joint and 1 cm limb shortening.

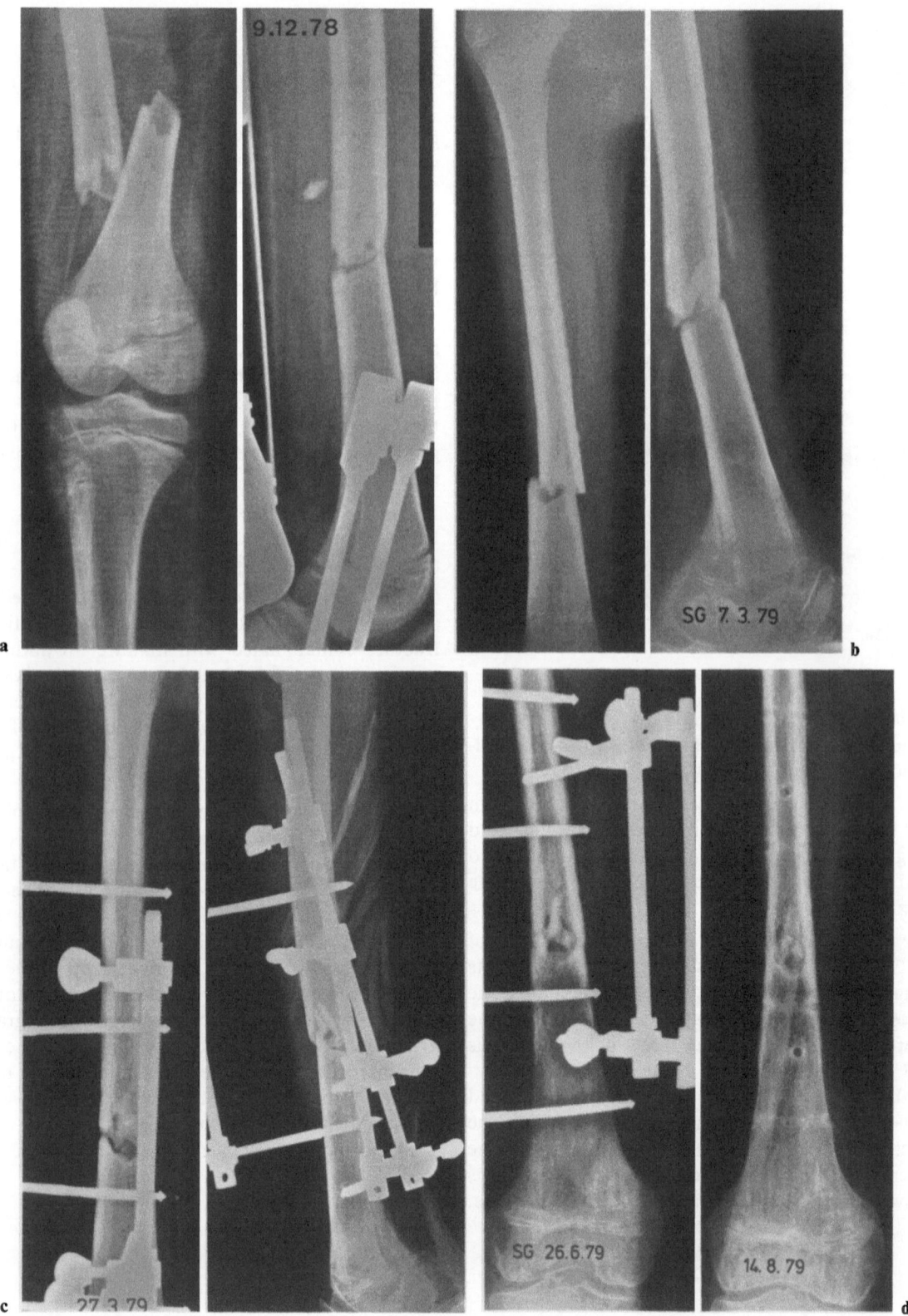

**Fig. 263a–d**

**Fig. 263 a–e.** Infected fracture following conservative treatment. M.R., 1964, 14 years, ♂, 227263.

**a** Closed fracture of right distal femoral shaft sustained in sledding accident. Treated by traction on supracondylar Kirschner wire. Wire removed due to wire track infection, hip spica applied.

**b** Three months postinjury: mobile, infected fracture with draining sinus.

**c** Operation: wound debridement, excision of sinus, suction irrigation for 2 weeks, 2 unilateral frames applied at right angles to each other, cancellous bone graft 2 weeks later.

**d** $3^1/_2$ months and 5 months after external fixation. Bony union, infection resolved.

**e** Two years postinjury: complete recovery

---

**Fig. 264 a–i.** Infected tibial nonunion with bone loss and arthritis of the ankle joint. G.E., 14 years, ♂, 142956.

**a** Grade II open tibial fracture with lacerated and contused wound over the lateral ankle joint.

**b** Calcaneus traction: initiation of *E. coli* infection in fracture and ankle joint.

**c** $2^1/_2$ weeks postinjury: debridement, bilateral frame with arthrodesis of ankle joint.

**d** Redebridement, frame is solidly in place.

**e** Eleven weeks postinjury: sequestrectomy is required.

**f** One month after sequestrectomy and cancellous bone graft: early consolidation.

**g** Five months postinjury: consolidation has progressed well enough to permit frame removal.

**h** Nine months postinjury: definitive cast removal.

**i** Two years postinjury, late follow-up: bony consolidation, good position of arthrodesis

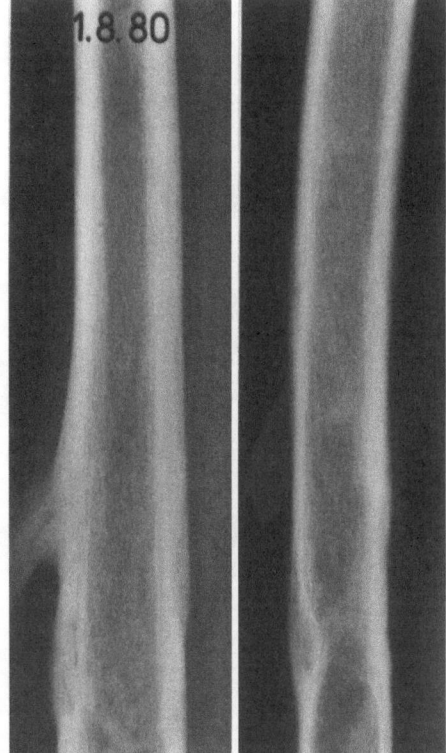

Fig. 263e

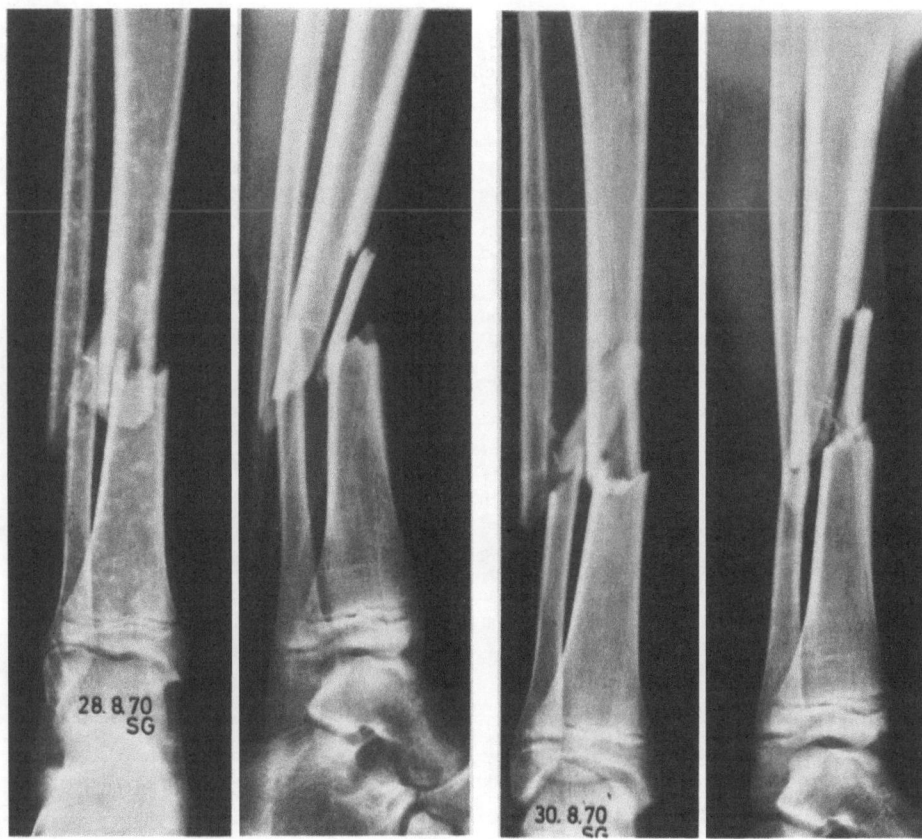

Fig. 264a, b

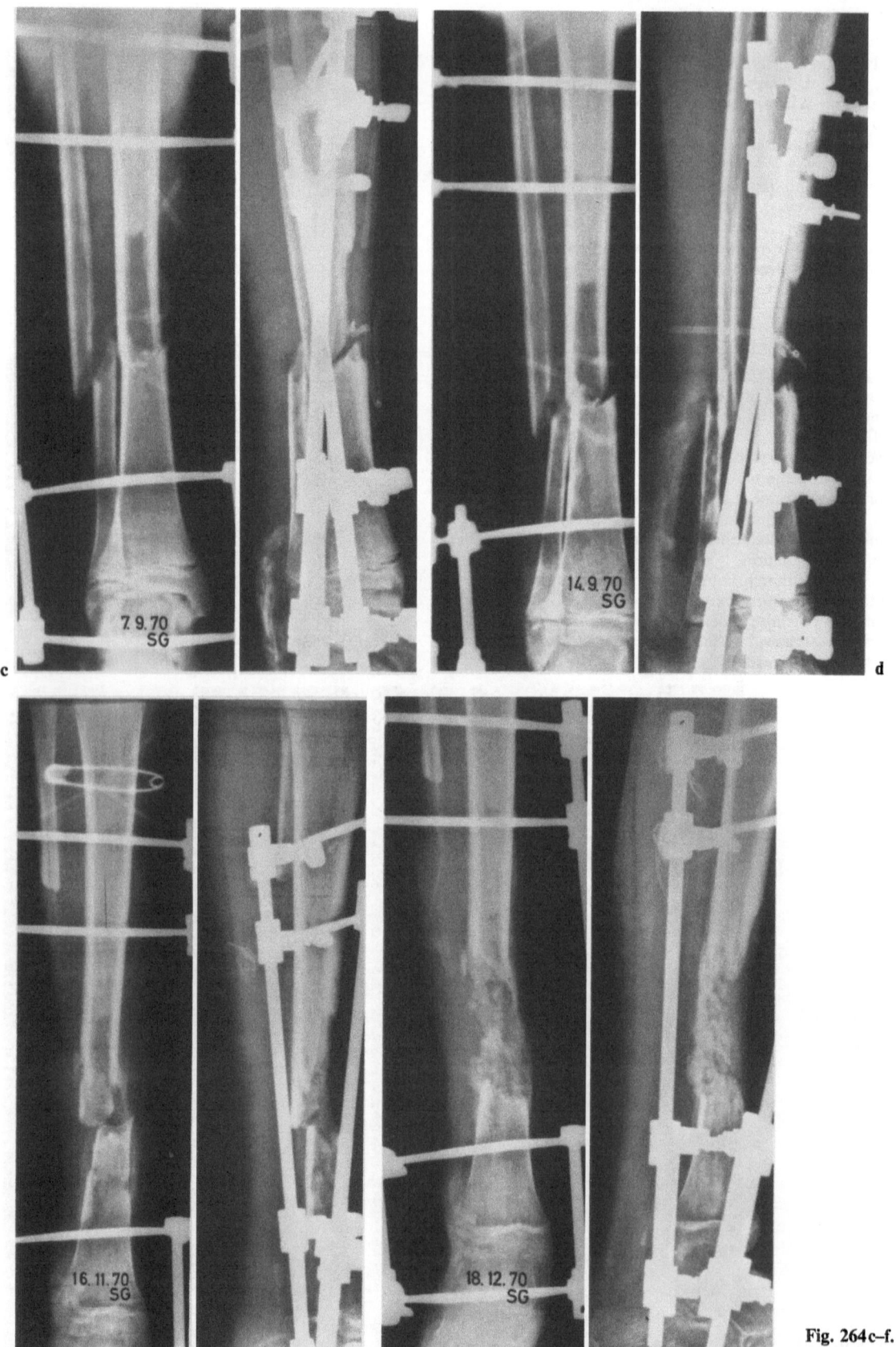

**Fig. 264c–f.**
Legend see p. 249

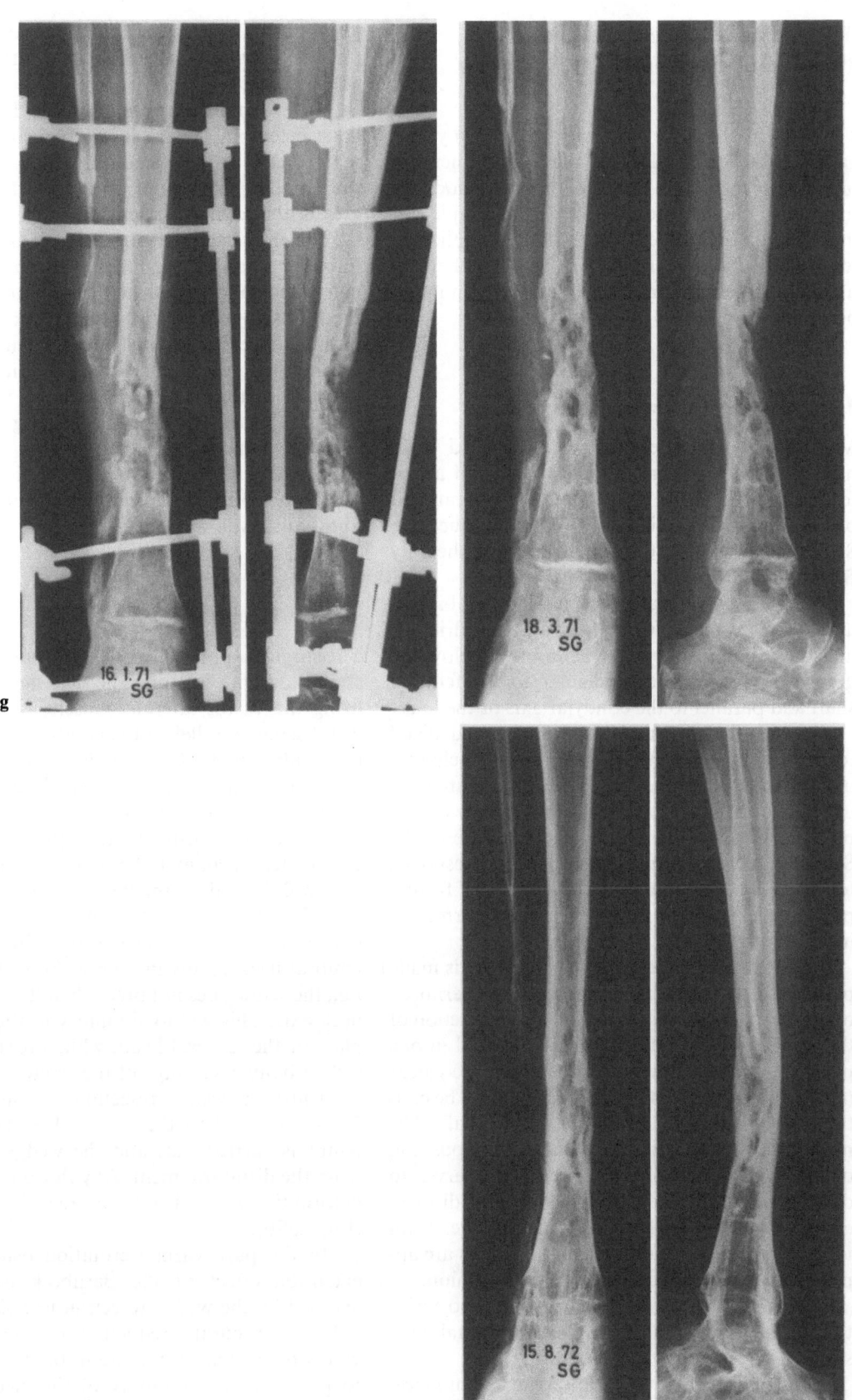

# 3 Corrective Osteotomies of the Proximal Femur in Small Children

The intertrochanteric corrective osteotomy has gained a definitive place in the management of hip joint dysplasias in small children. Methods for fixation of the osteotomy range from simple immobilization in plaster to the most complicated techniques of internal fixation. We feel that the unilateral external frame is an ideal fixation method in such cases.

## 3.1 Instrumentation and Technique

MÜLLER, in 1955, described the standard technique for the unilateral external fixation of an intertrochanteric varus osteotomy in the treatment of hip joint dysplasias. In this technique two Schanz screws and two threaded rods are the only fixation materials that are used.

*First,* the vastus lateralis muscle is mobilized, a pilot hole is predrilled with the 3.2-mm drill bit, and the distal Schanz screw is inserted below the greater trochanter, perpendicular to the femoral shaft and parallel to the condylar axis of the knee.

*Second,* the proximal screw is inserted distal to the epiphyseal plate of the greater trochanter in the direction of the femoral neck, its angle of insertion corresponding to the desired angle of correction. At this point the divergence angle of the Schanz screws relative to each other corresponds to the angle of varus correction in the frontal plane, and to the angle of rotational correction in the sagittal plane.

*Third,* the intertrochanteric osteotomy is made parallel to the proximal Schanz screw (Bernbeck osteotomy). Following reduction and impaction of the fragments, the Schanz screws are fixed in one plane by means of two threaded rods; the calcar (medial border of the femoral neck) should be continuous with the medial border of the shaft. The medial rod serves basically to maintain apposition of the fragments, while the lateral rod serves to distract the screw ends and thus exert additional compression across the osteotomy surface. With this technique the cancellous bone surfaces are apposed and compressed in an optimum fashion.

The Schanz screws are inserted just posterior to the operative wound through separate stab incisions.

While this technique affords an excellent placement of the external fixator in biomechanical terms, it results in two separate, indrawn, unsightly pinhole scars that may be particularly objectionable to adolescent girls.

A further disadvantage of the Bernbeck oblique osteotomy is the inevitable extension effect that occurs in the osteotomy itself. The greater the axial or rotational correction must be, the greater the resulting extension effect (Fig. 265 a).

It is interesting to note that MÜLLER has come to prefer small angled-blade plates over the external frame for fixation of the osteotomy, even in the 2–7 age group. While this method avoids the disadvantages mentioned above, it necessitates a second operation and a second hospitalization for removal of the plate. We continue to prefer the unilateral external frame in this age group because it obviates the need for readmission.

Additionally, the external fixation technique has been modified and improved to eliminate the above disadvantages.

## 3.2 The Technique Practiced at our Center

The surgical approach is made through a standard straight lateral incision. The *first step,* after mobilizing the vastus lateralis muscle, is to insert the distal screw parallel to the condylar axis and perpendicular to the femoral shaft. A 3.2-mm pilot hole is predrilled to facilitate the insertion.

*Second,* the drill bit for the proximal screw is introduced just distal to the epiphyseal plate of the greater trochanter. The orientation of the pilot hole will depend on the type and degree of correction that is required. For most varus derotation osteotomies the proximal screw should exit the femoral neck cortex in its posteromedial portion, i.e., the screw does not precisely follow the femoral neck axis. This will avoid injury to the epiphyseal plate of the femoral head, while providing an excellent bony anchorage of the screw.

*Third,* a wedge resection osteotomy is performed parallel to the screws. Derotation of the femur is carried out, and the wedge is removed from the distal fragment. Any flexion or extension deformities may also be corrected at this time (Fig. 265 b).

In the pure varus derotation osteotomy, the extension effect of the Bernbeck osteotomy is avoided by the wedge resection technique. It provides an accurate reduction of the fragments, which is secured by mounting the two rods so as to preserve the continuity of the medial cortical line. The screw-rod system is oriented parallel to

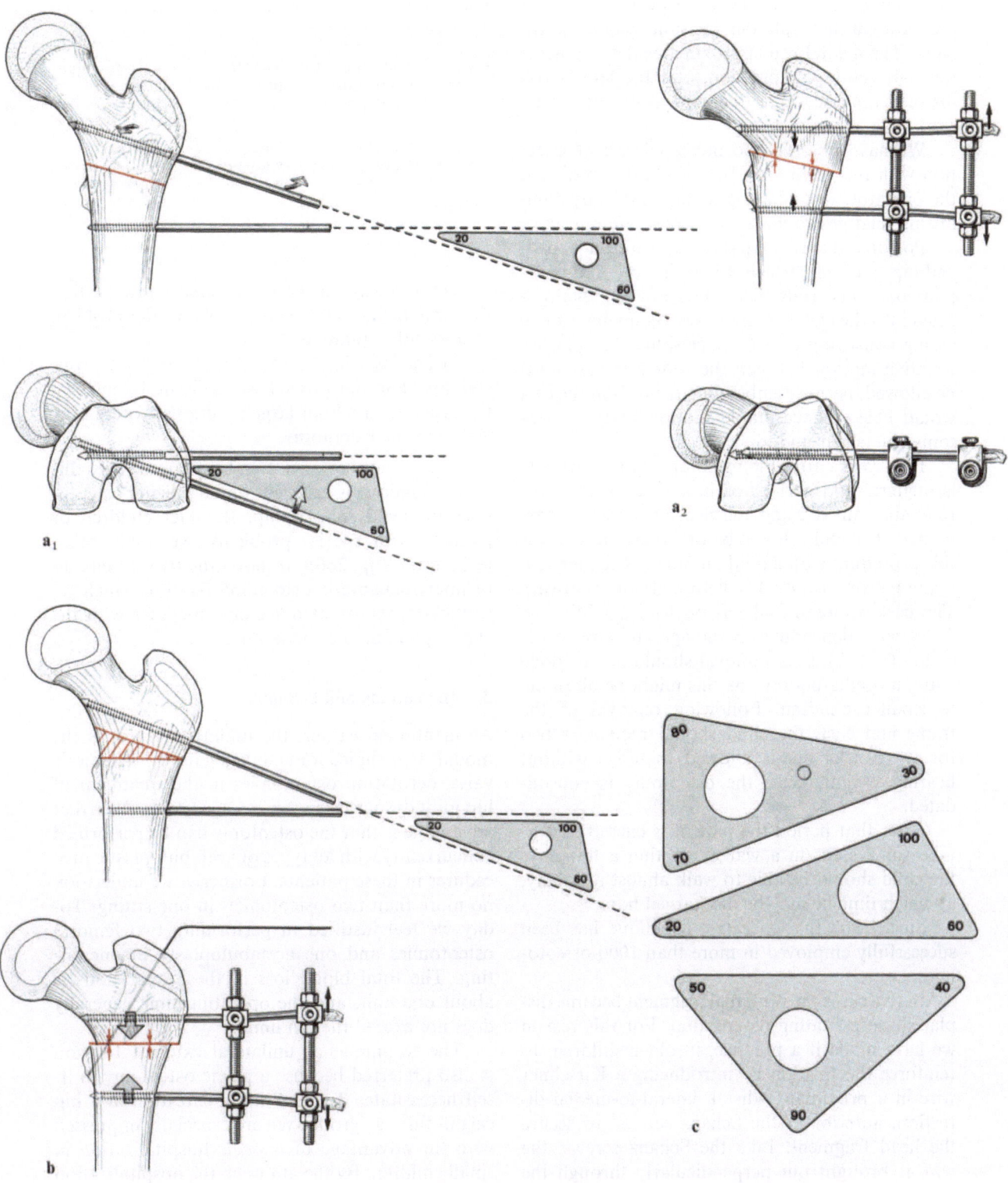

**Fig. 265 a–c.** The basic technique of the unilateral external fixation of an intertrochanteric corrective osteotomy in a small child. **a** The basic technique of MÜLLER (1955). **b** Current technique: wedge osteotomy, supplemental fixation with Kirschner wire. **c** Triangular positioning plates help to define the angle of correction

the frontal plane, and the screws can be brought out straight through the incision without difficulty. The medial rod approximates the fragments through gentle compression, and the lateral rod distracts the screw ends to compress the osteotomy site.

We have observed no increased risk of infection with this technique, because both screws exit the operative wound at right angles, thereby minimizing relative motion at the screw-skin interface.

Postoperatively the patient is placed in a padded hip spica cast which leaves the foot and ankle joint free. The rods themselves are not incorporated into the cast and are covered only by a small casing consisting of a Cramer splint and plaster. Relative motion between the rods and cast must be allowed, because embedding the rods in the cast would cause unacceptable motion at the osteotomy site (shear and torsion!).

Five weeks after the osteotomy, which usually is bilateral and performed in a single sitting, the rods are removed and the Schanz screws are extracted. The child should be well premedicated for this procedure with a mild anesthetic (we give Rohypnol drops orally 1 h before frame removal). The cast is closed and left on for an additional 2–4 weeks, depending on the age and size of the child (Table 2). Cast removal should not be done with an oscillating saw, as this might be alarming to smaller children. Following removal of the frame and cast, the child should remain in bed for two weeks but is allowed to move without bearing weight, since the osteotomy is consolidated.

After that period the patient is encouraged to take some steps in a walker. Within a few days the child should be able to walk almost normally, at which time he may be discharged home.

Since 1967 this operative technique has been successfully employed in more than 1000 osteotomies.

In five cases the proximal fragment became displaced, necessitating reoperation. For this reason we have made it a practice, in older children, to reinforce the fixation by introducing a Kirschner wire in a proximal-to-distal, lateral-to-medial direction, anterior to the Schanz screws, to secure the head fragment. Like the Schanz screws, the wire is brought out perpendicularly through the surgical incision and later is removed together with the screws. This supplemental fixation has entirely eliminated the problem of fragment dislodgement. We have made only two slight modifications in the original technique of MÜLLER:

**Table 1.** Scheme for the postoperative management of intertrochanteric osteotomies

| Age (years) | Time in external fixator after surgery | Time in plaster after surgery | Start of ambulation after surgery |
| --- | --- | --- | --- |
| 2–5 | 5 weeks | 7 weeks | 9 weeks |
| 5–6 | 5 weeks | 8 weeks | 10 weeks |
| 6 | 5 weeks | 9 weeks | 11 weeks |

a) We always place the Schanz screws within the straight incision, thereby solving the problem of unsightly "pinholes."

b) The insertion of a Kirschner wire to improve stability. This has proved especially useful in spastic patients, in whom large additional forces may act upon the osteotomy.

In children between 2 and 7 years of age, this basic technique is excellent for stabilizing osteotomies in the dysplastic hip. In older children or patients with special problems, we apply other techniques. Fig. 266a, b shows the five techniques of intertrochanteric osteotomy fixation which we routinely practice at our clinic, together with the classic plate fixation in adults.

### 3.3 Indications and Examples

As mentioned earlier, the unilateral frame is the modality of choice for stabilizing intertrochanteric varus derotation osteotomies in the treatment of hip joint dysplasias in the 2–6 age group. A further advantage is that the osteotomy can be performed concurrently with all types of acetabuloplastic procedures in these patients. Formerly, we undertook no more than two osteotomies in one sitting. Today we feel justified in performing two femoral osteotomies and one acetabuloplasty in one sitting. The total blood loss in these operations is about one unit, and the operating time generally does not exceed the 2-h limit.

The technique of unilateral external fixation is also preferred because a pelvic osteotomy in itself necessitates 7 weeks' immobilization in a hip cast in this age group. We are especially impressed with the advantage of a *single* hospitalization in small children. By the 4th week the hospitalization experience can no longer be considered to be a psychological insult, and the child still has sufficient time, after pain has subsided, to become fully integrated into his peer and preschool environment.

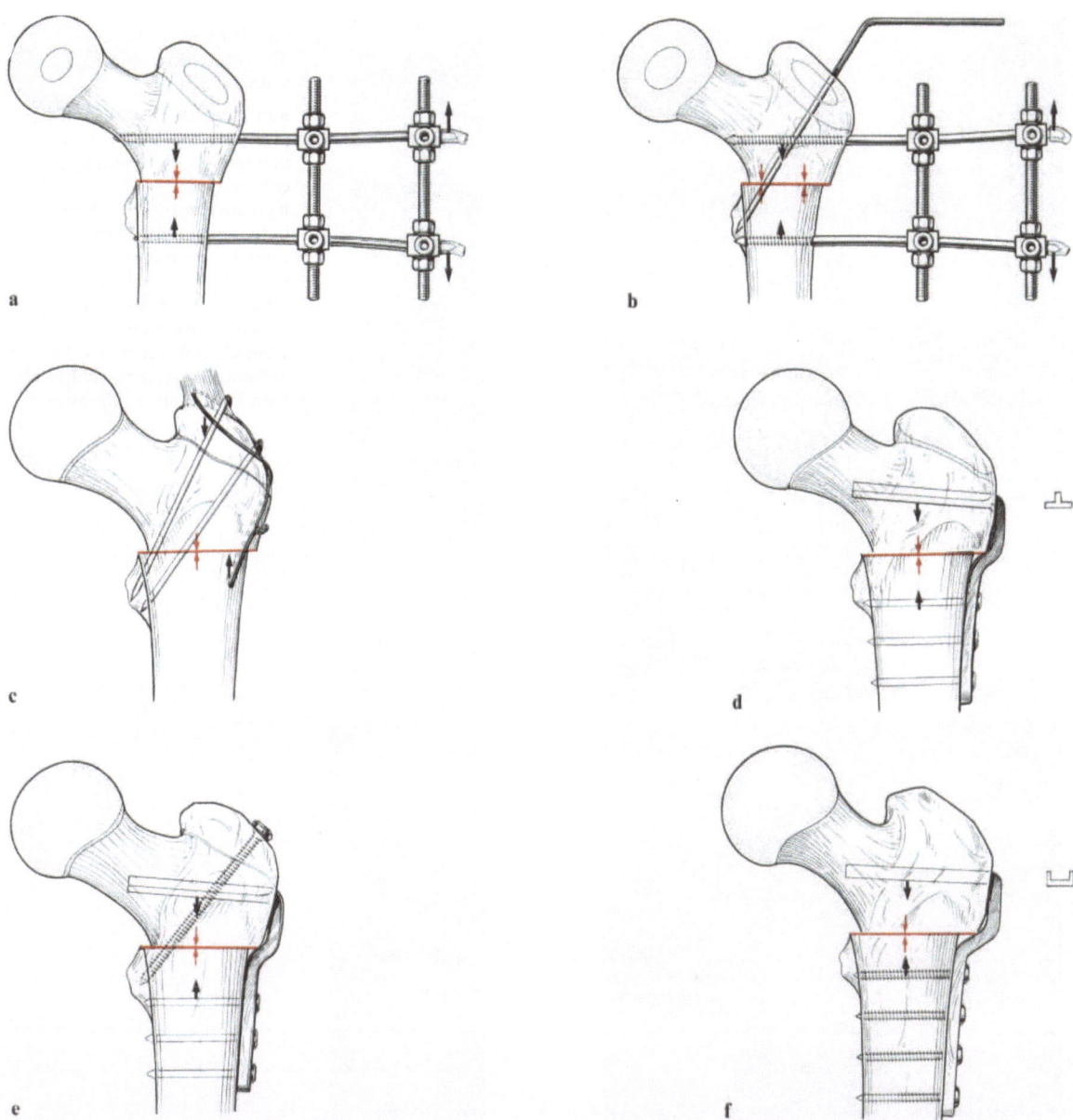

**Fig. 266a–f.** Different fixation techniques for intertrochanteric osteotomies. **a** Unilateral frame in a small child. **b** Unilateral frame and Kirschner wire for children of 2–6 years. **c** Tension-band fixation with Kirschner wires and cerclage (5–9 years). **d** Tension-band fixation with standard pediatric hip plate. **e** Standard pediatric hip plate and anteromedial lag screw. **f** Standard plate fixation (with angled-blade plate) in an adult

*Example 1* (Fig. 267)
The basic technique.

The patient, a boy 2 years and 3 months of age, exhibits a severe dysplasia of the left acetabular roof associated with a bilateral pathologic ante-

torsion and coxa valga. The aim of surgery is to alter the mechanics of the hip so as to relieve the acetabular dysplasia and restore normal joint motion. In the example shown, the left side is corrected in an initial sitting by acetabuloplasty and intertrochanteric osteotomy. The right side is corrected 15 months later by an intertrochanteric varus derotation osteotomy of the wedge-resection type. A unilateral external frame is applied. Nine weeks later consolidation is complete.

*Example 2* (Fig. 268)
Bilateral varus derotation osteotomy combined with acetabuloplasty in one sitting.

A boy 2 years and 7 months of age was treated conservatively for a congenital dislocation of the

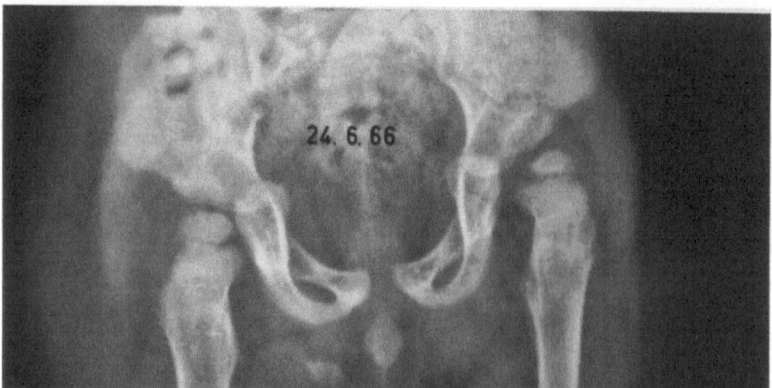

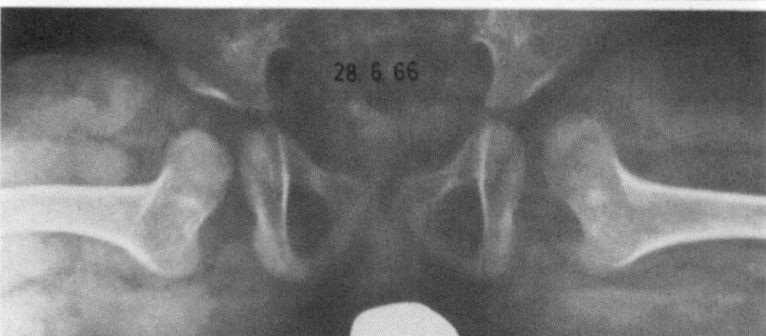

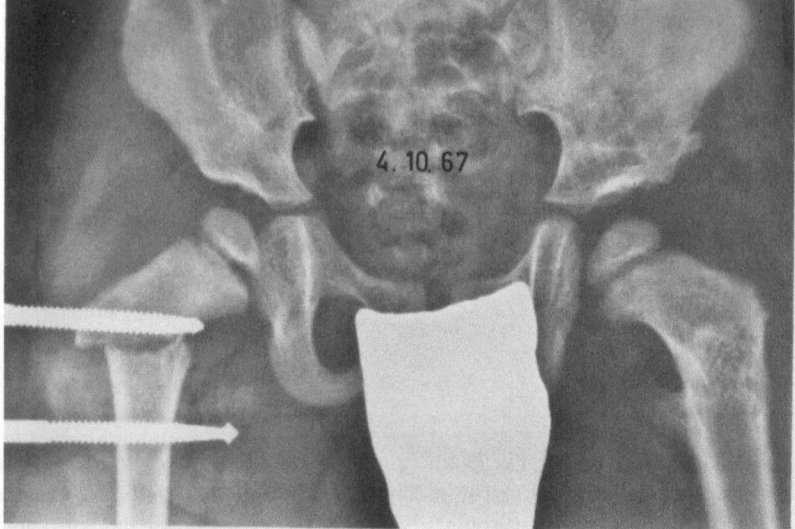

b

**Fig. 267 a–c.**
The basic technique. G.T., 1964, 3 years, ♂, 95470.

**a** Preoperative status: acetabuloplasty on left side, severe bilateral antetorsion of femoral neck and coxa valga.
**b** Operation on right side: technique of intertrochanteric osteotomy with unilateral frame. Operation on left side: status 15 months after acetabuloplasty and intertrochanteric osteotomy.
**c** Nine months after right-sided osteotomy: excellent consolidation with no fragment migration

left hip. He presented with a residual dysplasia of the left hip with marked pathologic antetorsion of the femora.

The operation corrects both the bilateral femoral deformity and the deformity of the left acetabulum (SALTER pelvic osteotomy).

Seven weeks later all three osteotomies are consolidated. At five months both hip joints are developing normally.

**Fig. 267c**

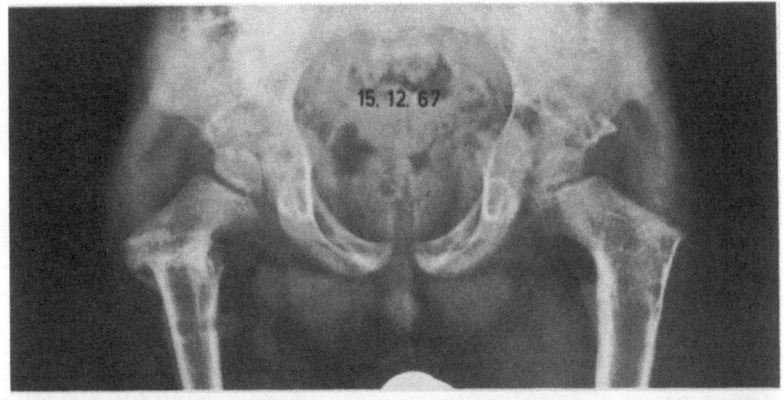

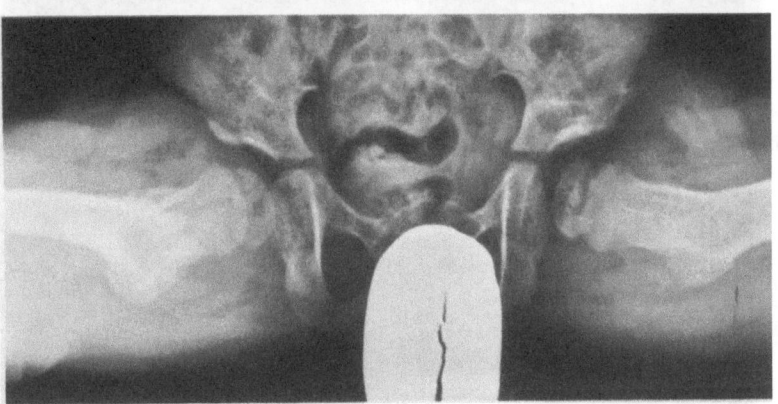

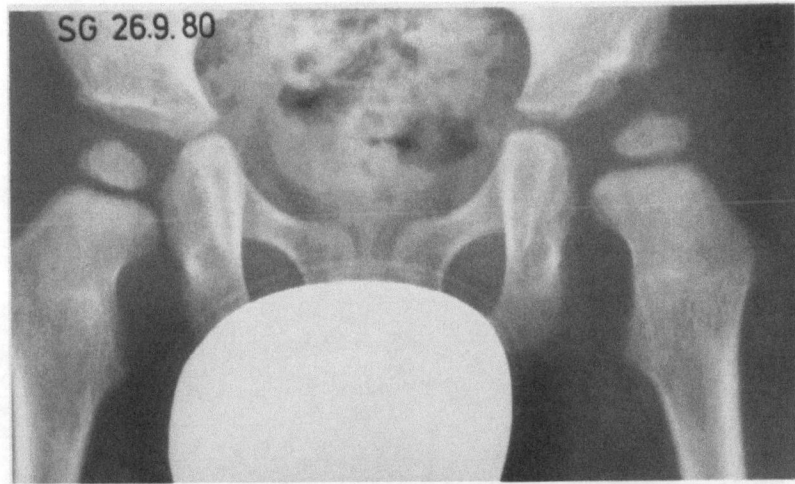

**Fig. 268 a–d.**
Technique for the unilateral external fixation of an intertrochanteric osteotomy combined with acetabuloplasty. B.B., 1978, 2 years 7 months, ♂, 245721.

**a** Preoperative status: severe bilateral coxa valga and femoral antetorsion with marked dysplasia of the left acetabular roof.
**b** Operation: bilateral intertrochanteric corrective osteotomy, supplemental Kirschner wire fixation; Salter pelvic osteotomy on left side.
**c** Seven weeks postoperatively: femoral osteotomy is well consolidated in desired position.
**d** Five months after osteotomy: normal bone structure in all osteotomized areas

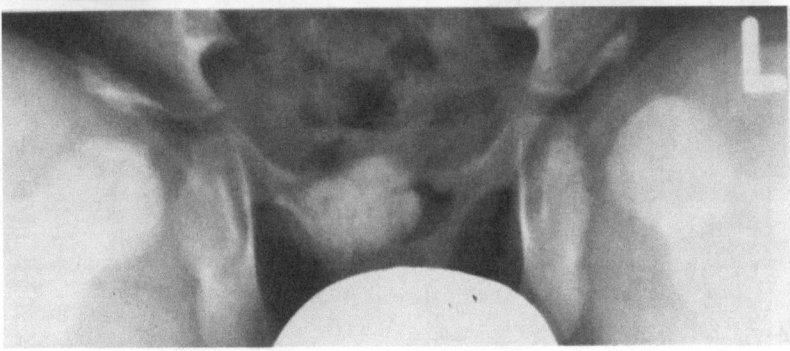

a

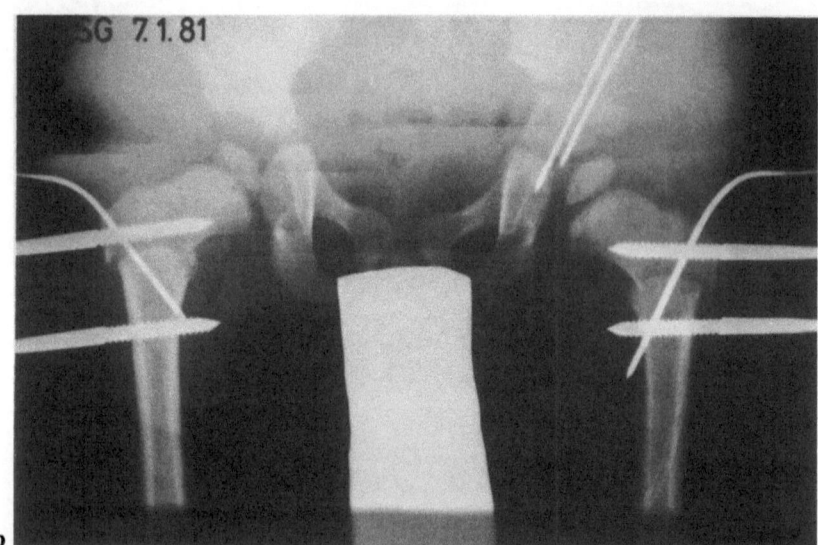

**Fig. 268b–d.** Legend see p. 257

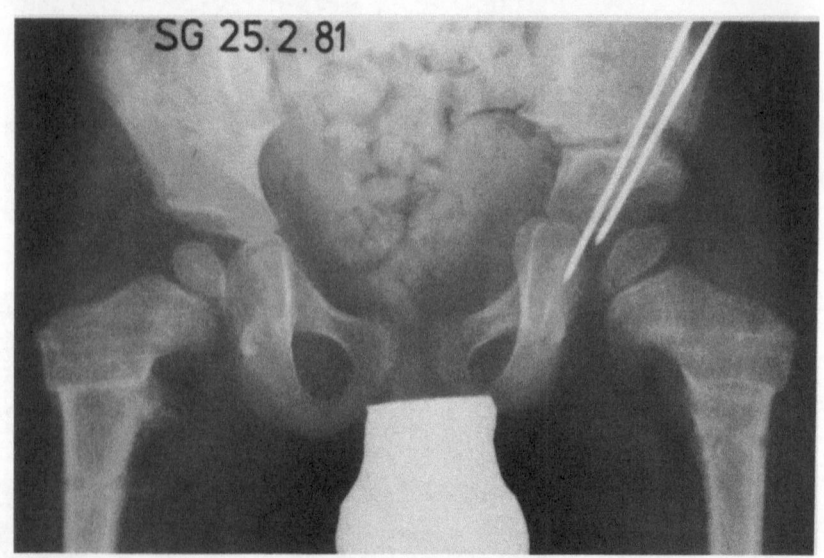

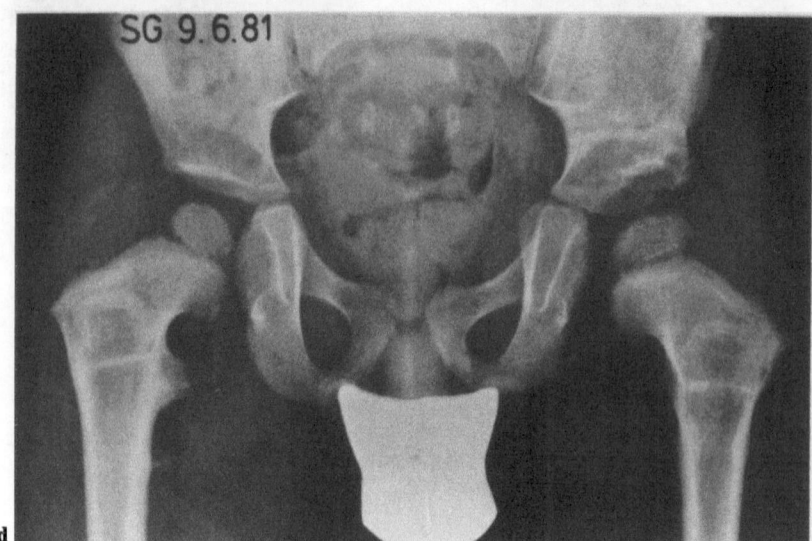

# 4 Lengthening Osteotomies in Children and Adolescents

## 4.1 Introduction

External fixation has become a standard part of limb lengthening procedures. Two types of external frame may be used, depending on the site of the lengthening and the age of the patient:

1. The bilateral frame, originated by ANDERSON.
2. The unilateral frame. This may be either a double threaded-rod frame or the telescoping apparatus of WAGNER.

The bilateral frame is best suited for thin bones. The main disadvantage is that the screws or pins often are embedded in large soft-tissue masses.

The unilateral frame is suitable for use on the femur in children and on the tibia in adolescents.

We divide all limb lengthening procedures into two stages:

a) The *distraction stage,* in which the limb is elongated slowly and continuously at a rate of no more than 1–1.5 mm per day.

b) The *consolidation stage:* In children, it is very often sufficient to leave the lengthening apparatus in place. The osteogenic potential in children is so good that complete consolidation can occur in just a few weeks. This is especially true of meta-physeal osteotomies, although the great majority of osteotomies must be performed in the midshaft region. In older children and adolescents, cancellous bone grafting and internal fixation are necessary once the desired degree of lengthening has been obtained.

The standard technique of the lengthening osteotomy was described extensively by WAGNER, and so here we shall examine it only on the basis of examples. Main attention will be given to any modifications that we have made in the WAGNER method, and to our own special techniques.

## 4.2 Lengthening Osteotomy of the Humerus

While lengthening osteotomies of the humerus are rarely indicated, it must be borne in mind that girls in particular may experience serious functional and cosmetic disability as a result of significant shortening.

*Example 1* (Fig. 269)
A juvenile aneurysmatic bone cyst in a 5-year-old girl caused extreme deformity of the proximal humeral epiphysis with destruction of the growth zone. Corrective osteotomy can restore the mechanics of the shoulder joint, but a discrepancy of limb length is inevitable. The patient presented with 8 cm of limb shortening. The WAGNER apparatus was applied anterolaterally, and the humerus

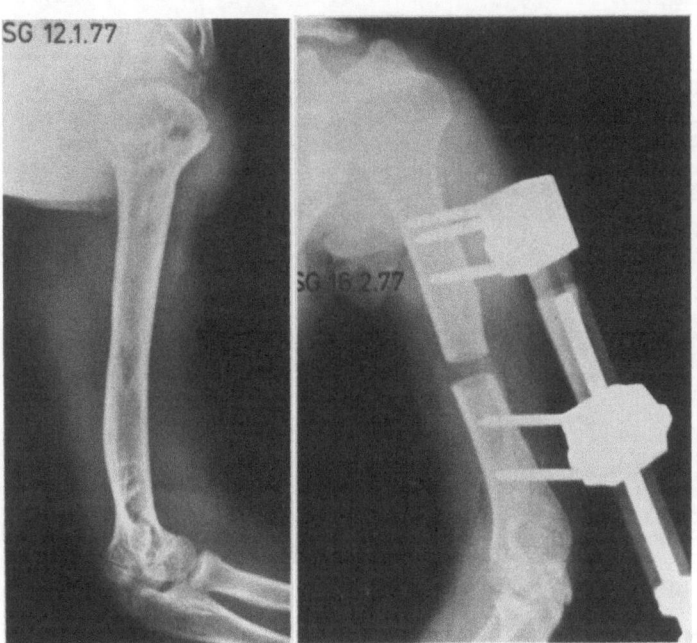

**Fig. 269 a–d.** Lengthening osteotomy of the humerus. L.A., 1965, 12 years, ♀, 138427.

**a** Humeral shortening (8 cm) secondary to surgery for juvenile aneurysmatic bone cyst of proximal humerus 7 years prior. Application of small Wagner lengthening apparatus, transverse subperiosteal osteotomy of humerus.
**b** Staged lengthening carried out over $2^1/_2$ months. External fixator left on for additional 2 months.
**c** Seven months after osteotomy: consolidation with 8-cm gain of limb length.
**d** Three years after lengthening: equal limb lengths, normal osseous structure

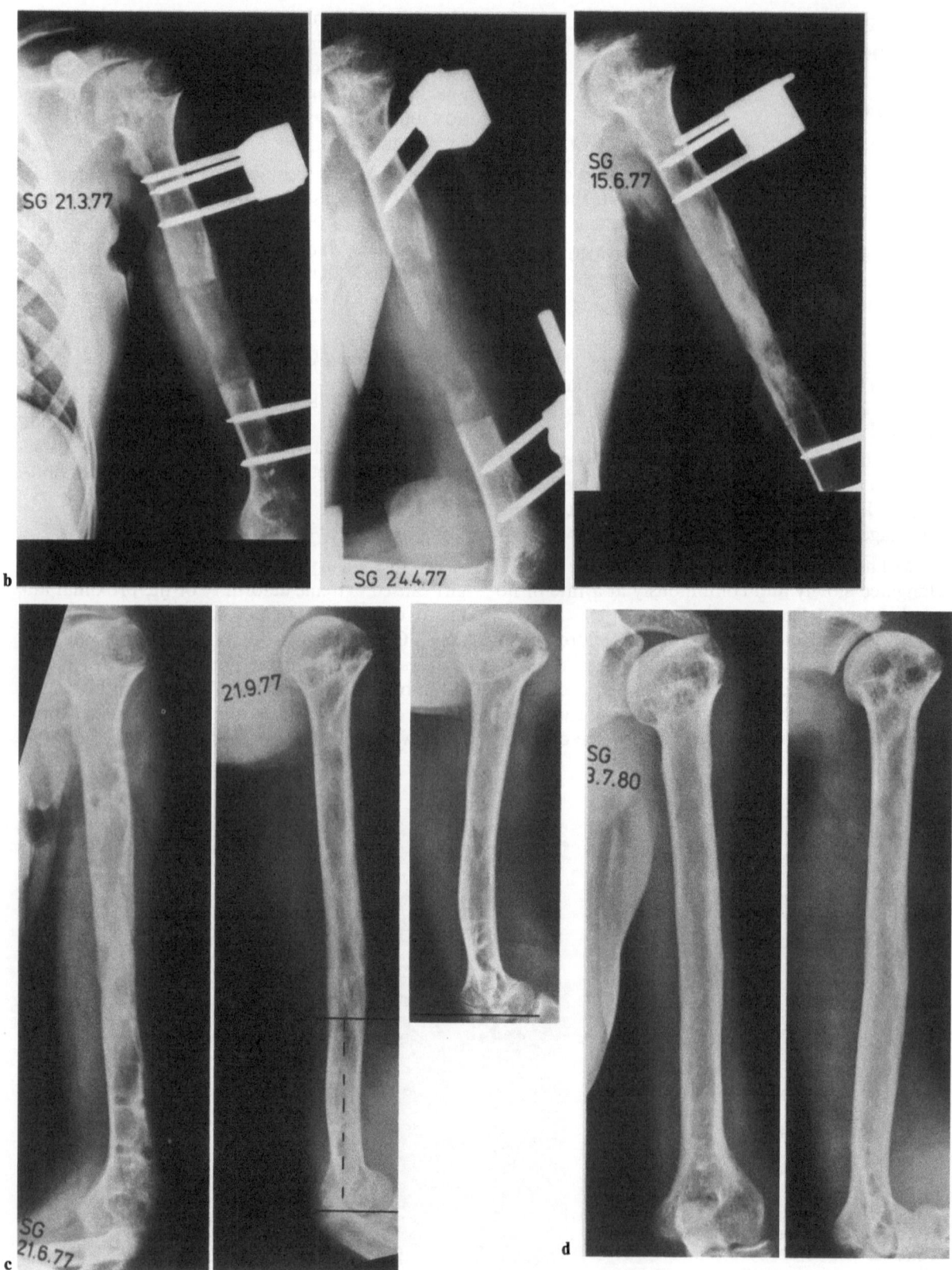

**Fig. 269 b–d.** Legend see p. 259

was osteotomized subperiosteally so that periosteal bone formation would not be impaired.

This obviated the need for a secondary internal fixation or cancellous bone graft of the humerus. Once length symmetry was obtained, the Wagner device was left on for an additional 8 weeks before removal. Late follow-up shows normal osseous structures with no visible bone scar.

## 4.3 Lengthening Osteotomy of the Femur

External fixation for limb lengthening is most commonly employed for the short femur. Either the threaded-rod fixator or the Wagner device may be used, depending on the size of the femur, the age of the patient, and the desired correction.

*Example 1* (Fig. 270)
Subtrochanteric lengthening for coxa vara with a pseudarthrosis of the femoral neck.

*The problem:* A 9-year-old girl has a marked limb length discrepancy as a result of a coxa vara deformity. Because of instability in the hip joint, supplemental fixation is desired.

*The solution:* First a hip spica cast patterned after the push-and-pull cast is applied. Then the threaded-rod external fixator is applied, and the subtrochanteric osteotomy is performed. Following the staged lengthening, internal plating is done as in a Schanz osteotomy, and a cancellous bone graft is applied. Secondary bending of the plate occurs during the protracted course of healing. At reoperation a tibial bone graft is interposed on the medial side, and a new, somewhat longer tension-band plate is fastened to the lateral side. Rapid, uneventful bone healing and remodeling ensue. Fourteen months after the second operation the bone is entirely sound.

*Example 2* (Fig. 271)
Posttraumatic femoral shortening with varus growth deformity of the distal femur.

*The problem:* Four years previously a 14-year-old boy sustained a transcondylar fracture of the distal femur with partial destruction of the epiphyseal plate. Despite accurate open reduction and internal fixation with screws, the injury resulted in impaired and arrested growth with 5 cm of limb shortening and a marked varus deformity of the knee.

*The solution:* The screws of the Wagner apparatus are inserted so as to effect a partial valgus correction of the limb axis.

A 6-cm lengthening osteotomy is performed, and a plate and cancellous bone graft are applied to the lengthened area to ensure a rapid consolidation. Eighteen months later the residual distal deformity is corrected by a closing-wedge osteotomy secured in standard fashion with a lateral angled-blade plate.

*Example 3* (Fig. 272)
Posttraumatic limb shortening and valgus deformity of the knee.

*The problem:* Two years earlier a girl of 12 years sustained a fracture of the distal femur and tibia that was managed with a condylar plate. She presented to us with a valgus deformity of the knee and an arrest of growth in the distal femur.

*The solution:* A closing-wedge varus supracondylar osteotomy is performed on the medial side and secured with a semitubular tension-band plate using our standard technique. In the same sitting a Wagner apparatus is applied anterolaterally across the transversely osteotomized shaft. After sufficient length is obtained, a posterior wave plate is applied with the patient in the prone position, and a bone block from the iliac crest is interposed anteriorly; cancellous bone grafts also are applied. Consolidation is rapid and uneventful. Two years postoperatively the axial and length symmetry of the limbs is excellent, and the patient is free of complaints.

---------------------------------------------→

**Fig. 270 a–h.** Lengthening osteotomy of the femur in coxa vara with femoral neck nonunion. R.A., 1967, 9 years, ♀, 198310.

**a** Preoperative status: 4 cm of shortening.
**b** Postoperatively: threaded external fixator + hip spica with incremental lengthening.
**c** Three weeks after lengthening: internal plate and cancellous bone graft (as in Schanz osteotomy).
**d** Four months postoperatively: equality of limb length.
**e** Ten months postoperatively: nonunion with bending of plate.
**f** Second operation: medial fibular bone graft + lateral tension-band plate.
**g** One year after 2nd operation: problem-free consolidation.
**h** Three years after lengthening osteotomy: perfect consolidation

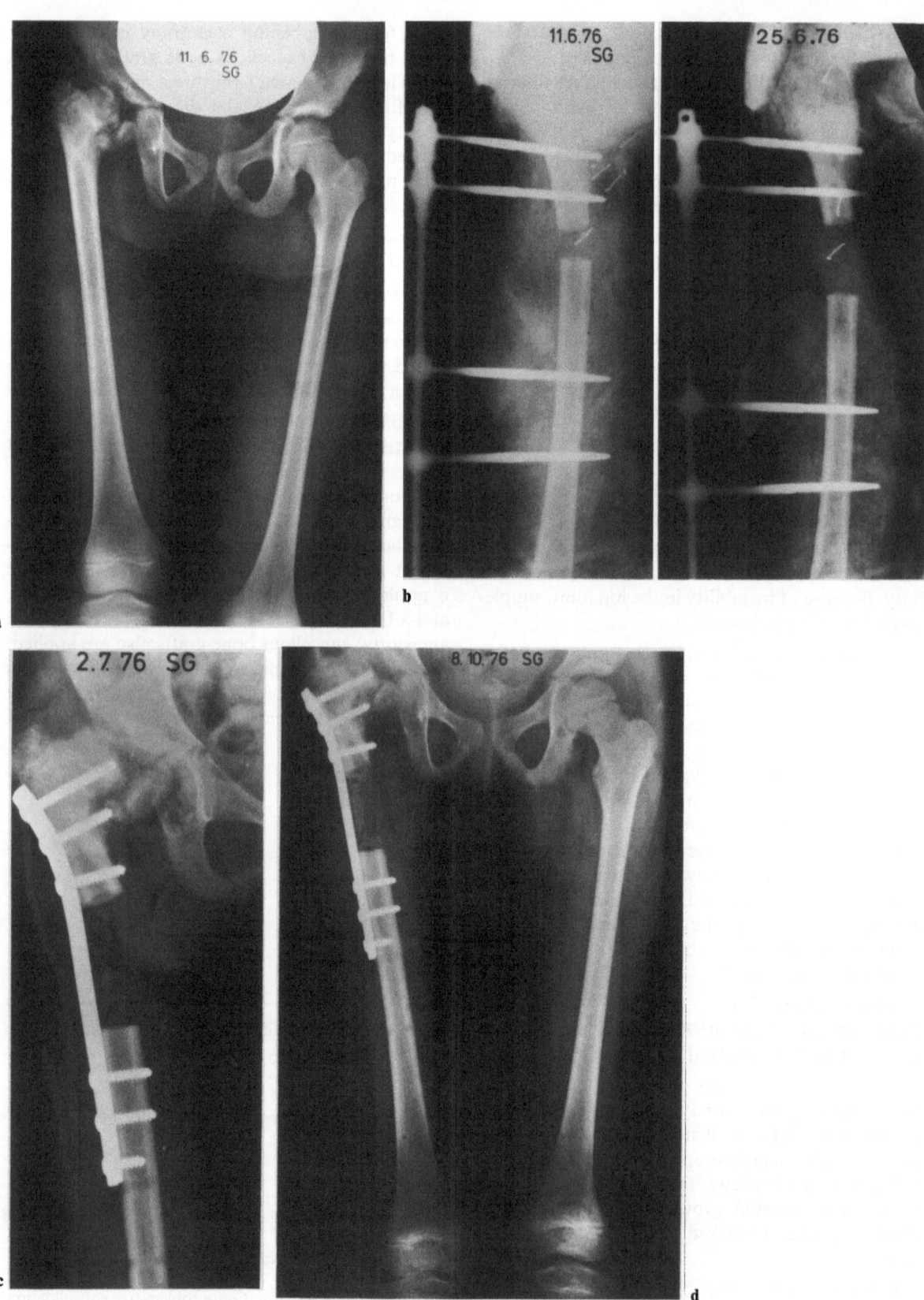

**Fig. 270 a–d.** Legend see p. 261

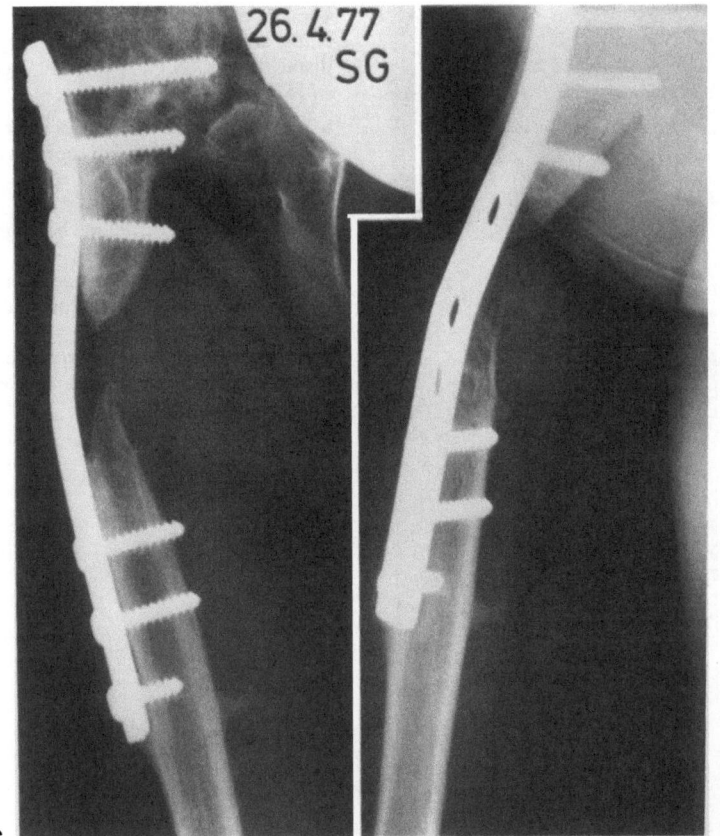

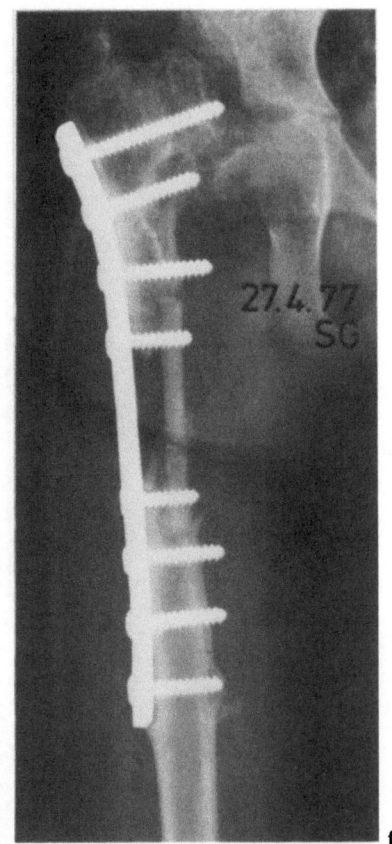

e                                                                          f

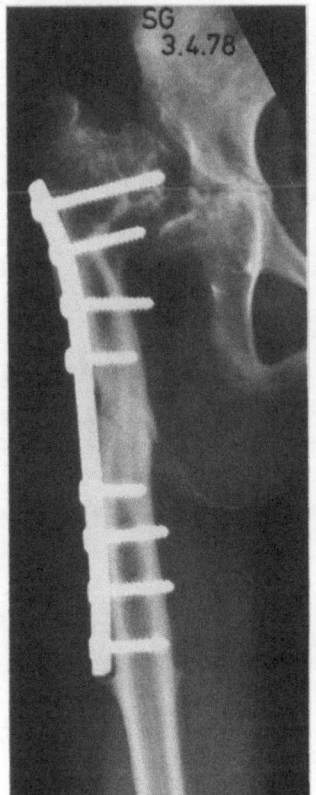

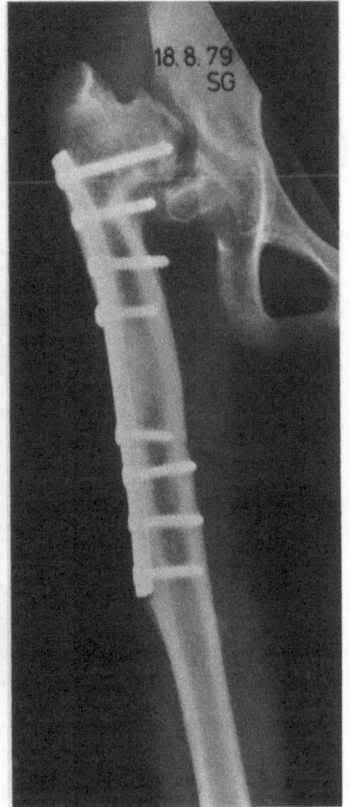

**Fig. 270e–h.** Legend see p. 261

g                                                                          h

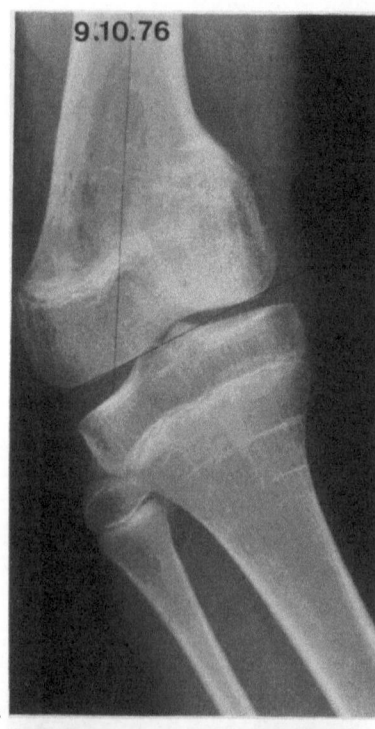
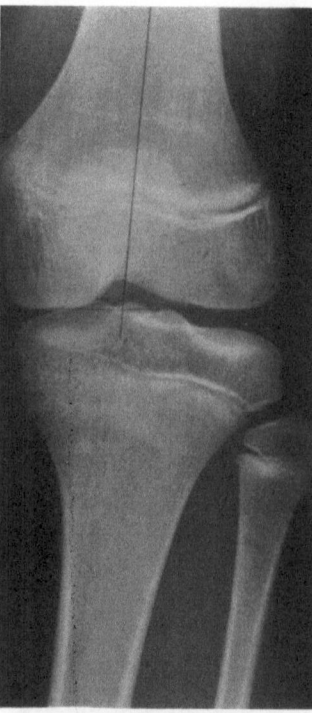

**Fig. 271 a–e.** Posttraumatic femoral shortening and varus growth deformity of the distal femur. S.P., 1964, 12 years, ♂, 174518.

**a** Preoperative status 4 years after condylar fracture causing epiphysiodesis and impaired growth.
**b** Lengthening: 6 cm.
**c** Plate fixation: cancellous bone graft, rapid consolidation.
**d** Eighteen months after fixation: perfect consolidation with residual distal deformity.
**e** Seven months after corrective osteotomy: normal femoral axis and equality of leg length

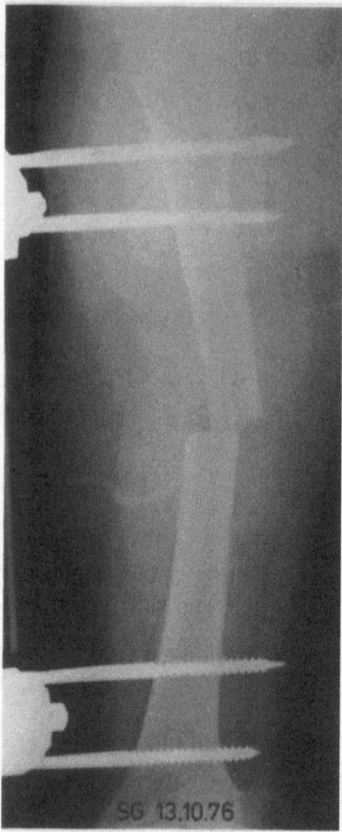
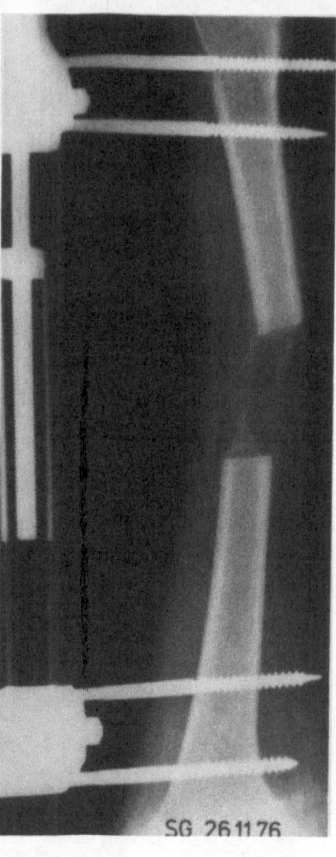
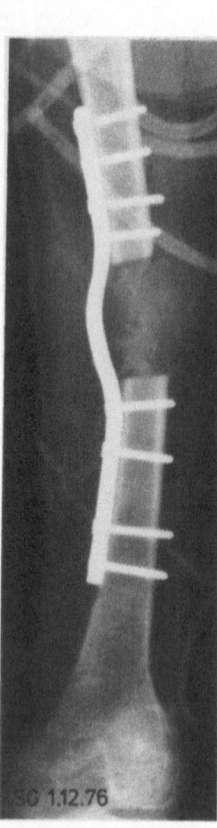

**Fig. 271d, e**

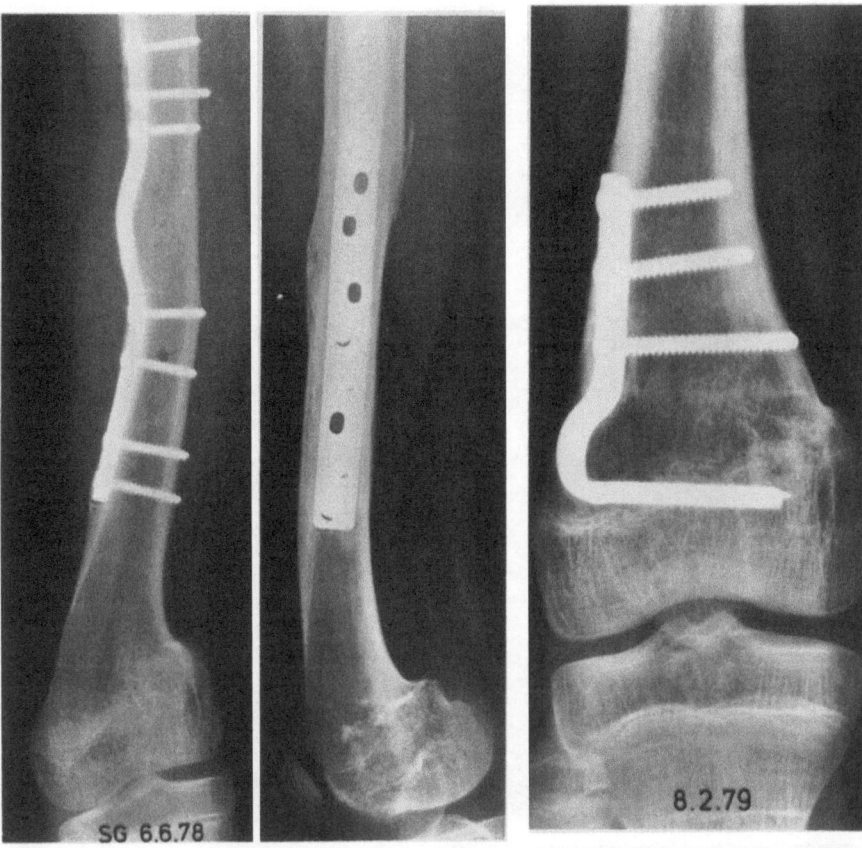

**Fig. 272a, b.**
Legend see p. 266
▼

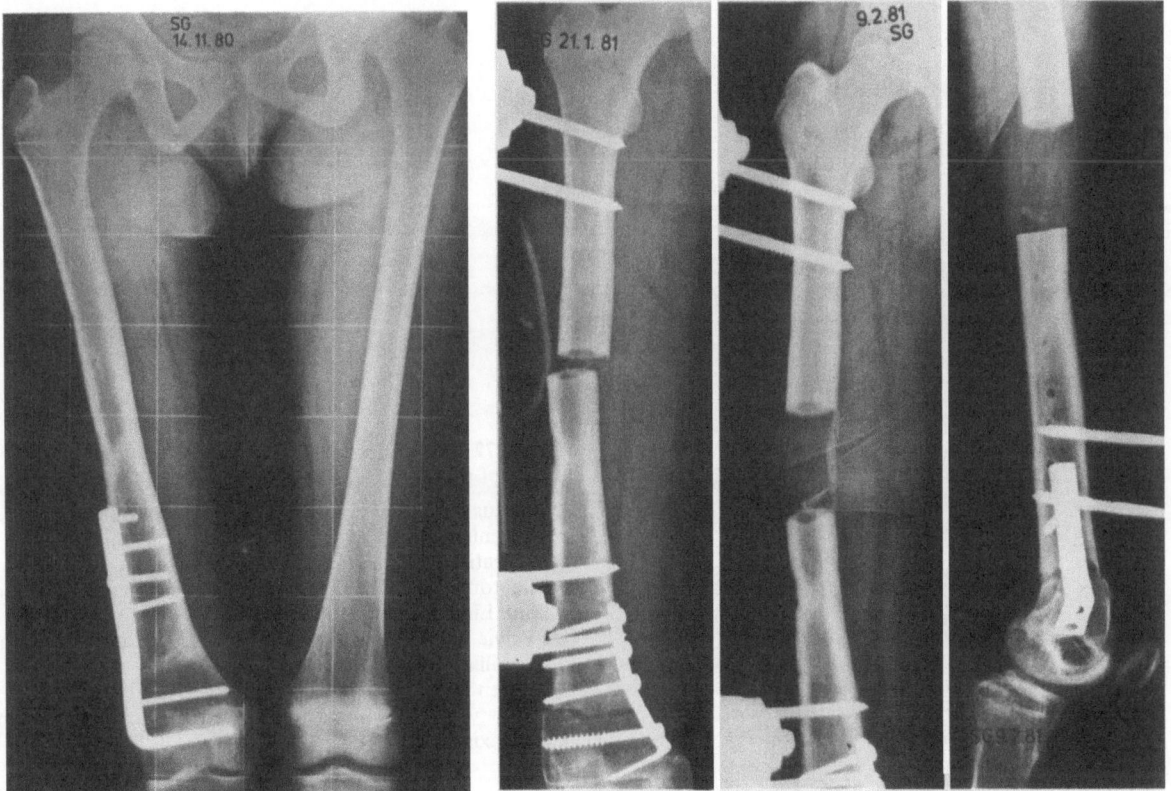

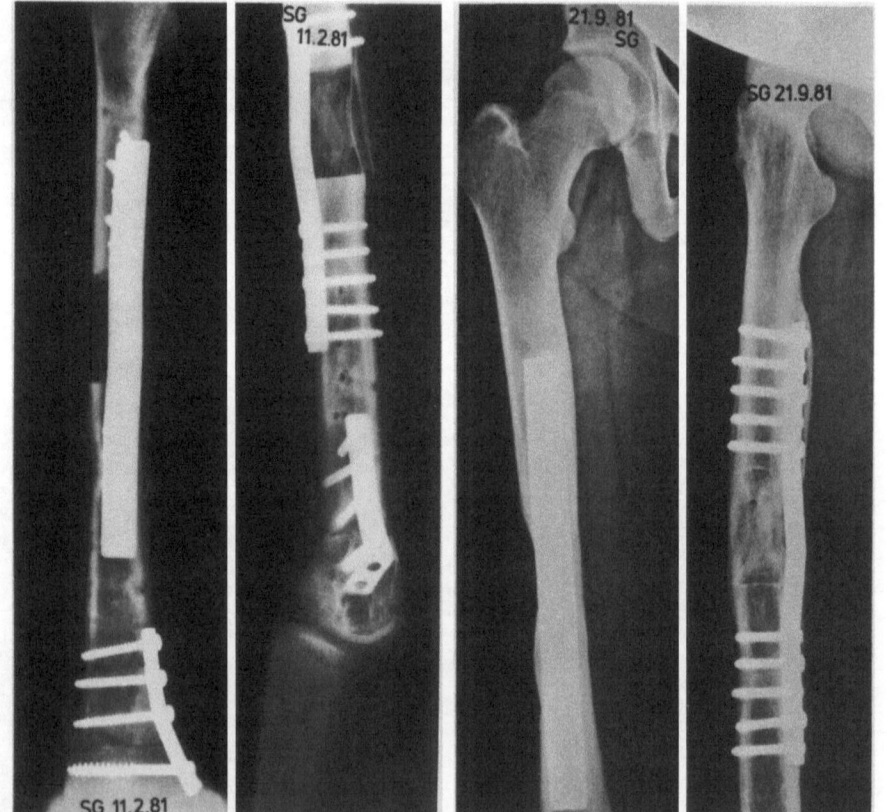

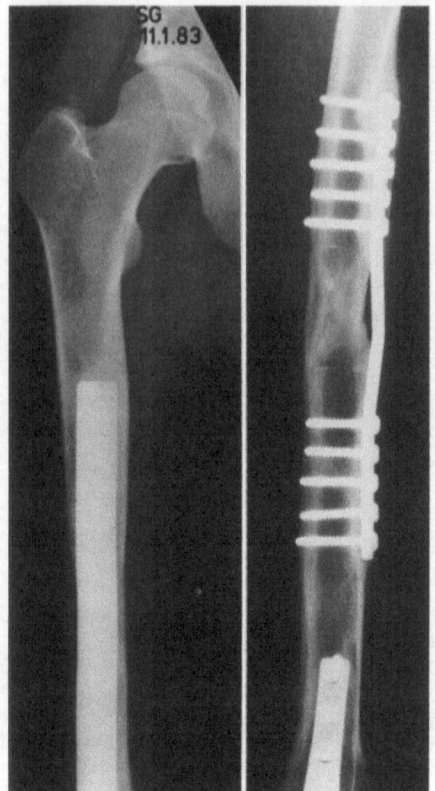

**Fig. 272 a–e.** Posttraumatic leg shortening and valgus deformity of the knee. S.A., 1968, 13 years, ♀, 246285.

**a** Status 2 years after fracture of femur and tibia: 2-cm leg shortening and 20° valgus deformity of the knee.
**b** Opeation: supracondylar varus osteotomy + lengthening osteotomy with Wagner apparatus on anterior aspect of limb. Limb was lengthened 5 cm in 12 days.
**c** Pelvic internal fixation: posterior wave plate + bone graft from iliac crest.
**d** Seven months after internal fixation: ideal consolidation.
**e** Two years postoperatively: normal bone structure and limb axis

*Example 4* (Fig. 273)

Femoral lengthening, biomechanically favorable placement of external fixation, and type of internal fixation.

*The problem:* An 18-year-old girl of short stature possesses a hypoplastic femur with a 3-cm length discrepancy. It would be inappropriate to shorten the normal limb or alter the axis of the femur. Problems of consolidation may be anticipated in this patient, who has been skeletally mature for three years.

*The solution:* The Wagner apparatus is applied to the anterior side of the femur to compensate for quadriceps traction. Despite the insertion of a strong medial bone graft and the application of a femoral plate of adequate length and width at a second operation, the fixation loosens within four months. At this time a wave plate, which is far more favorable biomechanically, is applied to the femur, and a second cancellous bone graft is undertaken. Within six months the femur is able to bear weight normally. A late follow-up at $1^1/_2$

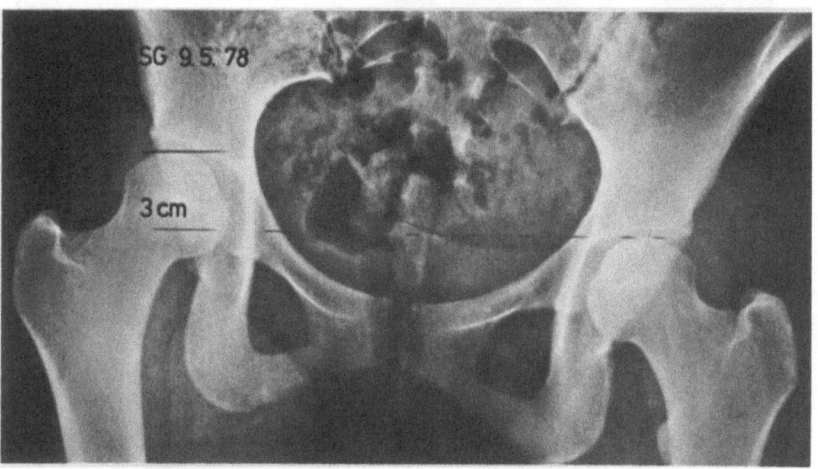

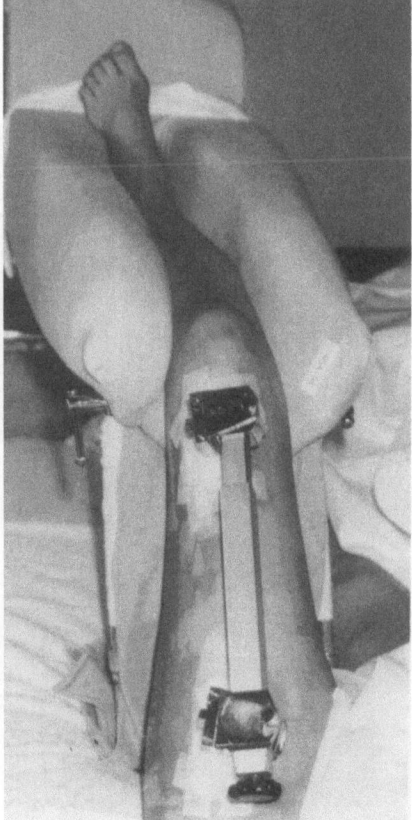

**Fig. 273 a–f.** Biomechanical placement of the external fixator and type of internal fixation. M.E., 1961, 17 years, ♀, 218163.

**a** Femoral hypoplasia with 3 cm of shortening.

**b** Anterior Wagner apparatus. 3 cm lengthening.

**c** Clinical photo showing the Wagner apparatus in place.

**d** One week after plate fixation, iliac bone graft and cancellous bone graft; loosening of metal and nonunion 4 months later; reoperation with wave plate and repeat cancellous bone graft.

**e** Three and 6 months after reoperation: healing is progressing well.

**f** Three years after lengthening osteotomy: perfect clinical and radiologic result

b

c

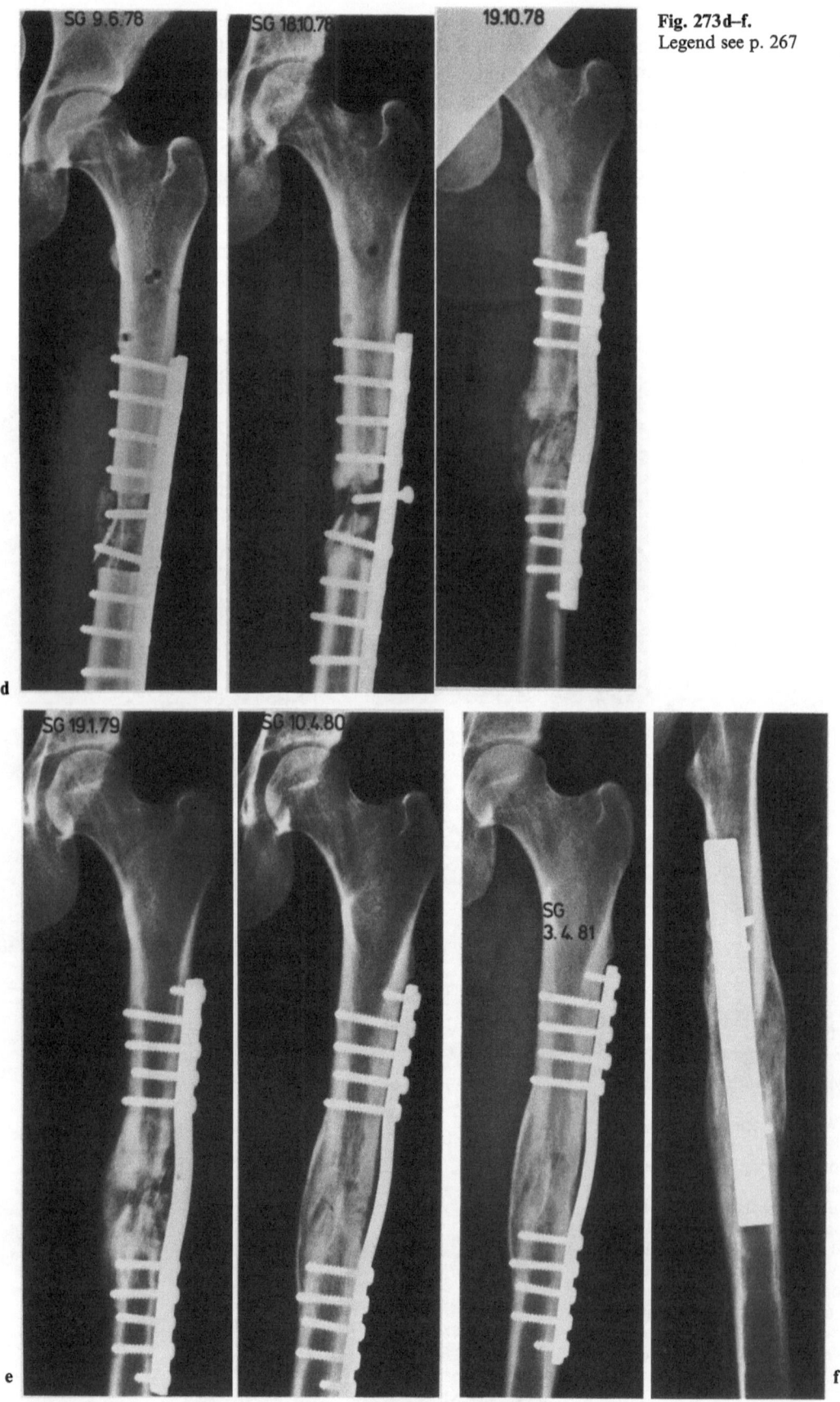

**Fig. 273d–f.**
Legend see p. 267

years after the third operation indicates an excellent result.

### 4.4 Lengthening of the Tibia

Both unilateral and bilateral frame configurations have applications in tibial lengthenings. Secondary cancellous bone grafting and internal fixation frequently are unnecessary in smaller children. Angular and rotational deformities may be corrected secondarily or at the time the fixator is applied.

*Example 1* (Fig. 274)
Varus deformity and posttraumatic shortening in a small child.

*The problem:* A 2-year-old girl sustained a fracture of the medial malleolus whose true significance was not appreciated. The result was a severe clubfoot deformity and limb shortening.

*The solution:* At age 5 a bilateral external frame is applied, at which time the varus deformity is partially corrected. The limb is lengthened by 4 cm. Two weeks before frame removal the Achilles tendon and flexor tendons are lengthened. Two months after the lengthening osteotomy a cancellous bone graft is performed, the frame is removed, and a long leg walking cast is applied. Consolidation at nine months postoperatively is excellent. The varus deformity is corrected by de-epiphysiodesis, open-wedge osteotomy and the interposition of bone cement into the curetted callus bridge. Eleven years postinjury, at skeletal maturity, there is equality of limb length owing to a 1.5-cm gain of length in the left femur combined with a 1.5-cm residual shortening of the ipsilateral tibia.

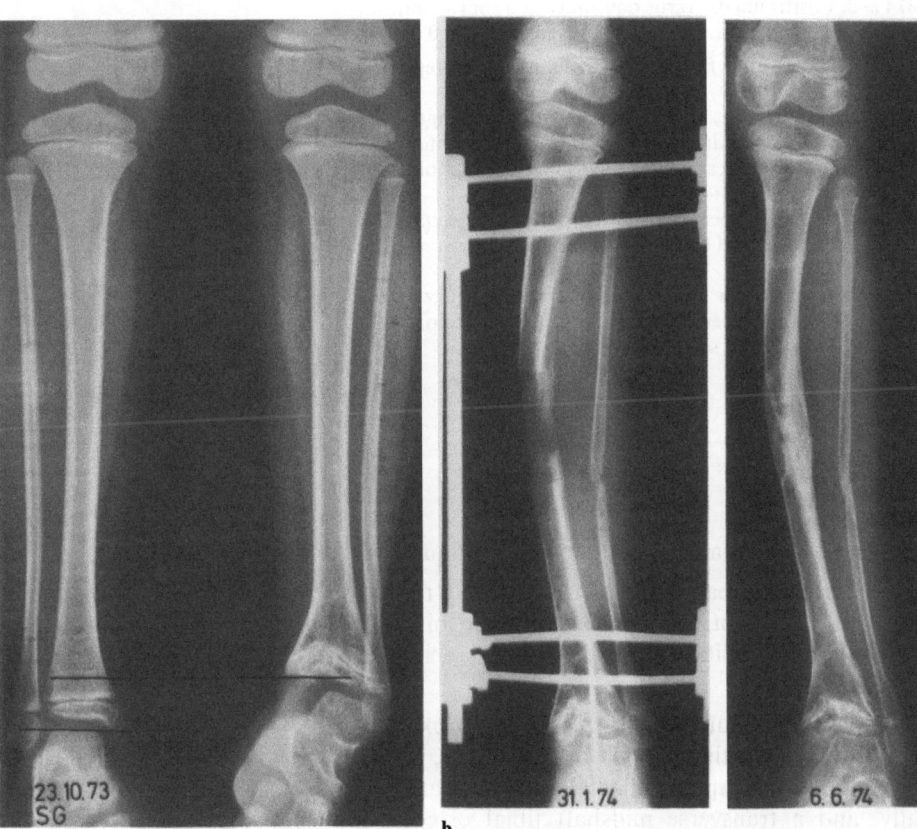

**Fig. 274a, b.**
Legend see p. 270

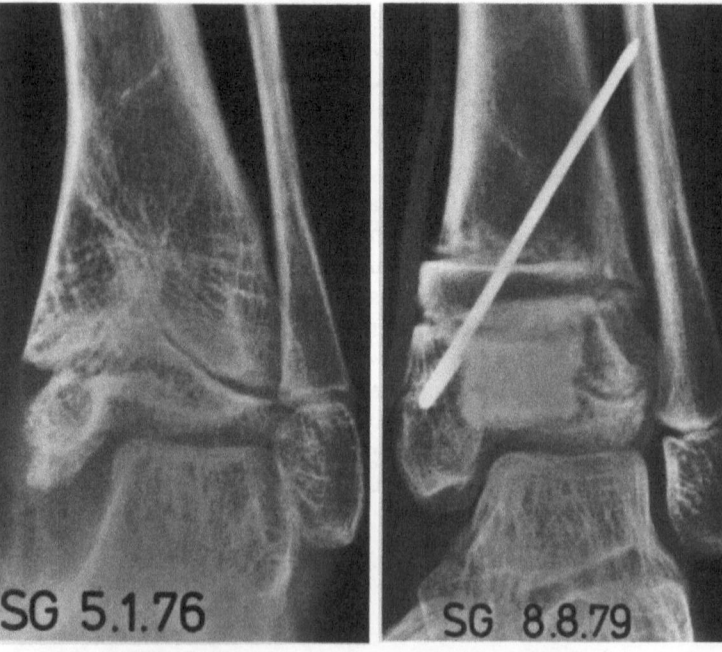

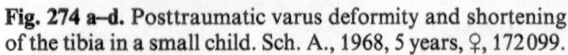

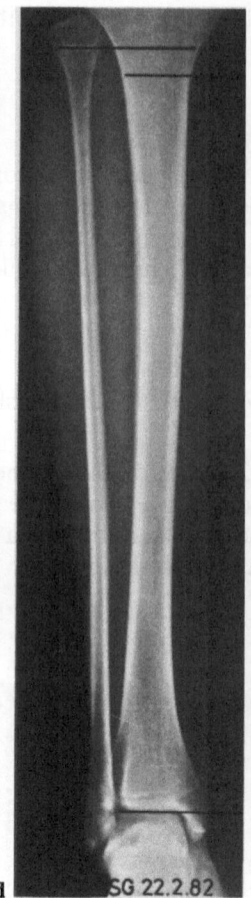

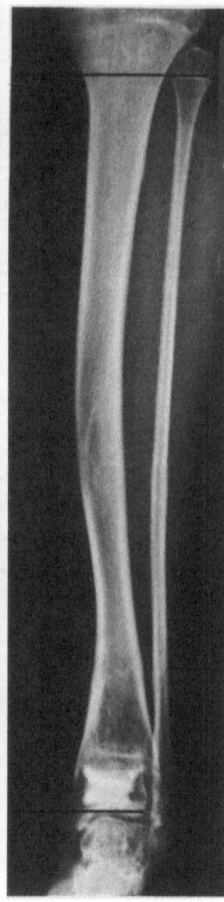

**Fig. 274 a–d.** Posttraumatic varus deformity and shortening of the tibia in a small child. Sch. A., 1968, 5 years, ♀, 172099.

**a** Status three years after fracture of medial malleolus (epimetatibial shortening).
**b** Lengthening osteotomy: bilateral frame with 6-cm lengthening, 2 weeks after lengthening of Achilles and flexor tendon. Three months later cancellous bone graft and immobilization in plaster.
**c** Correction of varus: open-wedge osteotomy with interposition of bone cement and bony wedge, Kirschner wire fixation.
**d** End result 9 years after lengthening osteotomy: There is equality of overall limb length owing to 1.5 cm of femoral lengthening. Limb axis is satisfactory

*Example 2* (Fig. 275)
Hypoplasia of the tibia and lengthening technique.

*The problem:* A 16-year-old girl exhibits a ray reduction of the left foot, a dome-shaped ankle joint due to subtalar coalition, and 3.5 cm of tibial shortening.

*The solution:* The fibula is fixed to the tibia proximal and distal to the proposed osteotomy, a Wagner apparatus is applied medially and subperiosteally, and a transverse midshaft tibial osteotomy is carried out. Valgus bowing develops due to the very large checking forces on the lateral side.

Once sufficient length has been obtained, the osteotomy is plated, and extensive cancellous bone grafting is performed. Eight weeks later the bone

graft is well incorporated. Sixteen months later biomechanical remodeling of the tibia is complete, with the line of weight bearing again passing through the bone. Aside from a thickening of the tibia, the result following removal of the metal is perfect.

*Example 3* (Fig. 276)
Marked hypoplastic shortening of the tibia.

*The problem:* A skeletally mature girl of 17 years developed a tibial shortening of 6 cm as a result of hypoplasia. Osseous union may be difficult to achieve in cases of this type. Nonunions are common and may necessitate a lengthy series of operations.

*The solution:* Tibial lengthening is effected with the Wagner apparatus in standard fashion, followed by cancellous bone grafting and internal fixation with two wave plates applied at right angles to each other. One year later there is solid consolidation across the defect, and a staged removal of the implants is planned.

**Fig. 275 a–f.**
Lengthening osteotomy for tibial hypoplasia. H.R., 1963, 16 years, ♀, 224834.

**a** Preoperative status: tibial hypoplasia, dome-shaped ankle joint, ray reduction of foot.
**b** Wagner apparatus in situ.
**c** Following distraction: plating + cancellous bone graft.
**d** Eight weeks after 2nd sitting: limb is stable on weight bearing.
**e** Nineteen months after lengthening: massive callus formation and correction of valgus angulation in shaft.
**f** Status after removal of metal: some thickening of tibia, otherwise perfect result

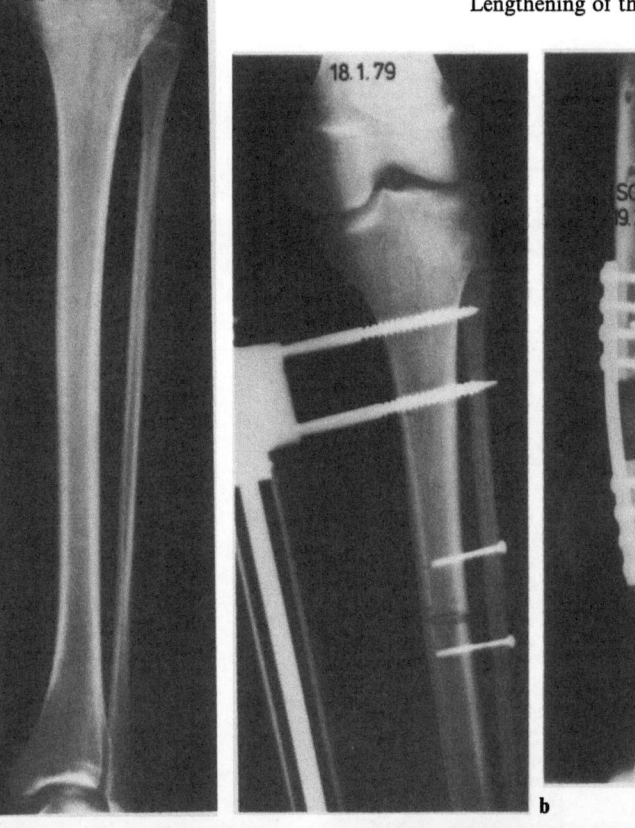

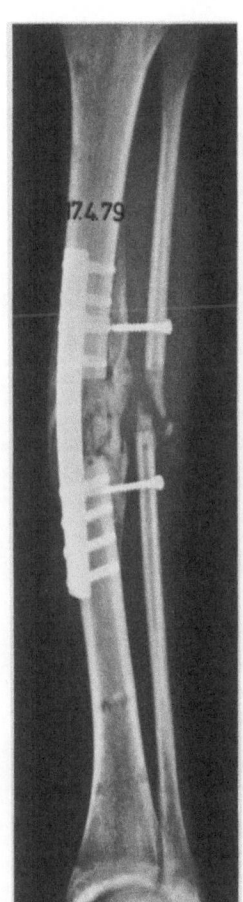

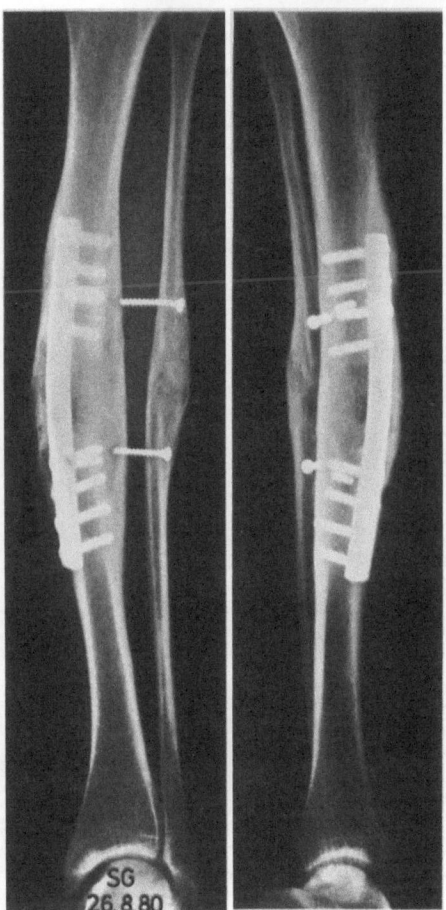

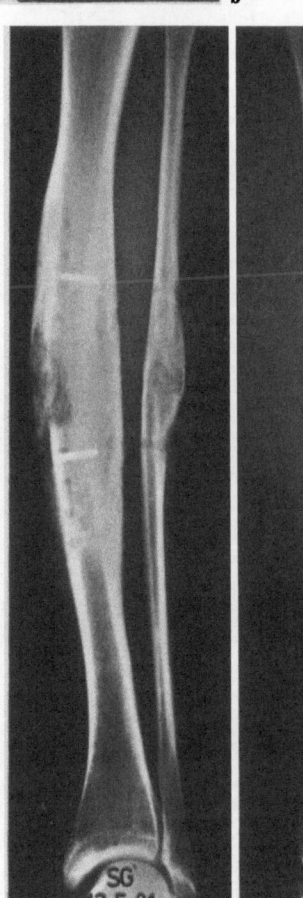

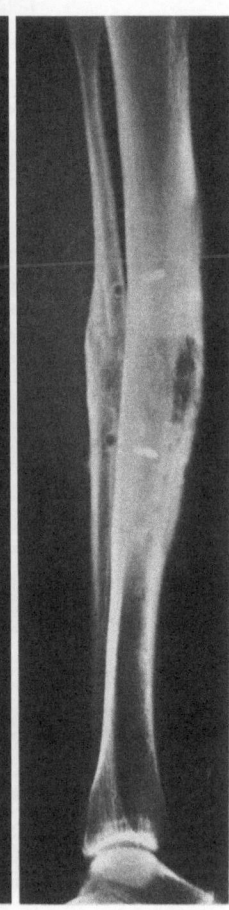

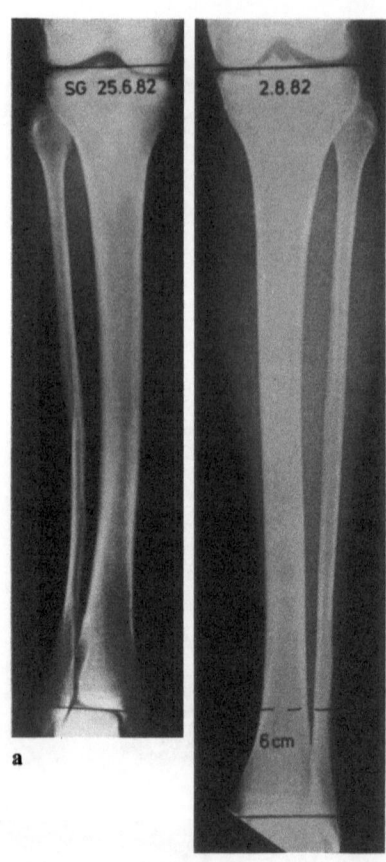

**Fig. 276 a–c.** Severe hypoplastic shortening of the tibia. A.B., 1965, 17 years, ♀, 261092.

**a** Preoperative status: marked hypoplasia of the right tibia with 6-cm shortening.
**b** Four weeks after application of Wagner apparatus by standard technique, dual osteotomy of the fibula and 6-cm lengthening: dual plate fixation (wave plates) and cancellous bone graft.
**c** One year postoperatively: defect is consolidated

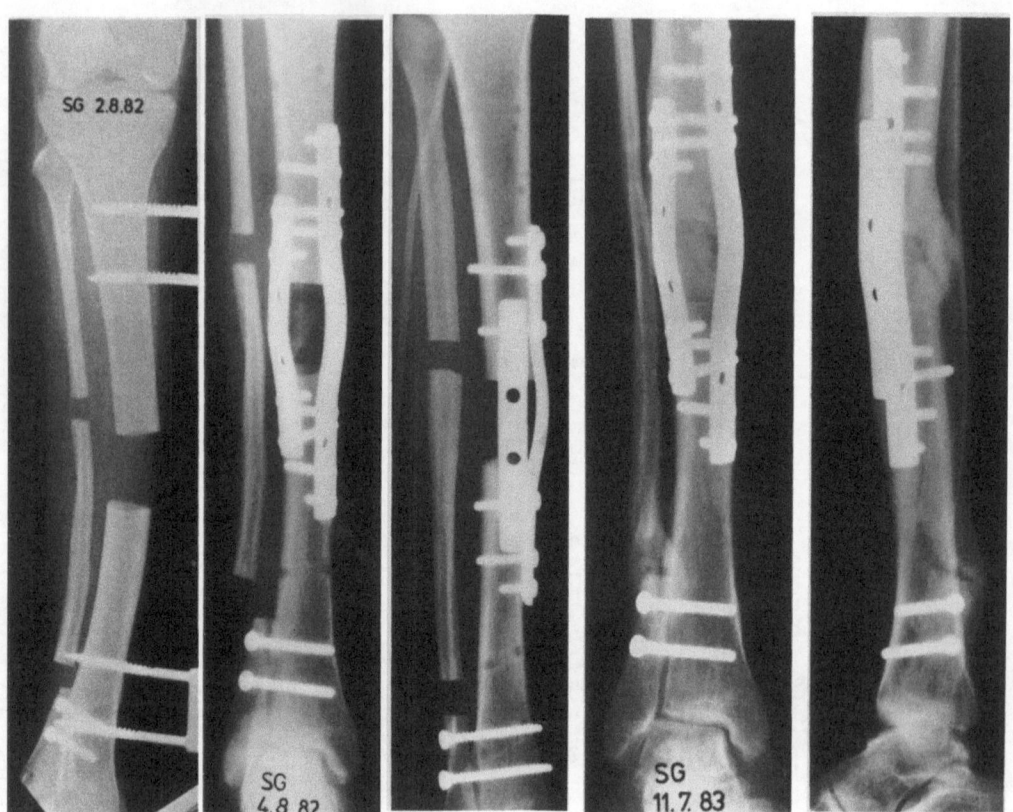

## 5  Corrective Osteotomy for Staged Limb Lengthening

The key to correcting posttraumatic soft-tissue contractures without risking necrosis lies in the gradual application of a distracting force. This is also indicated in areas where a one-stage lengthening would carry an unacceptable risk of injury to nerves, vessels and tendons. In such cases we conduct a staged lengthening in which the correction is effected gradually over a period of days. The unilateral external frame, either alone or combined with a bilateral frame, is very well suited for this procedure.

---

**Fig. 277 a–f.** Recurrent valgus deformity following trauma to the distal femur. V.J., 1964, 15 years, ♀, 215497.

**a** Status after lengthening and corrective osteotomy secured by plating: intentional overcorrection, heavy scar formation on lateral side.
**b** Oblique osteotomy and external fixation for staged correction.
**c** Scheme of frame assembly.
**d** Correction is achieved.
**e** Plate fixation.
**f** Eight months after internal fixation: limb axis and length are normal, osteotomy is healed

### 5.1  Staged Supracondylar Lengthening of the Femur

*Example 1* (Fig. 277)
Recurrent valgus deformity secondary to trauma.

*The problem:* A 15-year-old girl suffered a "sprained knee" three years prior, presumably involving an unrecognized epiphyseal plate injury above the lateral collateral ligament. A valgus deformity developed. One previous attempt was made to correct the deformity by plating. On referral to our care the valgus deformity was still present, accompanied by a limb length discrepancy and large cutaneous and muscle scars.

*The solution:* The special placement of the four Schanz screws permits the condition to be corrected gradually without touching the scar itself. At each incremental lengthening the fixation screws on the distal clamps are loosened, and the angled Schanz screws are progressively straightened with the plate bending pliers. When the correction has been achieved, internal plates may be applied with no risk of scar necrosis. Osseous union is prompt and complete.

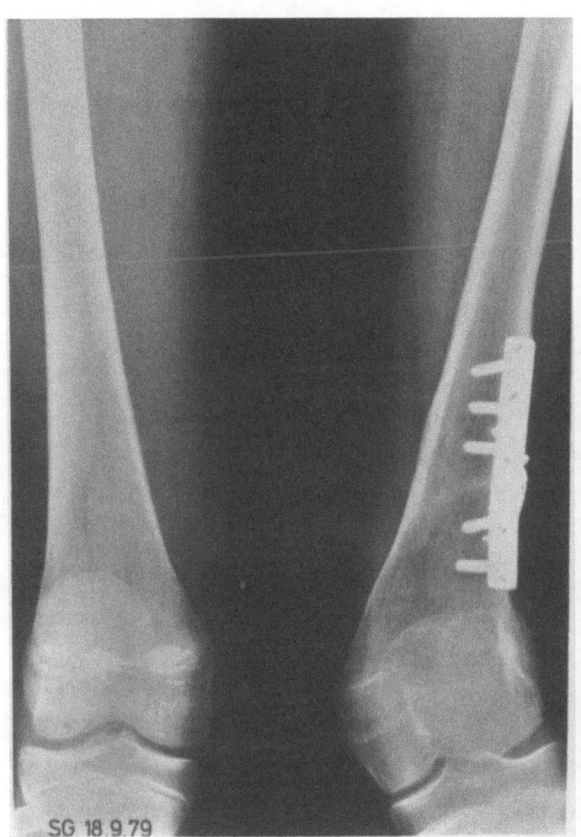

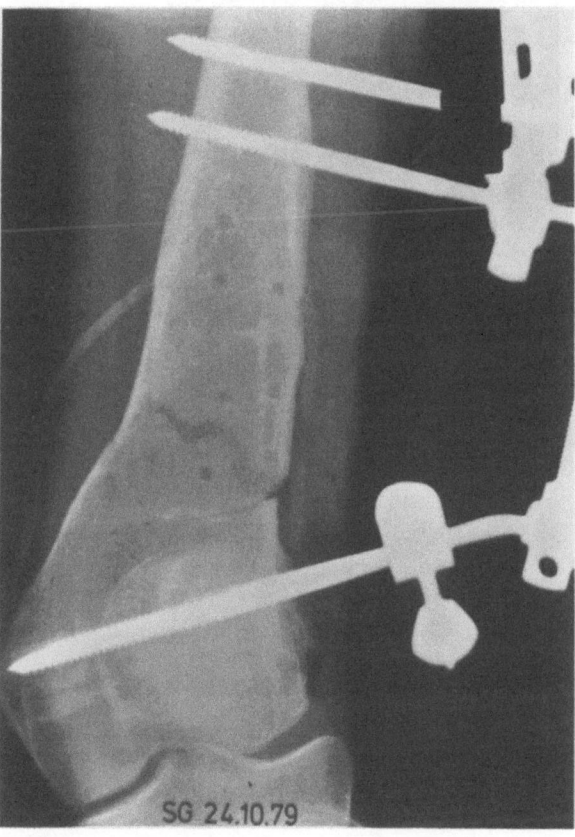

a  SG 18.9.79                                                    b

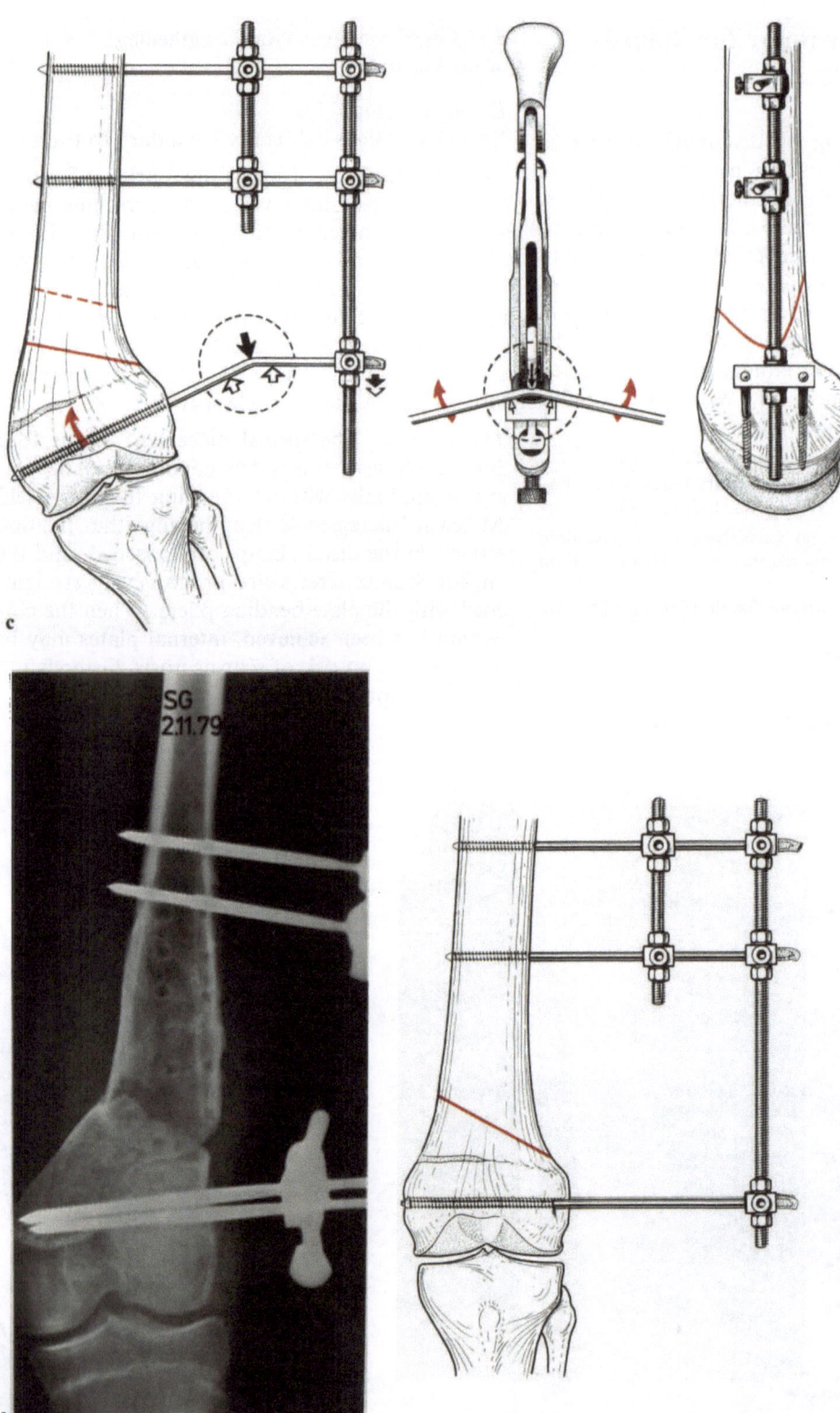

**Fig. 277c, d.** Legend see p. 273

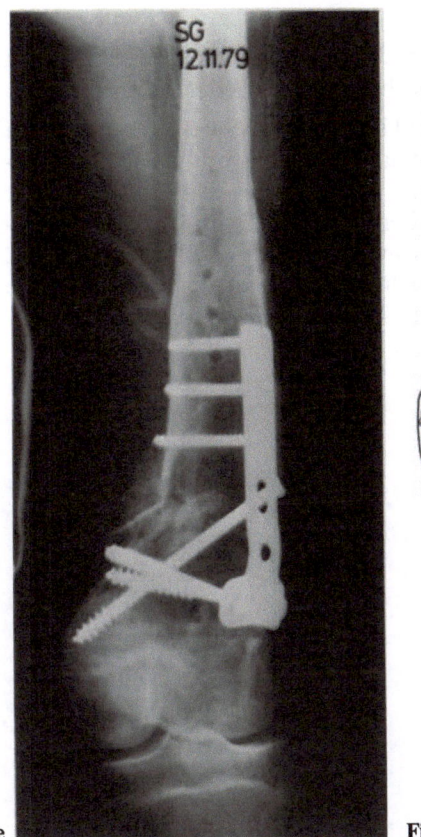
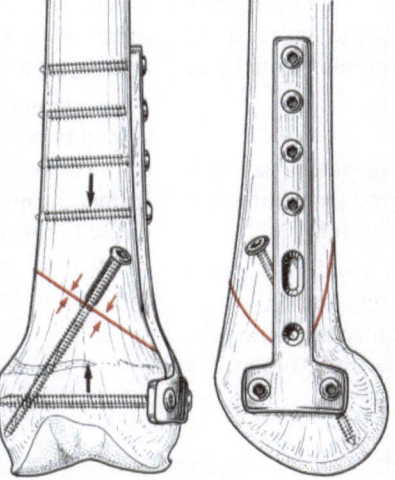
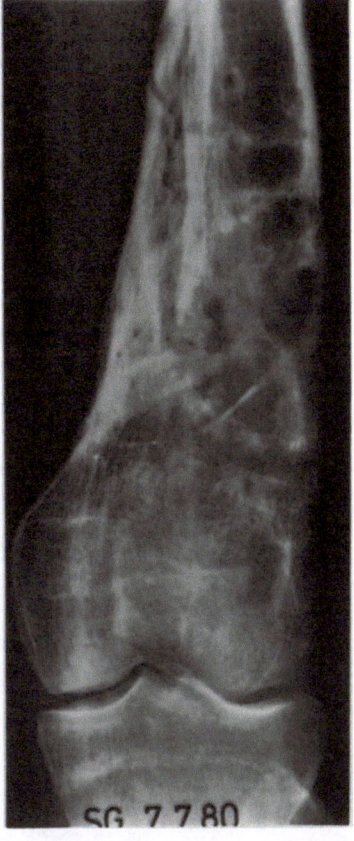

e

**Fig. 277 e, f.** Legend see p. 273

f

## 5.2 Corrective Osteotomy of the Proximal Tibia

Corrective osteotomies of the upper tibia and proximal tibial shaft always carry a risk of compartment syndrome due to the alteration of compartmental volume that accompanies a significant degree of lengthening. For this reason, axial and length corrections should always be carried out as staged procedures.

*Example 1* (Fig. 278)
Genu recurvatum secondary to an epiphyseal plate injury of the tibial tuberosity.

*The problem:* A 16-year-old girl sustained a femoral fracture at age 10, which was managed by traction on a Kirschner wire through the upper tibia. The traction damaged the epiphyseal plate of the tibial tuberosity, resulting in genu recurvatum and shortening. A closing-wedge osteotomy would exacerbate the shortening.

*The solution:* A bilateral external frame is applied anteriorly, a transverse tibial osteotomy is made just distal to the insertion of the patellar tendon,

and the tibialis anterior compartment is incised. Gradual distraction of the frame makes it possible to correct the angular deformity of the upper tibia and restore a normal limb length. When the desired amount of correction is obtained, two bone blocks from the iliac crest are interposed in the sagittal plane so that the same frame can be used to apply compression.

*Example 2* (Fig. 279)
Severe recurrent valgus deformity of the proximal tibia in the setting of Ellis van Crefeld syndrome.

*The problem:* A 10-year-old boy has severe genua valga with a maldeveloped tibial plateau. A varus osteotomy would place too much tension on the peroneal nerve, posing a danger of paralysis.

*The solution:* A bilateral frame is applied such that the angular limb deformity can be corrected through staged lateral distraction of the frame. This is combined with a unilateral frame system which permits a medialization of the distal fragment. Seven weeks after the osteotomy the frame is removed and a long leg cast is applied, in which the osteotomy goes on to union. This correction is not definitive, however, and the patient required a total of three corrective osteotomies to achieve normal limb axes in adulthood.

### Example 3 (Fig. 280)

Genu recurvatum and low-riding patella secondary to an etiologically unclear growth disturbance of the epiphyseal plate of the tibial tuberosity.

*The problem:* A 16-year-old boy developed a progressive genu recurvatum deformity over a 4-year period, greatly hampering his ability to participate in sports. In an initial sitting the tibial tuberosity was transposed proximally and fixed with a Blauth screw; also, a transverse osteotomy was performed and secured with an anterior bilateral frame.

*The solution:* The deformity was corrected in a staged fashion, and iliac bone grafts were implanted. To permit compression with the anterior frame, a unilateral frame was applied posteromedially to absorb varus, valgus and torsional forces. Uneventful healing of the grafts ensued, and knee function at late follow-up was normal.

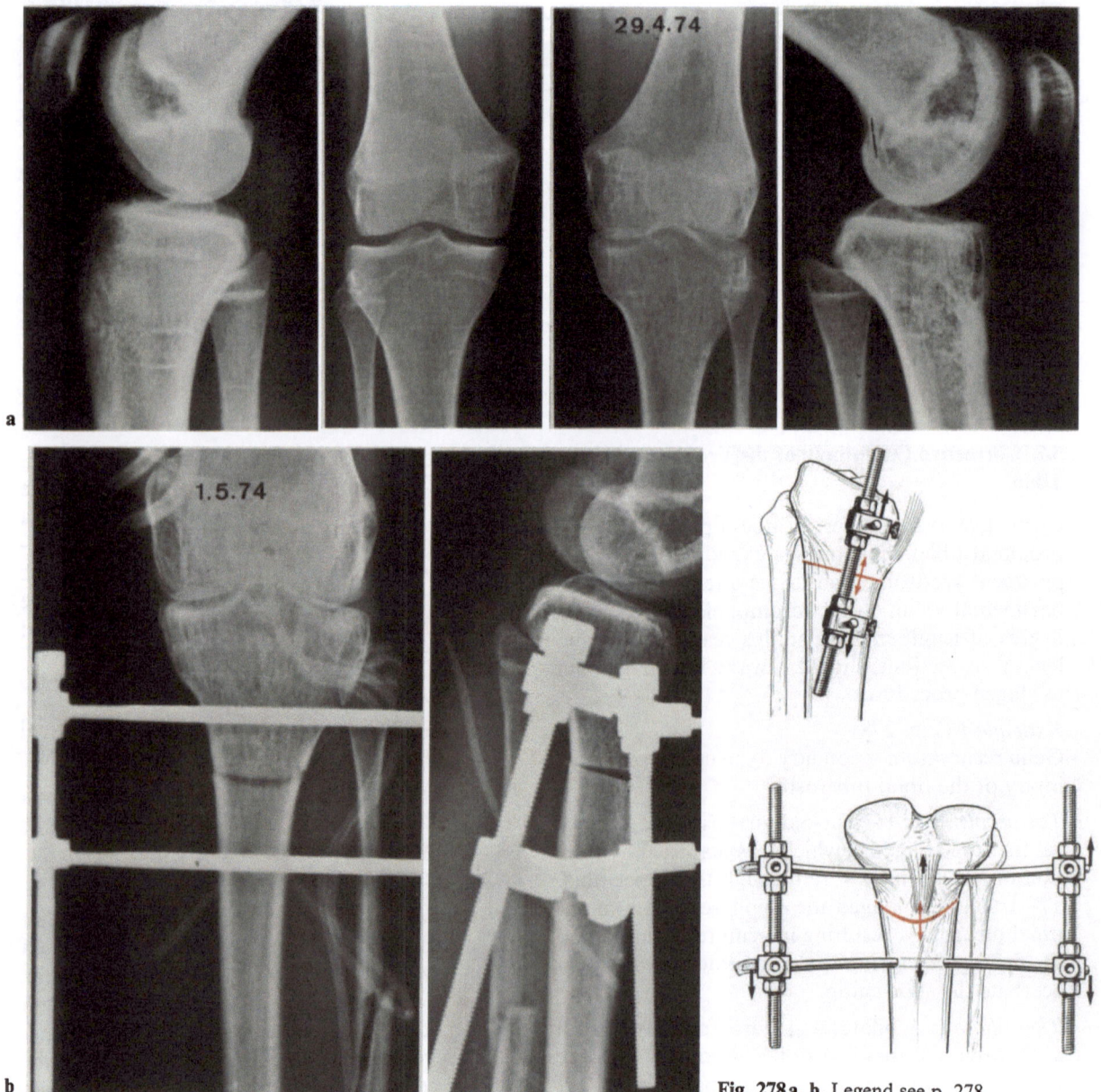

**Fig. 278a, b.** Legend see p. 278

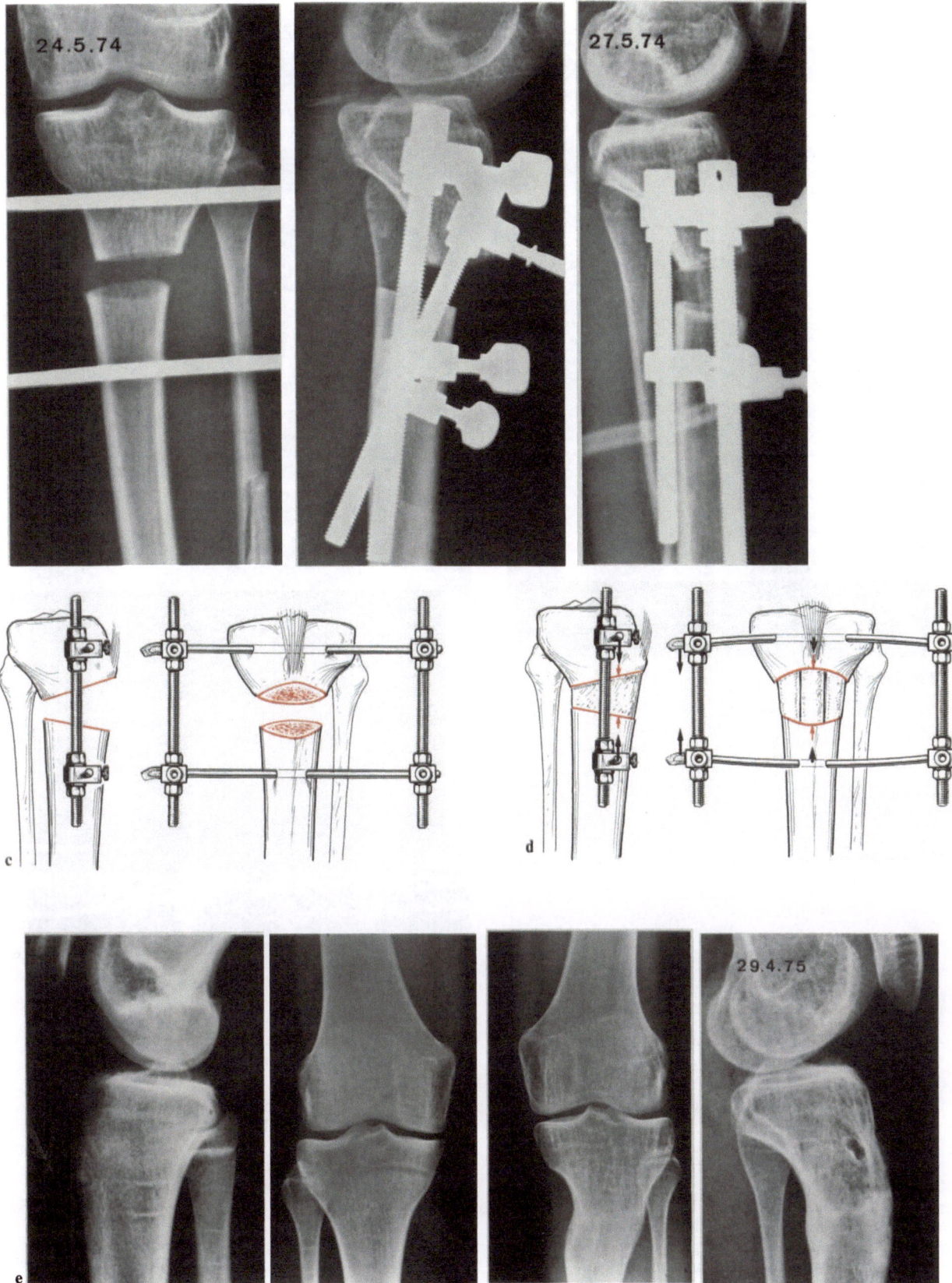

**Fig. 278 c–e.** Legend see p. 278

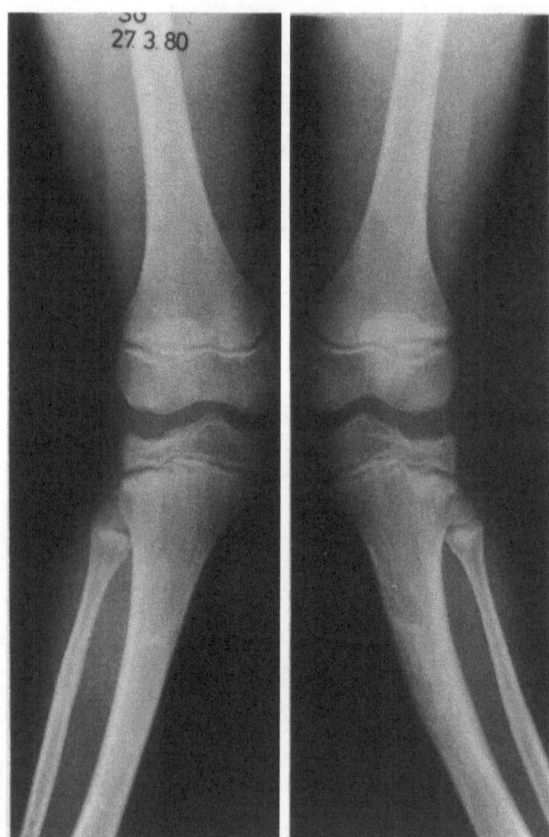

Fig. 279 a–c

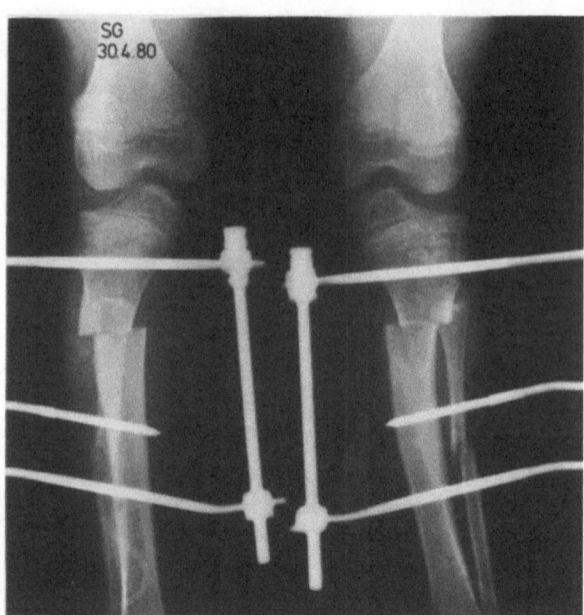

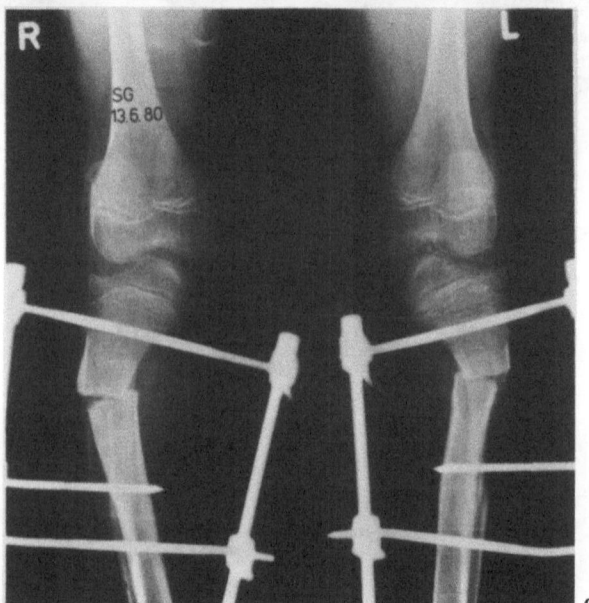

Fig. 278 a–e. Genu recurvatum secondary to epiphyseal plate lesion of tibial tuberosity. L.D., 1958, 16 years, ♀, 126128.

a Status 6 years after Kirschner wire traction on upper tibia: injury of upper epiphyseal plate, impaired growth, genu recurvatum and limb shortening.
b Application of a bilateral external frame.
c Scheme of staged correction.
d After correction is obtained, bone grafts from the iliac crest are interposed, and compression is applied with the bilateral frame. Six weeks after graft insertion: frame is removed, cast is worn for additional 6 weeks.
e One year postoperatively: good incorporation of grafts, correct limb length and axes

Fig. 279 a–e. Ellis van Crefeld syndrome with recurrent valgus deformity of the proximal tibia. S.A., 1970, 10 years, ♂, 196116.

a Three years after initial corrective surgery: recurrence.
b Upper tibia osteotomy: bilateral frame + unilateral half frame.
c Six weeks postoperatively: correction is achieved. Excellent callus formation, removal of frame and fixation in plaster.
d Check film in plaster.
e $3^1/_2$ months after osteotomy: good consolidation

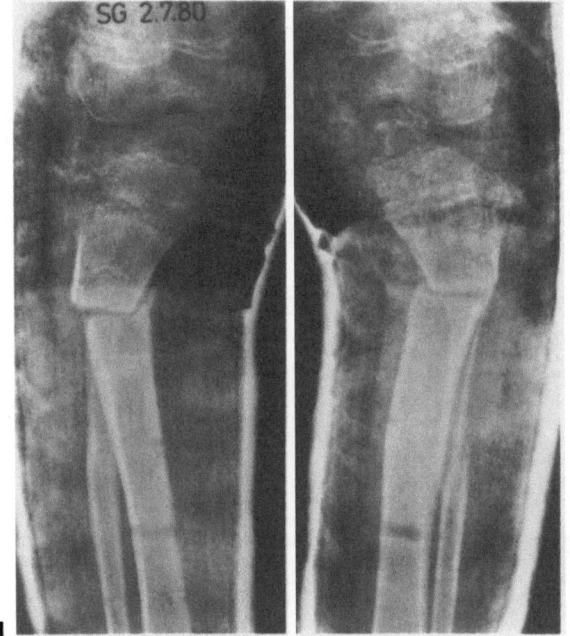

**Fig. 279 d, e**

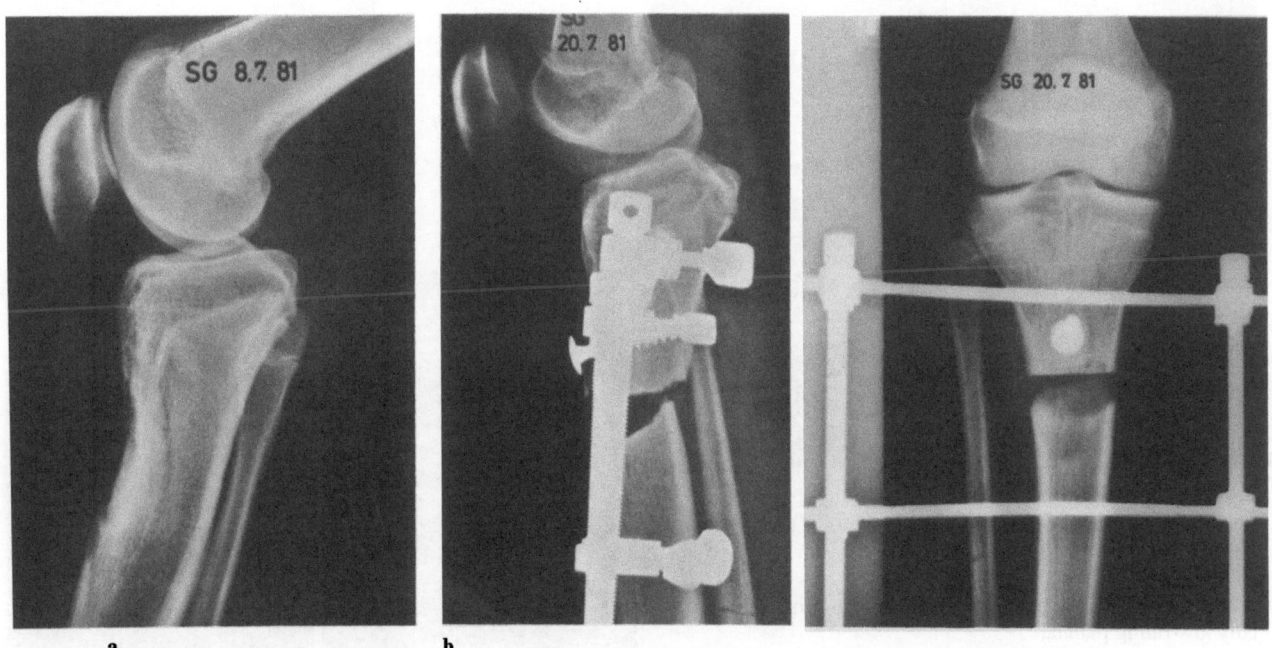

**a**    **b**    **Fig. 280 a, b.** Legend see p. 280

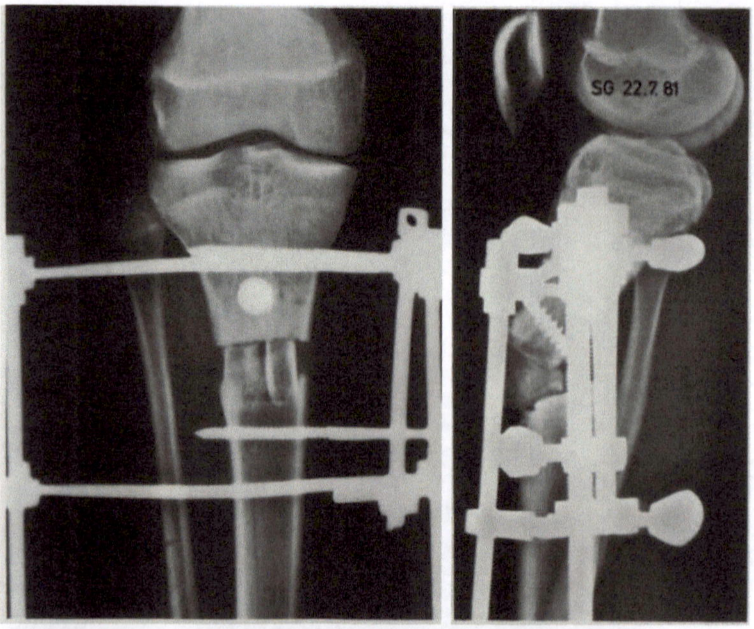

**Fig. 280 a–e.** Genu recurvatum and low-riding patella secondary to unexplained growth disturbance of the epiphyseal plate of the tibial tuberosity. F.C., 1965, 16 years, ♂, 240 768.

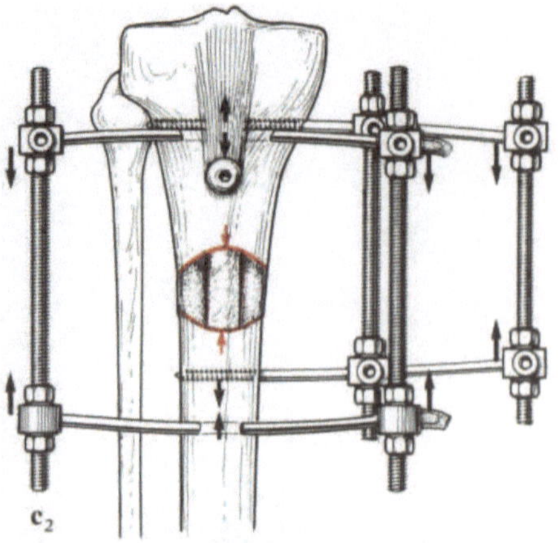

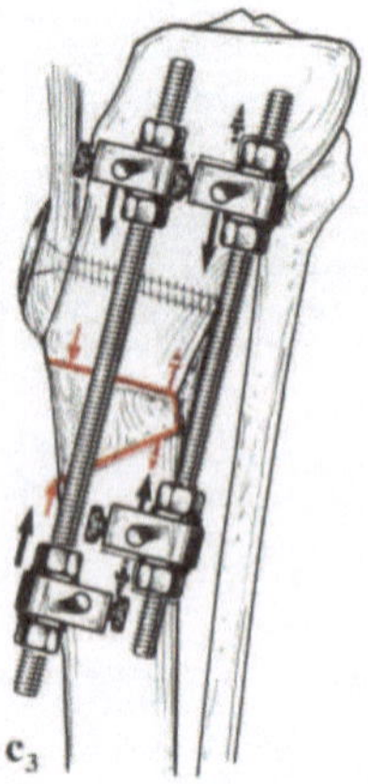

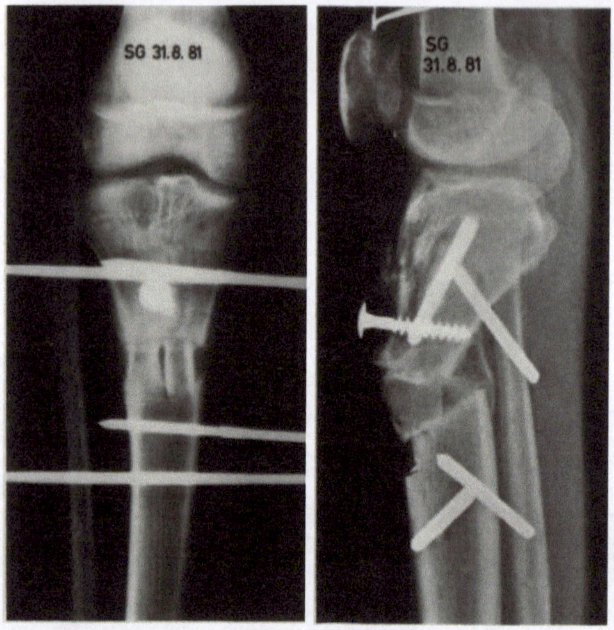

**a** Preoperative status: severe genu recurvatum with a markedly low-riding patella.

**b** Operation: application of anterior frame for staged correction, proximal transfer and screw fixation of tibial tuberosity.

**c** Technique of bone graft interposition: Given its mechanically unfavorable placement, the bilateral frame exerts a tipping force when compression is applied; hence a unilateral frame must be applied medially to neutralize this force and to serve as a spacer.

**d** Six weeks after graft insertion: the osteotomy is solid. The external fixation is removed, and a cast is applied for 5 weeks.

**e** Six weeks postoperatively: perfect end result

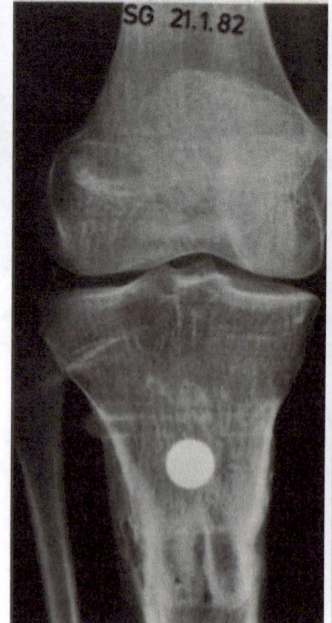
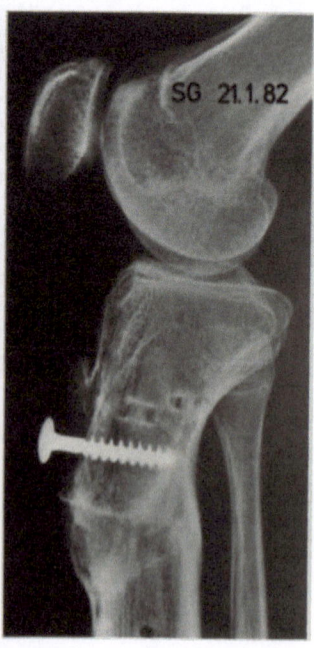

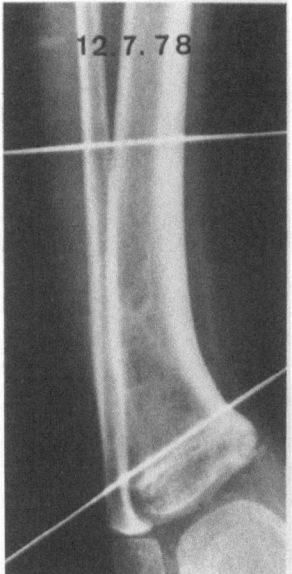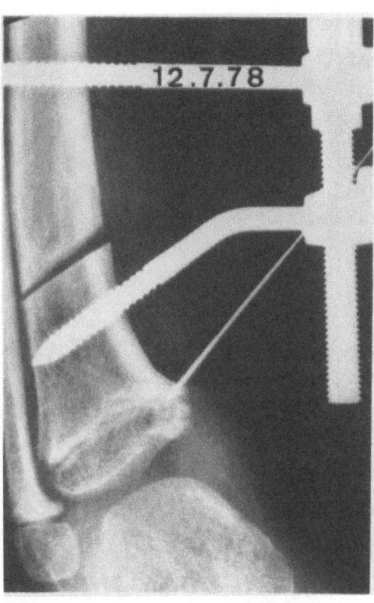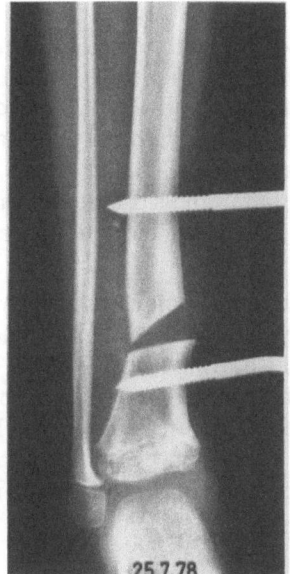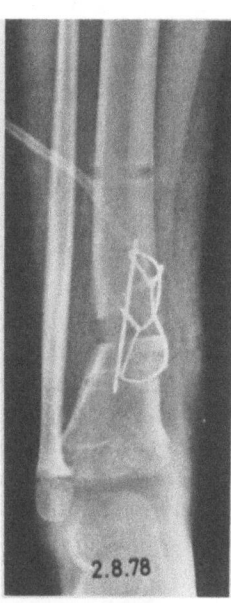

a, b

c

d

**Fig. 281 a–e.** Sequela of medial distal tibial epiphyseal plate injury with clubfoot deformity and shortening. Z.A., 1973, 5 years, ♂, 194006.

**a** Preoperative status: varus deformity and shortening.
**b** Staged correction with external frame. The angled distal Schanz screw is progressively straightened each time the frame is adjusted.
**c** Distraction and correction are not yet complete.
**d** Three weeks after external fixation: autogenous bone graft inserted and secured with tension band.
**e** Bone graft is incorporated

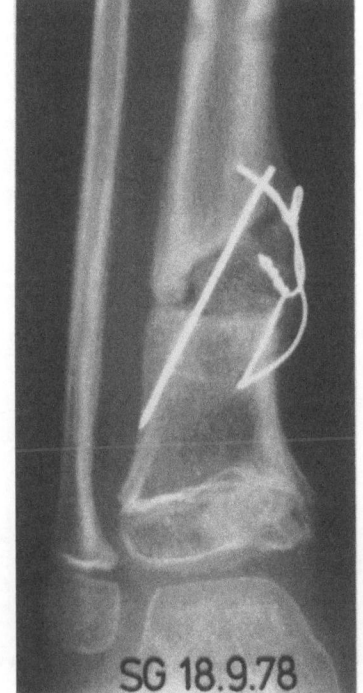

e

## 5.3 Supramalleolar Corrective Osteotomy of the Tibia

In supramalleolar open-wedge osteotomies of the tibia, large cicatrizing forces can act against the correction, leading to treatment failure, nerve injury or impaired blood flow. Staged corrections can eliminate these difficulties.

*Example 1* (Fig. 281)
Posttraumatic clubfoot deformity secondary to medial epiphyseal plate injury.

*The problem:* Prior rickets and a series of corrective operations left this 5-year-old boy with a clubfoot deformity, marked scarring and soft-tissue contracture.

*The solution:* A unilateral external frame can relieve the soft-tissue contracture in a staged fashion without provoking blood flow disturbances or paralysis. The angled Schanz screw is progressively straightened with the plate bending pliers. At final correction both Schanz screws are parallel, and

a normal length is restored. The iliac bone graft is fixed with a small tension band and immobilized in plaster. Healing is uneventful.

*Example 2* (Fig. 282)
Clubfoot deformity following medial posttraumatic epiphysiodesis. Status following a high supramalleolar corrective osteotomy and lateral deviation of the ankle joint.

*The problem:* Six years previously a 16-year-old boy sustained a malleolar fracture with subsequent epiphyseodesis of the medial malleolus and partial ischemic necrosis of the epiphysis. A corrective osteotomy resulted in a varus deformity and lateral deviation of the ankle joint relative to the line of weight bearing. A pure valgus osteotomy would further remove the joint from the line of weight bearing.

*The solution:* A unilateral frame is used to move the distal osteotomy fragment medially, placing it back into the weight-bearing line. When the correction is completed, the bone graft can be compressed with the frame to ensure rapid union. Five years later there is no evidence of degenerative change, and the patient remains free of complaints.

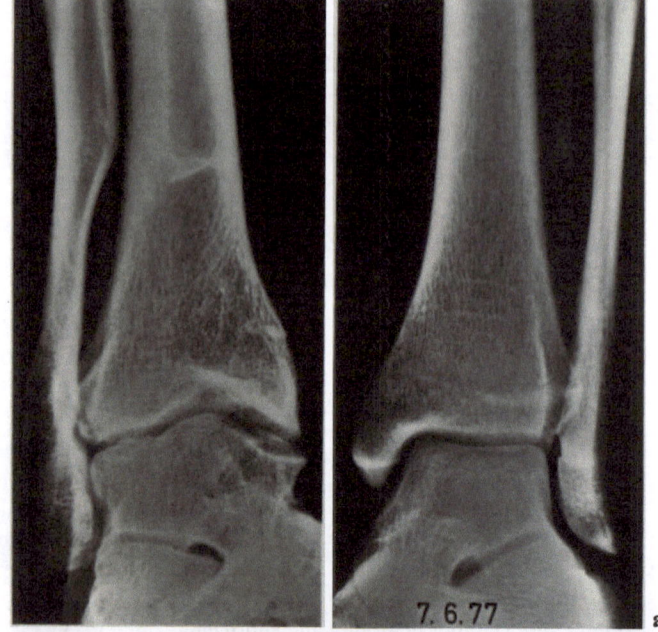

7. 6. 77    a

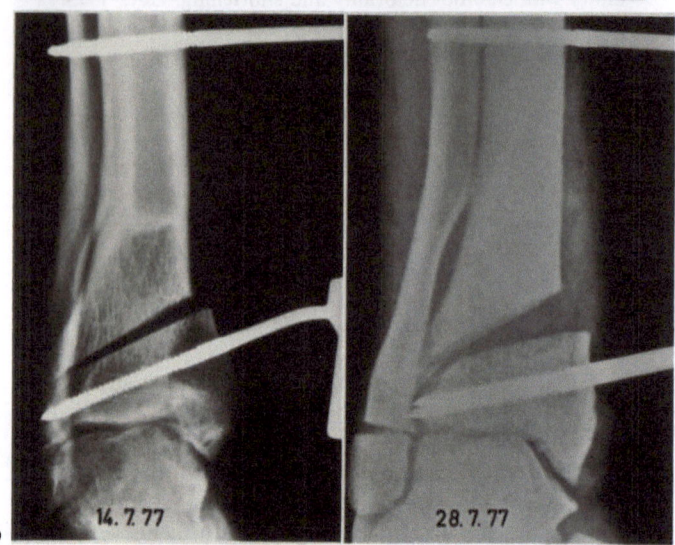

b    14. 7. 77    28. 7. 77

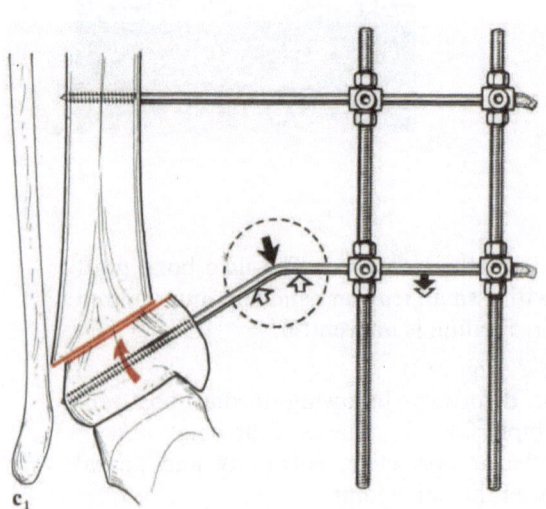

c₁

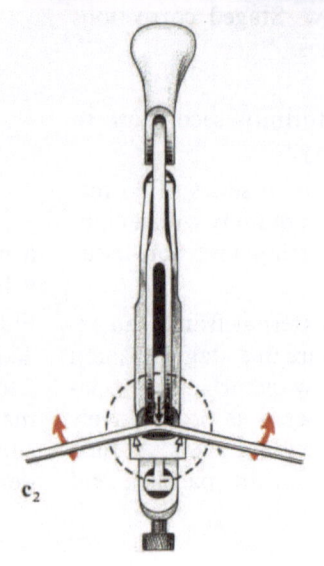

c₂

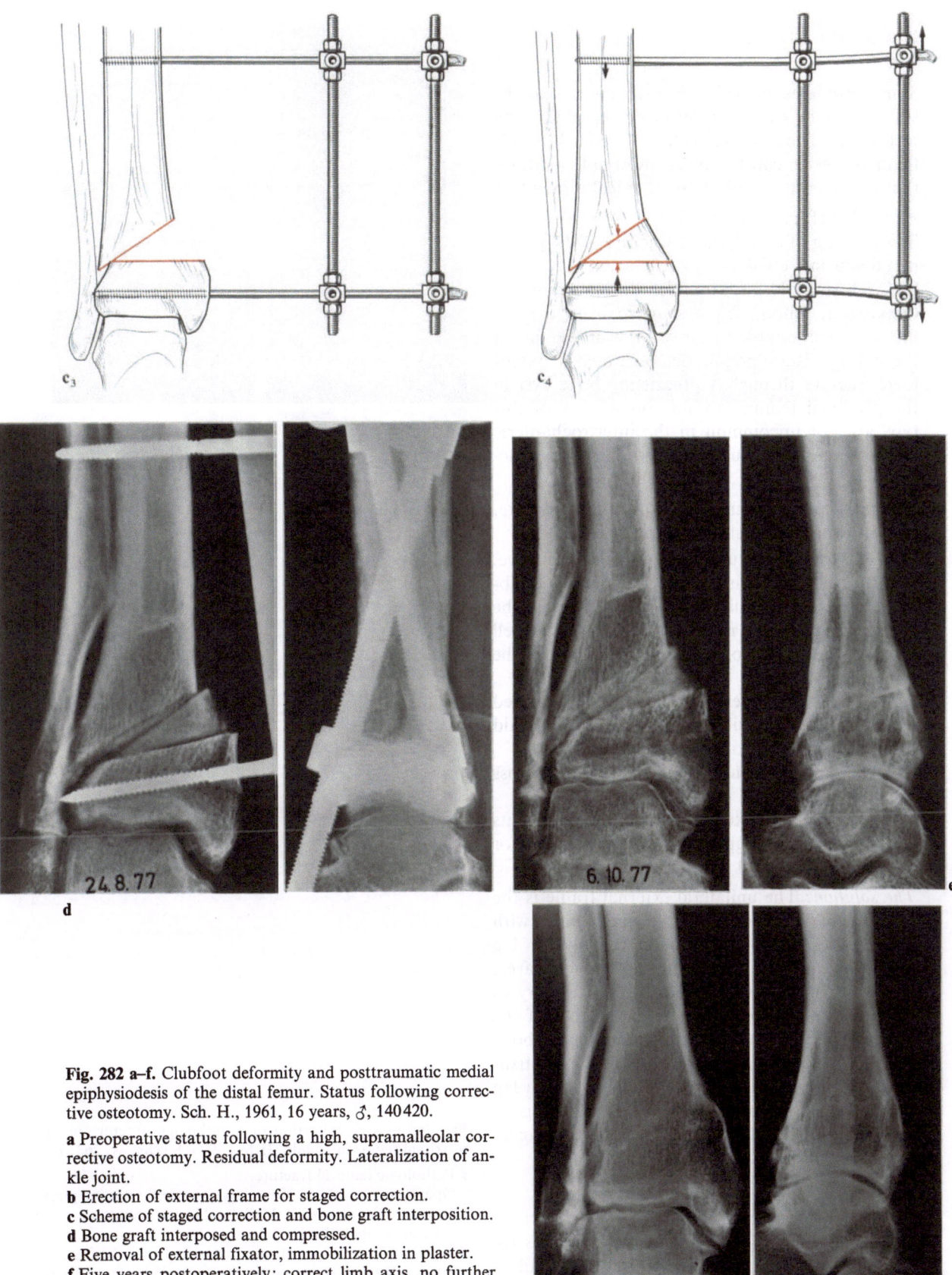

**Fig. 282 a–f.** Clubfoot deformity and posttraumatic medial epiphysiodesis of the distal femur. Status following corrective osteotomy. Sch. H., 1961, 16 years, ♂, 140420.

**a** Preoperative status following a high, supramalleolar corrective osteotomy. Residual deformity. Lateralization of ankle joint.
**b** Erection of external frame for staged correction.
**c** Scheme of staged correction and bone graft interposition.
**d** Bone graft interposed and compressed.
**e** Removal of external fixator, immobilization in plaster.
**f** Five years postoperatively: correct limb axis, no further degenerative change; patient is asymptomatic

# 6 Special Problems

Some problems in pediatric orthopedics can be solved only by the use of special external fixation techniques. The examples below illustrate how difficult problems can be solved by simple methods that are consistent with biomechanical principles.

*Example 1* (Fig. 283)
Stabilization of a pathologic fracture of the proximal femur in a child.

An 8-year-old boy stumbled during gymnastic exercises at school, felt a sharp pain in the left hip, and was unable to move or bear weight on the left leg. Radiographs demonstrated a pathologic fracture through a preexisting bone cyst in the proximal femur. Juvenile bone cysts of this type are not uncommon in the intertrochanteric area and are highly susceptible to pathologic fracture.

*The problem:* In the management of this fracture, the following points should be noted:

a) *Biopsy:* An accurate diagnosis is imperative. A histologic diagnosis is of value only in the absence of fracture healing processes. Otherwise the callus can easily be mistaken for malignant cell species. Thus, the biopsy must be done while the fracture is still fresh.

b) The proximal femur should be reconstructed as accurately as possible, and the fracture should be able to unite without significant deformity.

c) Screws and plates should not bridge or cross growth zones if at all possible.

It is highly unlikely that these requirements could be met through conservative treatment or conventional internal fixation methods.

*The solution:* The unilateral external frame is the modality of choice, especially when combined with a Kirschner wire, tension-band cerclage or lag screw. Because the cyst in question is very large, extensive cancellous bone grafting is necessary to ensure union of the fracture. The mother of the patient makes a suitable donor (homologous bone graft). Open reduction, curettage of the cyst, fixation with a unilateral frame combined with a lag screw and tension band, and massive homologous cancellous bone grafting create conditions highly conducive to osseous union.

*Example 2* (Fig. 284)
Shortening osteotomy of the tibia.

*The problem:* A 16-year-old girl has an excessive limb length of 3.5 cm, almost entirely in the tibia, 4 years subsequent to an open tibial fracture and

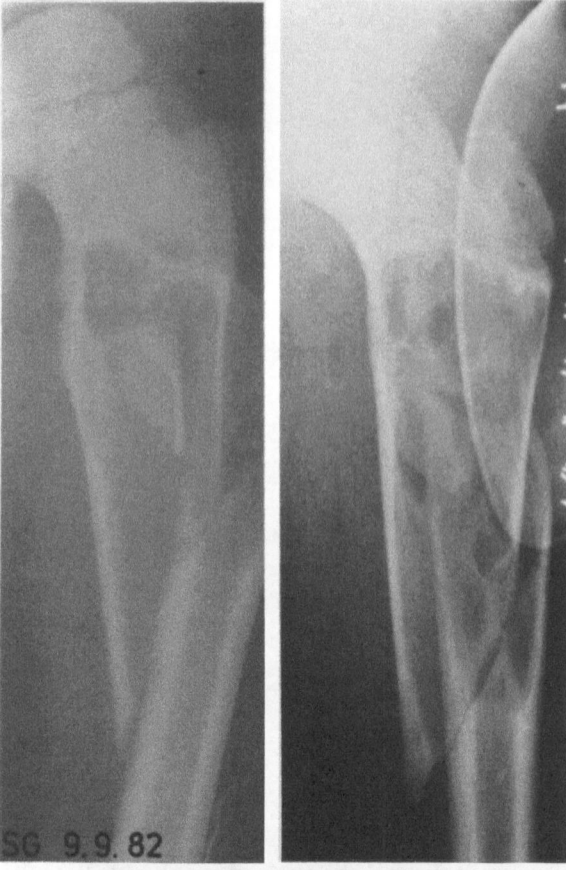

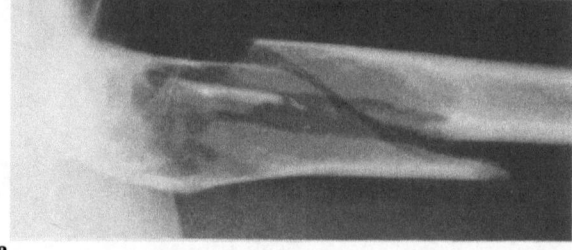

a

**Fig. 283 a–e.** Stabilization of a pathologic fracture of the proximal femur in a child. H.M., 1974, 8 years, ♂, 263 578.

**a** Pathologic femoral fracture.
**b** Operation: curettage. Homologous cancellous bone graft. Lag screw. Tension band. Unilateral frame as buttress.
**c** Scheme of operative fixation.
**d** Eight weeks postoperatively: removal of external frame.
**e** Six months and 1 year postinjury: normal healing of bone and cyst

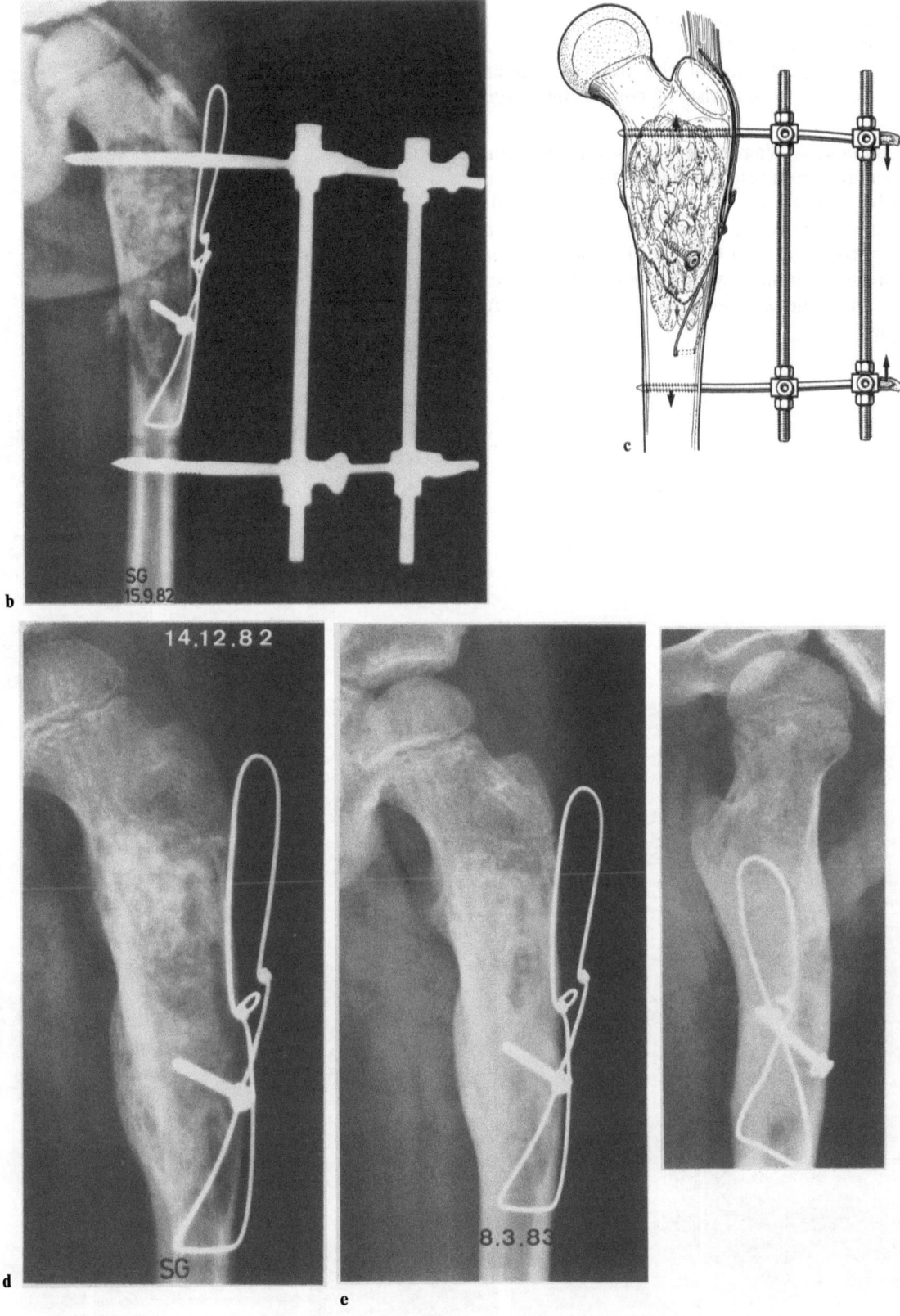

Fig. 283b–e

internal fixation. The patient refuses a shortening osteotomy of the femur on cosmetic grounds. A single-stage shortening of the tibia by 3.5 cm would carry a serious risk of compartment syndrome.

*The solution:* A Wagner apparatus is applied, and a 3.5-cm resection osteotomy is performed on both the tibia and fibula using parallel oblique cuts. The patient gradually adjusts the apparatus until the desired length is obtained. Subsequent internal compression plating supplemented by a lag screw across the oblique osteotomy ensures uneventful healing.

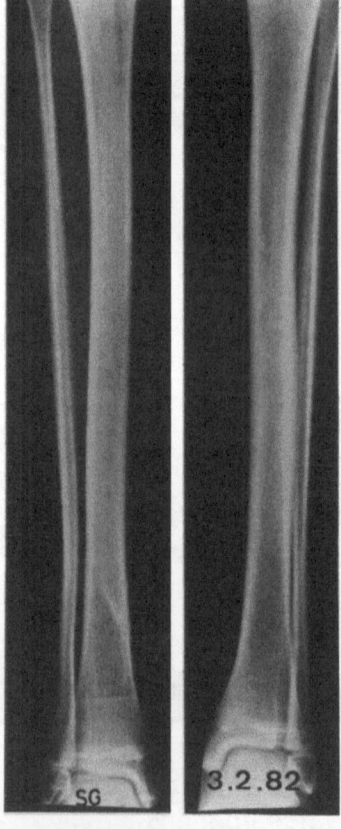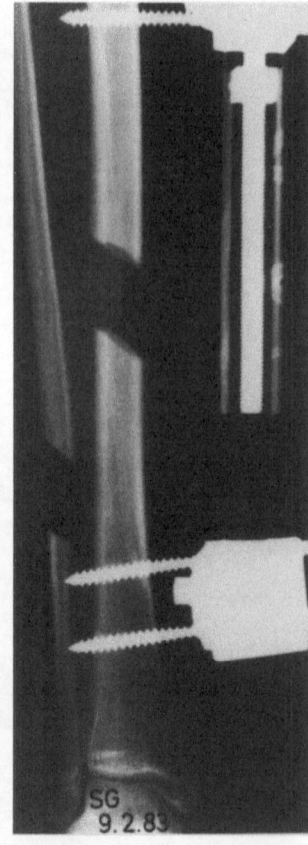

**a, b**

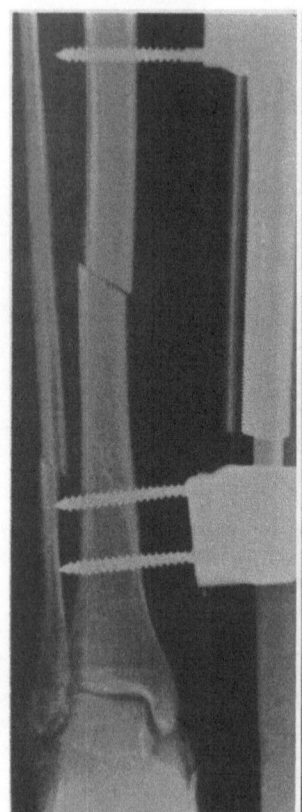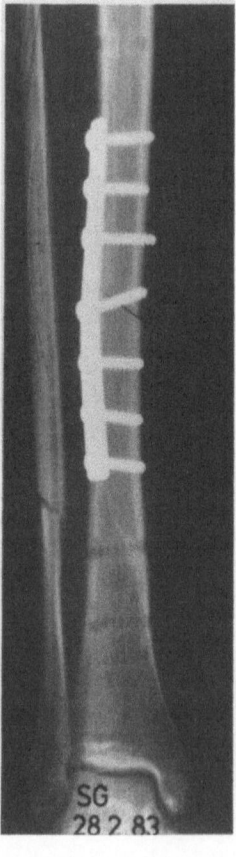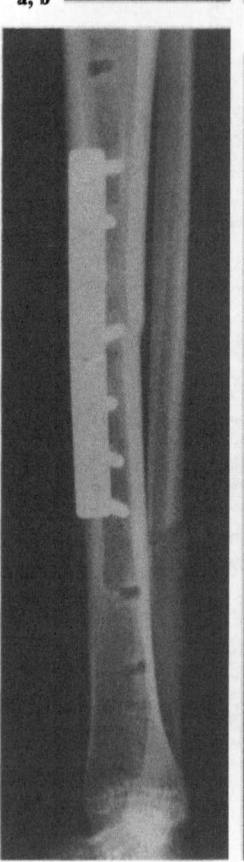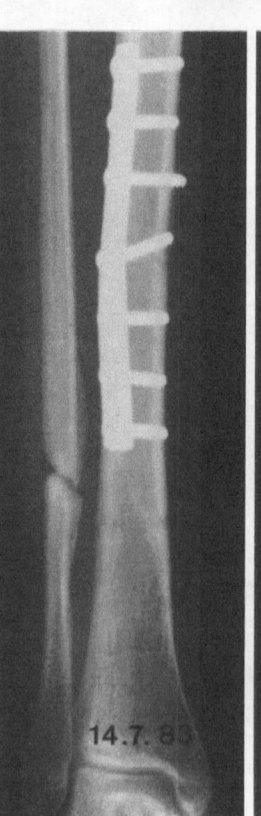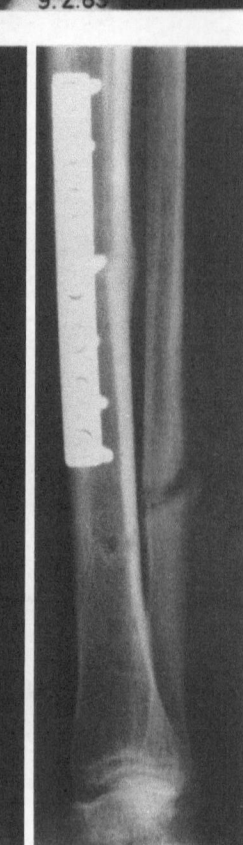

c                                    d

# N Concluding Remarks

B.G. WEBER

In this book we have examined the applications of the threaded external fixator of the ASIF. In so doing, it was our intention to address the problems of external skeletal fixation in the broadest possible scope, and thus in terms that would be of interest to the clinician.

The modern external fixation device must meet a number of requirements, the foremost being:

1) a simple, logical and trouble-free design;
2) availability of components which enable the elasticity or rigidity of the assembly to be modified as needed;
3) adaptability to all skeletal regions (excluding the skull and the spine);
4) adaptability to problems both in trauma surgery and in corrective orthopedics;
5) patient acceptability (a "humane" device).

In the preceding chapters we have demonstrated that the ASIF threaded external fixator satisfies these requirements.

At the same time, it should now be clear that the external fixator is not an easy device to use. This is due to the fact that the best indications for the device involve challenging situations in which the external fixation itself does not represent the greatest problem. The difficulty of the external fixator lies not so much in its technical handling as in the necessity of managing the circumstances which necessitate its use.

Success with the external fixator is largely a matter of case selection. Thus, the surgeon must possess sufficient mastery of all operative and non-operative treatment modalities relating to the musculoskeletal system in order to be able to select a modality which is optimum for a given case. This process of deliberation and selection has not been described here, or elsewhere, in such a way as to spare the reader the necessity of acquiring his own experience. In this sense the surgeon is advised to proceed as cautiously with external fixation as he would with any other operative fixation method.

The external fixator is neither good nor bad in itself – only in its application. Its value, then, is decided entirely by the competence of the physician.

---

**Fig. 284 a–d.** Shortening osteotomy of the tibia. W.A., 1967, 16 years, ♀, 247250.

**a** 3.5-cm limb length discrepancy following open tibial fracture, internal fixation and plastic surgery.

**b** Application of Wagner apparatus to intact tibia, resection osteotomy.

**c** Shortening effected in 16 days: frame removal, internal plating.

**d** Five months after plating: good consolidation of bone, normal limb function

# External Spinal Skeletal Fixation

F. Magerl

# 1 Introduction

The thoracolumbar junction is by far the most frequent site of injury to the vertebral column. At the same time, the frequency of neurologic complications diminishes in a cranial-to-caudal direction. We personally have observed a 37% incidence of significant neurologic complications in patients with cervical spine injuries, as opposed to 22% of patients with thoracic injuries and 8% with lumbar injuries (MAGERL 1980).

Statistics at our center also underline the predominant role of nonoperative methods in the management of thoracic and lumbar spine injuries. From 1961 to 1979 we treated only 8% of thoracic and 10% of lumbar injuries by surgical means. However, in recent years there has been a marked increase in these percentages, and a similar trend is apparent elsewhere. The main reasons for this are improved knowledge of the nature and consequences of the various types of spinal injury, as well as progress in the development of surgical techniques.

Cases that are not amenable to conservative treatment mainly consist of unstable injuries associated with a neurologic deficit. In these cases the capabilities of modern surgical methods are most clearly demonstrated. Due to the instability itself, patients who are treated conservatively are confined to a protracted course of bed rest and nursing care. However, when adequate stabilization is provided the patient is able to be mobilized or ambulated within a matter of days and can be rehabilitated more quickly (cf. BRADFORD et al. 1977).

In spinal surgery as elsewhere, the goal of treatment is to effect the most complete recovery possible using methods that are acceptable to the patient both physiologically and psychologically. This goal can be met only by satisfying the following: effective decompression of neural structures, healing of the spine without deformity and instability, early mobilization and functional aftercare, improved patient comfort, and facilitation of nursing care and rehabilitation. Any operative technique must be able to satisfy these goals; otherwise its benefit would be questionable.

A central priority in spinal trauma is stabilization. Various options are available at the present time, such as the Harrington rod instruments (BRADFORD et al. 1977; FLESCH et al. 1977; YOSIPOVITCH et al. 1977; DICKSON et al. 1978; CONVERY et al. 1978; GERTZBEIN et al. 1982), posterior plates (ROY-CAMILLE et al. 1976, 1977, 1980; LESOIN et al. 1982), fusion by means of posteriorly anchored coil springs (WEISS 1975), anterior fusions (KOSTIUK 1983), and the fairly new "segmental spinal instrumentation" (LUQUE 1982; FERGUSON et al. 1982; BRYANT and SULLIVAN 1983). WHITESIDES and GHAZANFAR ALI SHAH (1976) recommend that a posterior stabilization be combined with anterior decompression and fusion.

The treatment of an unstable low thoracic or lumbar fracture by a conventional posterior technique requires that a minimum of five vertebrae be immobilized. Even so, it is seldom possible to mobilize these patients without a plaster jacket or rigid brace. The necessity of immobilizing a number of vertebrae and the additional need for external immobilization are by no means favorable from a functional point of view. On the other hand, anterior or combined operations on the thoracic and lumbar spine are highly invasive and thus may be inappropriate for emergency situations.

It was the author's concern to find a method which was free of these disadvantages, and yet would enable the surgeon to perform all necessary measures, including decompression, dural closure and stabilization, through a single exposure in any situation. Therefore, the posterior approach seemed the only reasonable option.

Experience with plate fusions has demonstrated the very strong bony purchase that is gained by screws driven through the pedicles into the vertebral body. The weakness of plate fixation lies in the mobility at the plate-screw junction. It appeared necessary, to find a fixation device which possessed a stronger connection between the solidly anchored screws and the longitudinal stabilizing elements. The external fixation device seemed an obvious choice. By eliminating mobile connections in the system, it is possible to achieve a more secure stabilization while the number of immobilized healthy vertebrae may be reduced as well. A system of this type requires no more than two intact vertebrae, one cranial and one caudal to the injury, to be included in the fixation, regardless of the degree of instability. Thus, with injury to a single vertebra, the fixation device spans only three segments instead of the customary five to seven.

We know from the investigations of SAILLANT (1976) that the pedicles can accommodate screws 5 mm in diameter, even in the lower thoracic spine. At the level of the ninth thoracic vertebra the pedicles are approximately 7 mm wide and 14 mm high. From the third lumbar vertebra on, the cross-sectional area of the pedicles increases rapidly. At the fifth lumbar vertebra the pedicles are 16–17 mm wide and about 15 mm high.

The greatest diameter of a pedicle is not oriented vertically, but is directed laterally and caudally at an oblique angle, corresponding to the angle of emergence of the spinal nerves. At the thoracolumbar junction the pedicle has a more upright orientation, thereafter becoming more oblique in the lumbar spine. The pedicle of the fifth lumbar vertebra has roughly a transverse oval shape.

The author first treated a vertebral fracture with an external fixation device in 1977. The operating technique and outcome have been reported in several publications (MAGERL 1979, 1980, 1982, 1983, 1983, 1984). While the principle of the stabilization has not changed significantly since 1977, the surgical technique and indications have naturally been modified somewhat. Mr. F. SCHLAEPFER contributed greatly to the technical development of the external spinal skeletal fixation (ESSF) device.

Injuries of the lower thoracic and lumbar spine vary widely in their pathomorphology, mechanics and prognosis. Hence, no single surgical technique is ideally suited for coping with all types of injury. At our center, stabilization with the ESSF device is only one of a number of treatment options, and its application depends upon the nature of the presenting injury.

Of course, operative stabilizations of the spine also play an important role in the treatment of many spinal diseases. The goals of treatment mentioned earlier apply with equal validity to these cases. Some techniques that are currently used in trauma surgery were originally developed for orthopaedic purposes. The Harrington instrumentation and Gruca-Weiss springs, for example, were initially applied in the treatment of scoliosis. By the same token, the advantages of the ESSF device may easily be utilized in the management of orthopaedic conditions such as spondylitis.

## 2 Classification and Prognosis of Spinal Injuries and Their Relevance to Stabilization

As yet there is no standard nomenclature and classification for injuries of the spinal column. It is hoped that the new insights provided by computed tomography and surgical techniques into the pathomorphology of spinal trauma will help a common "language" to evolve.

We have classified cases treated with the ESSF device according to McAFEE et al. (1983). Based on the work of DENIS (1982, 1983), McAFEE et al. regard the spine as consisting of three osseoligamentous columns. The anterior column is formed by the anterior and middle portions of the vertebral bodies and intervertebral discs and by the anterior longitudinal ligament. The middle column is composed of the posterior portions of the vertebral bodies and discs, as well as the posterior longitudinal ligament. The posterior column is formed by the laminae, joints and ligaments (Fig. 285).

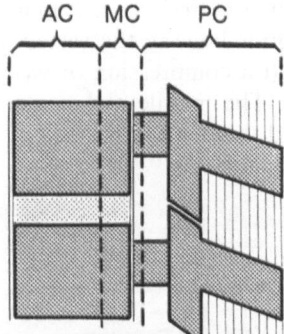

**Fig. 285.** The three osseoligamentous columns of the spine (cf. text). AC – anterior column; MC – middle column; PC – posterior column

The middle osseoligamentous column is of key importance, because the nature of the injury to this column determines the type of injury present. The authors ascribe all injuries to the middle column to three basic mechanisms: axial compression, axial distraction, and shifting in the transverse plane. McAFEE et al. differentiate six types of injury:

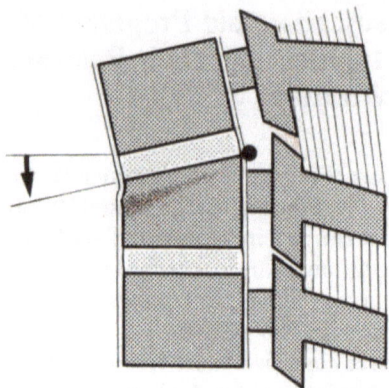

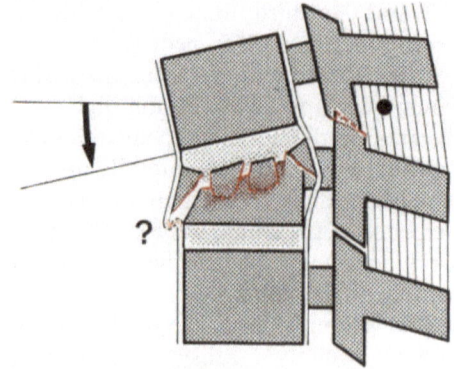

**Fig. 286.** Stable wedge-compression fracture. Only the anterior column is fractured. The cancellous bone of the vertebral body is compressed and compacted. The axis of rotation is located in the posterior wall of the vertebral body

**Fig. 287.** Incomplete burst fracture. Both the anterior and middle columns are fractured by compression. The cancellous bone of the vertebral body is compressed. An upper posterior edge fragment has been driven into the spinal canal. Possibly the anterior longitudinal ligament is torn; the posterior longitudinal ligament is intact. The axis of rotation is posterior to the articular processes. The compression resistance of this fracture is questionable; tension resistance is preserved

## 2.1 Wedge-Compression Fracture (Fig. 286)

This is an isolated injury of the anterior column caused by a flexion force which compresses the vertebral body roughly into the shape of a wedge. Because the major effect consists in a compression of the cancellous bone in the vertebral body, this injury is called a compression or wedge-compression fracture. The middle and posterior columns are intact, and the fracture is stable.

## 2.2 Stable Burst Fracture or Incomplete Burst Fracture (Fig. 287)

The anterior and middle columns are destroyed by compressive forces, leaving the posterior column intact. Because the compression resistance of this fracture is questionable, we prefer to call it "incomplete" rather than "stable".

A bony fragment from the upper posterior edge of the vertebral body may be driven into the spinal canal.

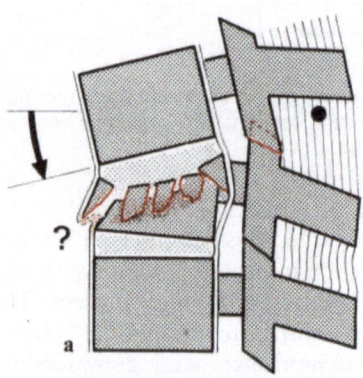

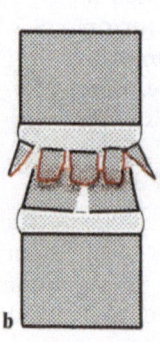

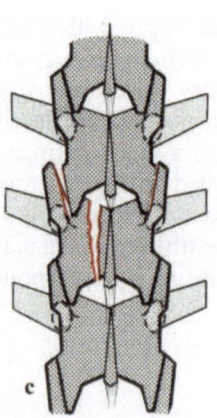

**Fig. 288 a–c.** Complete burst fracture, of the crush-cleavage type. All three columns are fractured by compression. The cancellous bone of the vertebral body is compressed. The neural arch fragments are still joined to the two lower vertebral body fragments by the pedicles. No compression resistance, rotational stability is questionable, tension resistance is intact. **a** The upper posterior edge fragment is displaced into the spinal canal. The anterior longitudinal ligament

may be torn; the posterior longitudinal ligament is intact. The axis of rotation is located farther posteriorly than in incomplete burst fractures. **b** The superior half of the vertebral body is comminuted, and there is a split fracture of the inferior half. **c** Split fracture of the lamina with impaction of the superior facets. Note the separation of the pedicles

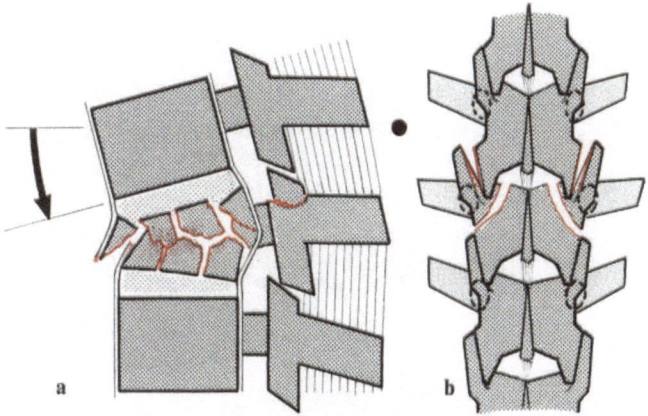

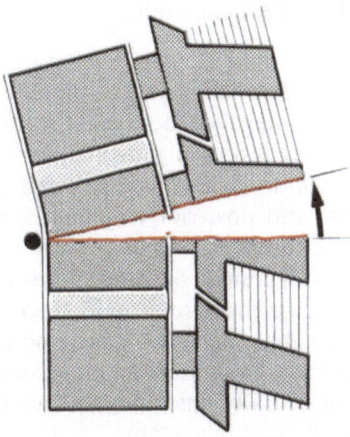

**Fig. 289 a, b.** Complete burst fracture, comminuted type. All three columns are fractured by compression. The cancellous bone of the vertebral body is compressed. The neural arch fragments are not joined to the vertebral body fragments. No compressive and rotational stability, tension resistance is intact. **a** Comminution of the vertebral body, probable tear of the anterior longitudinal ligament, intact posterior longitudinal ligament. The upper posterior edge fragment is displaced into the spinal canal. The axis of rotation is located still farther posteriorly. **b** Fracture of articular processes or split fracture of the lamina. Separation of the pedicles is marked

**Fig. 290.** Classic Chance fracture. All three columns are fractured by distraction. The posterior longitudinal ligament is torn or severely strained. The axis of rotation is located in the vicinity of the anterior longitudinal ligament. The reduced fracture is compression-resistant. Posterior tension resistance and rotational stability are nil

## 2.3 Unstable Burst Fracture or Complete Burst Fracture (Figs. 288 and 289)

The anterior and middle columns are destroyed by compressive forces, and the posterior column is fractured. We call this a complete burst fracture. The posterior column may be damaged by compression, lateral angulation or rotation. These injuries predispose to posttraumatic kyphosis and progressive neurologic deficits. A posterior edge fragment usually is driven to a varying extent into the spinal canal, and neurologic complications are not infrequent.

## 2.4 Chance Fracture (Figs. 290 and 291)

The classic Chance fracture is a horizontal fracture through the entire vertebra. Other forms have also been described. Chance fractures are caused by flexion about an axis situated anterior to the spine. Distraction forces act over the entire cross section of the spine, and a rotatory component may also be involved (GUMLEY et al. 1982) (Fig. 291). The fracture is unstable.

This injury typically occurs in persons wearing a lap belt in vehicular accidents ("lap belt fracture"). The localization is from T12 to L3. Associated intraabdominal injuries are frequent (GUMLEY et al. 1982).

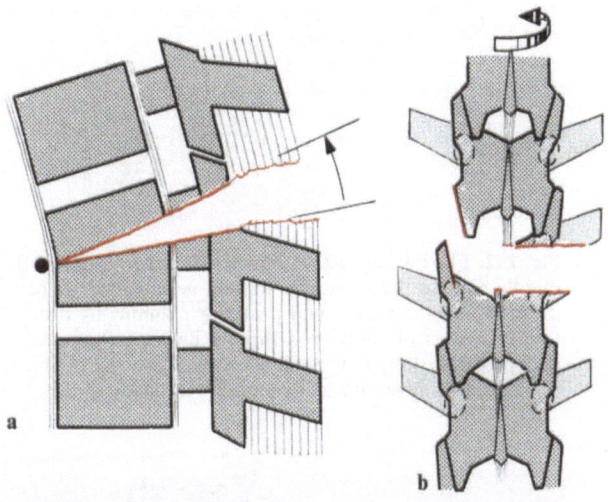

**Fig. 291 a, b.** Chance fracture with a rotational component. Both anterior columns are fractured, the injury to the posterior column may be osseo-ligamentous. The posterior longitudinal ligament is torn or severely strained. The supraspinal and interspinal ligaments are torn. The stability is the same as in classic Chance fractures. **a** Semioblique distraction fracture of the vertebra. The axis of rotation is located in the vicinity of the anterior longitudinal ligament. **b** Fracture through the pedicle and transverse process on one side with dislocation of the contralateral facet joint. The spinous processes have been displaced somewhat by the rotation

## 2.5 Flexion-Distraction Injury
(Figs. 292–294)

In a flexion-distraction injury the axis of flexion is located somewhere between the anterior and posterior longitudinal ligaments. As a result, the anterior column is destroyed by compression, and the middle and posterior columns by distraction. Distraction forces stretch or rupture the posterior longitudinal ligament, and the supraspinal and interspinal ligaments are usually torn. The facet joints may subluxate or dislocate, and the articular processes may fracture. Flexion-distraction injuries are potentially unstable, and we believe that some may be highly unstable.

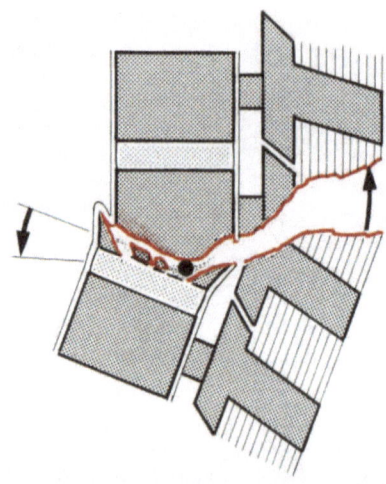

**Fig. 294.** Flexion-distraction injury, caudal type with fractures of all three columns. The mechanism of injury is the same as in Fig. 293

## 2.6 Translational Injuries (Figs. 295–299)

The somewhat heterogenous group of translational injuries are characterized by an interruption in the axis of the spinal canal at the level of injury, caused by a shifting of the principal fragments in the transverse plane. The mechanism of this injury, which affects all three osseoligamentous columns, involves a combination of rotary and shear forces. This group includes slice fractures (HOLDSWORTH 1963, 1970), rotatory burst fractures, fracture-dislocations and pure dislocations (see Sect. 2.7). These injuries are unstable. Indeed, translational injuries represent the least stable of all spinal injuries, and often lead to neurologic complications.

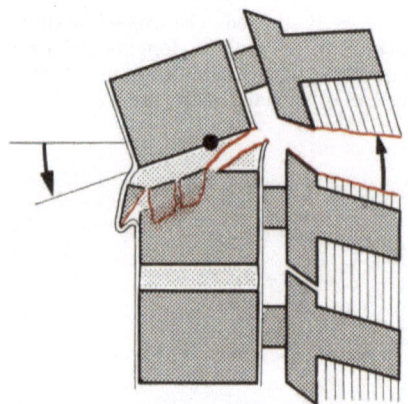

**Fig. 292.** Flexion-distraction injury without fracture of the middle column. The anterior column is damaged by compression and the middle and posterior columns by distraction. The axis of rotation is located between the anterior and posterior longitudinal ligaments. This type of injury resists compression. Posterior tension resistance is nil

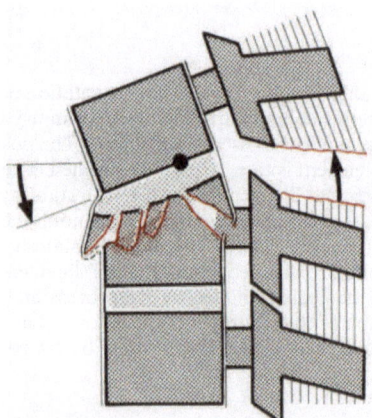

**Fig. 293.** Flexion-distraction injury with fracture of the middle column. The mechanism of injury is the same as in Fig. 292. An upper posterior edge fragment is torn out and protrudes into the spinal canal. The injury lacks compression resistance, rotational stability and posterior tension resistance

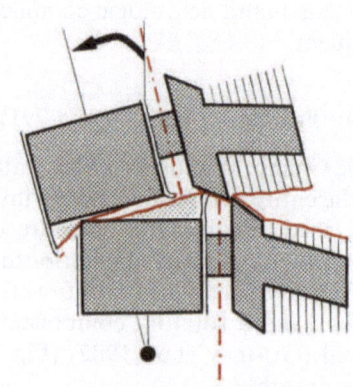

**Fig. 295.** Translational injury, pure dislocation. The injury is caused by a combination of shear and distraction. The axis of the spinal canal is interrupted. The intervertebral disc and ligaments are ruptured. When reduced, the injury is compression-resistant. Tension resistance and rotational stability are nil

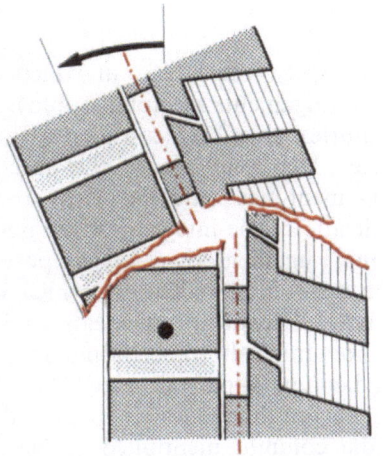

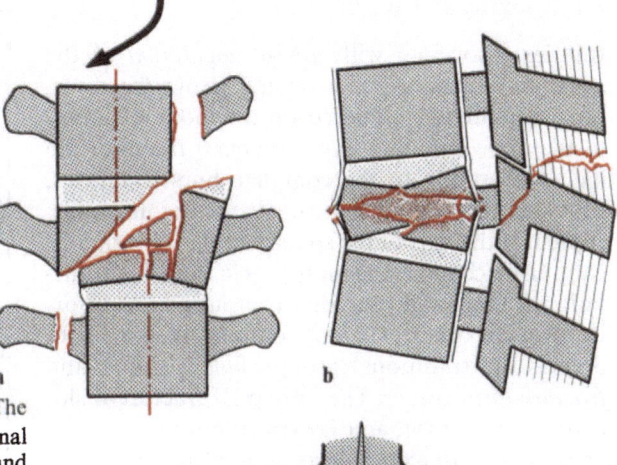

**Fig. 296.** Translational injury, fracture-dislocation. The mechanism of injury is shear. The axis of the spinal canal is interrupted. The disc and ligaments are ruptured, and the articular processes are fractured. The injury is still compression-resistant but is completely unstable in other respects

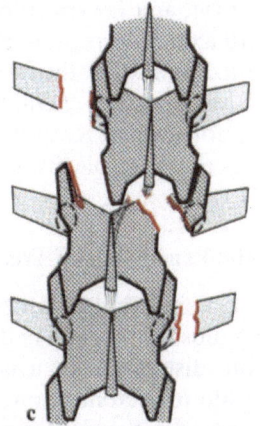

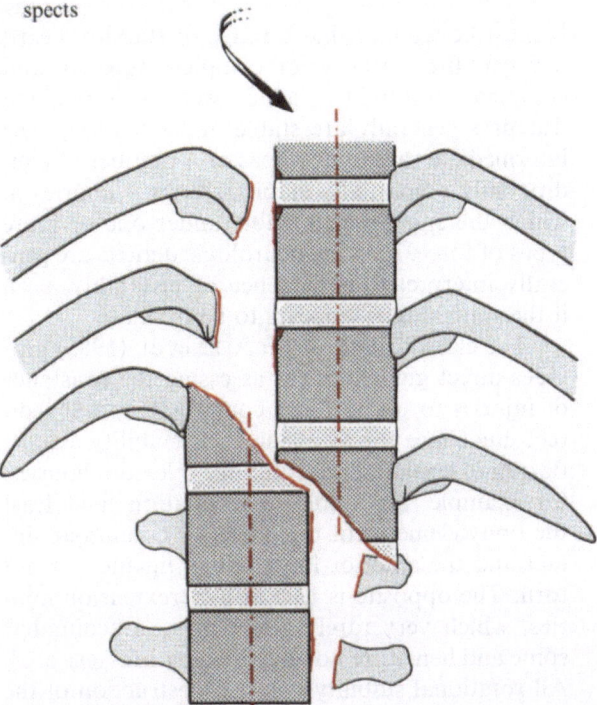

**Fig. 297 a–c.** Translational injury, rotatory burst fracture. The mechanism of injury is a combination of rotation and strong axial compression. All three columns are fractured, and all ligaments are torn. Instability is complete. **a** The axis of the spinal canal is interrupted. The avulsion of transverse processes is characteristic of rotatory injuries of this type. **b** The severity of the injury may not be fully appreciated in the lateral view. **c** Fracture of an articular process with dislocation of the contralateral facet joint

**Fig. 298.** Translational injury, rotatory compression fracture. The injury is caused by a combination of rotation and moderate axial compression. We have seen this injury on several occasions at the thoracolumbar junction. It is characterized by an interruption of the spinal canal axis and the avulsion of transverse processes with displacement of the corresponding ribs. The three columns are fractured, and all intervertebral ligaments are torn. Instability is complete

**Fig. 299.** Translational injury, slice fracture. The mechanism ▶ of injury is rotation. This type of injury is peculiar to the thoracolumbar junction. Besides the features of the translational and rotatory injury, there is a characteristic disc-shaped vertebral body fragment. All three columns are fractured, and all intervertebral ligaments are ruptured. The "ideal" slice fracture has reasonably good compression resistance when reduced. In other respects the injury is completely unstable

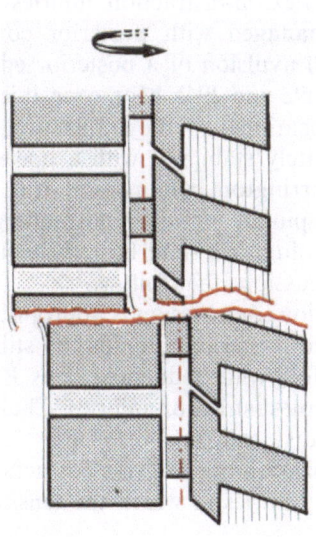

## 2.7 Remarks on Classification

Injuries associated with *lateral angulation* of the spine may be classified as lateral wedge fractures, burst fractures, etc., based on the mode of injury to the three columns. *Rotatory burst fractures* are included among to the complete burst fractures, provided the axis of the spinal canal is not interrupted. If the axis of the spinal canal shows significant displacement, the injury is classified as translational. One might say that translation has priority over all other classification criteria. This subdivides the traditional group of *dislocations* and *fracture-dislocations*. The Group III fracture-dislocations of KAUFER and HAYES (1966) that are not associated with axial interruption of the spinal canal are classified as flexion-distraction injuries in the system of McAFEE et al. (1983). Classification of the subluxations which KAUFER and HAYES assign to the class of "unstable dislocations" is more problematic.

## 2.8 Classification and Mode of Treatment

We favor the classification of McAFEE because it is simple and it aids the surgeon in deciding whether compression, distraction or a neutral mode is most appropriate for stabilization. McAFEE et al. (1983) have devised a simple formula, tailored to the Harrington and segmental spinal instrumentation, which takes into account the residual stability of an injury. According to this formula, compression injuries should be stabilized in distraction, distraction injuries in compression, and translational injuries by segmental spinal instrumentation.

However, certain fractures do not fit into this surprisingly simple formula. For example, we know of flexion-distraction injuries that should not be managed with posterior compression – those with avulsion of a posterior edge fragment (cf. Figs. 293 and 294). Moreover, it is known that pure dislocations, of the translational type may be adequately stabilized with a posterior tension band (Harrington compression rod, wire loop), since the spinal column cannot undergo appreciable shortening. We shall bear these facts in mind in the discussions that follow.

Posterior compression is appropriate when the middle and posterior columns can still resist compression following reduction. This is the case in most flexion-distraction injuries, Chance fractures and pure dislocations.

Stabilization by posterior distraction is indicated for all injuries in which the tension resistance of the spine is largely intact, i.e., in which the powerful posterior ligaments are not disrupted. All compression injuries, then, are considered to be tension resistant. The condition of the anterior longitudinal ligament has little relevance to the posterior stabilization. The integrity of the posterior longitudinal ligament has an important bearing on the distraction–reduction, which will be discussed later. Except for dislocations and "ideal" slice fractures, all translational injuries lack tension and compression resistance. The same applies to the flexion-distraction injuries with a fractured middle column, mentioned earlier. In these cases the spine should ·be splinted and protected against shortening.

## 2.9 Degree of Stability

It must be realized that a range of stabilities exist between the extremes of complete stability and complete instability. Mild wedge-compression fractures generally are stable under loading. The intermediate range encompasses a number of conditionally or partially stable injuries – injuries in which the spine is still stable under one or more types of force. Existing neurologic deficits are generally interpreted as evidence of instability, even if the spinal injury appears to be trivial.

The classification of McAFEE et al. (1983) provides direct guidelines for assessing the resistance of injuries to tension and compression, and indirect guidelines for assessing their stability against flexion-extension and rotation. Flexion injuries, for example, are stable in reclination if at least the bony elements of the posterior column are intact and the anterior longitudinal ligament is not torn. The opposite is true in hyperextension injuries, which very rarely affect the thoracolumbar spine and hence are not classified by McAFEE et al. All rotational stability is lost if destruction of the anterior and middle columns is combined with a complete division of the posterior column. These injuries, like most translational injuries, are completely unstable in all respects.

The degree of instability of complete burst fractures, like other injuries, depends on the condition of the lamina and facet joints. Complete burst fractures in which there is a vertical split through the inferior half of the vertebral body and the lamina (Fig. 288), known as crush-cleavage fractures (LINDAHL et al. 1983), are more stable than complete burst fractures with fractures of articular processes or the pars interarticularis (comminuted burst fractures, Fig. 289). This is because a split fracture of the lamina does not impair the longitudinal splinting function of the posterior column as much as a transverse bony division of that column. Also, the laminar fragments cannot displace significantly, at least distally, because there they are held together by the inferior facet joints, which usually are undamaged.

## 2.10 Type of Instability and Prognosis

KAUFER, in 1975, made an important contribution to our understanding of spinal instability by making a distinction between acute and chronic instabilities.

The spine is *acutely unstable* if, in the early postinjury period, the fragments can displace in a manner which jeopardizes neural structures. Both angular deformities and translational displacements are potentially dangerous in this regard. Translational displacements are the most hazardous, because they cause the greatest luminal reduction of the vertebral canal. The danger decreases as healing progresses.

*Chronic instability* is characterized by a deformity which gradually progresses over a period of months or years. Both dislocations and fractures of the thoracic and lumbar vertebrae are potential causes of chronic stability. A progressive angular deformity of the spine can cause neurologic deficit even years after the initiating event.

KAUFER indicates the importance of *prognosis* when he says that it would be useful, from a therapeutic standpoint, to know the instability of an injury. In the case of an acute instability, this is fairly simple: Any translational displacement is regarded as a sign of acute instability. Chronic instability is by far more difficult to predict. It may develop secondarily to the destruction of the anterior and middle columns, but it is more likely to result from the destruction of all three columns. Regular follow-ups are necessary to identify this condition.

BRADFORD et al. (1977), expanding on the work of KAUFER, cite severe burst fractures and serial compression fractures as causes of chronic instability. They also point to laminectomy as having causal significance. It should be added that a laminectomy can transform a partially stable injury into an acutely unstable one.

LOUIS (1977) further elucidates the nature of instabilities by pointing out two factors which should be considered when designing a plan of treatment. The first is *iatrogenic instability*. The surgeon invariably introduces instability when he reduces a fracture or dislocation and when he performs a laminectomy or another decompressive procedure that involves the removal of elements which contribute substantially to spinal stability.

The second factor is the *type of tissue* involved. It is important to differentiate between *osseous* and *ligamentous* (discoligamentous) *instability* because of their different prognostic significance. Pure osseous injuries or instabilities carry a favorable prognosis owing to the good healing potential of cancellous bone. Pure discoligamentous injuries have a less favorable prognosis. The bradytrophic ligamentous and disc tissue heals slowly. Also, the scar tissue that develops is a poor substitute for the highly differentiated tissue that was destroyed.

When we consider spinal injuries in terms of LOUIS' concept of transitory osseous instability versus permanent ligamentous instability, we find that the pure osseous injuries of the wedge-compression fracture and classic Chance fracture are located at one end of the scale, while pure dislocations, being solely discoligamentous injuries, are located at the other. Between these extremes are the mixed osseous and discoligamentous forms of injury. The incomplete burst fractures represent a predominantly osseous type of injury. Even here, however, involvement of the superior intervertebral disc (Fig. 287) is considered as an unfavourable prognostic sign. It remains unclear how splitting of the inferior half of a vertebra in the crush–cleavage fractures affects the inferior intervertebral disc. In theory, the disc should lose its turgor and thus its function if significant portions of the nucleus pulposus can herniate into the vertebral body. In follow-ups we have seen several instances where the inferior disc collapsed in the wake of crush–cleavage fractures.

## 2.11 Prognostic Significance of Angular Deformities

*Angular deformities of the spine* should be mentioned in connection with prognosis. It is known that marked angular deformities imply an unfavorable prognosis. Scoliotic deformities are more notorious in this regard than kyphotic deformities.

Tolerance toward kyphotic deformities varies greatly from one individual to the next and depends on the compensating ability of the spine in question. Even large kyphotic deformities are well tolerated if spinal mobility is good. For example, if a kyphosis at the thoracolumbar junction can be compensated by extension of the thoracic spine and lordosis of the lumbar spine within its physiological limits. On the other hand, if a more or less fixed kypholordosis is already present, or if the lumbar capacity for compensatory lordosis is limited, even a relatively mild kyphosis at the thoracolumbar junction may lead to subsequent complaints. Quantitative data on the tolerance for kyphosis, and the often great diversity of opinion concerning that tolerance, should be viewed in this light.

On the average, the tolerance limit for kyphosis at the thoracolumbar junction appears to be 15 to 20° (TROJAN 1972), or a relative loss of about 50% in the anterior height of a vertebral body. WHITESIDES (1977) states a figure of 60%. Beyond this point realignment of the fracture site should be considered.

# 3 The ESSF Device and Instrument Set

In the first 12 cases we used the original external fixator of the ASIF with threaded rods. Two longitudinal threaded rods were cross-connected by Steinmann pins to form a rigid, rectangular external frame. Because this device was too difficult to handle and adjust, we had to seek a different solution. The current ESSF device, as well as several preliminary versions, were developed in cooperation with Mr. F. SCHLAEPFER of the Laboratory for Experimental Surgery in Davos, Switzerland.

The ESSF device (Figs. 173 and 300) consists of four Schanz screws and an adjustable external frame. Two transverse bars (or carrier plates) and three longitudinal threaded rods form the external frame. The threaded rods are connected to the transverse bars by ball and socket joints (Fig.

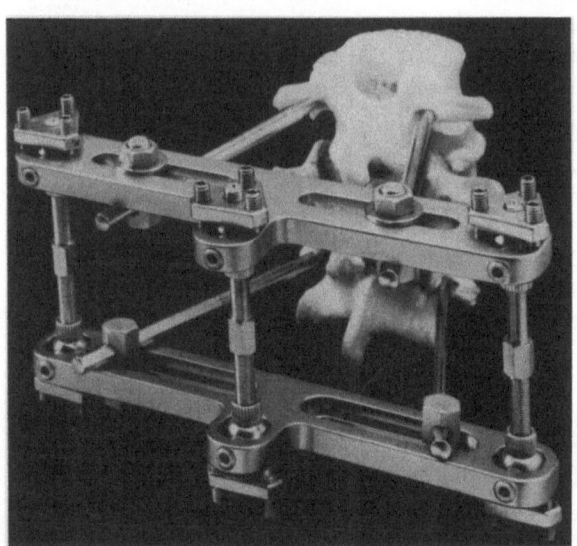

**Fig. 300.** The ESSF device (cf. text)

**Fig. 301 a, b.** Connection between the transverse bars and threaded rods. **a** Ball and socket joint with set screw. **b** Lock plate (cf. text)

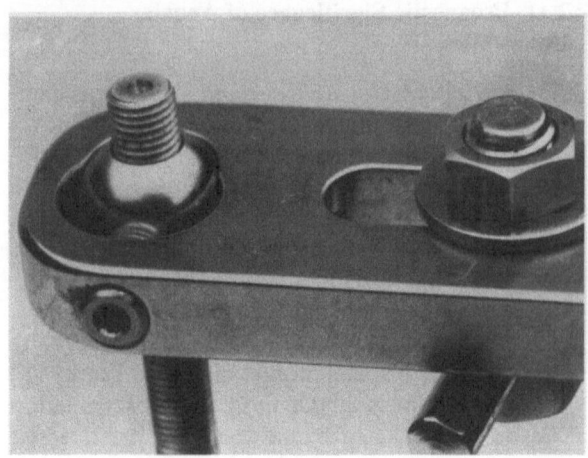
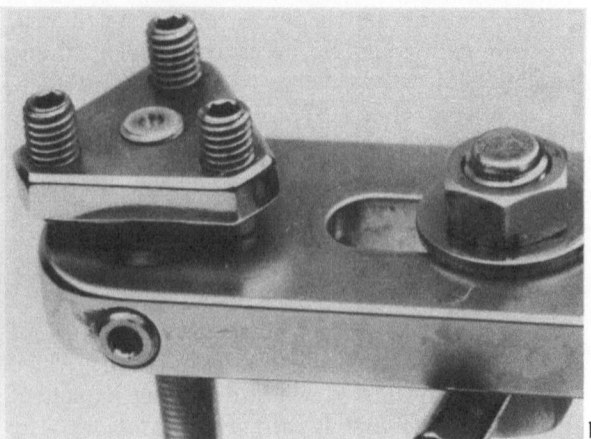

a                                                                                                    b

301a), thereby providing an external frame with a high degree of adjustability.

To assemble the device, the threaded rod with the balls attached is introduced through the larger, posterior portion of the holes in the transverse bars, such that the balls become seated in the sockets. Set screws hold the balls in place. Because the set screws cannot secure the relative positions of the fixation elements by themselves they are supplemented by small triangular lock plates (Fig. 301b) which are threaded onto the ends of the rods. Each lock plate is equipped with three set screws. Just as three points define a plane, the three points of the set screws define the plane of the transverse bars relative to the long axis of the threaded rods. Once the set screws are tightened, the angles between the rods and transverse bars can no longer be altered.

All the rods have counter-rotated threads. Each ball and lock plate is provided with both a right-hand and a left-hand thread so that they can be screwed onto the rods without regard to the direction of the thread.

The Schanz screws are connected to the transverse bars by means of screw clamps. Slots in the bars make it possible to vary the transverse distance of the Schanz screws.

The versatility and adjustability of the ESSF device can be expressed in numeric terms as follows:

– Minimum transverse spacing of the Schanz screws at the level of the transverse bars = 30 mm.
– Maximum transverse spacing of the Schanz screws at the level of the transverse bars = 85 mm with short and 110 mm with long transverse bars.
– The threaded rods come in a variety of lengths, permitting the longitudinal spacing of the Schanz screws to be varied from a minimum of 18 mm to a maximum of 145 mm. For small spacings the Schanz screws are fixed to the inside surfaces of the transverse bars; for larger spacings, to the outside surfaces.
– The inclination of the transverse bars in the sagittal plane (flexion-extension) may be varied over a range of 100° (Fig. 302).
– The bars may be inclined up to 35° in the frontal plane (scoliosis).
– The threaded rods have about a 30° range of mobility in the transverse direction.
– The mobility of the rods in the AP direction is about 40°.

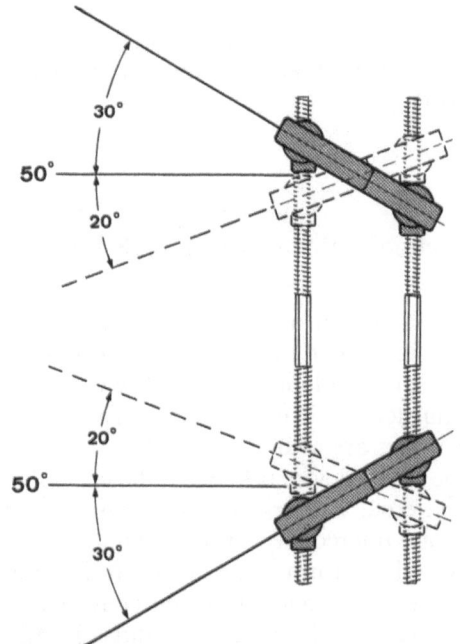

**Fig. 302.** The ESSF device has 100° of adjustability in the sagittal plane (flexion-extension)

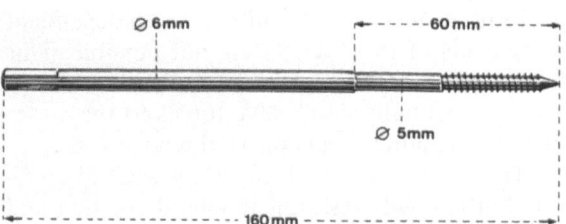

**Fig. 303.** Modified Schanz screw with self-tapping thread

– The transverse bars can be rotated 33° relative to each other around the middle threaded rod.

The modified Schanz screws (Fig. 303) are 160 mm long and have sharp, self-tapping points to allow percutaneous insertion without predrilling. The shaft of each screw is 6 mm in diameter, and the anterior 60 mm is 5 mm in diameter.

The instrument set for the ESSF device (Fig. 173) includes 2 pairs of transverse bars in different lengths; threaded rods (3 each) in lengths of 90, 120 and 150 mm; and distraction forceps. The adjustable distraction forceps shown in Fig. 173 is an improved version which replaces the model previously used.

Threaded rods 250 mm in length and double screw clamps are also available as accessories. The 250-mm threaded rods are intended for cases where the transverse bars are spaced very far apart, or a straight coupled fixation assembly is employed (cf. Fig. 313). The double screw clamps are used for angled coupled assemblies (cf. Fig. 314).

# 4 Biomechanics of the ESSF Device

In our discussion of positions and directions, we shall assume that the ESSF device is mounted on the spinal column. This will allow us to use anatomic terms whenever positional and directional references are made.

The ESSF device belongs to the class of "half-pin" external fixators. The two pairs of Schanz screws are interconnected both longitudinally and transversely to form a rectangular frame. Because the screw pairs occupy three different planes, the device may be classified as a three-dimensional half-pin external fixator.

The horizontal pairs of screws are interconnected by the fixed vertebrae and transverse bars to form a mechanical unit. Thus independent movements of these screws are not possible. This means that the Schanz screws cannot transmit opposite, potentially destructive forces to the vertebrae during adjustments of the threaded rods.

The ESSF device is elastic in the sagittal direction but is highly resistant to lateral bending and axial rotation.

At one time we regarded the sagittal elasticity of the device as a disadvantage, but since then we have found cause to revise that opinion. We have found that this elasticity is in no way detrimental to either the retention of the fracture or its healing. Indeed, it has proved extremely useful in preventing breakage of the Schanz screws and protecting their anchorage. The few cases of screw loosening that have occurred to date are due entirely to technical errors during insertion which weakened the surrounding bone. It is reasonable to assume that the sagittal elasticity of the device serves to cushion the transmission of shock loads to the screw sites in the bone. Excellent screw retention has also been documented in laboratory experiments.

## 4.1 Open or Percutaneous Application of the ESSF Device

In open application, it is possible to increase the primary stability of the fixation and to secure the long-term stability of the injured region. Primary stability is improved by implants, while long-term stability is ensured by the insertion of bone grafts.

Definitive fusions with bone grafts are performed across damaged motion segments. Therefore, the need for a definitive fusion will depend on the prognosis of the injury.

For some time we believed that every damage to the discs or facet joints warranted a primary definitive fusion on prognostic grounds so that secondary operations could be avoided. The validity of this policy will be examined later on.

When the device is applied percutaneously, the long-term stability of the injured area, and thus the end result of treatment, depends entirely on the quality of healing of the injured structures.

## 4.2 The Importance of Prestressing

Mechanically the ESSF device may be used in three different modes: the neutral mode without prestressing, the distraction mode with prestressing in distraction, and the compression mode with prestressing in compression. The mode of application chosen depends on the residual or restored stability of the injured area.

With "prestressing" the load-bearing capacity of the spine-fixator system is increased by the application of a primary stress. This is essentially based on the elastic deformation of the Schanz screws. The force necessary for this deformation is produced by the threaded rods. In simplified terms, we may regard the posterior rod as providing the deforming force, while the proximal rods serve as a fulcrum around which the Schanz screws are deformed. The counterpressure arising in the spine is a function of the pressure and tension resistance of the injured area. When the Schanz screws are prestressed in distraction, part of the counterpressure is provided for by the muscle tone. The situation described is comparable to three-point bending; it exists whenever the device is applied percutaneously or by open technique I (see Sect. 4.4.1 and 4.4.2).

When the device is applied by the open methods II and III, a second fulcrum on the posterior column is created by means of implants or solid bone grafts (cf. Figs. 306, 307). In this case the mechanical situation is one of four-point bending.

When elastically deformed, the Schanz screws act as taut springs, resisting loads for which the injury is unstable. In the case of a compression fracture, for example, the screws are prestressed in distraction, producing a force that is directed against the load of the upper body. The distance between the fixed vertebrae remains constant as long as the primary stress is greater than the upper body load. If the latter exceeds the primary stress, the intervertebral distance will be reduced.

In many cases we have measured the primary distracting stresses that had been applied "by feel." The highest values were around 180 Nm per Schanz screw, with 10 cm as the average length of the lever arm formed by the screw fulcrum and vertebra. It would be useful to be able to measure the primary stress by simple means, and to establish standard values for the amount of stress that should be applied in the specific situation. Unfortunately, research and technology have not yet progressed to the point where this is possible. For the time being, therefore, the surgeon must still rely on guidelines and feeling. Our experience indicates that good results can be achieved in this way.

One way of judging, the magnitude of the primary stress is by watching the degree of bowing of the Schanz screws and twisting of the transverse bars. At the upper limit of 180 Nm there will be a distinct bowing of the Schanz screws and an incipient twisting of the transverse bars. Also, the turning resistance of the posterior threaded rod increases greatly in this range. Stresses higher than 180 Nm per Schanz screw were not required to date.

If the second fulcrum at the spinal column is lacking, overdistraction may occur. Therefore, during prestressing the intervertebral distance should be monitored closely using an image intensifier. This distance should increase by no more than one-fourth the normal value. Overdistraction could delay healing, increase kyphotic deformity in the event of a subsequent disc collapse, and lead to neural injury.

## 4.3 Use of the ESSF Device in the Neutral Mode

If the spine possesses good tension and compression resistance, the ESSF device can be applied in the neutral mode in order to neutralize unfavorable bending and rotatory forces. However, this combination of circumstances is rare (cf. Sect. 9.1).

## 4.4 Use of the ESSF Device in Distraction

Prestressing in distraction is indicated in cases where the tension resistance of the spine is intact or restored, but compression resistance is lacking. This mode is by far the most frequently employed in clinical practice.

When prestressing in distraction, a technical detail must be observed: We assume that the cor-rect intervertebral distance is restored by distraction and secured by screw fixation of the facet joints or by a pressure resistant bone graft.

At prestressing, the Schanz screws deform elastically. Under prestress in distraction, the Schanz screws are bent in such a way that their anterior ends converge. Through this convergence, a slight but usually undesirable kyphosis may result.

In order to keep the anterior ends of the Schanz screws parallel, the threaded rods close to the skin must be approximated as well (Fig. 304).

### 4.4.1 Percutaneous Application

Because the tension resistance of the injured area depends entirely on the intervertebral ligaments, and these ligaments tend to elongate under traction due to their viscoelasticity, percutaneous application of the device requires that a smaller primary stress be used than in open techniques.

For the percutaneous stabilization of injuries that lack both compression and tension resistance (e.g., translational fractures), it would seem reasonable to apply the device in the neutral mode. However, these injuries are highly susceptible to shortening due to the axial load imposed by body weight and muscular tension, and consequently they should be stabilized in distraction as well. Because of the absence of tension resistance, overdistraction is a particular danger in these cases.

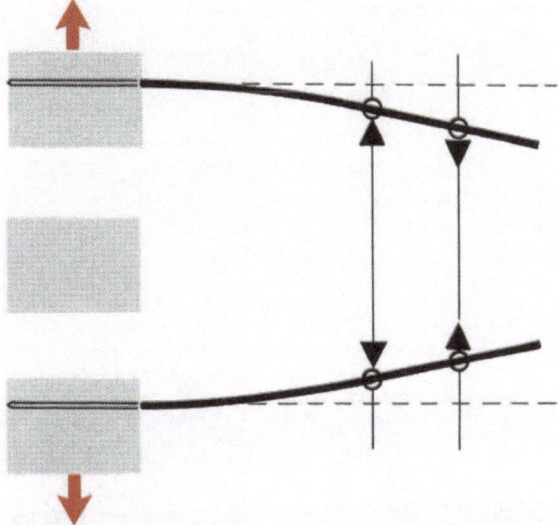

**Fig. 304.** Schematic illustration of the prestress in distraction. The actual distraction has already been carried out. At prestressing, the Schanz screws are bent elastically (exaggeratingly demonstrated). In order to keep the anterior ends of the Schanz screws parallel, the threaded rods close to the skin must be approximated as well during application of the prestress

### 4.4.2 Open Application

Three techniques are available, depending on the type of injury:

*Technique I* (Fig. 305). The middle and/or anterior columns are destroyed, the lamina may be split but still allows translaminar screw fixation. Intervertebral damage is confined to the upper motion segment.

The superior facet joints are fixed with translaminar screws. Only the upper motion segment is fused with cancellous bone grafts; the lower motion segment remains unfused. To avoid overdistraction of the unfused level, a smaller primary distraction stress is applied than in the following two techniques.

*Technique II* (Fig. 306). The anterior and middle columns are destroyed, and the condition of the posterior column permits translaminar screw fixation. Both adjacent motion segments are damaged.

Screw fixation of all four facet joints creates both a tension- and compression-resistant column extending from the upper to the lower fixed verte-

bra. Now a large primary stress may be applied. Both motion segments are fused with cancellous bone.

*Technique III* (Fig. 307). All three columns are destroyed, and there is damage to both adjacent motion segments. Translaminar screw fixation is not possible.

A second posterior fulcrum has to be created by a combination of bone grafting and wiring. The corticocancellous bone graft inserted between the spinous processes of the fixed vertebrae provides compression resistance, and the wire loop provides tension resistance. Supplementary cancellous bone grafts are applied to ensure a solid fusion of the damaged motion segments.

### 4.5 Use of the ESSF Device in Compression

Following pressure resistant interbody fusion, the ESSF device should be used in compression. A primary compressive stress will prevent anterior gaping of the fusion during reclination. This will

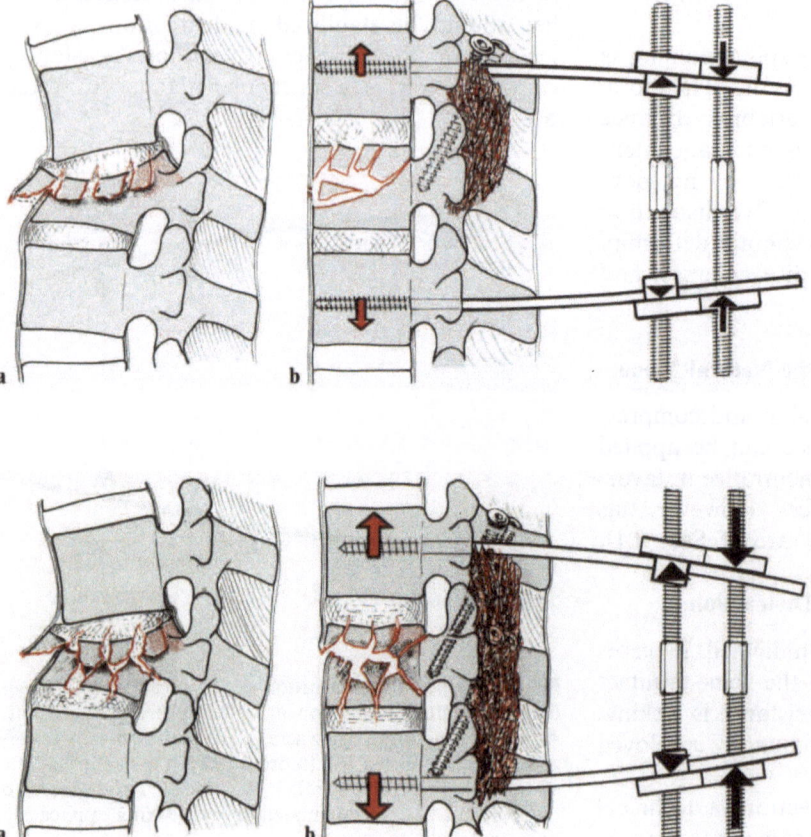

**Fig. 305 a, b.** Application of the ESSF device in distraction, open method, technique I (see text). **a** Incomplete or crush-cleavage fracture. The upper disc is damaged, and the posterior edge fragment encroaches upon the spinal canal. **b** Translaminar screw fixation of the superior facet joints. Cancellous bone is applied across the upper motion segment, and the injury is stabilized in moderate distraction. The posterior edge fragment is reduced. A defect persists in the vertebral body due to compression of the cancellous bone

**Fig. 306 a, b.** Application of the ESSF device in distraction, open method, technique II (see text). **a** Comminution of the vertebral body with damage to both adjacent discs. The spinal canal is narrowed by the posterior edge fragment. The condition of the posterior elements permits translaminar screw fixation. **b** Translaminar screw fixation of the superior and inferior facet joints with cancellous bone grafting of both motion segments and stabilization in strong distraction. The posterior edge fragment is reduced; a defect persists in the vertebral body

**Fig. 307a, b.** Application of the ESSF device in distraction, open method, technique III (see text). **a** Comminution of the vertebral body with damage to both discs and narrowing of the spinal canal. Destruction of the posterior elements precludes translaminar screw fixation. **b** After resection of the spinous process, a compression- and tension-resistant posterior fusion is performed with an H graft, cancellous bone and a wire loop. The fusion is stabilized in strong distraction. The posterior edge fragment is reduced, and a defect is present within the vertebral body

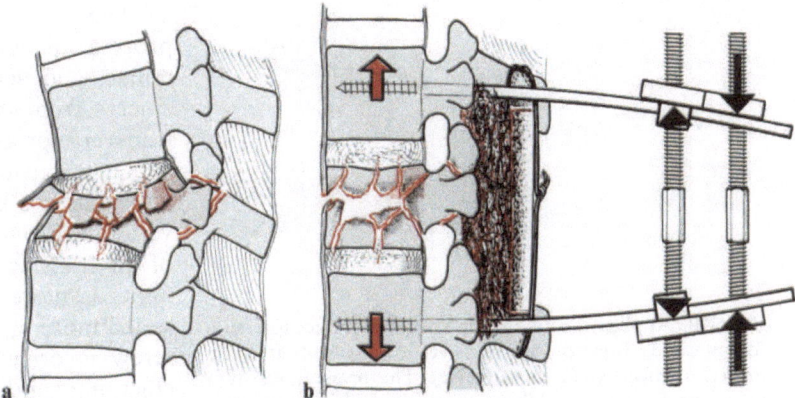

prevent healing impairment due to motion caused by "cycling" between compression and tension.

Again, it is important that the anterior parts of the Schanz screws remain parallel while the primary stress is imposed. This is accomplished by slightly increasing the distance between the Schanz screws at the level of the threaded rods near the skin as well (Fig. 308).

In all cases only a small amount of compression will be needed (Figs. 309 and 310), because some axial pressure is already being exerted by the weight of the upper body and by muscle tension. High axial compression could place excessive loads on interbody grafts or, in the case of percutaneous stabilization, could cause extrusion of disc material into the spinal canal. For the few instances where compression is warranted, we feel that the percutaneous mode of application is the most appropriate.

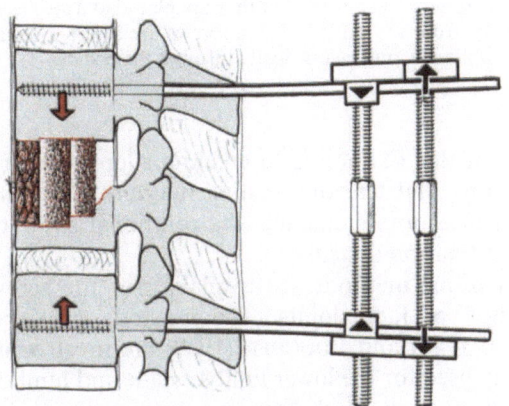

**Fig. 309.** Application of the ESSF device in compression (see text). The initial situation is comparable to that in Fig. 305a. The defect is filled with solid bone grafts and cancellous bone chips, followed by percutaneous stabilization in mild compression

### 4.6 Stabilization of Fractures of the Fifth Lumbar Vertebra

Fractures to the fifth lumbar vertebra, like all other fractures, are managed with one of the three techniques described above. The normal sacrum will afford adequate purchase for the Schanz screws despite the absence of pedicles. Anchorage in the osteoporotic sacrum, on the other hand, is precarious. Placement of the Schanz screws may also prove difficult in very muscular or obese patients, because the image intensifier may not demonstrate the sacrum in the lateral projection. In such cases it is safer to anchor the caudal pair of screws in the iliac wings (Fig. 311).

### 4.7 Translaminar Screw Fixation of Facet Joints

The advantages and effect of the screw fixation of facet joints were discussed above. The main pur-

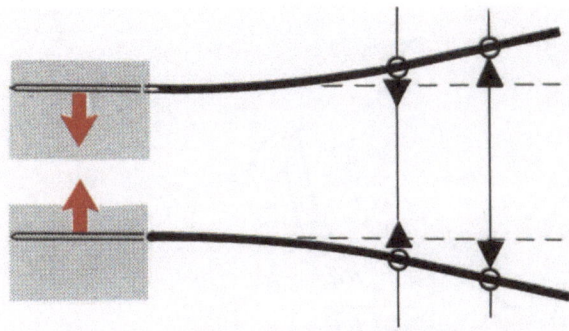

**Fig. 308.** Schematic illustration of the prestress in compression. While prestressing in compression, elastic bending of the Schanz screws (exaggeratingly demonstrated) must be considered in principal as well. In order to keep the anterior ends of the Schanz screws parallel, the distance between the screws must be slightly enlarged at the site of the threaded rods close to the skin as well

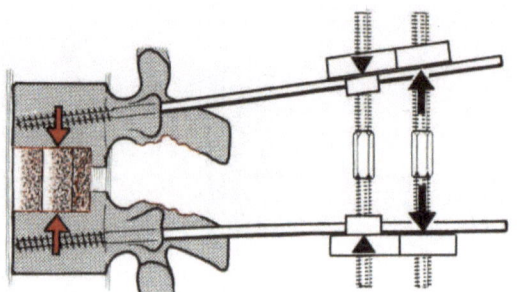

**Fig. 310.** Application of the ESSF device in compression for interbody fusions with massive dorsal instability (e.g. posterior infection or its sequelae). The pressure-resistant interbody fusion is stabilized percutaneously in moderate compression. To provide a greater spacing between the Schanz screws and ensure that they are placed at a sufficient distance from the graft bed, the screws are inserted somewhat obliquely and eccentrically through the pedicles

pose of this fixation is to create a supplementary pressure- and tension-resisting fulcrum. Also, the fixed facet joints enhance the rotational stability of the fixation system.

Various methods are available for the screw fixation of facet joints. The methods of King (1944, 1948) and Boucher (1959) are most commonly used for the lower lumbar spine and lumbosacral junction. Both have the disadvantage of a relatively weak screw anchorage in the laminae, especially when the bone is osteoporotic.

The translaminar screw fixation recommended by the author (Magerl 1980; Fig. 312) provides a better screw anchorage and may also be used in the region from T11 to the lumbosacral joints:

The screws are inserted through the spinous process, through the inferior portion of the laminae, and across the facet joints. Their points emerge from the caudal part of the bases of the transverse processes.

Owing to their placement in the laminae, the screws have a secure anchorage even in the upper vertebra. From a mechanical standpoint the angle of the translaminar screws in relation to the facet joints is more favorable than that of screws inserted more sagitally. Also, since the translaminar screw is oriented approximately parallel to the emerging spinal nerve, the danger of nerve injury is reduced.

Given their diverging direction, the translaminar screws cannot be used as lag screws. An attempt to do this could destroy the spinous process of the upper vertebra. Translaminar screws function as threaded bolts which prevent motion but do not exert compression.

### 4.8 Coupled ESSF Assemblies

The standard ESSF device spans one or two vertebral segments. Longer distances may be spanned by using the special, long threaded rods. However, the stability of the fixation system declines as the distance increases. In these circumstances stability

**Fig. 311 a, b.** Stabilization of the fifth lumbar vertebra (see text). **a** The caudal Schanz screws are driven into the ilia. Technique III is illustrated. **b** Position of the Schanz screws in the ilia

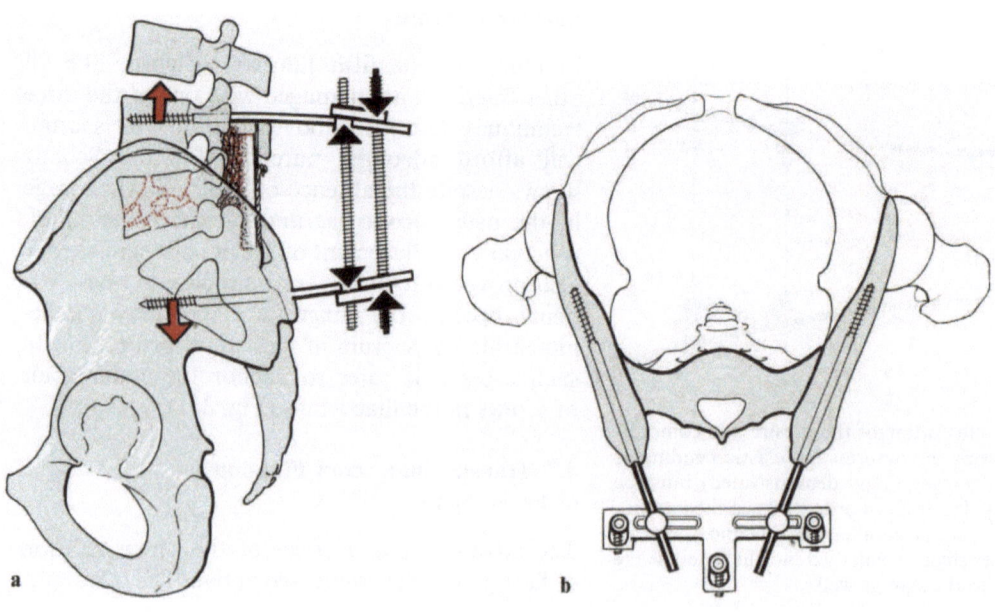

a                                              b

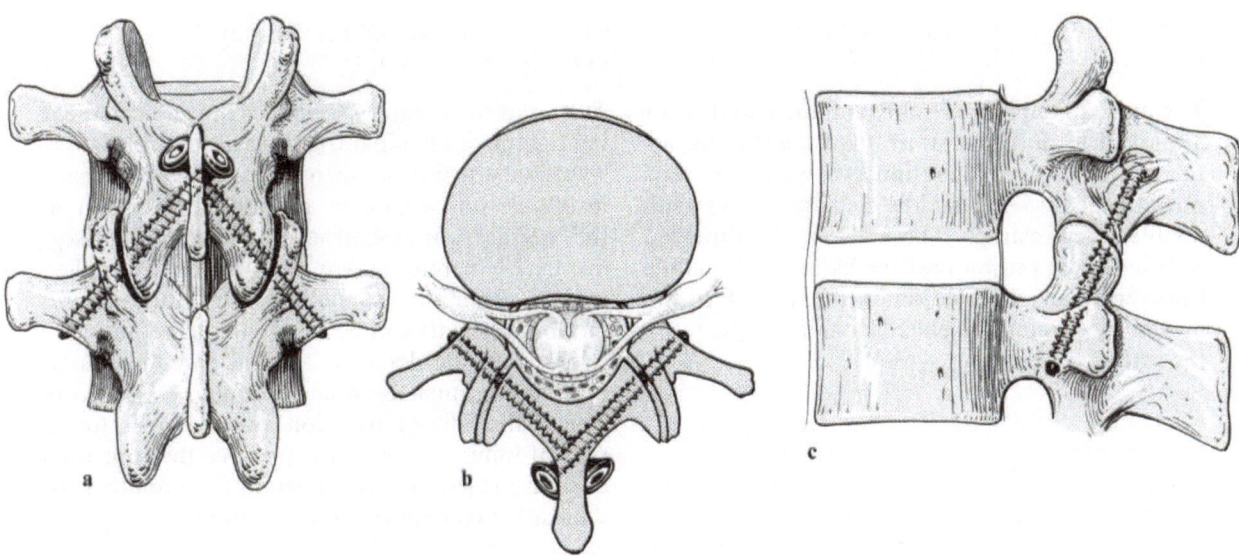

can be improved by incorporating a third vertebra into the system. This may be done in one of two ways:

### 4.8.1 The Straight Coupled Assembly (Fig. 313)

This assembly is appropriate for spinal regions without significant sagittal curvature. It requires special long threaded rods with an eccentric hexagonal component (cf. Fig. 173).

First the two outermost bars are mounted on the Schanz screws, which are arranged approximately in a straight line. The middle bar is mounted loosely. The threaded rods are then introduced through all three bars. The ball joints of the outermost bars are tightened with the set screws first, and then the joints of the middle bar. Only now is the middle pair of Schanz screws definitively clamped to the middle bar.

Turning the threaded rods moves only those two transverse bars between which the threads of the rods run in opposite directions. The third bar can be moved toward the middle bar only by rotating the balls on the stationary rods.

**Fig. 312 a–c.** Translaminar screw fixation of the facet joints (see text). The screws immobilize the joints but do not produce compression! **a** Posterior view. **b** Position of the screws in the posterior spinal elements and their relation to the facet joints. The screws roughly parallel the course of the emerging spinal nerves. **c** The point of the screw penetrates the inferior border of the transverse process near its base

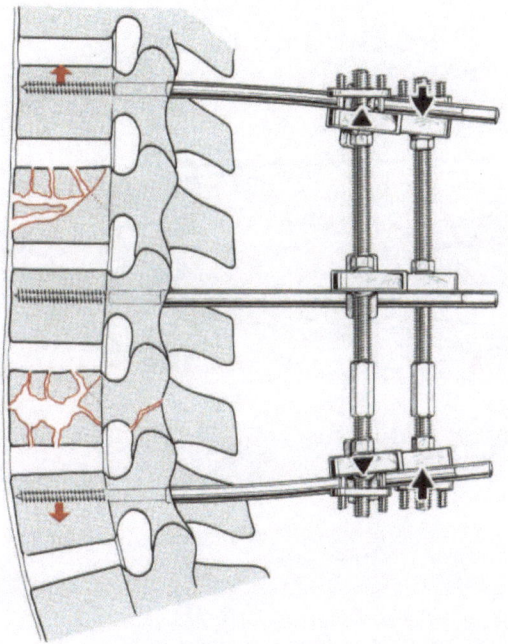

**Fig. 313.** The straight coupled fixation assembly, used here to treat a two-level fracture in a straight spine. Moderate primary distraction is applied (see text)

### 4.8.2 The Angled Coupled Assembly (Fig. 314)

The angled coupled assembly is more suitable for a marked lordotic curvature than the straight assembly. In this configuration two transverse bars are attached to the middle Schanz screws with double screw clamps. The ends of the threaded rods must not project past the balls of the middle transverse bars. The two outer transverse bars are moved by turning the balls belonging to them on the stationary rods.

### 4.8.3 Application and Prestressing of Coupled Assemblies

The coupled fixation assemblies are indicated for the treatment of spinal fractures at multiple levels. A primary fusion in such cases, though perhaps justifiable on prognostic grounds, may result in the needless immobilization of uninjured segments. We therefore favor the ESSF device applied by the percutaneous method. Unstable, painful motion segments can be fused later as required.

Because the device is applied percutaneously, prestressing must be done carefully, as stated in Sect. 4.4.1. Special attention must be given to the type of injury present. It is possible that one level of injury is less tension-resistant than another, or that one even requires compression.

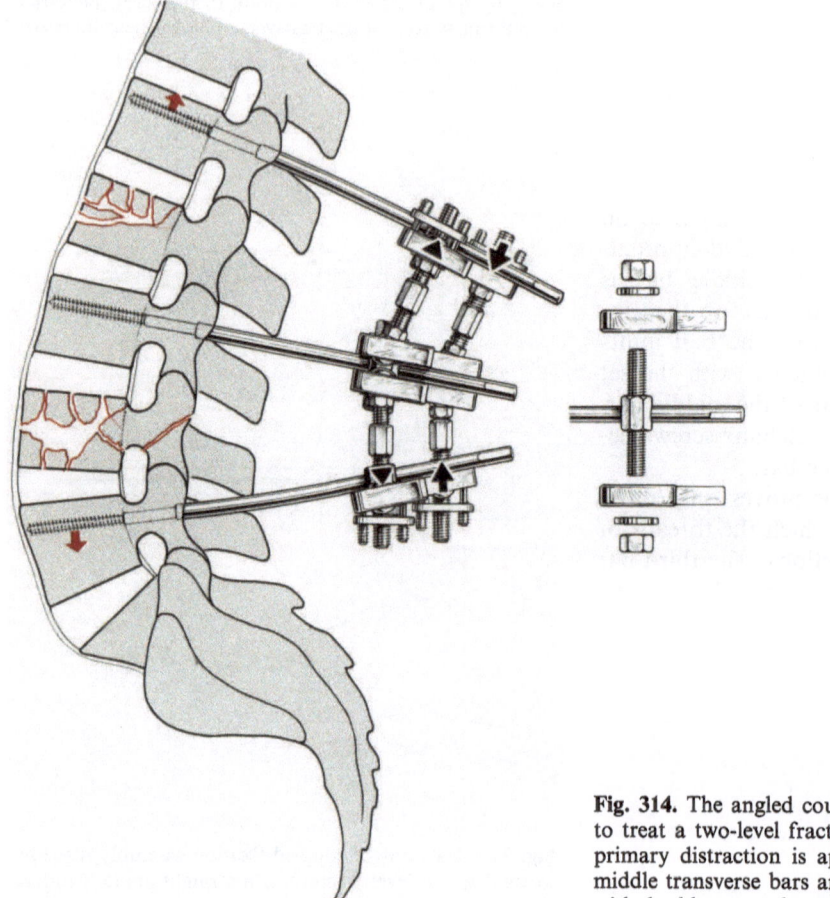

**Fig. 314.** The angled coupled fixation assembly, used here to treat a two-level fracture in a lordotic spine. Moderate primary distraction is applied (cf. text). *Detail:* The two middle transverse bars are connected to the Schanz screws with double screw clamps

# 5 Experimental Investigations

Comprehensive experimental investigations were conducted in cooperation with the Laboratory for Experimental Surgery in Davos, Switzerland. Some results of these studies have been published in journals (SCHLÄPFER et al. 1980, 1982, in press). WÖRSDÖRFER (1981) has reviewed the studies in detail in a qualifying thesis submitted to the University of Ulm.

The laboratory studies had the following objectives:

– Investigate the mechanical properties of the Schanz screws and the ESSF device.
– Investigate the anchorage of the Schanz screws in deep-frozen cadaveric specimens. Tests were done to determine the pull-out and push-in strength of the screws and their resistance to bending moments. The correlation between bone density and pull-out strength was analyzed.
– Investigate the effect of prestressing in distraction on the stability of the ESSF device.
– Conduct a comparative in-vitro investigation of the stability achieved with the ESSF device, the original Harrington distraction rods, the modified distraction rods of JACOBS et al. (1980), and plate fixation. The studies were carried out on fracture models (deep-frozen cadaveric specimens) with and without severed anterior longitudinal ligaments. The ESSF device immobilized three vertebrae, and each of the internal fixation systems immobilized five vertebrae. Using a special test machine, the stabilizing systems were subjected to pure bending in the sagittal plane without axial compression.

Here we shall only summarize the results of the laboratory investigations, rather than present a detailed account. Details may be found in the publications cited above.

Both the ESSF device and the Schanz screw anchorage proved to be sufficiently stable for clinical use. Prestressing increases the load-bearing capacity of the spine-fixator system. Stability is further enhanced by translaminar screw fixation.

Evidence from the in-vitro investigations (SCHLÄPFER et al. 1982) demonstrates that the ESSF device affords a stability of greater reliability than that obtained with the internal fixation systems tested (Fig. 315). The rigidity of the spine-fixator system achieved with the ESSF device is lower than that obtainable with plates or Jacobs rods. However, stabilization with the Jacobs rods failed at a bending moment of 19.5 Nm, and the

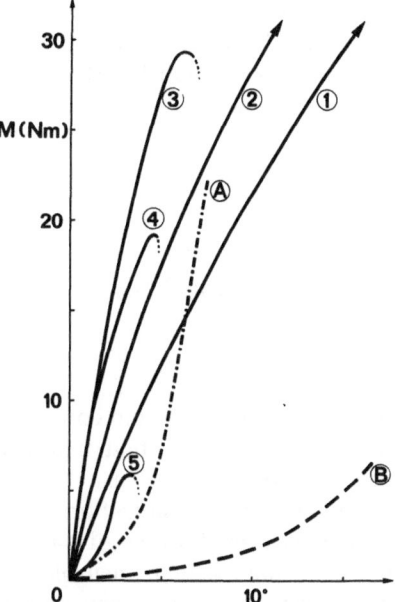

**Fig. 315.** Load-bearing capacity and deformation of different fixation systems, measured in a lumbar fracture model with an intact anterior longitudinal ligament (see text). Fixation systems: ESSF device without (*1*) and with (*2*) screw fixation of the facet joints; plate fixation (*3*); Jacobs distraction rods (*4*); and original Harrington distraction rods (*5*). Comparative investigation of the intact spine (*A*) and the fracture model (*B*). The plate fixations provide the highest rigidity. Loosening of the screws occurred at a bending moment of 29.5 Nm. The hooks of distraction systems 4 and 5 dislodged at 19.5 Nm and 5.9 Nm, respectively. The loads applied in this experiment produced only an elastic deformation of the ESSF device. Plastic deformation of the Schanz screws occurred in other experiments at 50–60 Nm

Harrington rods failed at 5.9 Nm due to dislodgement of the upper hooks. In the plate fixations the screws loosened at a bending moment of 29.5 Nm. With the ESSF device, on the other hand, elastic deformation was the only effect observed over a large range of loads. Loads of 50–60 Nm had to be imposed before plastic deformation of the Schanz screws occurred. Even in this range, the anchorage of the Schanz screws remained intact. With severance of the anterior longitudinal ligament, the Harrington and Jacobs systems failed at substantially smaller loads. The mechanical behavior of the ESSF device was not affected by severance of the anterior longitudinal ligament. It should be pointed out that the experimental setup was highly unfavorable for both the Harrington and Jacobs distraction systems, because a pure bending load can dislodge the hooks fairly easily in the absence of axial compression.

Application of the ESSF device in the ambulant patient provides an excellent opportunity to measure the loads acting on the spine. Investigations in this area have been initiated, and preliminary results have been published (SCHLÄPFER et al. 1980, in press; WÖRSDÖRFER 1981).

# 6 Indications for the ESSF Device

## 6.1 Trauma

Without discussing the pros and cons of operative treatment, we shall assume that treatment is administered according to the usual criteria, and shall outline the principal indications.

*Absolute indications* for operative treatment are increasing neurologic deficits, neurologic involvement of delayed onset, and open spinal injuries (rare).

*Relative indications* are unstable injuries and injuries that have an unfavorable prognosis. Neurologic complications tend to favour operative treatment. A spinal fluid block caused by narrowing of the vertebral canal is, we believe, an unfavorable prognostic sign. In general, then, the acutely unstable injury with a poor prognosis (e.g., dislocation) and neurologic complications constitutes the strongest relative indication for operative intervention.

Because the aftercare is relatively demanding, the patient should be reliable and cooperative and should be able to present for regular follow-ups. We do not treat complete cord lesions with the ESSF device on the basis of nursing considerations.

As before, we generally limit the use of the ESSF device to the region from T9 to L5. Above that level the device would hamper the excursion of the scapulae, while the movements of the scapulae and soft tissues could precipitate a pin track inflammation.

Within these limits, the indications for the ESSF device are practically identical to the indications for operative stabilization. In open stabilizations, however, preference is given to a simpler method if at all possible. Thus, all injuries that are compression resistant upon reduction are stabilized by a posterior tension-band fusion (wire loop, Harrington compression rods, short plates) followed by treatment with a plaster jacket or stable brace for about eight weeks. These injuries include flexion-distraction injuries in which the bony elements of the posterior and middle columns are intact and pure dislocations.

In open application of the ESSF device, the differentiation between tension- and compression-resistant injuries is purely academic. Because tension resistance can be restored by screw fixation of the facet joints or with a wire loop, it is always possible to prestress the device in distraction. The situation is different with percutaneous application. Here attention must be given to the type of injury, and residual stability will have a crucial bearing on the type and amount of primary stress that is applied.

## 6.2 Other Indications

In the treatment of *spondylitis,* external skeletal fixation offers the same advantages as in the treatment of infected fractures and nonunions of the extremities: immobilization of the affected skeletal region is ensured even with early mobilization and functional aftercare; no implant is in contact with infected tissues; and ample space is available for bone grafting.

These advantages apply particularly to the treatment of infections secondary to posterior operations on the spine, such as herniated disc surgery. The safety of external stabilization is also highly advantageous for the direct anterior debridement and fusion of spondylodiscitis of other aetiology.

In addition, external skeletal fixation offers two new treatment options: the indirect treatment of spondylodiscitis by percutaneous stabilization, and the semidirect treatment by posterior fusion and suction irrigation. The prerequisites for the three modes of treatment are discussed in Chap. 9.

Stabilization with the ESSF device is basically an option for nonspecific forms of spondylitis. Tuberculous spondylitis is an indication only in problem cases.

*Posterior fusions* for degenerative disease are *not* an indication for the ESSF device. They can and should be stabilized by simpler means.

The fixation device is definitely an option for any *difficult stabilization problems,* provided there is a sufficient amount of bony material that can unite and recover its supportive function. It must be borne in mind that the fixation device is only a temporary aid to stabilization. We know of cases at other centers in which the external fixation device provided a last recourse after attempts to stabilize the spine by other methods had failed due to infection or other causes.

# 7 Timing of Surgery

A basic distinction is made between immediate or emergency surgery, early surgery, and late surgery.

It is generally agreed that whenever an absolute indication exists, surgical intervention should be instituted without delay.

Surgery for relative indications should be done early. Whenever possible, we operate immediately for relative indications. If immediate surgery is not deemed possible, we put off the operation until the patient's condition is stable and bowel activity has normalized. Immediate and early operations are less risky and technically simpler than late operations for several reasons:

- Reduction is safer while the hematoma is still liquid and before scar tissue has formed. We are very reluctant to reduce an injury if more than three weeks have elapsed, because firm reparative tissue could cause pressure injury to neural structures as severely dislocated fragments are reduced.
- Reduction becomes more difficult with time. It is easiest in immediate operations, especially with regard to the closed reduction of posterior wall fragments by distraction. After three to four weeks, scar tissue and callus bridges can make the correction of deformities extremely difficult. In fact, it is highly unlikely that the closed reduction of posterior wall fragments will still be possible at that time.
- The structure of the bone has an important bearing on the reduction of the injury and the anchorage of implants. Both are safer in the absence of reactive osteoporosis.

Apart from these considerations, it should be asked at what time an operation should be performed whose intent it is not only to stabilize the spine, but also to aid neurologic recovery. Research indicates that the earlier neural structures are decompressed, the better the prognosis for neurologic recovery. The outlook is best when the neural tissue is decompressed and its blood flow restored in the first hours following injury (TARLOV 1972; WHITE 1975; RUGE 1977).

The arguments described above underscore the importance of early surgery. Moreover, when one considers the pain that is caused by an unstable spine, much can be said in favor of immediate intervention.

Another factor to be considered in connection with the timing of surgery is its effect upon fracture healing.

In all compression fractures, i.e., in wedge and burst fractures and to some extent in flexion-distraction fractures, the cancellous bone in the vertebral body is compressed to some degree. This causes cavities to form within the vertebral body when the fracture is reduced. BÖHLER (1982, personal communication) pointed out that osseous defects of this kind will fill spontaneously with new bone if two conditions are met: the absence of motion between the fragments, and the presence of a liquid hematoma to serve as a matrix for new bone formation in the cavities. The reossification process always progresses slowly. Small defects, of course, are closed more rapidly than large ones. In addition, our experience indicates that the period of time elapsing between the injury and the operation has an important bearing on reossification. The earlier the injury is reduced and stabilized, the more rapid the rate of reossification. BÖHLER also noted that the capacity for spontaneous reossification is lost at about three weeks after injury. Presumably these empirical facts relate to the state of the fracture hematoma. As long as the hematoma is liquid, it is able to permeate the resulting defect. But once the hematoma has become organized, probably only fluid without significant osteogenic potential enters the cavities. Thus, early surgical intervention also appears beneficial for fracture healing.

# 8 Operative Technique: Trauma

## 8.1 Open Technique

### 8.1.1 Operating Table, Closed Reduction, Positioning

The operating table must be tiltable and radiolucent and should have a break so that lordotic adjustments of spinal alignment may be made during the operation.

The anesthetized patient is placed in a prone position, and a careful closed reduction of the spine is carried out under image intensification. Due to the associated risk of spinal cord or root injury, a closed reduction is not attempted if it would necessitate undue force or cause additional kyphotic deformity.

It is always safest to initiate the reduction by the application of longitudinal traction. Fractures associated with shortening require simple longitudinal traction, while those associated with both shortening and kyphotic deformity will require a combination of axial realignment and traction. Flexion-distraction injuries will require some degree of longitudinal traction, but reduction is effected predominantly by axial realignment.

The advantages of a preliminary closed reduction are early decompression of neural structures and the facilitation of surgery, particularly in terms of providing the distraction needed for intraoperative reduction maneuvers. This is important because of the large frictional resistance between the body and the table that may be encountered.

Bolsters are placed under the chest and pelvis to remove pressure from the abdominal viscera and keep the lower spine in mild lordosis. Greater lordosis would make surgery more difficult.

### 8.1.2 Approach (Fig. 316)

The surgical approach is performed through a vertical midline incision extending over three to four vertebrae. The soft tissues over the fractured vertebra and the two adjacent vertebrae are dissected away from the midline to the middle of the transverse processes. Bleeding in the vicinity of the spine is controlled with bipolar coagulation.

### 8.1.3 Intraoperative Reduction

At this stage the fracture may be reduced in standard fashion with the aid of distraction forceps, prying, instruments, or large towel clips applied

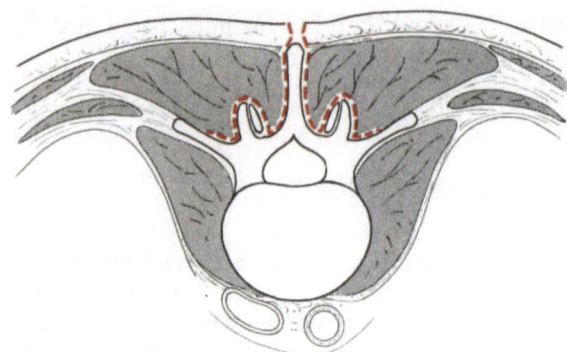

**Fig. 316.** Open technique: approach. On each side the soft tissues are stripped away from the midline to the middle of the transverse process

to the spinous processes. If counterpressure makes the distraction difficult, an assistant can pull the patient's upper body cranially to lessen the resistance. Loose fragments are removed to improve visualization of the fracture site.

### 8.1.4 Insertion of the Schanz Screws

The insertion of the Schanz screws is one of the most critical stages of the operation. The effectiveness of the operation and stabilization will depend upon the position of the Schanz screws in the vertebrae and soft tissues.

#### 8.1.4.1 Determining the Position of the Screws

The pedicles are short bony tubes with an oval cross-section. The objective is to insert the Schanz screws through the center of the pedicles, approximately parallel to the upper end plate or angled slightly downward. The screws should converge about 10° toward the midline at the thoracolumbar junction, and up to 15° in the lower lumbar region (Fig. 317). A purely sagittal insertion would place the screws too close to the lateral wall of the vertebral body, with a consequent risk of perforation.

The long axis of the pedicle can be identified either by direct exposure or image intensification. Though each method is reliable by itself, it is best to use a combination of the two.

At practically all levels in the thoracolumbar junction and lumbar spine, the long axis of the pedicle pierces the lamina at the intersection of two lines (Fig. 317): a vertical line tangent to the lateral border of the superior articular process, and a horizontal line bisecting the transverse process. Their point of intersection lies in the angle between

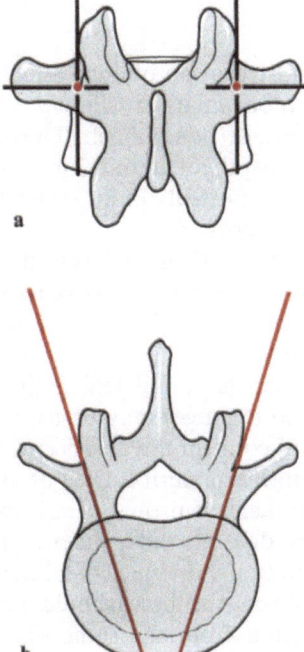

**Fig. 317 a, b.** The point of entry and direction of the Schanz screws (cf. text). **a** The point of entry is at the intersection of two lines. The vertical line touches the lateral border of the superior articular process, and the horizontal line bisects the transverse process. **b** The screws converge 10–15° toward the midline, depending on the level of the segment

the superior articular process and the base of the transverse process. In all cases it is necessary to identify and expose these sites, even if a purely radiologic localization of the peduncular axes and screw sites is proposed.

After the point of intersection has been identified, a 1.5-mm Kirschner wire is driven several millimeters into the bone at that location, taking care to keep the wire approximately in line with the pedicular axis. The position and direction of the Kirschner wire is then checked by image intensification. This is done by placing the sterile draped image intensifier in the vertical position and centering it over the pedicle in question. Then either the table or intensifier is tilted until the pedicle appears as a distinct oval at the center of the monitor screen. At this point the central axis of the pedicle will lie within the central beam of the image intensifier. Normally the table or intensifier will be tilted 10–15° in the transverse plane and may also be tilted longitudinally depending on the obliquity of the pedicle in the sagittal plane (cf. Fig. 330). Now the Kirschner wire is seized with a clamp and manipulated until it aligns precisely with the central beam and appears as a point at the center of the pedicle on the monitor screen.

If the point is not centered within the pedicle, the Kirschner wire must be removed and reinserted. After correct positioning, it may be driven somewhat deeper into the lamina.

When all Kirschner wires have been introduced, their placement is checked in the lateral projection, and any errors of orientation in the sagittal plane are corrected. To avoid losing orientation in the horizontal plane at this time, we recommend marking the angle of inclination to the median plane with a second Kirschner wire before any corrections are carried out.

Naturally any perforation of the medial wall of the pedicle must be strictly avoided so that the spinal canal is not violated. Lateral wall perforations are also unfavorable because they weaken the anchorage. Therefore, if there is any doubt, it is wise to double-check the position of the Kirschner wires by surgical exposure of the pedicles.

In the absence of extensive degenerative changes, the cranial or caudal aspect of the pedicles may be exposed by dissecting anteriorly from the angle between the articular and transverse process, always keeping beneath the periosteum. A small dissector is used for this purpose. The inferior border of the pedicle is more easily visualized than its superior border. Following this exposure, the medial and lateral aspects of the pedicle may be probed with a curved dissector to double-check the position of the Kirschner wire (Fig. 318). This extra check is particularly worthwhile if there is a preexisting scoliosis, because even a slight neural arch asymmetry can result in the perforation of a pedicle.

It is also possible to demonstrate the entire lateral aspect of the pedicle by osteotomizing the transverse process near its base. However, an osteotomy at that location will weaken the site of entry of the Schanz screw. Exposure of the caudal aspect of the pedicle is generally sufficient.

### 8.1.4.2 Drilling of the Pedicles

The laminae and pedicles are predrilled using a 3.2-mm drill bit (Fig. 319). Repeated drilling through a pedicle should be avoided, as this would weaken the anchorage of the Schanz screw. Before the Kirschner wire is removed, a second wire should be inserted into an adjacent part of the lamina, exactly parallel to the first, to serve as a directional guide during drilling. Also, to keep the bit from slipping off the bone surface, which usually is sharply inclined, the drilling either

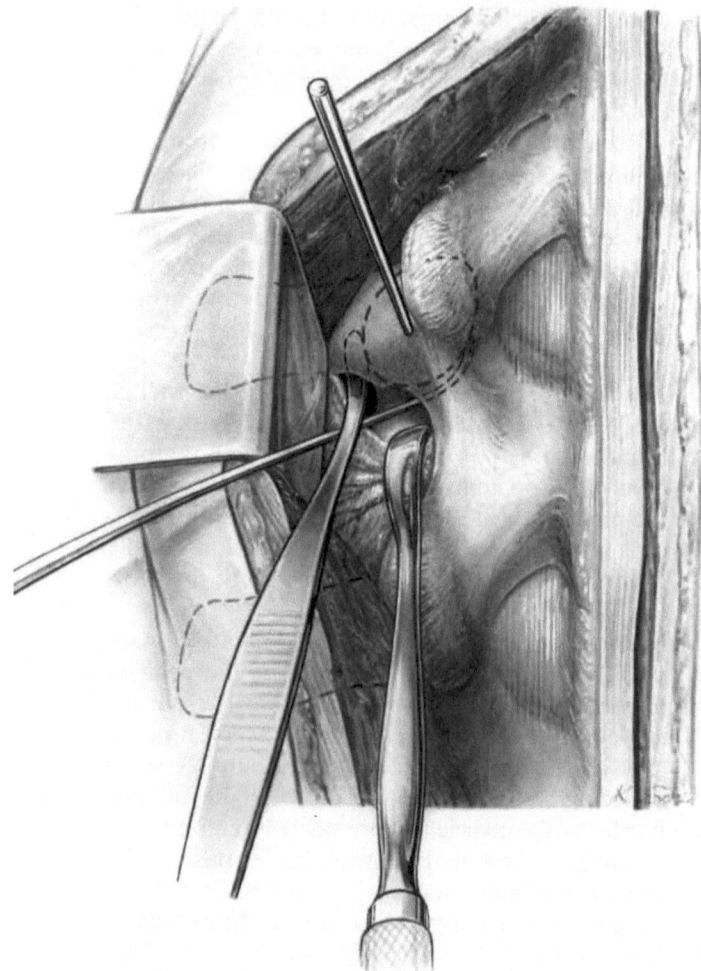

should be started at an oblique angle, or the pilot hole should be enlarged slightly with a larger Kirschner wire or bone punch. The drill bit is advanced to a depth of about 3 cm. A depth stop or mark on the bit will aid in controlling the drilling depth. Deeper drilling is unnecessary and would be problematic in the event that subsequent correction of the drill hole is required. It would weaken the cancellous bed of the Schanz screws unnecessarily.

After drilling is completed, a fine hook (e.g., the screw depth gauge) may be used to probe the drill hole and confirm the absence of perforations. A small tangential perforation of the pedicle is of no consequence if proper care is taken that the Schanz screw does not enter the perforation during the insertion. In the presence of a larger wall perforation, however, the hole should be redrilled in a new direction from the same site. The second drilling will not seriously compromise the anchorage of the Schanz screw if the cancellous bone of the vertebral body was not drilled too deeply initially.

Next the Schanz screw is driven into the predrilled hole to a depth of about 4 cm, whereupon its position is reconfirmed by image intensification in two planes. It is now possible to effect a definitive reduction by manipulation of the Schanz screws.

**Fig. 318.** Open technique. Determining the position of a screw in the lumbar spine by caudal exposure of the pedicle (seen in a slightly laterocaudal view). The inferior aspect of the pedicle, visible deep in the field, was exposed by dissecting subperiosteally from the base of the transverse process. The soft tissues with the spinal nerve branches and blood vessels were carefully retracted with a curved dissector. A small, curved dissector is used to probe the lateral and medial wall of the pedicle (projection of pedicle shown in red). The Kirschner wire marking the direction of the screw should follow the central axis of the pedicle in regions where the pedicles are narrow. But if the pedicle is sufficiently broad, as pictured here, it is better to shift the screw placement slightly laterally and caudally to avoid damaging the superior facet joint

**Fig. 319.** Open technique. The screw hole is predrilled to a depth of 3 cm (see text)

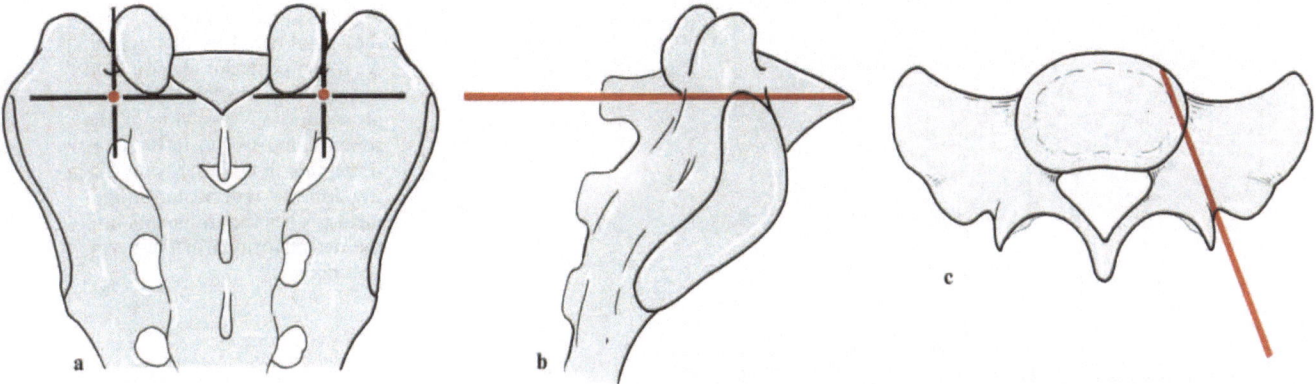

### 8.1.4.3 Screw Placement in the Sacrum and Ilium

*Sacrum:* The sites of entry and position of the Schanz screws are shown in Fig. 320. The orientation of the screws is 15–20° convergent toward the midline, and the screw tips are within the promontory. Image intensification is essential for correct positioning of the screws. The canal of the first sacral nerve is usually well demonstrated in the a.p. projection by the image intensifier and must be avoided.

*Ilia* (cf. Fig. 311): The Schanz screws are introduced just above the posterior superior iliac spine in the direction of the anterior inferior iliac spine (iliac tubercle), parallel to the outer wall of the ilium. Placement of the Schanz screw on the side where the bone grafts are to be harvested is relatively easy, for the outer wall is well exposed in that area. Care should be taken, however, that the screw bed is not weakened when the grafts are taken, and that the Schanz screw does not lie in the skin incision.

On the opposite side a short skin incision is made lateral to the posterior superior iliac spine, and the outer wall of the ilium is exposed subperiosteally to the necessary extent.

### 8.1.5 Instrumental Reduction, Distraction–Decompression

In most cases all gross displacements will have been reduced at this stage, and it remains only to restore the anatomic dimension of the spinal canal and the physiologic curvature of the spine in the sagittal plane. If a great deal of force has to be applied during the reduction maneuvers, the Schanz screws should be driven somewhat deeper into the bone under image intensifier control.

Any residual narrowing of the spinal canal at this stage is almost invariably caused by bone frag-

**Fig. 320 a–c.** Sacrum. Points of entry and position of the Schanz screws. **a** The point of entry is at the intersection of two lines – a vertical line tangent to the lateral border of the articular process, and a horizontal line tangent to its inferior border. **b** The screws point toward the promontory. **c** They converge 15–20° toward the midline

ments from the posterior wall of the vertebral body. Experience with many cases has taught us that these fragments may generally be reduced by strong distraction if the continuity of the posterior longitudinal ligament is intact (Fig. 321). The reduction and distraction decompression are carried out under image intensification.

The distraction is effected by means of distraction forceps inserted between the Schanz screws (Fig. 322). Opening the forceps produces a distraction of the vertebrae as well as a certain degree of kyphotic angulation. Since this angulation is generally undesired, it is necessary to approximate the posterior ends of the Schanz screws. When the distraction reduction is completed, the handles of the forceps are locked in place, and the posterior ends of the Schanz screws are wired together.

The distraction reduction of posterior wall fragments may also be accomplished with the external fixation device, inserted through the open wound. However, distraction forceps are easier to handle and more versatile.

Residual displacements of the spine in the sagittal plane are corrected simply by tipping the distraction forceps (Fig. 322). Lateral displacements are corrected by turning both forceps as required, lateral angulations by asymmetric distraction of the forceps, and rotational deformities by tipping one of the forceps.

During instrumental distraction it is helpful to have an assistant pull the upper body cranially if much resistance is felt. This will relieve the strain on the anchorage of the Schanz screws.

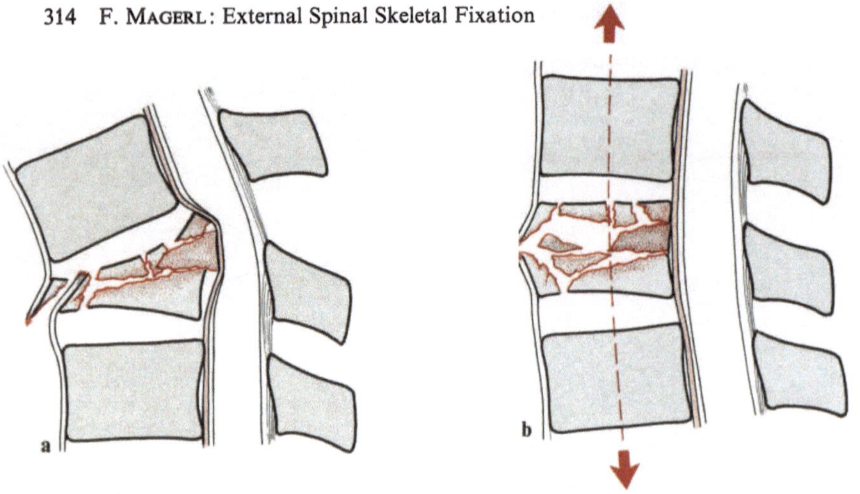

**Fig. 321 a, b.** Decompression of the spinal canal by distraction. An intact posterior longitudinal ligament is necessary for this procedure. **a** Narrowing of the spinal canal by posterior edge fragments. **b** Under strong distraction, the taut posterior ligament pushes the fragments into the defect formed in the vertebral body

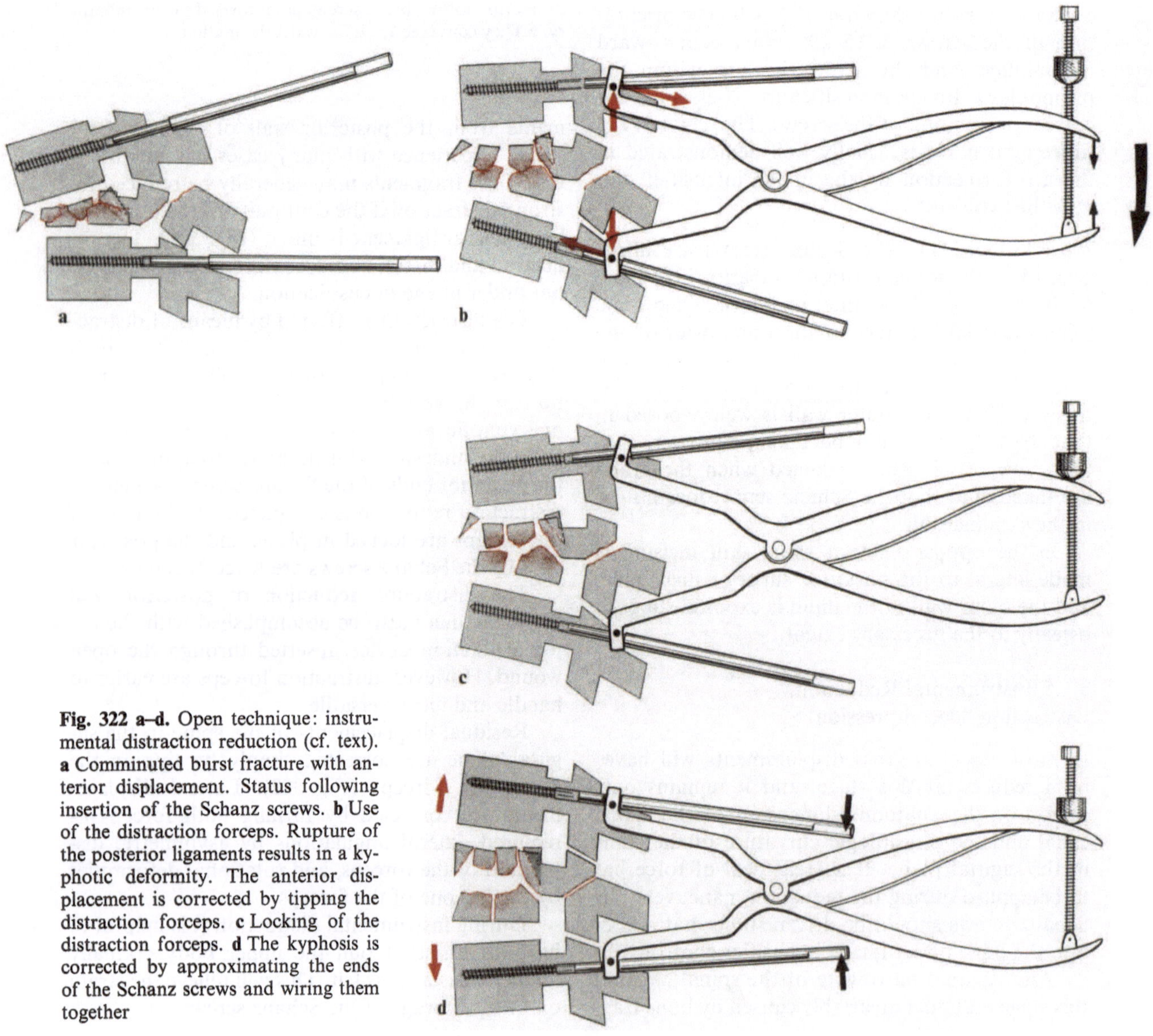

**Fig. 322 a–d.** Open technique: instrumental distraction reduction (cf. text). **a** Comminuted burst fracture with anterior displacement. Status following insertion of the Schanz screws. **b** Use of the distraction forceps. Rupture of the posterior ligaments results in a kyphotic deformity. The anterior displacement is corrected by tipping the distraction forceps. **c** Locking of the distraction forceps. **d** The kyphosis is corrected by approximating the ends of the Schanz screws and wiring them together

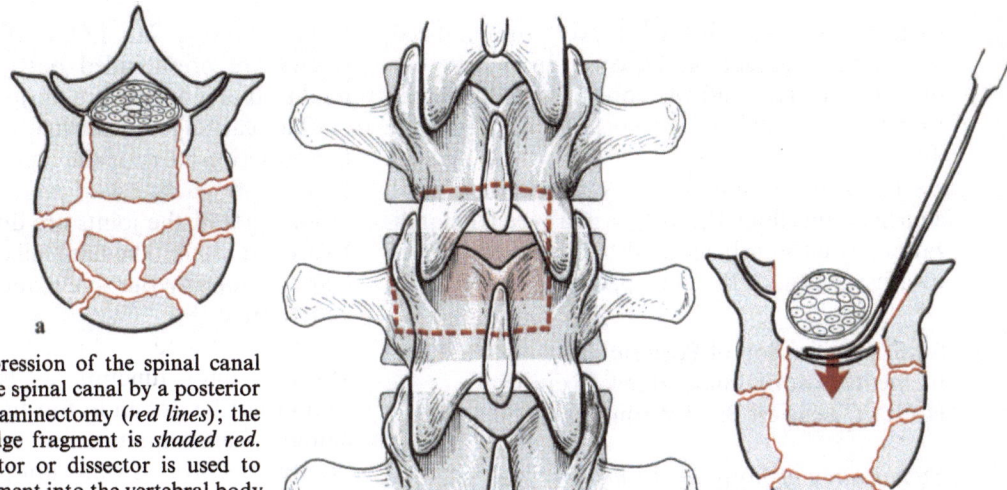

**Fig. 323 a–c.** Open decompression of the spinal canal (see text). **a** Narrowing of the spinal canal by a posterior edge fragment. **b** Extended laminectomy (*red lines*); the location of the posterior edge fragment is *shaded red*. **c** A curved periosteal elevator or dissector is used to push the posterior edge fragment into the vertebral body defect created by the reduction (cranio-caudal view)

### 8.1.6 Intraoperative Myelography

The reduction of fragments intruding into the spinal canal cannot always be adequately evaluated by fluoroscopic means. For this reason, and in order to detect a disc prolapse or dural laceration, intraoperative myelography is indispensable in patients with a neurologic deficit. In all cases treated to date, myelography has enabled us to accurately assess the patency of the subarachnoid space.

We currently use 10 cm$^3$ of the water-soluble, nonionic contrast agent iopamidol (Iopamiro 200®, Bracco) to visualize the subarachnoid space. If a spinal fluid block cannot be excluded with certainty, the effect of additional distraction and hyperextension should be evaluated. If the fluid block is not relieved by this manoeuver, or if significant leakage of contrast medium into the epidural space is observed, indicating the presence of a relevant dural laceration, the spinal canal is opened. However, we have not found this to be necessary in the last 45 cases treated. We have always been able to proceed directly to the second operative step in Sect. 8.1.8.

### 8.1.7 Laminectomy, Open Decompression, Repair of Dural Lacerations

When an open decompression becomes necessary under the circumstances discussed (Fig. 323a), the spinal canal must be opened broadly at the level of the fractured vertebra so that the surgeon will have sufficient exposure and room to work safely. Thanks to the adaptable and secure stabilization, the loss of intrinsic stability caused by the resection of facet joints will be of little consequence for the outcome.

At the thoracolumbar junction and in the upper lumbar spine, the following elements of the vertebral arch may be resected to gain access to posterior vertebral body fragments or extruded disc material (Fig. 323b): the superior half of the lamina of the fractured vertebra, together with the superior articular process and medial part of the pedicle on one side; the inferior articular process of the ipsilateral upper vertebra, together with a portion of the lamina; and the medial parts of the contralateral facet joint if required. If necessary, this exposure also permits slight retraction of the dural sac without undue risk.

Posterior wall fragments are reduced by introducing a curved periosteal elevator past the dural sac and pushing the fragments anteriorly into the cancellous bone defect left by the reduction (Fig. 323c). Bony fragments that may redisplace, as well as extruded disc material, are removed.

If this does not provide an adequate clearance, the exposure is extended by resecting the entire predicle. Then the posterior portion of the vertebral body may be excavated and the fragments pressed into the space thus created.

A broad laminectomy is generally sufficient to decompress the spinal canal in the mid- to lower lumbar spine.

Dural lacerations with spinal fluid leakage are closed by continuous watertight suture. The suture may reduce the circumference of the dural sac to some degree. While this is of no consequence in the region of the cauda equina, it may cause significant compression when done over a traumatized, edematous segment of the cord. In these areas, therefore, a free graft of lyophilized dura is used to achieve a tension-free repair by enlarging the dural sac.

The laminectomy defect is covered later with a corticocancellous H-graft, as in a type III stabilization. A tension band is also applied to prevent overdistraction of the interspace (cf. Fig. 307).

### 8.1.8 Stabilization of Posterior Elements, Translaminar Screw Fixation, H-Graft, Tension Band Wiring

*Stabilization of Posterior Elements*

At this stage normal lordosis is supported by elevating the torso (e.g., by placing an additional bolster under the chest or manipulating the break in the table). Essential elements of the neural arch are repositioned and secured, if possible, with lag screws of the appropriate size. Fragments that may displace into the spinal canal are cut up into graft material.

It is assumed that these steps have been undertaken, all reductions have been carried out, and the Schanz screws and distraction forceps are in place. No the facet joints are fixed with translaminar screws or the spine is stabilized with an H graft and tension band, depending on the condition of the lamina and articular processes.

*Translaminar Screw Fixation of Facet Joints* (cf. Figs. 312, 305, 306). The principles of translaminar screw fixation were discussed in Sect. 4.7. Each fixation screw requires an intact articular process and pars interarticularis.

Insertion of the screws can be quite difficult in the presence of thick soft-tissue masses or if the Schanz screws or distraction forceps obstruct the field, but we have always found it possible. Soft tissues are retracted by means of a short-pointed Hohmann retractor placed subperiosteally below the upper articular process of the lower vertebra to be included in the screw fixation. If a Schanz screw is in the way, it is usually better to insert the facet screw at a slightly more horizontal angle; a steeper angle might compromise the screw anchorage in the lower vertebra.

The holes for the screws are predrilled with a long 3.2-mm drill bit protected by a long tap sleeve. The sleeve also aids in soft-tissue retraction. The length of the drill hole is measured with the depth gauge in standard fashion, using the hook on the gauge as a probe to confirm the absence of perforations. The holes for the 4.5-mm cortex screws are prethreaded only in hard bone that might otherwise fracture during screw insertion.

The cartilaginous surfaces are removed from the posterior parts of the facet joints, which additionally are packed with cancellous bone. The anterior parts of the joints are difficult to reach and so are left alone. The hard subchondral bone layer helps to solidify the screw anchorage and should be left intact.

It was stated in Sect. 4.7 that translaminar screws cannot function as lag screws, and so should not be driven in too tightly. Indeed, tightening a translaminar screw could easily fracture the spinous process while not producing any compression across the facet.

At one time we routinely placed a wire loop around the spinous processes perforated by the screws. We abandoned this practice when we learned that these processes are too weak to provide an effective abutment for wire fixation.

Once the translaminar screws are in place, the distraction forceps and Schanz screws may be removed. This is followed by the step described in Sect. 8.1.9.

*H Graft, Tension Band* (cf. Figs. 307 and 311). After laminectomies, or in cases where translaminar screw fixation is precluded by the configuration of the neural arch fracture, a compression-resistant H graft may be inserted between the spinous processes to provide an additional posterior fulcrum.

For this purpose we use an autogenous corticocancellous graft taken from the posterior iliac crest. Before the graft is applied, the wire loops are secured, and the spinous process of the fractured vertebra is resected. Normally we attach the wire loops to the intact spinous processes above and below the fracture site. But if a spinous process is so weak that it might fracture during prestressing of the fixation device, the wire is secured around a lamina or pars. The wire is twisted over the H graft to secure it in place. The distraction forceps and Schanz screws may now be removed.

This part of the operation should be done prior to definitive reinsertion of the Schanz screws (see below), because access to the spine is more difficult thereafter.

### 8.1.9 Definitive Insertion of the Schanz Screws, Cancellous Bone Grafting, Wound Closure

The Schanz screws must not tether the soft tissues of the back, i.e., they should not exert tension on the skin and muscles. Therefore, each screw must be reinserted with meticulous care. This is done as follows:

First the location of the skin incision is ascertained. This is done by inserting a Kirschner wire into the screw hole and measuring the distance from the Kirschner wire to the midline at the level of the skin (Fig. 324). The soft tissues are then repositioned. The skin and muscle fascia should be retracted toward the midline instrumentally and the muscles well apposed against the spine. A vertical, 8- to 10-mm-long skin incision is made at the measured distance, and the Schanz screw is advanced through the soft tissue until it touches the bone (Fig. 325). The soft tissues are then retracted, and the screws are inserted under direct vision to a depth of 4 cm (Fig. 326). The step in the screw shaft is a useful landmark during this procedure. Insertion of the screws is completed under image intensification in the lateral projection (Fig. 327). The screw tips should touch the anterior wall of the vertebral body.

Following the insertion of the Schanz screws, the cancellous bone harvested from the posterior ilium is applied over the motion segments that are to be fused (Fig. 328). Finally, drainage tubes are inserted and the wound is closed (Fig. 329).

## 8.1.10 Assembly and Prestressing of the ESSF Device

The image intensifier should remain in place while the ESSF device is assembled so that the effect of the prestressing can be accurately monitored.

During assembly of the device, close attention should be given to the maintenance of symmetry. After the transverse bars have been mounted, the threaded rods with balls attached are introduced through the bars, and the balls are fixed loosely in their bearings with the set screws. Rigid fixation of the balls would hamper the final adjustment of the fixation device and also would bend the threaded rods.

If an adjustment of the device is necessary to a greater extent at this stage, we insert the two anterior rods first and use them to apply distraction or compression until the position of the transverse bars is approximately correct. Only then is the posterior rod inserted and used to correct the sagittal spinal curvature or apply the desired primary stress. If additional corrections are required after all the threaded rods are in place, the three rods must be turned in an alternating fashion; otherwise potentially adverse forces could be transmitted to the spine or transverse bars. After the system is prestressed, the alignment of the spine

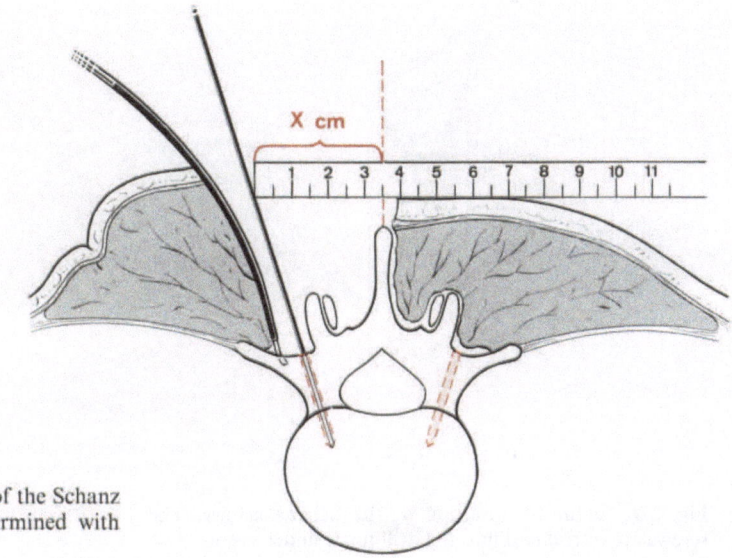

**Fig. 324.** Open technique: definitive insertion of the Schanz screws. The site for the skin incision is determined with the aid of a Kirschner wire

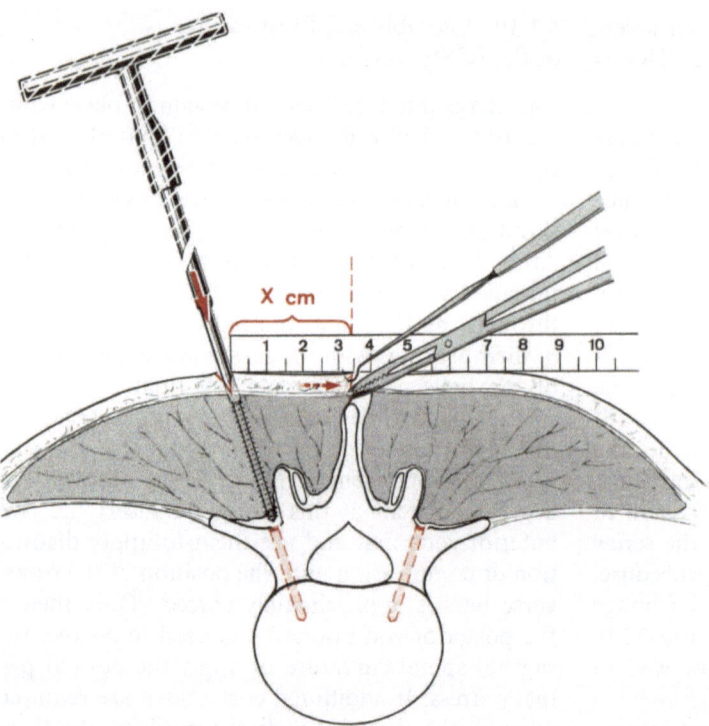

**Fig. 325.** Open technique: definitive insertion of the Schanz screws. The muscles, skin *and* fascia are carefully replaced, and the Schanz screw is advanced through them in the direction of the screw hole. The screw must not exert pressure on the soft tissues

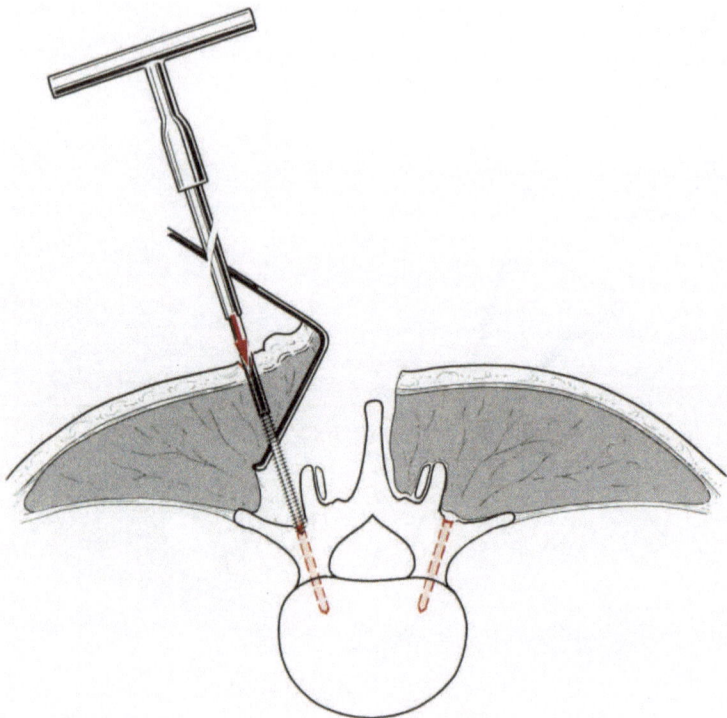

**Fig. 326.** Definitive insertion of the Schanz screws. The screws are introduced into the drill holes under vision

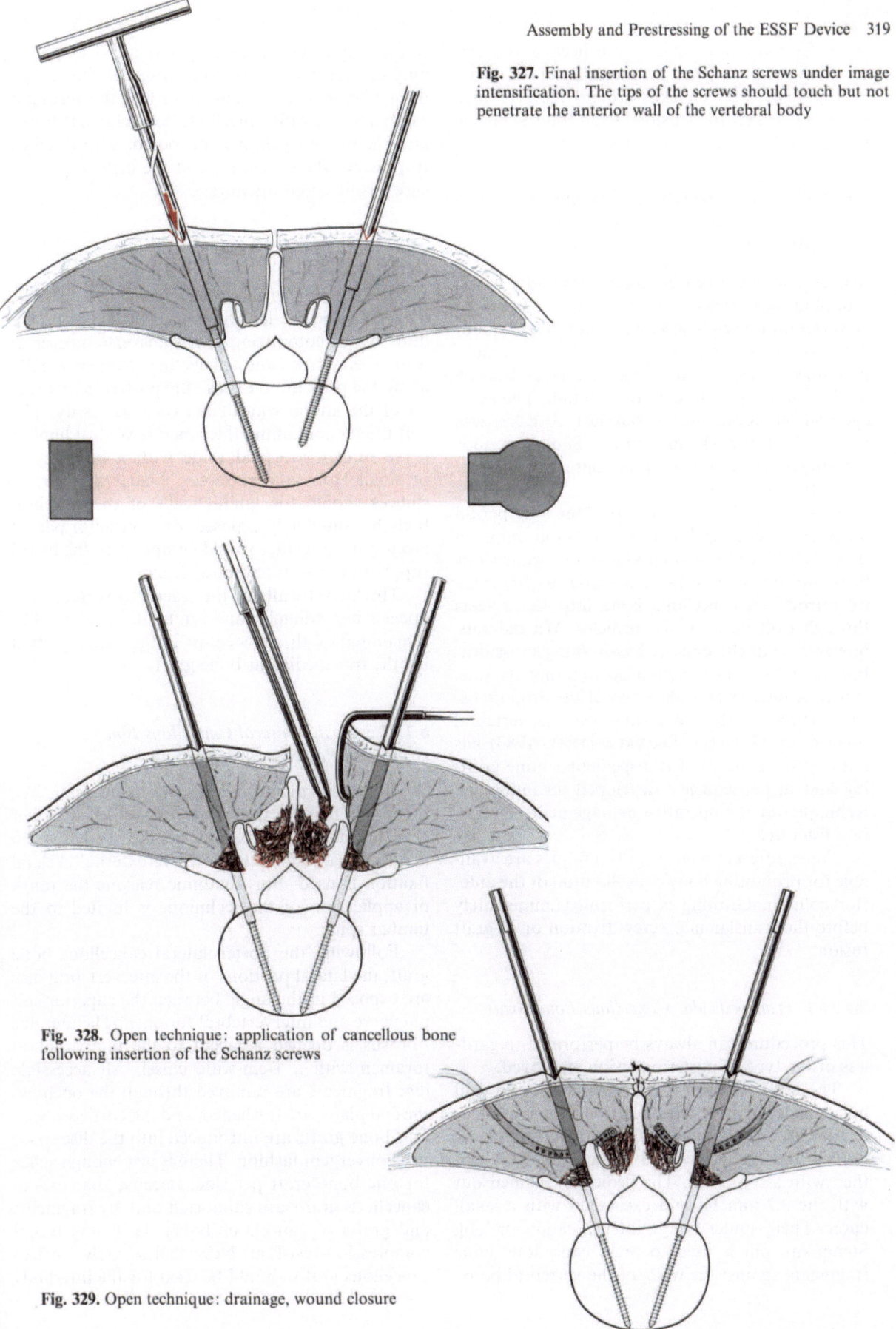

**Fig. 327.** Final insertion of the Schanz screws under image intensification. The tips of the screws should touch but not penetrate the anterior wall of the vertebral body

**Fig. 328.** Open technique: application of cancellous bone following insertion of the Schanz screws

**Fig. 329.** Open technique: drainage, wound closure

in the frontal plane should be rechecked and corrected as required. Then the assembly of the device is completed, and the skin around the stab incisions is checked for tension. Even mild skin tension should be released with a scalpel.

### 8.1.11 Open Technique with Cancellous Grafting of the Vertebral Body, Posterior Interbody Fusion

In Sect. 7 we described the conditions under which cancellous bone defects formed by the realignment of vertebral-body compression fractures may undergo spontaneous reossification. The consolidation time of these defects has a crucial bearing on the duration of the external fixation. The average consolidation time in our last 20 cases was 18.5 weeks (28 weeks in 2 cases). Similar periods are known to be necessary in conservative treatment (BÖHLER 1951).

It is reasonable to assume that the long period of reossification and external fixation may be shortened by transplanting autogenous cancellous bone into the defects. In three of our earlier cases we introduced cancellous bone into the defects through drill holes in the pedicles. We did this, however, with the object of promoting reossification in general rather than accelerating its rate. When we later learned that the defects would reossify spontaneously, we abandoned the vertebral body graft. However, DANIAUX (1981, 1983) has pursued the concept of transpedicular bone grafting and in consequence developed an individual technique for the operative management of vertebral fractures.

Three different bone graft techniques are available for promoting bony consolidation of the anterior column. Grafting is performed immediately before the translaminar screw fixation or H-graft fusion.

#### 8.1.11.1 Transpedicular Cancellous Bone Graft

This procedure can always be performed, regardless of the type of posterior fusion employed.

The graft material is introduced through drill holes made at those sites described for the introduction of Schanz screws. The cortex at this location is first opened with a 3.2-mm drill bit and then with a 6-mm bit. The pedicle is reamed out with the 3.2-mm bit and excavated with a small curet. Then, under image intensification, a long Steinmann pin is used to press cancellous bone fragments against the walls of the vertebral body.

If the end plate has not been reduced as yet, it may be elevated at this time with the Steinmann pin under image intensification and the resultant cavity packed with cancellous bone chips. If translaminar screw fixation is proposed, care is taken to preserve the cortex around the drill site to ensure a solid screw anchorage.

#### 8.1.11.2 Posterolateral Cancellous Bone Graft

If screw fixation of the facet joints is not possible, one can avoid the laborious transpedicular procedure by osteotomizing the transverse processes near their base and dissecting subperiosteally along the pedicles to expose the posterior centimeter of the lateral wall of the vertebral body. The soft tissues containing the superior ventral lumbar nerve branch are held aside with a blunt hook or small Hohmann retractor. Under no circumstances should the lateral walls of the vertebral body be completely exposed, or a retractor passed around them. Either would compromise the blood supply of the vertebral body fragments.

The lateral walls of the fractured vertebra are opened immediately anterior to the pedicle. The remainder of the procedure is the same as that for the transpedicular bone graft.

#### 8.1.11.3 Posterolateral Cancellous Bone Graft with Posterior Interbody Fusion

We have used this technique on one occasion. We mention it here for the sake of completeness rather than to advocate it, because its cost-benefit ratio is questionable in settings where external skeletal fixation is used. For anatomic reasons the range of application of the technique is limited to the lumbar spine.

Following the posterolateral cancellous bone graft, the lateral portions of the intervertebral disc are exposed in the angle between the superior spinal nerve and intervertebral foramen. The annulus fibrosus is opened adjacent to the intervertebral foramen with a 1-cm-wide chisel. All accessible disc fragments are removed through the opening, the end plates are freshened, and the corticocancellous bone grafts are introduced into the disc space in a convergent fashion. There is just enough space for one bone graft per side. Because the corticocancellous grafts are supported only by fragments and grafts of cancellous bone, the fusion is not compression-resistant. Nevertheless, only corticocancellous grafts should be used for the interbody fusion; cancellous bone chips could extrude through the opening in the annulus and impinge on the spinal nerve.

## 8.2 Percutaneous Application of the Fixation Device (Fig. 330)

This technique should be practiced only by surgeons who are quite experienced in the use of the ESSF device.

Preparations for surgery are the same as for the open procedure (see Sect. 8.1.1). Particular emphasis is placed upon an accurate closed reduction.

### 8.2.1 Introduction of the Schanz Screws

The position of the screws is determined by image intensification as described in Sect. 8.1.4 for the placement of the Kirschner wires. In the sacrum, care is taken to avoid the canal of the first sacral nerve. A plastic handle is available for adjustments of the screws under radiologic control while avoiding irradiation of the surgeon's hand (see Fig. 173).

The skin is incised over the centers of the pedicles, whereupon the Schanz screws are inserted and advanced to the bone. Because the area of bone in contact with the screw tip is sharply inclined (angle between joint and transverse process or inferolateral border of articular process), the screw will have a tendency to slip despite its sharp point. Therefore the screw is simply held against the bone, tilted slightly laterally and caudally, and its tip is driven several millimeters into the bone with blows from a mallet. At this point the screw is realigned with the axis of the pedicle, hammered in another millimeter or so, and then inserted an additional 2 cm with the T-handled screwdriver.

The correct placement of the Schanz screw is again checked by image intensification in two planes before it is advanced to its definitive position with the tip just touching the anterior cortex of the vertebral body.

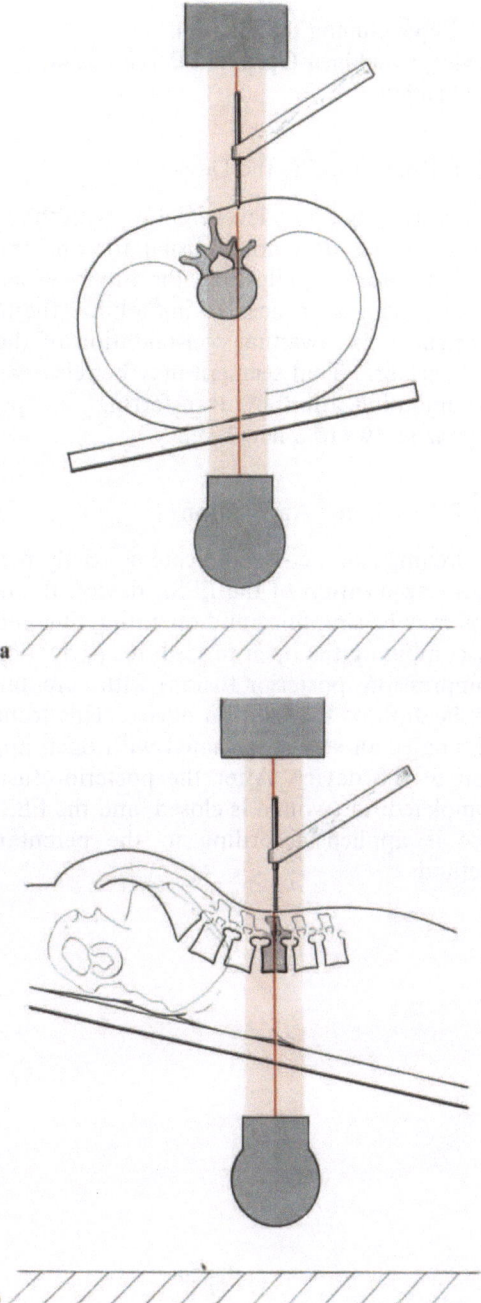

**Fig. 330 a, b.** Percutaneous application of the Schanz screws. The axis of the pedicles is located by image intensification. The table is tilted until the long axis of the pedicle aligns with the central beam of the image intensifier, causing the pedicle to appear as a sharply defined oval on the monitor screen. The same principle is applied in the open technique (see text). **a** Alignment in the horizontal plane. **b** Alignment in the sagittal plane

## 8.2.2 Assembly of the Fixation
Device, Final Reduction, Prestressing

These steps are carried out as described in Sect. 8.1.10. In the present case, however, final instrumental reduction is performed entirely with the fixation device. As in the open technique, any doubts concerning the patency of the spinal canal are resolved by myelography.

Any skin tension caused by final reduction maneuvers should be released by incision.

## 8.3 Repositioning the Fixation
Device, Combined Open and Percutaneous
Application

### 8.3.1 Repositioning the Device

When treating a two-level fracture with the simple ESSF device, it is not unusual for one fracture to unite more rapidly than the other. When this occurs, there is no need to immobilize the healed segment while awaiting consolidation of the second vertebra. That segment may be released from the immobilization by transferring one pair of Schanz screws to a new level.

### 8.3.2 Combined Application

If circumstances contraindicate a strictly percutaneous application of the ESSF device, the operation may be simplified and operating time reduced by combining the open procedures (reduction, decompression, posterior fusion) with percutaneous application of the fixation device. This technique eliminates all steps associated with open application of the device. After the posterior fusion is completed, the wound is closed, and the ESSF device is applied according to the percutaneous method.

# 9 Operative Technique: Spondylitis

We shall assume that the general condition of the patient, the local situation and the causative organism necessitate an operative approach to treatment, or at least an efficient technique of immobilization.

In order to obtain a specimen for microbiological testing, in all cases the affected disc is punctured prior to surgery through the posterolateral approach (OTTOLENGHI 1954, 1969) or through the pedicle (KÄGI et al. 1983) under image intensification. In this way the operation may be carried out under specific antibiotic protection, and an effective antibiotic irrigating solution may be administered. To confirm the correct placement of the needle and also evaluate the extent of destructive changes and abscessation, we first inject a water-soluble contrast medium (Hexabrix®, Guerbet or Ronpacon®, Cilag) into the disc space. After the microbiologic specimen is obtained, a neomycin-B-base bacitracin solution (Nebacetin, Lundbeck) is instilled. When bilateral needles are used, the disc space may be flushed during puncture.

The ESSF device has three main applications in the treatment of spondylitides. In all cases early ambulation is assured.

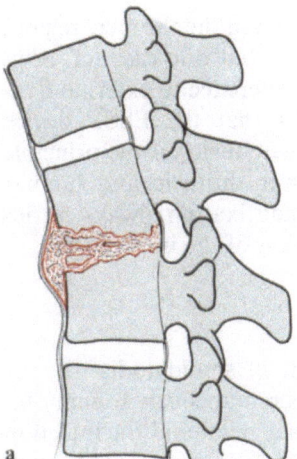

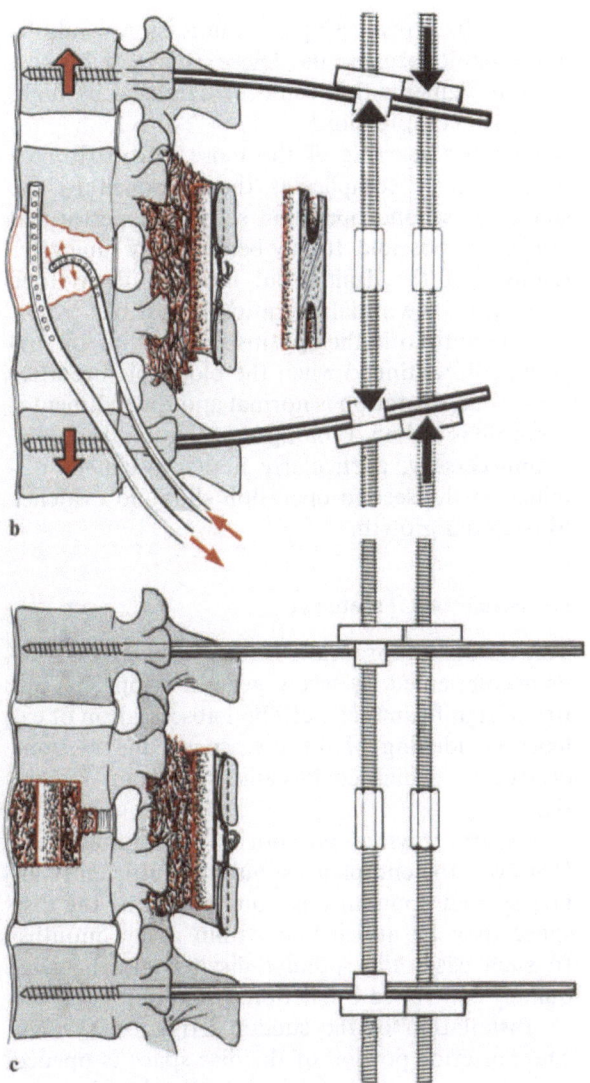

**Fig. 331 a–c.** Treatment of spondylitis: two-stage procedure with direct focal treatment (see text). **a** Extensive bone destruction; sequestrum, abscess and kyphotic deformity. **b** First sitting: posterior fusion, application of the ESSF device in distraction. Patient is repositioned for debridement and placement of suction-irrigation drains. **c** Second sitting: When infection has subsided, an interbody fusion is done with cancellous bone and compression-resistant bone grafts. Neutral stabilization is employed (no prestressing)

## 9.1 Two-Stage Procedure with Direct Focal Treatment (Fig. 331)

This procedure is indicated for spondylitides associated with soft-tissue abscesses, extensive destruction of vertebral bodies and sequestra – situations in which evacuation of the abscess, debridement and the implantation of bone grafts are crucial to restoration of the anterior and middle columns.

In the first sitting the affected motion segment(s) are fused posteriorly with autogenous bone and wire fixation, and the fixation device is applied to the healthy adjacent vertebrae. The device may be applied either by the open technique or percutaneously following wound closure; it is prestressed in moderate distraction.

The patient is now moved to the lateral position for debridement and installation of the suction irrigation system through a retroperitoneal approach. All infected cavities are irrigated continuously for approximately 48 h. Then suction drainage is maintained for as long as appreciable amounts of exudate are obtained. Usually the drains may be removed on the 6th to 8th postoperative day.

In the second sitting the intervertebral defect is bridged with autogenous, compression-resistant corticocancellous bone grafts, utilizing the same operative approach. In a few cases (cf. Fig. 359)

we have inserted hydroxylapatite blocks impregnated with an antibiotic solution instead of corticocancellous grafts, and then packed autogenous cancellous bone around the blocks (MAGERL et al., in press). For the present, we feel that hydroxyl apatite blocks should be applied only in elderly patients in whom the extent of surgery must be limited or suitable autogenous graft material is unavailable.

The reestablishment of suction irrigation should be considered if organisms are found in direct smears taken during the second operation. Otherwise simple suction drains are inserted.

After the interbody fusion is completed, the distraction is released, and the fixation device is set in the neutral mode so that muscular tone and upper body weight can compress and secure the bone grafts. Prestressing in compression would be unfavorable, because the device usually spans two motion segments that could be damaged by high, sustained compression.

Because scarring of the loose retroperitoneal layers greatly complicates the approach to the spine, the second operation should be performed as soon as possible. It may be done any time after removal of the drains, but no later than three weeks after the initial operation if possible.

The antibiotic therapy instituted prior to surgery is discontinued when the blood picture after the second operation is normal and the sedimentation rate is falling. Prolonged antibiotic treatment is unnecessary, particularly if the specimens obtained at the second operation show no evidence of bacterial growth.

## 9.2 Semidirect Treatment

This mode is appropriate for acute spondylodiscitis accompanied by severe general symptoms but free of significant paravertebral abscessation or extensive widening of the disc space due to bone destruction which could cause significant kyphosis.

Central cavities are not a contraindication. However, the end plates should be sufficiently intact so that spontaneous bony fusion of the disc space may be anticipated within a few months. In such cases the spondylodiscitis may be adequately controlled by suction irrigation.

Installation of the suction irrigation system: The posterior portion of the disc space is opened with a transpedicular drill bit introduced under image intensification. Redon drains with very short perforated sections are advanced into the disc space through the drill holes – a small-gauge irrigating tube on one side and a large-gauge suction tube on the other. To prevent posterior leakage of the irrigating solution, the drill holes should accommodate the tubes as snugly as possible and should be sealed with cancellous bone.

After suction irrigation has been established, a posterior fusion is performed as described in Sect. 9.1 and stabilized in mild distraction with the ESSF device. Drainage is conducted according to the guidelines stated above. Antibiotic therapy is continued for about three weeks after the blood picture has normalized.

The principle of semidirect treatment with instrumental stabilization and transpeduncular suction irrigation was devised by the author and has to date been applied in several cases. Because the spondylitides were localized in the thoracic region, however, up to now in all but one case (cf. Sect. 13) plates were used in preference to external fixation. There is no doubt·that the ESSF device would be superior to a plate fusion if the principle were applied to the lower thoracic and lumbar spine, inasmuch as internal fixation always carries some risk of contamination of the implant bed.

## 9.3 Indirect Treatment

In the indirect treatment of spondylodiscitis, the ESSF device is applied percutaneously to immobilize the affected motion segment, and the infection is cured by long-term antibiotic treatment. The advantage of this therapy over conventional methods is its more efficient immobilization, which is beneficial both for the control of infection and for spontaneous bony fusion of the affected motion segment.

Indirect treatment is indicated for spondylodiscitides with minimal bone destruction, relatively mild constitutional symptoms, and no paravertebral abscesses. The causative organisms should be sensitive to several antibiotics that are suitable for long-term use.

# 10 Postoperative Care and Postoperative Course

### 10.1 General Remarks

At the end of the operation a sterile pressure dressing composed of slotted compresses, artificial cotton and wooden tongue depressors is applied (Fig. 332). The pressure dressing is an important part of the postoperative regimen, because it prevents the occurrence of "window edema" caused by lying on the fenestrated mattress. One result of this edema is an increased discharge of transudate from the screw tracks, producing a saturated dressing that is conducive to bacterial growth.

Normally the pressure dressing is changed daily during the first two-thirds of the treatment period; later it is changed every other day. The Schanz screws and surrounding skin are thoroughly cleansed with hydrogen peroxide. Any crusts around the screws that might obstruct the discharge of transudate are removed; damming back of this fluid would allow rapid bacterial proliferation.

Before discharging the patient, we instruct relatives or other responsible third parties in the technique for dressing changes and care of the fixation device.

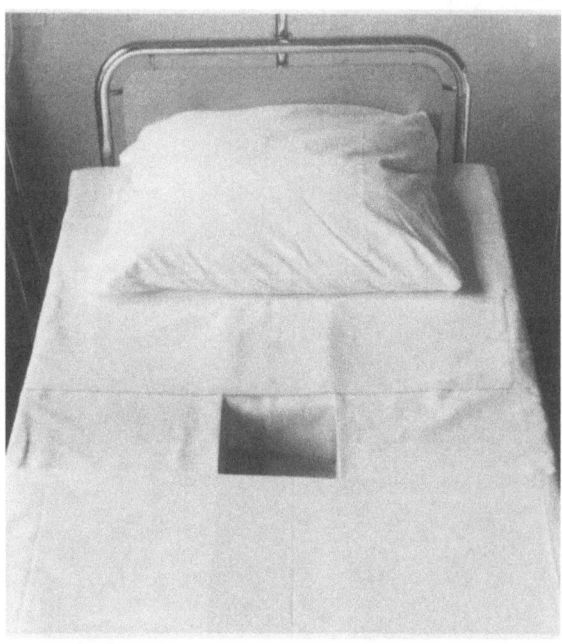

**Fig. 333.** Postoperative care. A foam mattress with a cutout enables supine positioning of the patient

The patient is provided with a thick foam mattress with an individually sized cutout (Fig. 333) so that he may lie in the supine position. As an additional precautionary measure against window

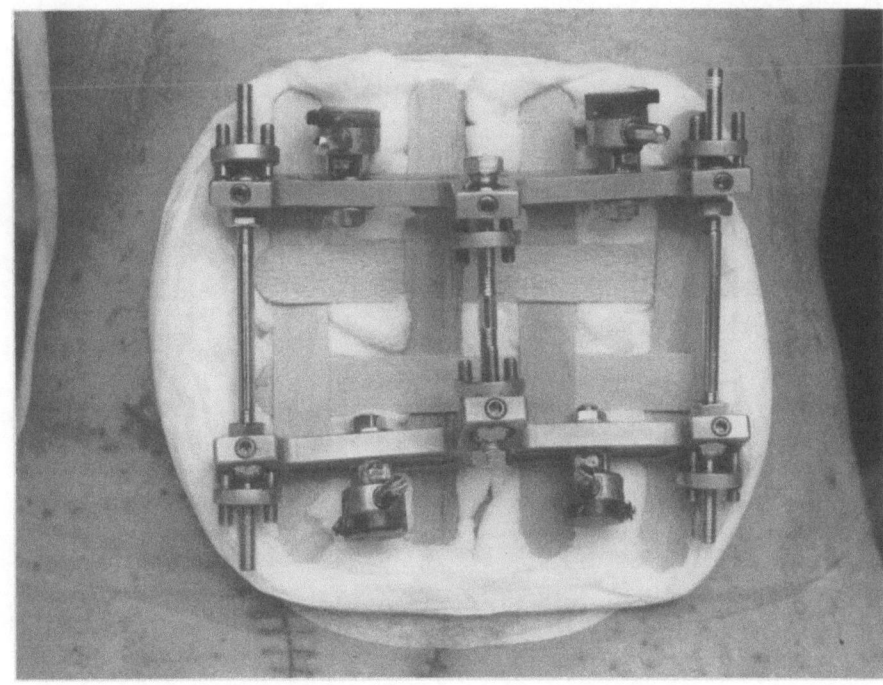

**Fig. 332.** Postoperative care. A pressure dressing is applied to prevent window edema. The compresses and artificial cotton are compressed against the skin by wooden tongue depressors

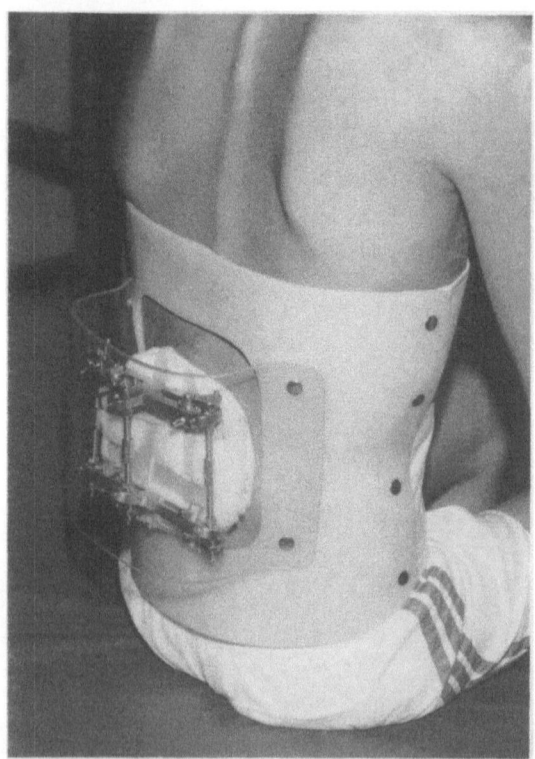

**Fig. 334.** Postoperative care: protective brace. To protect the ESSF device, ambulatory patients must wear a brace consisting of a posterior shell with a rigid cover for the device, and a flexible anterior part with adjustable straps

**Fig. 335.** Postoperative care: Early ambulation with the protective brace. Crutches are used only if ambulation is impaired by paralysis or if the patient feels unsecure

**Fig. 336.** Postoperative care: physical therapy. An active exercise program is instituted concurrently with ambulation (cf. text)

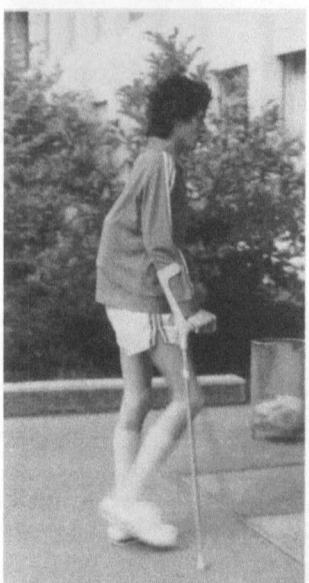

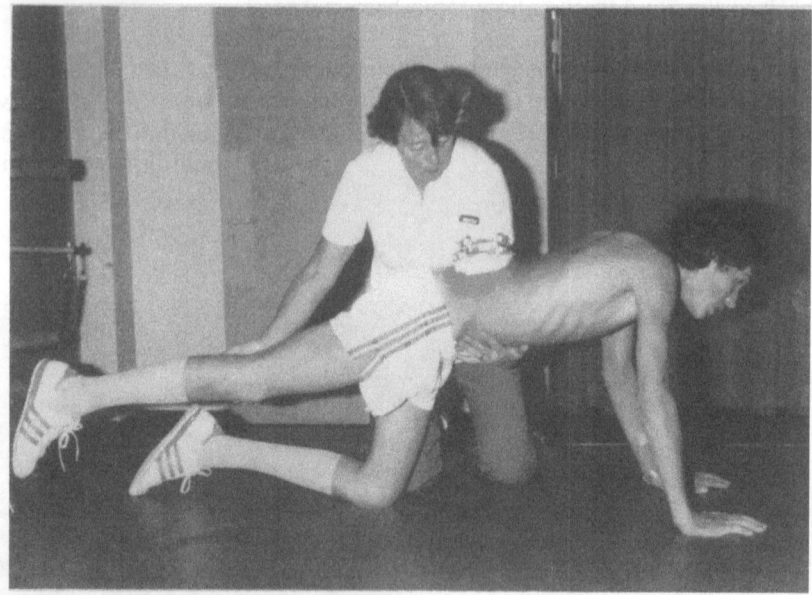

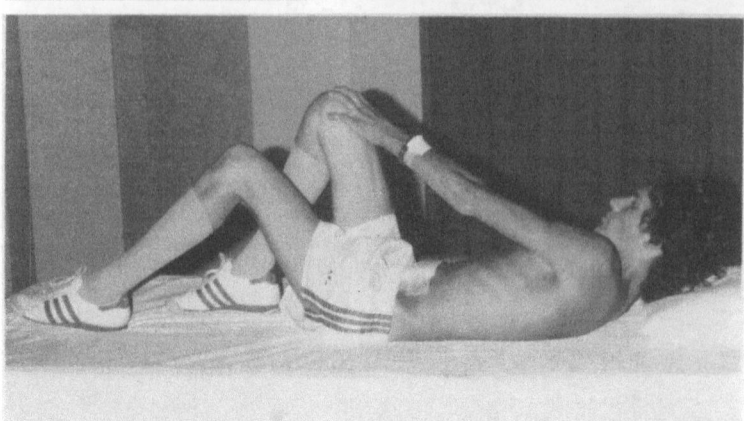

**Fig. 337.** Postoperative care: physical therapy. Supine exercises are performed on the windowed mattress

edema, the patient is encouraged to lie frequently on his side or stomach. He takes the mattress home when discharged.

The patient is allowed to be up as soon as his general condition permits. Our fracture patients were able to start full ambulation after six days on the average. Because a fall onto the fixation device can have serious consequences, the patients wear a protective brace while ambulating (Figs. 334, 335). This brace consists of a posterior plastic shell with a rigid casing for the fixation device, and a textile anterior part with adjustable straps.

Active exercises are initiated along with ambulation (Figs. 336, 337). Up to the time of discharge, the patients are taught isometric muscle strengthening exercises, postural exercises and breathing exercises. Special exercises mobilizing the spine are not performed. The patient continues his exercises independently after discharge.

Ordinarily the fixation device is removed as an outpatient procedure without anesthesia. Before removal of the external frame, all primary stresses are released by turning the threaded rods. The Schanz screws would cause considerable pain if allowed to spring back under their own tension. Removal of the Schanz screws is normally accompanied by sharp, radiating pains, especially if the screws are turned quickly or abaxially. Generally the pain is well tolerated if the patient is first given an analgesic and is told what to expect. To date only 1 patient out of 70 has required a general anesthetic for removal of the fixation device.

After wound pain has subsided, complaints referable to the spine diminish rapidly. Local pain on motion, especially when localized in the flank or buttock and accompanied by increased discharge from an ipsilateral screw track, usually indicates loosening of the involved screw. In three of the four cases of loosening seen to date, the pains were accompanied by transitory bouts of fever, sometimes lasting only a few hours.

If symptoms are not alarming, a wait-and-see approach is justified. However, the patient should limit his activities somewhat.

On the other hand, if pain increases and the discharge becomes purulent, it is necessary to remove the fixation device, irrigate the screw track, and stabilize the spine with a hyperextension body cast that is windowed over the operated area. The patient should be hospitalized for monitoring of temperature, sedimentation rate and blood picture, and suitable antibacterial agents should be administered.

Pressure on soft tissues by Schanz screws will be characterized by less severe but nonetheless troublesome pain, and by an increased discharge.

Frequently the patients complain of pain which originates from the graft donor site and radiate laterally or posterolaterally down the leg. Simple analgetics will relieve the pain, but usually it is sufficient to explain to the patient the cause of the discomfort and reassure him that it is harmless.

Fortunately we have not yet witnessed postoperative spondylitis in any of our patients. Thus, we can approach this problem only in theoretic terms and would offer this advice: If doubt exists, evaluate by means of scintigraphy ($^{67}$Ga-citrate, $^{111}$In-labeled leukocytes) or another suitable technique. If spondylitis is confirmed and operative treatment is warranted, proceed as described in Sect. 9.

## 10.2 Postoperative Management of Fractures

Biweekly follow-up visits are scheduled. Barring complications, the first radiographic follow-up occurs at three months after surgery. Thereafter the progress of fracture healing is followed at 4- to 6-week intervals. Special attention is given to the consolidation of the vertebral body defect. The fixation device is removed after consolidation of the fracture has been confirmed radiographically. In our last 20 cases the device was removed after 18.5 weeks on the average. In the presence of large vertebral body defects, or if surgical intervention has been delayed, a considerably longer period may be required for fracture union.

If the fixation device is removed earlier than scheduled, the collapse of a vertebral body may be prevented by applying a hyperextension body cast from the manubrium of the sternum to the symphysis. In the regular case, however, the vertebral body is solid enough to bear weight normally. There is no effective prevention against narrowing of the disc, and so there is no need to apply a lumbar corset or three-point brace after removal of the fixation device. Today we consider muscular insufficiency to be the only valid indication for these aids. Before we had sufficient experience with the ESSF device we often removed it relatively early and frequently splinted the spine externally for several weeks as a precautionary measure.

### 10.3 Postoperative Management of Spondylitis

The antibiotic therapy of spondylitis is discussed in Sect. 9.

Clinical follow-ups are scheduled biweekly. Radiographs, sedimentation rate and blood picture are obtained at four-week intervals. Laboratory tests may be discontinued when normal values are obtained on two successive visits and the patient is feeling well.

In most cases, and especially following interbody fusions with solid bone grafts, the ESSF device may be removed somewhat earlier in spondylitis than in fractures.

The majority of elderly patients who have been debilitated by their illness will show insufficiency of the back and abdominal muscles. In addition to a suitable orthosis, these patients will require a sound program of therapeutic exercise for their rehabilitation.

## 11 Clinical Examples

### 11.1 Trauma

#### 11.1.1 Open Procedure, Technique I (Figs. 338–341)

*Prerequisite:* Significant damage to the upper motion segment with little or no damage to the lower motion segment. Restoration of the longitudinal continuity of the posterior column by screw fixation of the facet joints is feasible and rational.

*Principle:* Translaminar screw fixation of the superior facet joints, fusion of the upper motion segment with autogenous cancellous bone. Open or percutaneous application of the ESSF device prestressed in moderate distraction.

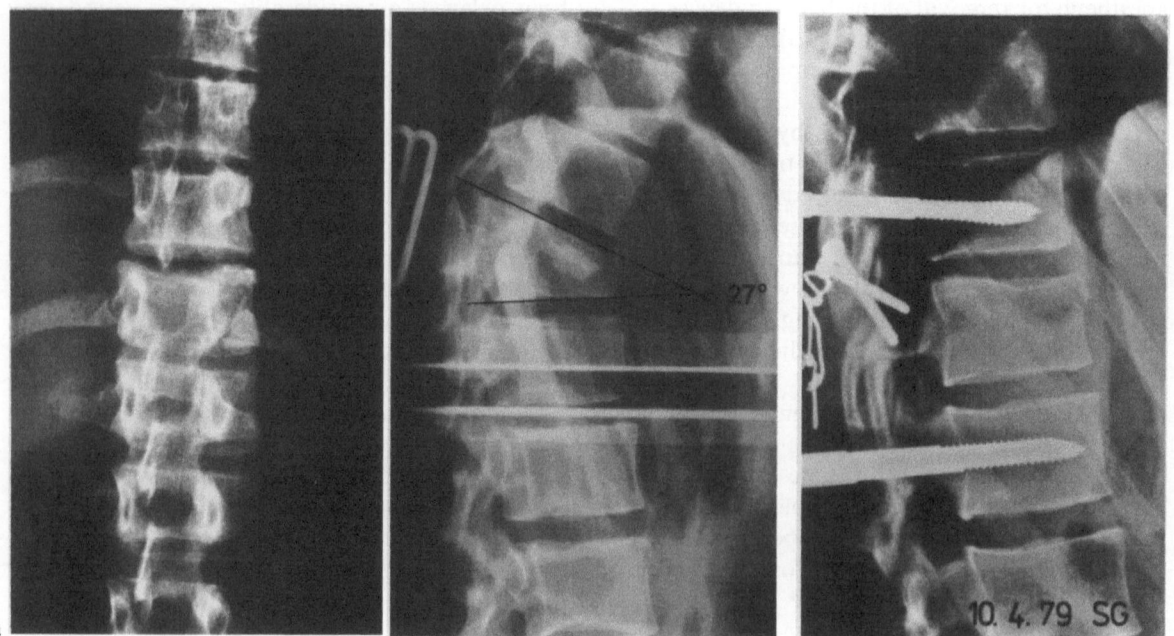

**Fig. 338a, b**

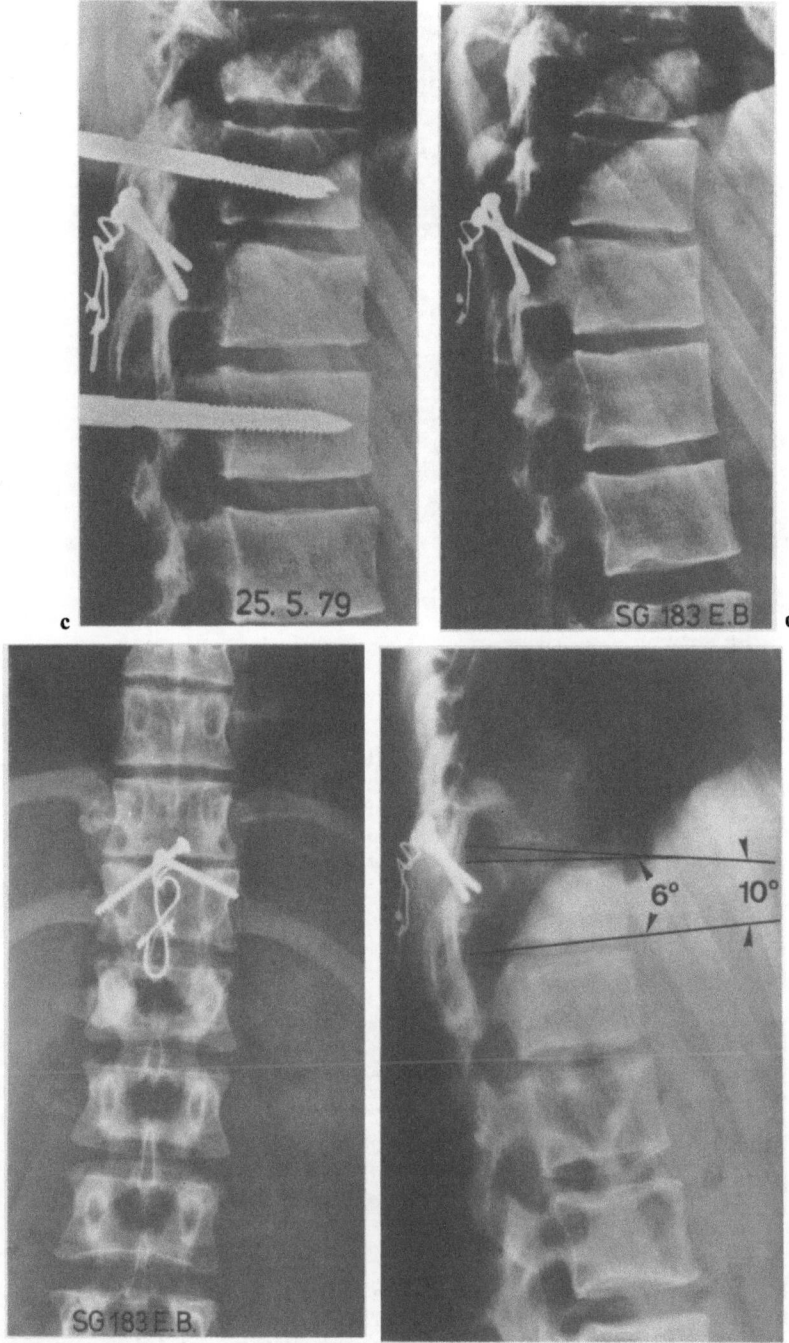

**Fig. 338 a–e.** Application of technique I for a wedge-compression fracture of T12. E.B., 1955, 24 years, ♀, 227179.

**a** The patient jumped from a height of 7 m in a suicide attempt, sustaining a wedge-compression fracture of T12 with a facet dislocation at T11–T12, 27° anterior wedging of the vertebral body, and a sensory deficit in the right foot.

**b** Surgery was done two days postinjury. Reduction produced a defect in the cancellous bone of the vertebral body. The wire fixation from T11 and T12 is now believed to be unnecessary. Ambulation was begun five days after surgery.

**c** Initial filling of the vertebral body defect is apparent at four weeks.

**d** The ESSF device was removed at 13 weeks, by which time the vertebral body defect had been obliterated. The T11–T12 disc already showed some narrowing. No special aftercare was necessary.

**e** By 53 months postinjury normal sensory function has returned. There is a residual 6° wedging of the vertebral body and a total kyphosis of 10° due to collapse of the upper disc. The patient is free of complaints and is able to engage in sports

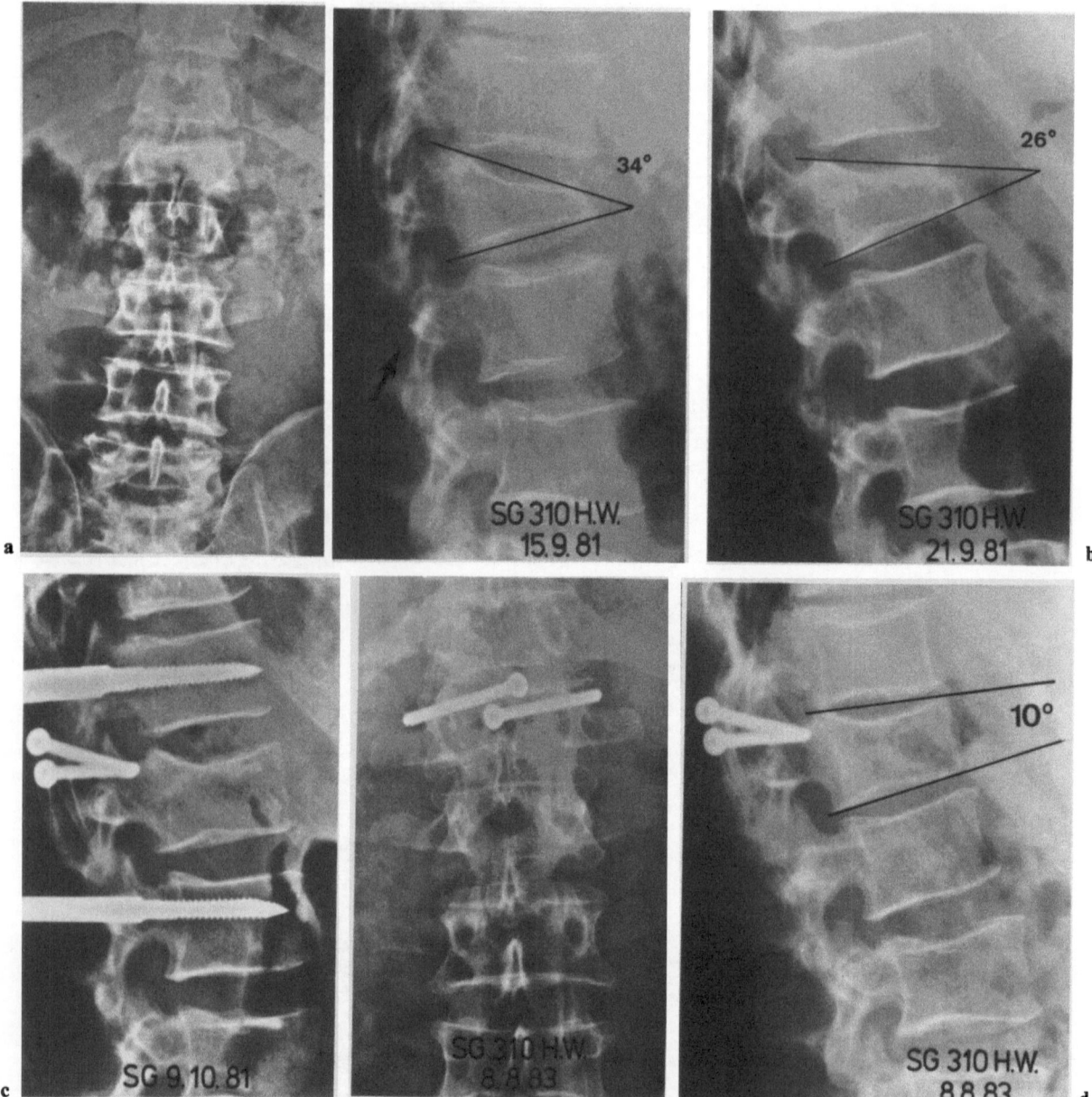

**Fig. 339 a–d.** Application of technique I for a crush-cleavage fracture of L1. H.W., 1945, 36 years, ♂, 120956.
**a** In a fall from a tree, the patient sustained a crush-cleavage fracture of L1, a rupture of the interspinous ligament at T12–L1, an avulsion of the L2 spinous process, and 34° anterior wedging of L1. Pedicular diastasis is evident in the AP projection due to the laminar split fracture.
**b** The wedging is reduced to 26° after 1 week of supine rest.

**c** Surgery was done eight days postinjury, with reduction creating a vertebral body defect. Ambulation was started at 4 days postoperatively, the ESSF device was removed at 16 weeks, and a body cast was worn for 4 weeks.
**d** At 23 months postinjury there is 10° residual wedging and a parallel collapse of both discs. The patient has mild complaints during strenuous labor but has been able to fully resume farming work

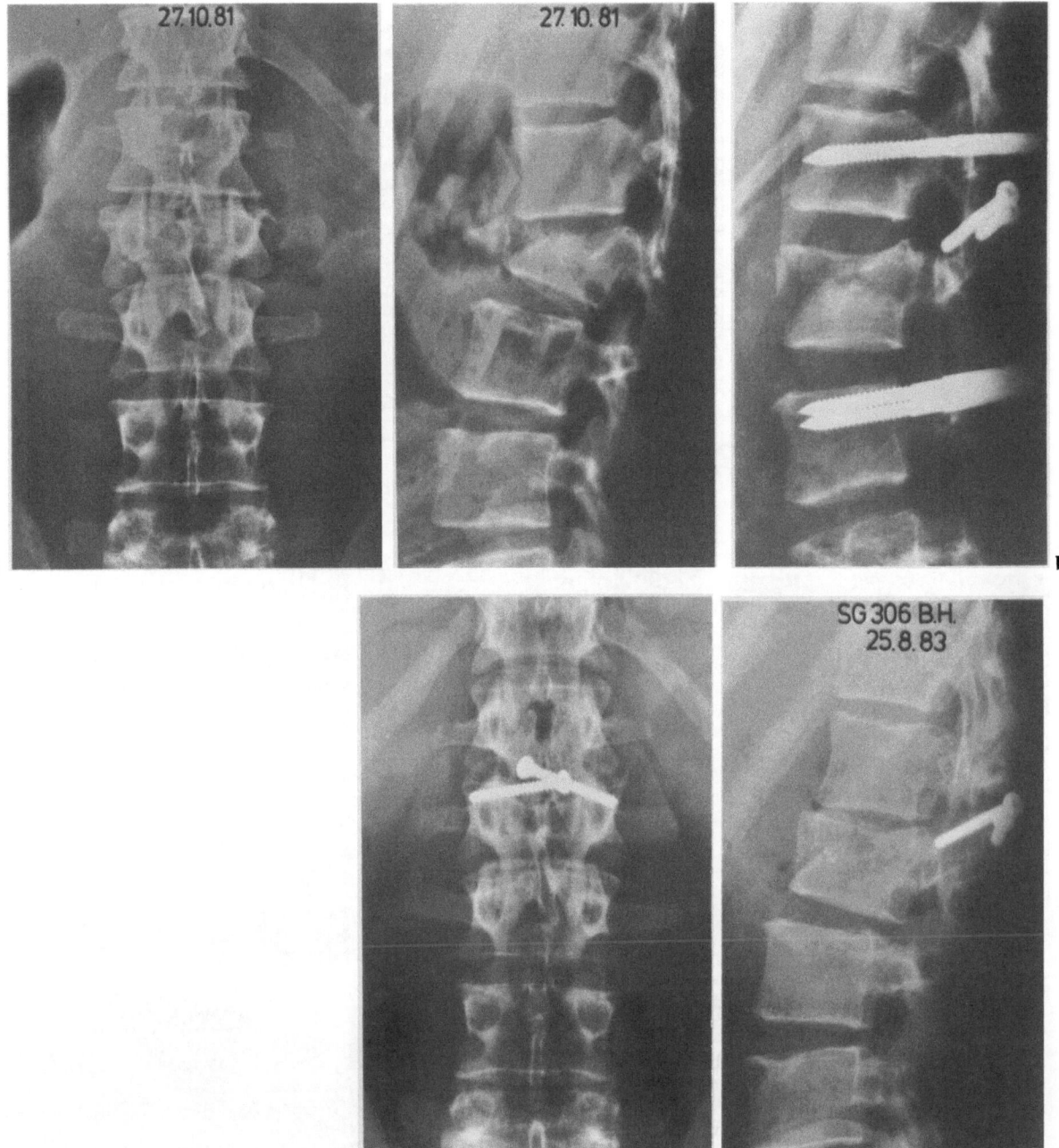

**Fig. 340 a–c.** Application of technique I for a crush-cleavage fracture of L2 with marked narrowing of the spinal canal. B.H., 1954, 27 years, ♂, 254279.

**a** The patient fell from a height of 10 m to incur a crush-cleavage fracture of L2, fractured transverse processes at L1 and L2, and a fracture of the L2 spinous process. A cerebral concussion also was sustained. Motor and sensory deficits are present in both legs, especially the right. The split fracture of the lamina is evidenced by an obvious diastasis of the pedicles at L2. The spinal canal is markedly narrowed by a displaced upper posterior edge fragment from the vertebral body, which shows 36° of anterior wedging.

**b** Surgery was done eight days postinjury. The offending fragment was reduced indirectly by distraction, accompanied by formation of the usual vertebral body defect. The patient was ambulated at seven days after surgery. The ESSF device was removed at 21 weeks, and a body cast was worn for 6 weeks.

**c** At 16 months postinjury there is 6° residual deformity of the vertebral body with collapse of the upper disc. The patient has mild residual neurologic symptoms and no complaints referable to the spine

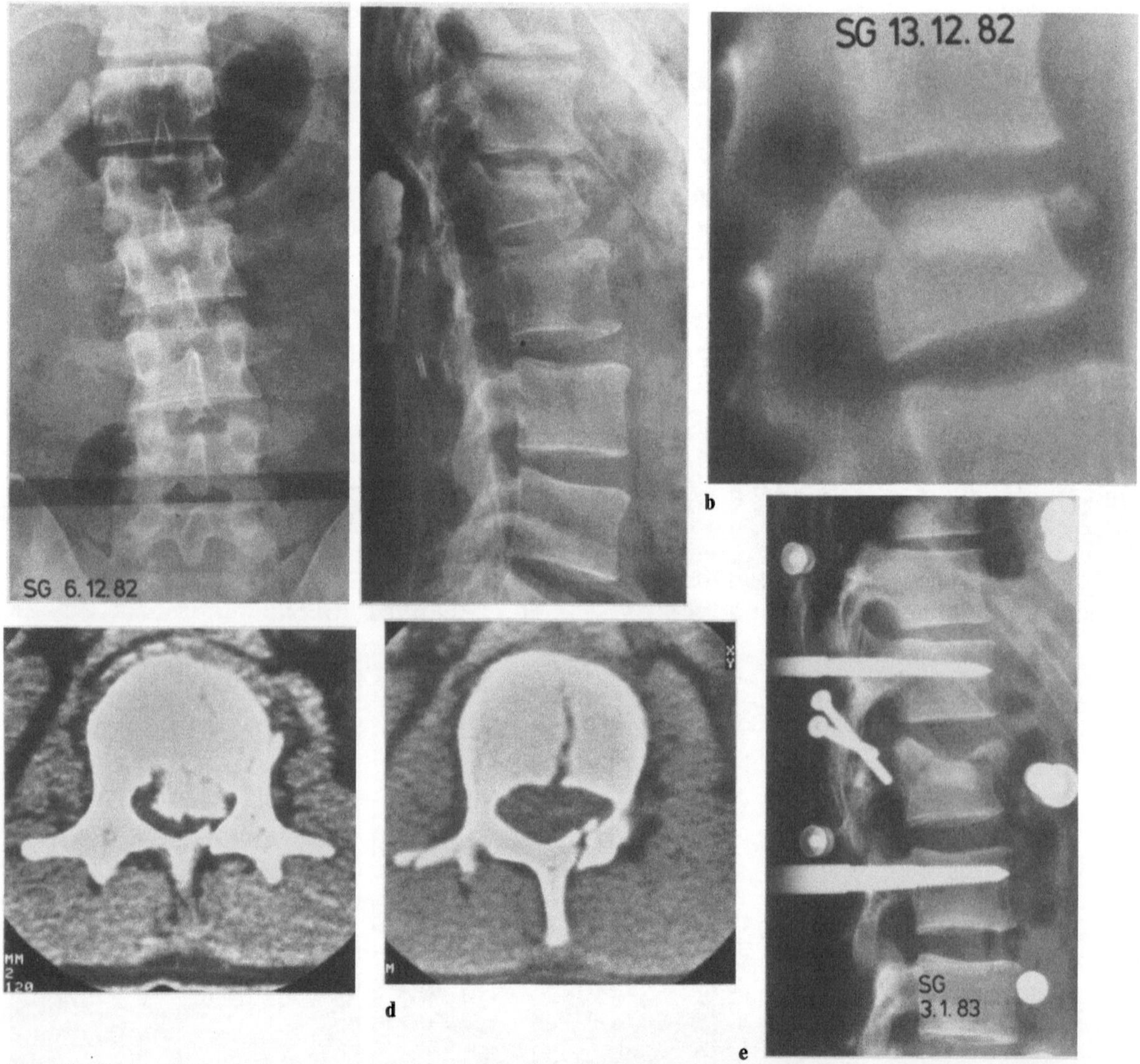

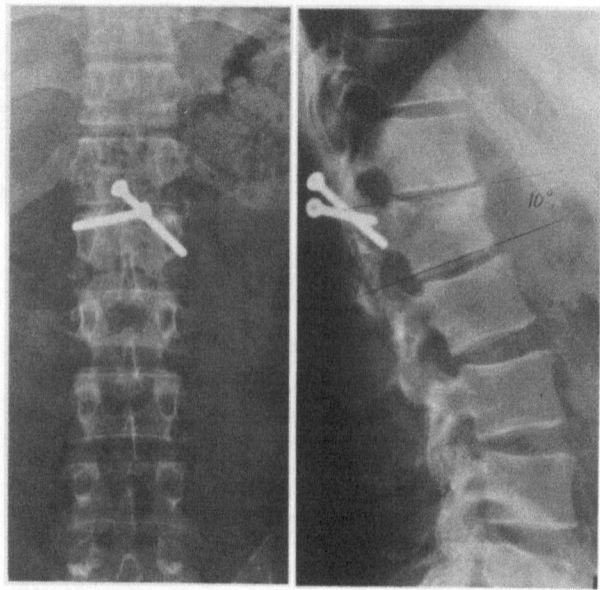

**Fig. 341 a–f.** Application of technique I for a crush-cleavage fracture of L1 with marked narrowing of the spinal canal. C.W., 1951, 31 years, ♂, 266729.

**a** The patient fell from a bridge into a brook while jogging, sustaining a crush-cleavage of L1 and a fracture of the left superior articular process of L1.

**b** An upper posterior edge fragment was driven into the spinal canal.

**c** A CT scan through the superior half of the vertebra shows marked narrowing of the spinal canal by the posterior edge fragment, as well as a split fracture of the lamina.

**d** A CT scan through the inferior half of the vertebra shows a longitudinal split fracture of the vertebral body and lamina.

**e** Surgery was done 12 days postinjury. The fragment was reduced indirectly by distraction. Ambulation was begun 3 days postoperatively, the ESSF device was removed at 15 weeks, and a lumbar corset was worn for 3 additional weeks.

**f** At 14 months postinjury there is 10° residual deformity of the vertebral body with collapse of both adjacent discs. The patient is free of complaints and is able to engage in sports

## 11.1.2 Open Procedure, Technique II (Figs. 342–345)

*Prerequisite:* Significant damage to both motion segments. Restoration of the longitudinal continuity of the posterior column by screw fixation of the facet joints is feasible and rational.

*Principle:* Translaminar screw fixation of the superior and inferior facet joints, fusion of both motion segments with autogenous cancellous bone. Open or percutaneous application of the ESSF device prestressed in strong distraction.

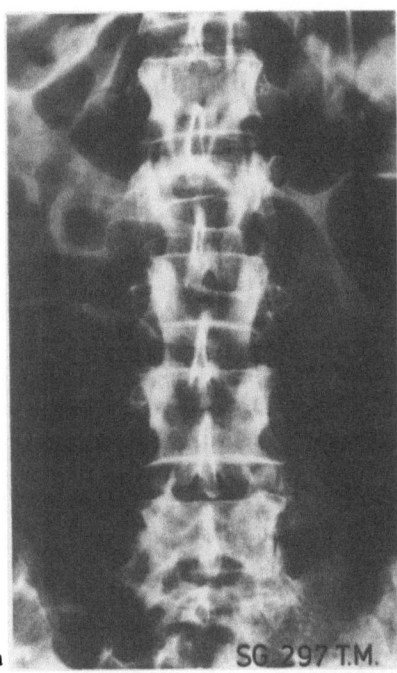
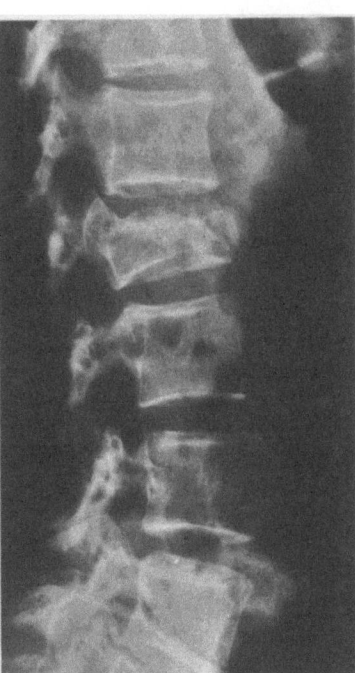
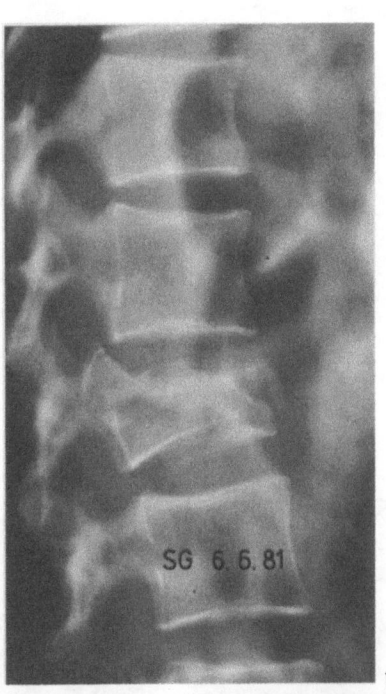

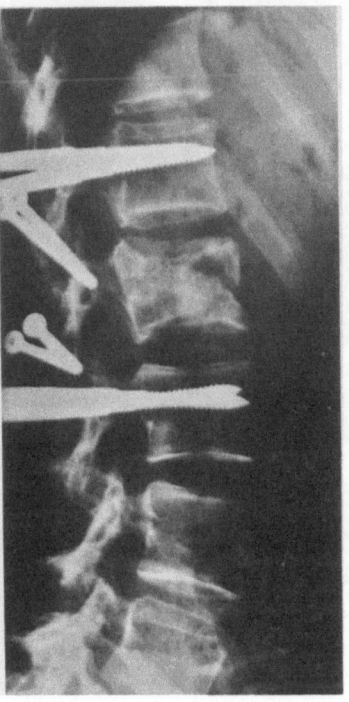
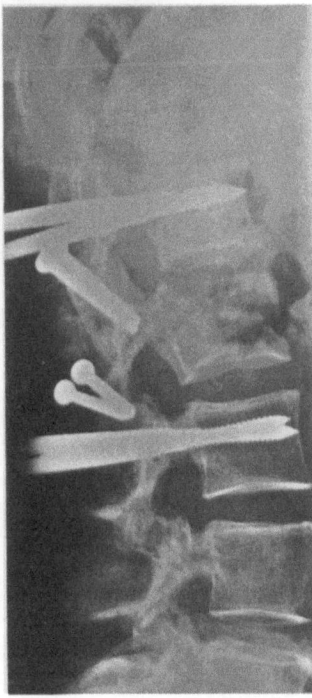

**Fig. 342 a–e.** Application of technique II for a comminuted burst fracture of L2. T.M., 1939, 42 years, ♀, 249 752.

**a** The patient sustained a comminuted burst fracture of L2 as a result of a traffic accident. There is very little displacement of the inferior vertebral body fragment, but an upper edge fragment encroaches on the spinal canal. The vertebral body shows wedging, broadening, and a reduction in height. A fracture of the lamina has produced marked pedicular separation. The clavicle is also fractured.

**b** Tomogram showing displacement of the upper posterior edge fragment.

**c** Surgery was done 12 days postinjury. The vertebral body was realigned, creating a cancellous bone defect, and the posterior edge fragment was reduced indirectly by distraction. Ambulation was begun two days after surgery.

**d** The defect shows little consolidation two months postoperatively. The ESSF device was removed at 16 weeks, and a lumbar corset was worn for 4 weeks.

**e** At 26 months postinjury the vertebral body shows no further deformity. Both discs are collapsed. The patient has pain at the graft donor site but reports no spine-associated complaints other than sensitivity to weather changes

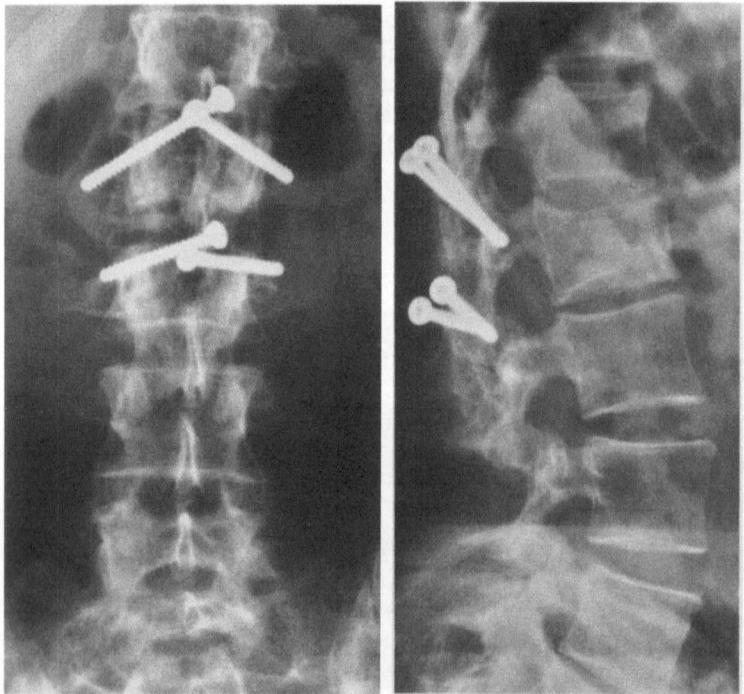

Fig. 342e. Legend see p. 333

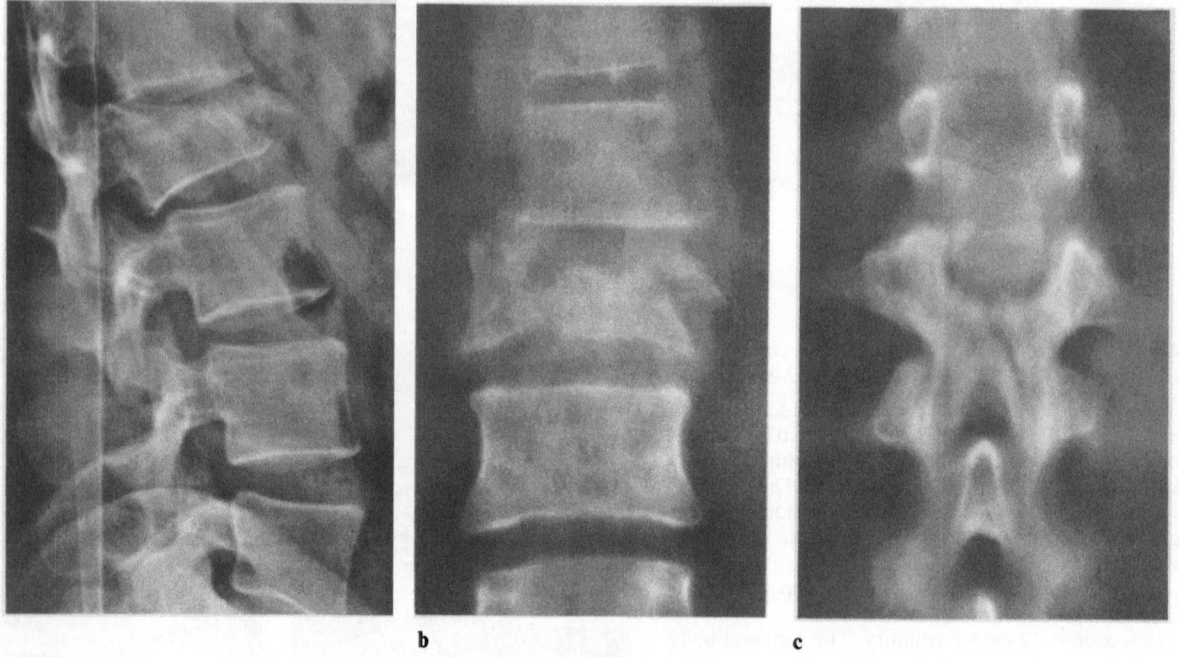

a

b

c

Fig. 343a–c

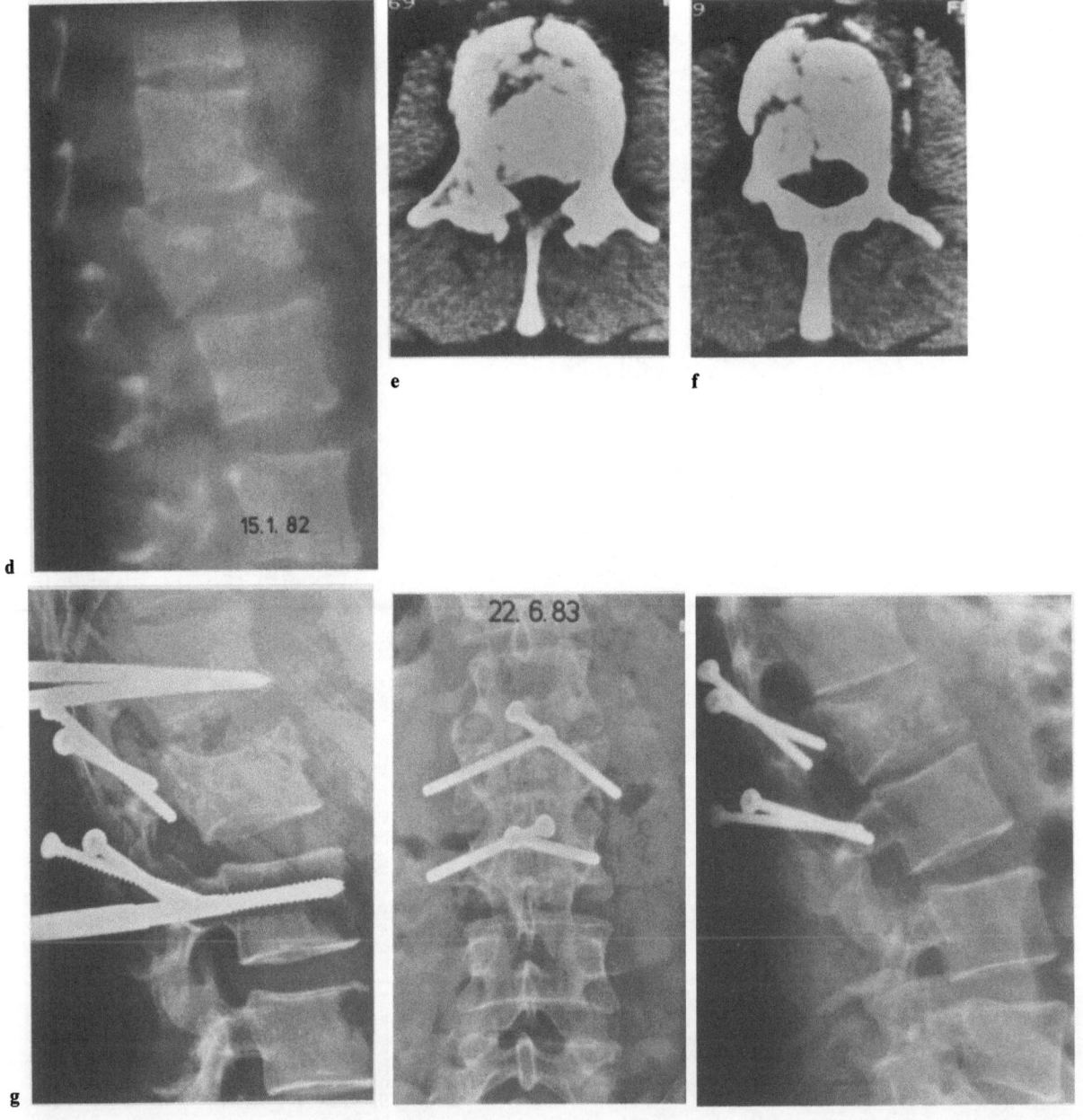

**Fig. 343 a–h.** Application of technique II for a comminuted burst fracture of L2. G.W., 1939, 42 years, ♂, 256604.

**a** The patient fell during skiing to sustain an injury having the appearance of a crush-cleavage fracture (AP projection is not available). There is wedging of the vertebral body, and narrowing of the spinal canal appears to be minimal. A mild cauda equina syndrome was present.
**b** Tomography of the vertebral body confirms the presence of a comminuted burst fracture.
**c** Split fracture of the lamina.
**d** The lateral tomogram discloses the true nature of the injury and the encroachment on the vertebral canal.
**e** A CT scan through the superior half of the vertebra demonstrates narrowing of the spinal canal by an upper posterior edge fragment.

**f** A CT scan through the inferior half of the vertebra demonstrates a stellate fracture, narrowing of the spinal canal on the right side, and a fissure fracture of the spinous process.
**g** At operation 10 days postinjury the vertebra was realigned, and the lumen of the spinal canal was restored by distraction. The patient ambulated 4 days after surgery, and the ESSF device was removed at 16 weeks without further special treatment.
**h** At 17 months postinjury the shape of the vertebral body is maintained, both discs are collapsed, and a bony bridge has formed across the right side of the L1–2 disc space. There is anesthesia of the S2 dermatome and paresthesia of the L4 dermatome; spinal complaints are very mild

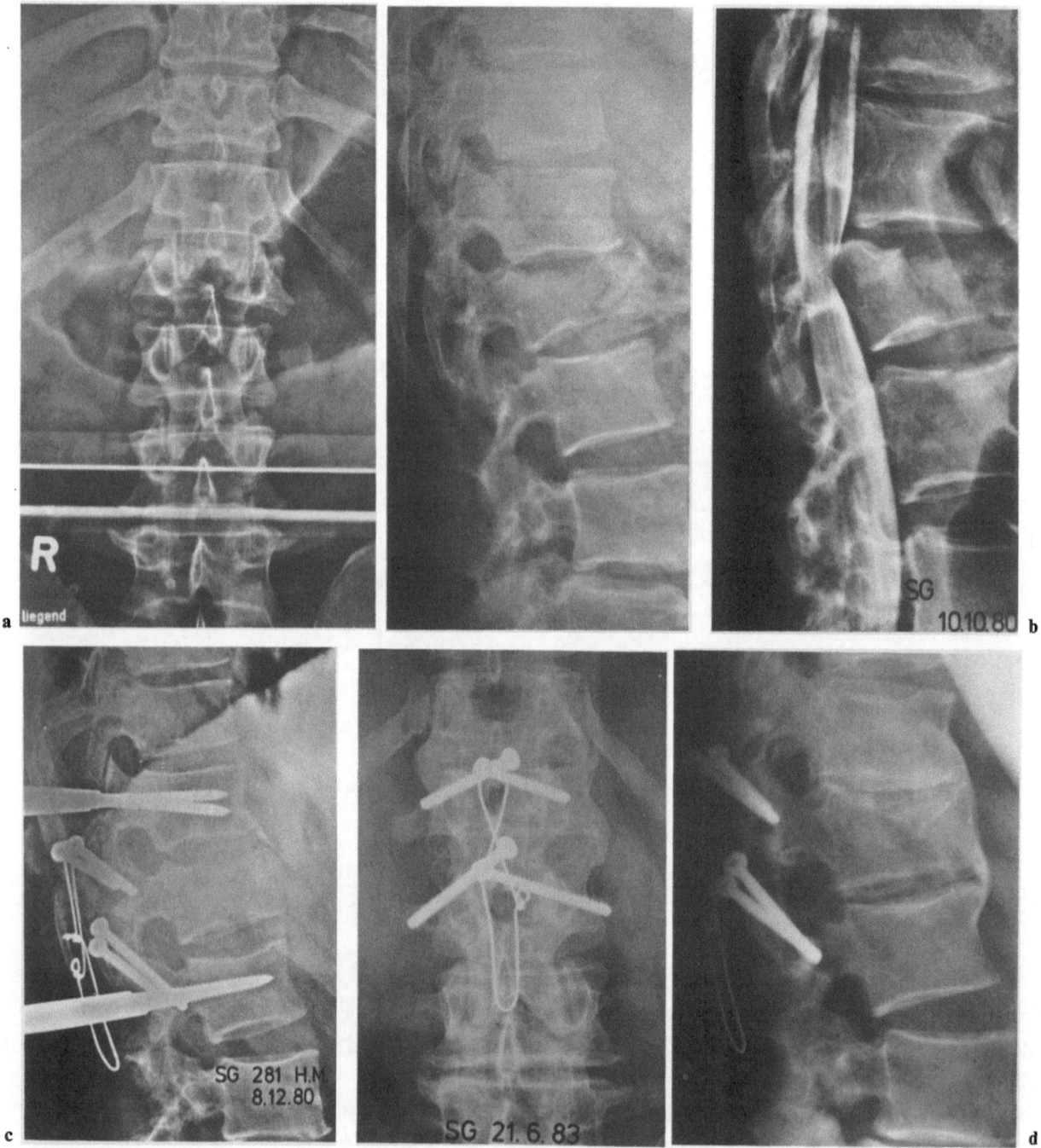

**Fig. 344 a–d.** Application of technique II for a comminuted burst fracture of L1. H.M., 1940, 40 years, ♂, 243222.

**a** The patient sustained a comminuted burst fracture of L1 in a fall from a tree. The vertebral body shows mainly a reduction of height, and pedicular separation is minimal. Bladder paralysis is present.
**b** Myelography demonstrates narrowing of the spinal canal by an upper posterior edge fragment.
**c** At operation seven days postinjury the vertebral body was realigned, and the edge fragment was reduced indirectly by distraction. The wire fixation would be unnecessary according to current opinion. The patient ambulated three days after surgery. A superficial wound infection was managed operatively.
**d** Status at 33 months postinjury. The vertebral body shows no change after removal of the ESSF device, and spontaneous fusion has occurred across both affected disc spaces. The residual kyphosis is due equally to the incomplete realignment of the vertebral body and to an eccentric collapse of the upper disc, with a parallel collapse of the lower disc. Bladder function has returned. The patient has little spinal discomfort but is handicapped in his work as a farmer. The clinical result was rated as fair

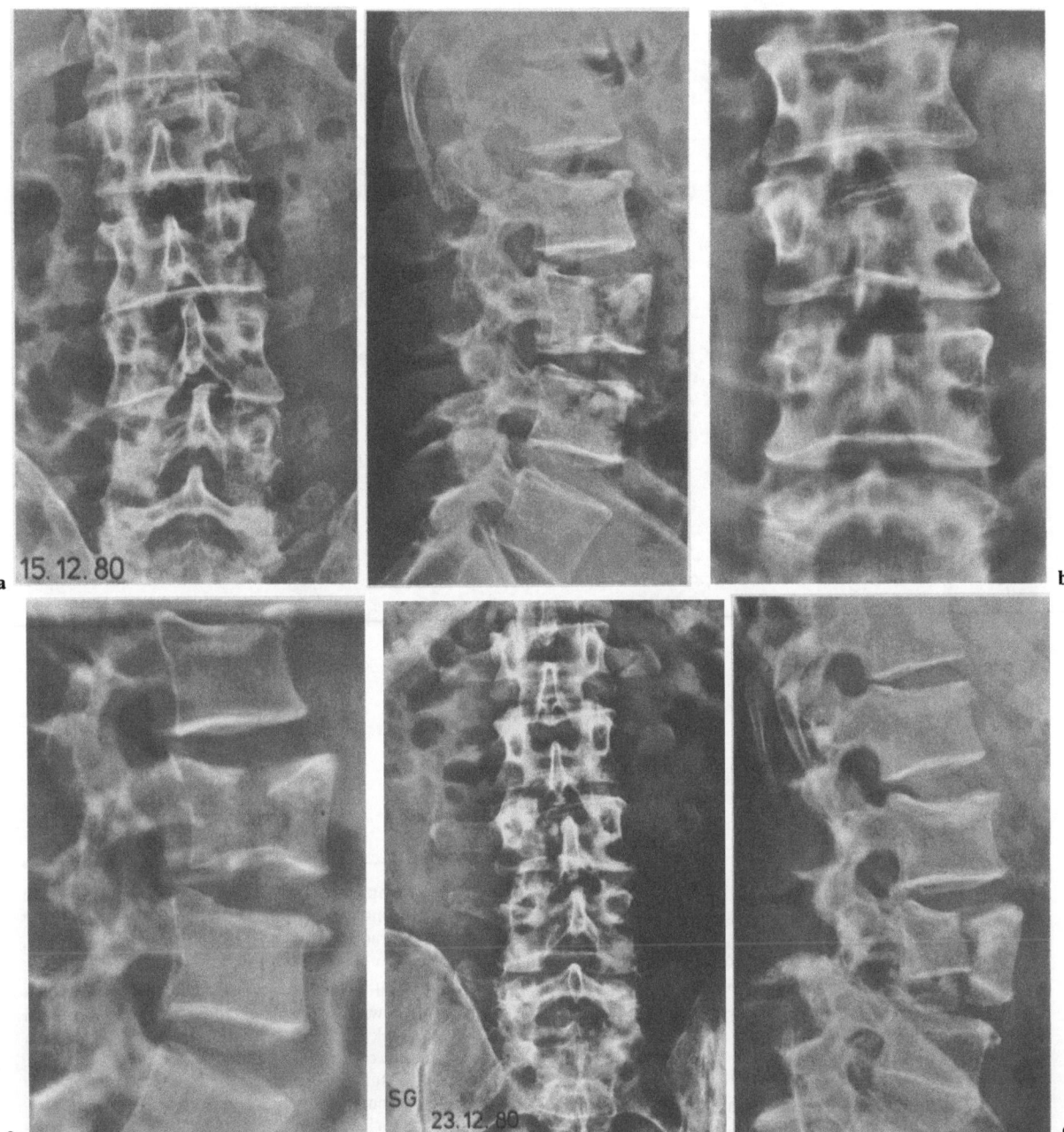

**Fig. 345 a–f.** Application of technique II for a multilevel fracture with bursting and comminution of L3. H.P., 1939, 41 years, ♂, 245 512.

**a** The patient was injured by a falling object, suffering mild compression fractures of L1, L2 and L4 and a rotatory-type comminuted burst fracture of L3 with little displacement. The serial fracture of the L1–3 transverse processes is typical of injuries with a rotatory component. At a hospital abroad the injury was misdiagnosed as a stable burst fracture, and L3 root paresis developed following early ambulation in a 3-point brace.

**b** The configuration of the fracture in the tomogram is typical of a rotatory lesion.

**c** The undamaged posterior wall of the vertebral body in the paramedian section is misleading.

**d** The displacement of the vertebral body fragments was exacerbated by ambulation.

**e** Surgery was done 29 days postinjury. Only the unstable fracture at L3 was bridged. A tension band was applied due to the precarious anchorage of the lower translaminar screws (fractured articular process). Ambulation was started two days after surgery, and the ESSF device was removed at 16 weeks without further special treatment.

**f** At 19 months postinjury the vertebra and fusion are consolidated. The remaining vertebral body fractures show no secondary displacement. The L3 root paresis has regressed completely. The patient has frequent moderate complaints which do not limits his physical activities

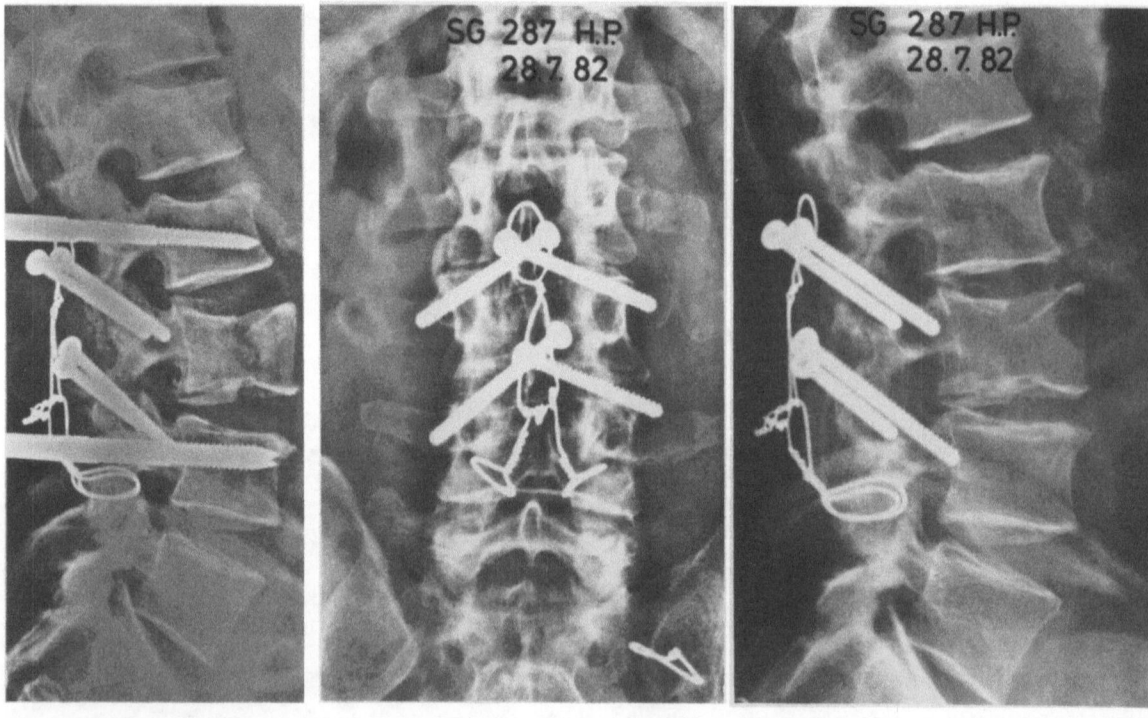

**Fig. 345e, f.** Legend see p. 337

## 11.1.3 Open Procedure, Technique III
(Figs. 346–349)

*Prerequisite:* Significant damage to both motion segments. Translaminar screw fixation is not feasible due to the destruction of posterior elements.

*Principle:* Reinforcement of the posterior column over two motion segments with a compression-resistant interspinous H graft and a tension-resistant wire loop. Open or percutaneous application of the ESSF device prestressed in strong distraction.

**Fig. 346 a–e.** Application of technique III for a fracture of L1. Transitional form between crush-cleavage fracture and flexion-distraction injury. L.W., 1954, 26 years, ♂, 201 034.

**a** The patient fell from a height of 10 m and sustained a fracture of L1, with a posterior edge fragment displaced upward and backward into the spinal canal. There is an avulsion fracture of both superior articular processes of L1 and a small diastasis of the L1 pedicles. In the lateral view the fracture presents as a flexion-distraction injury. The patient has an associated compression fracture of L3, a fracture of the right tibial pilon, and rib fractures.
**b** CT scan of the superior half of the vertebra shows narrowing of the spinal canal by the upper posterior edge fragment.
**c** CT through the inferior half of the vertebra shows longitudinal disruption of the vertebral body as in a crush-cleavage fracture. However, the lamina is not split.
**d** Twelve days postinjury a posterior fusion was performed with an H graft and wire loop from T12 to L1 (not visible). The vertebral body was not completely realigned. The patient ambulated 4 days postoperatively, the ESSF device was removed at 23 weeks, and a lumbar corset was worn for 4 weeks.
**e** At 16 months postinjury there is residual kyphotic deformity, collapse of both intervertebral discs, and spontaneous fusion of T12–L1 on the right side. The patient is free of complaints

**Fig. 346 a–e**

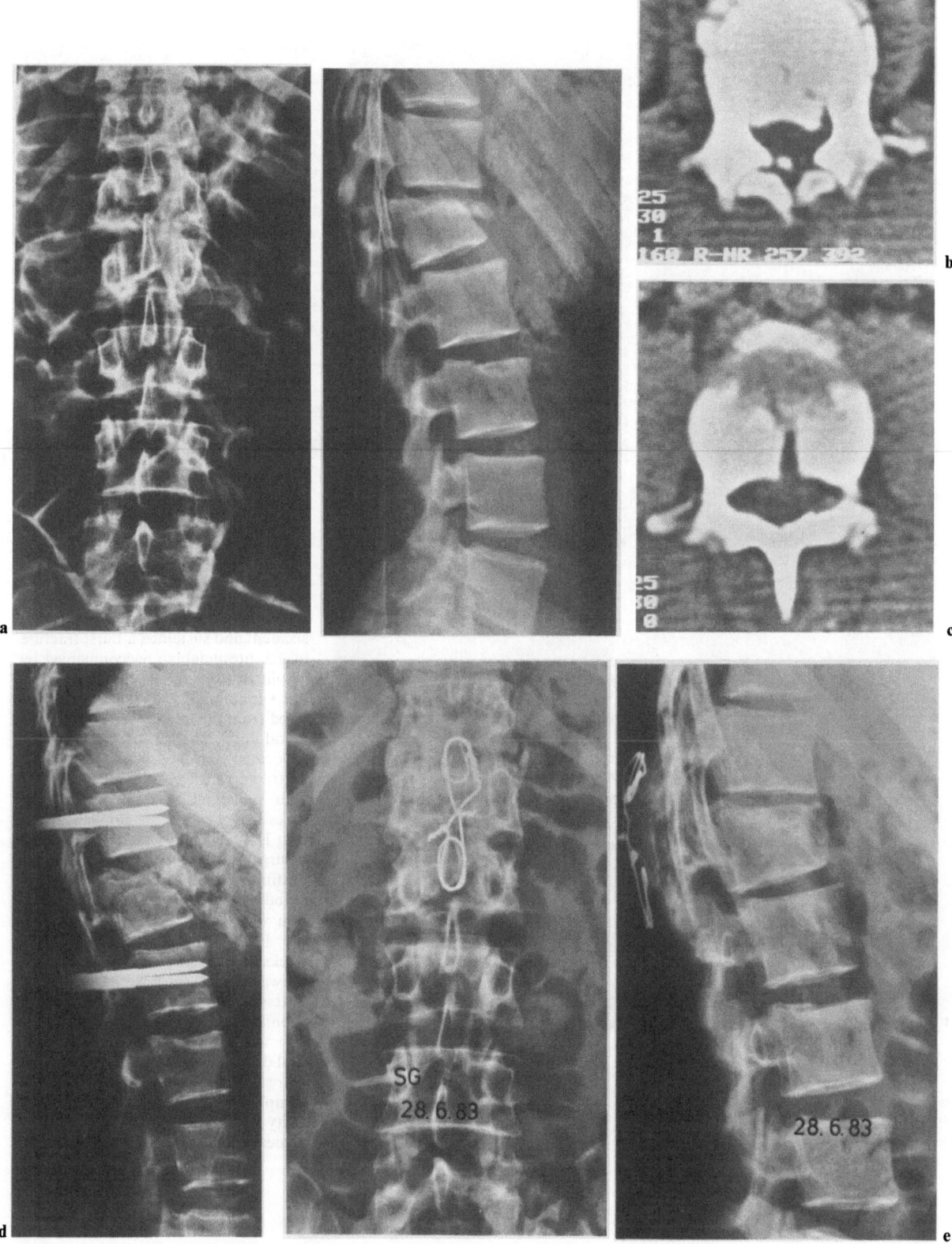

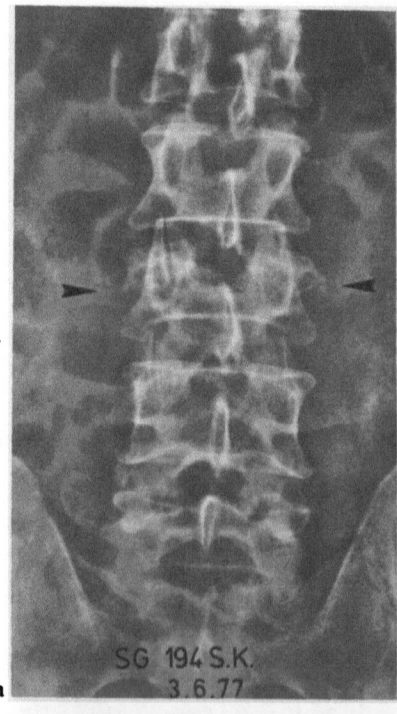
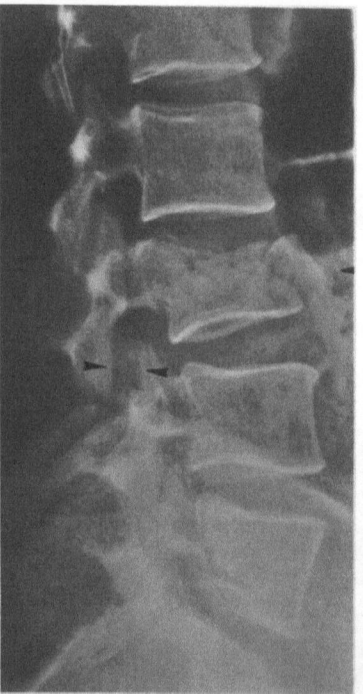
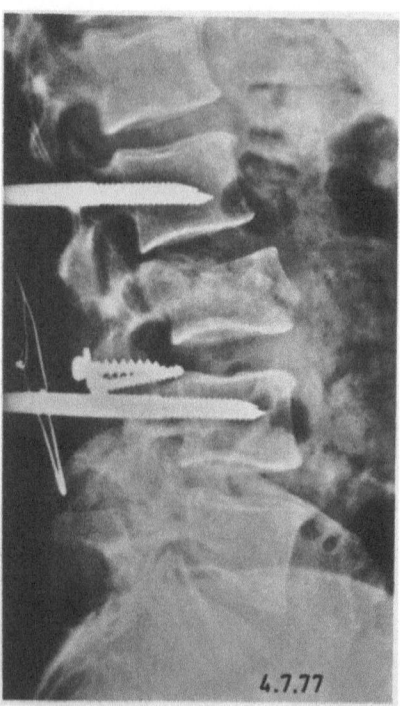
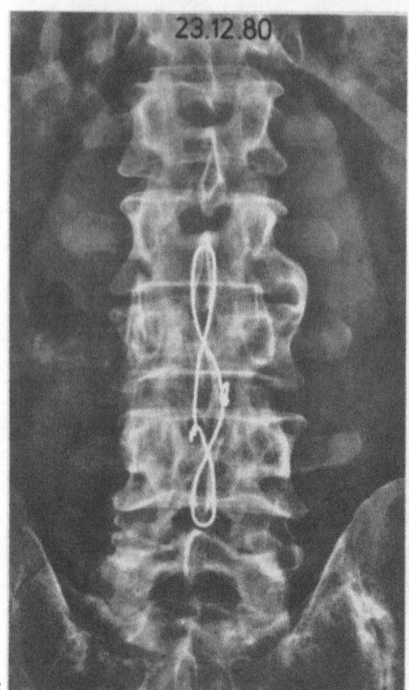
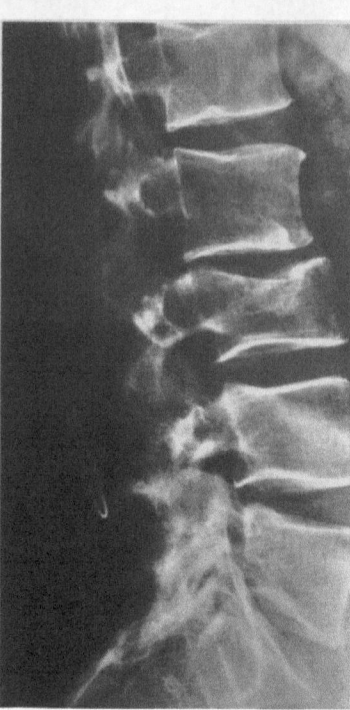

**Fig. 347 a–c.** Application of technique III for an atypical burst fracture of L3 with dislocation of the L3–4 facet joints. The first case treated with the ESSF device. S.K., 1933, 44 years, ♂, 139899.

**a** The patient was involved in a traffic accident and sustained a burst fracture of L3, presumably unaccompanied by a split fracture of the inferior half of the vertebra. The pedicles are separated from the inferior part of the vertebral body. The L3–4 facet joints are dislocated, and the L4 spinous process is fractured. The patient presented with unilateral sensory deficits and paresis of the muscles supplied by the root L5.

**b** Surgery was carried out five days postinjury. The facet joints were immobilized by screw fixation. Ambulation was begun 7 days after surgery, the ESSF device was removed 14 weeks after surgery, and a lumbar corset was applied for 6 weeks.

**c** At 43 months postfracture there is spontaneous fusion of L2–3 on the left side with collapse of both intervertebral discs. The neurologic deficits have regressed completely. The patient has complaints during certain types of activity and cannot do heavy work. The clinical result is fair

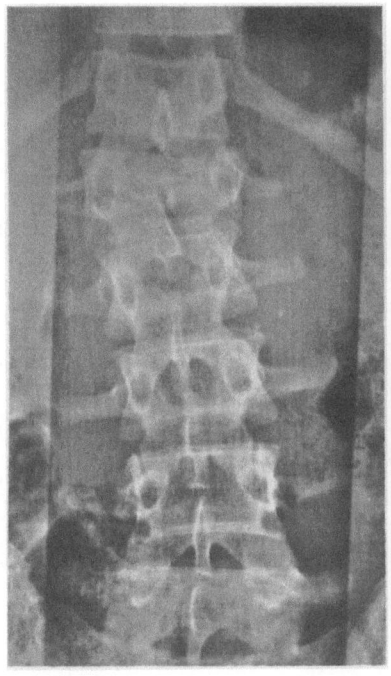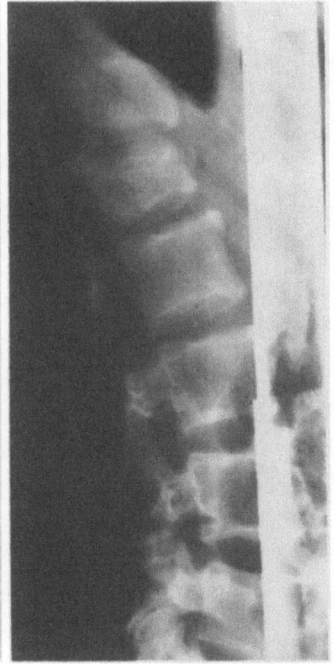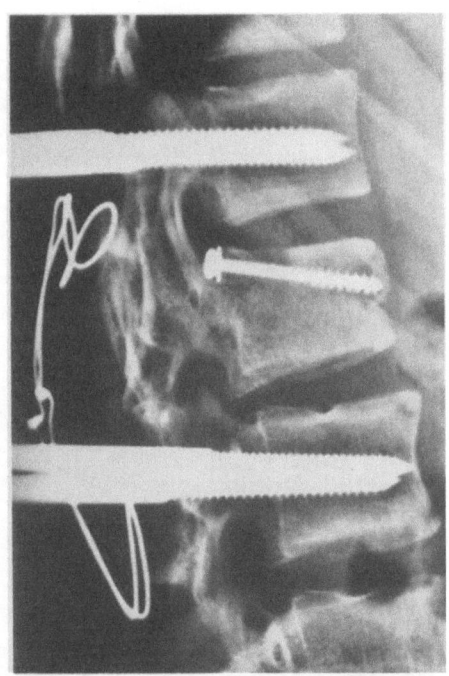

a                                                                        b

**Fig. 348 a–c.** Application of technique III with open decompression for a lateral comminuted burst fracture of L1. B.A., 1960, 19 years, ♂, 230 541.

**a** In a traffic accident the patient sustained a lateral comminuted burst fracture of L1 with a fracture of the right pars and diastasis of the pedicles. The patient exhibits an incomplete cauda equina syndrome, and dural lacerations are present.
**b** On the day of the injury an extensive laminectomy was performed, and the dural lacerations were repaired by suture. An upper edge fragment was prone to redisplacement, probably due to interposed disc tissue, and so was fixed with a lag screw lateral to the dural sac. The patient ambulated 5 days after surgery, and the ESSF device was removed at 15 weeks without further treatment.
**c** At 23 months postinjury there is residual kyphosis and scoliosis and collapse of both discs. The cauda equina syndrome has regressed completely. The patient can do light physical work without much discomfort and is 33% disabled in his capacity as a construction worker

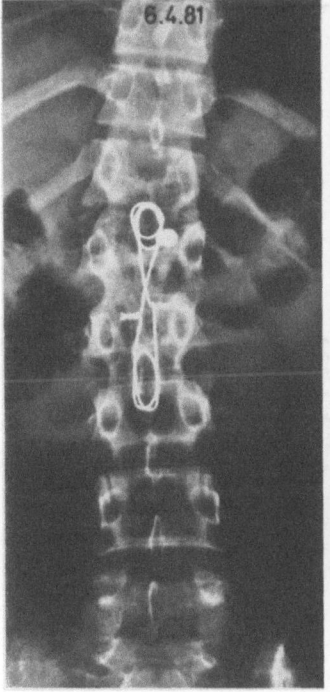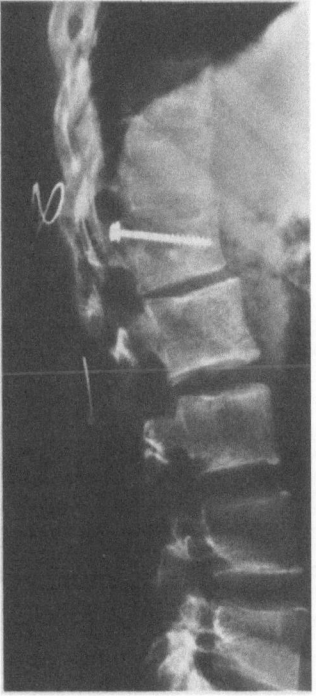

c

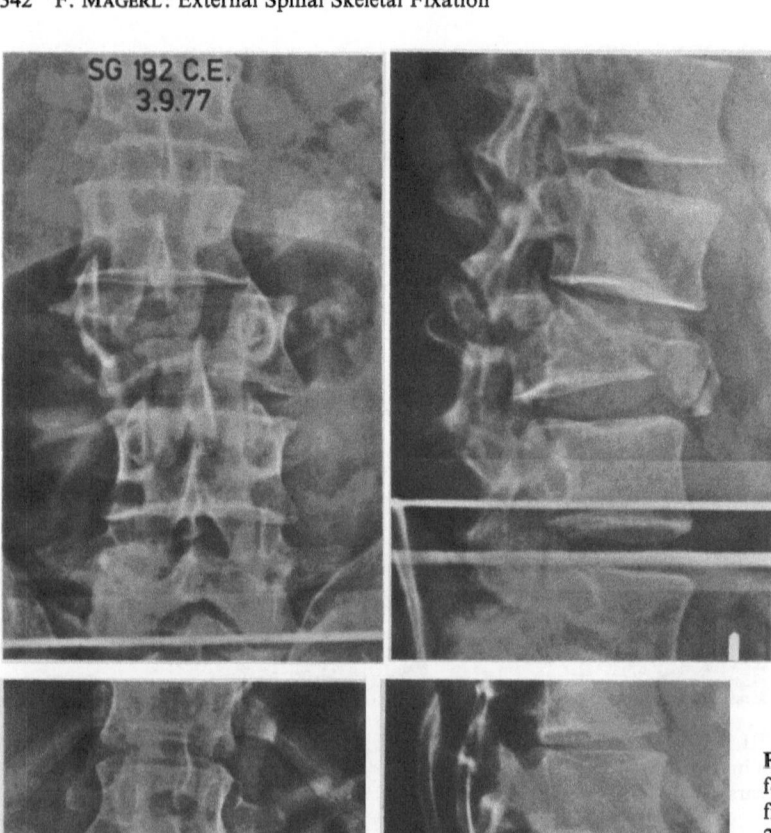

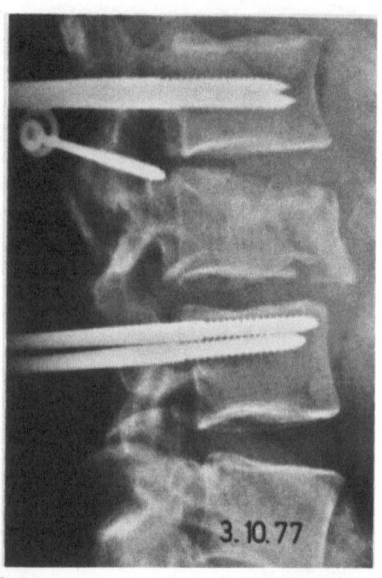

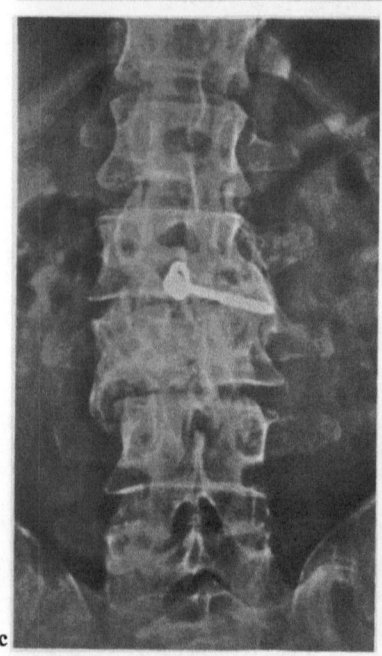

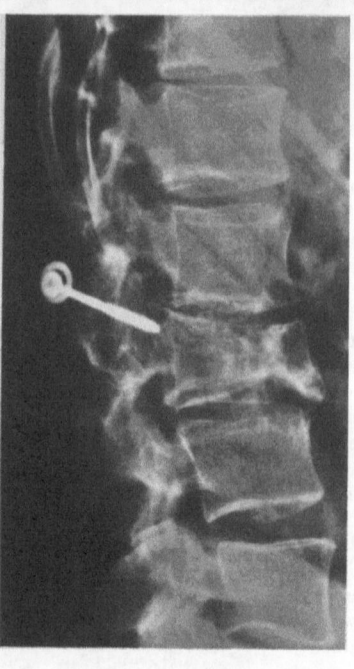

**Fig. 349 a–c.** Application of technique III for a translational injury (rotatory burst fracture) of L3. Early case. C.E., 1950, 27 years, ♂, 211093.

**a** A traffic accident resulted in a rotatory burst fracture of L3 with dislocation of the L2–3 left facet joint and a fracture of the left transverse processes of L2–3 and the right transverse process of L4.

**b** Surgery was performed on the day of the injury. The L2–3 facet joint was immobilized by screw fixation; wire fixation was not employed at that time. Ambulation was initiated three days after surgery. A wound seroma was treated by aspiration. The ESSF device was removed 12 weeks postoperatively, and a hyperextension body cast was worn for 5 weeks.

**c** At 43 months postinjury there is residual kyphosis, spontaneous fusion of L2–3 on the left side, and collapse of both discs. The patient is free of complaints

### 11.1.4 Stabilization of the 5th Lumbar Vertebra with the ESSF Device (Fig. 350)

*Principle:* Open or open-percutaneous procedure using techniques I–III or percutaneous application of the ESSF device. The caudal Schanz screws are anchored in the sacrum or ilia.

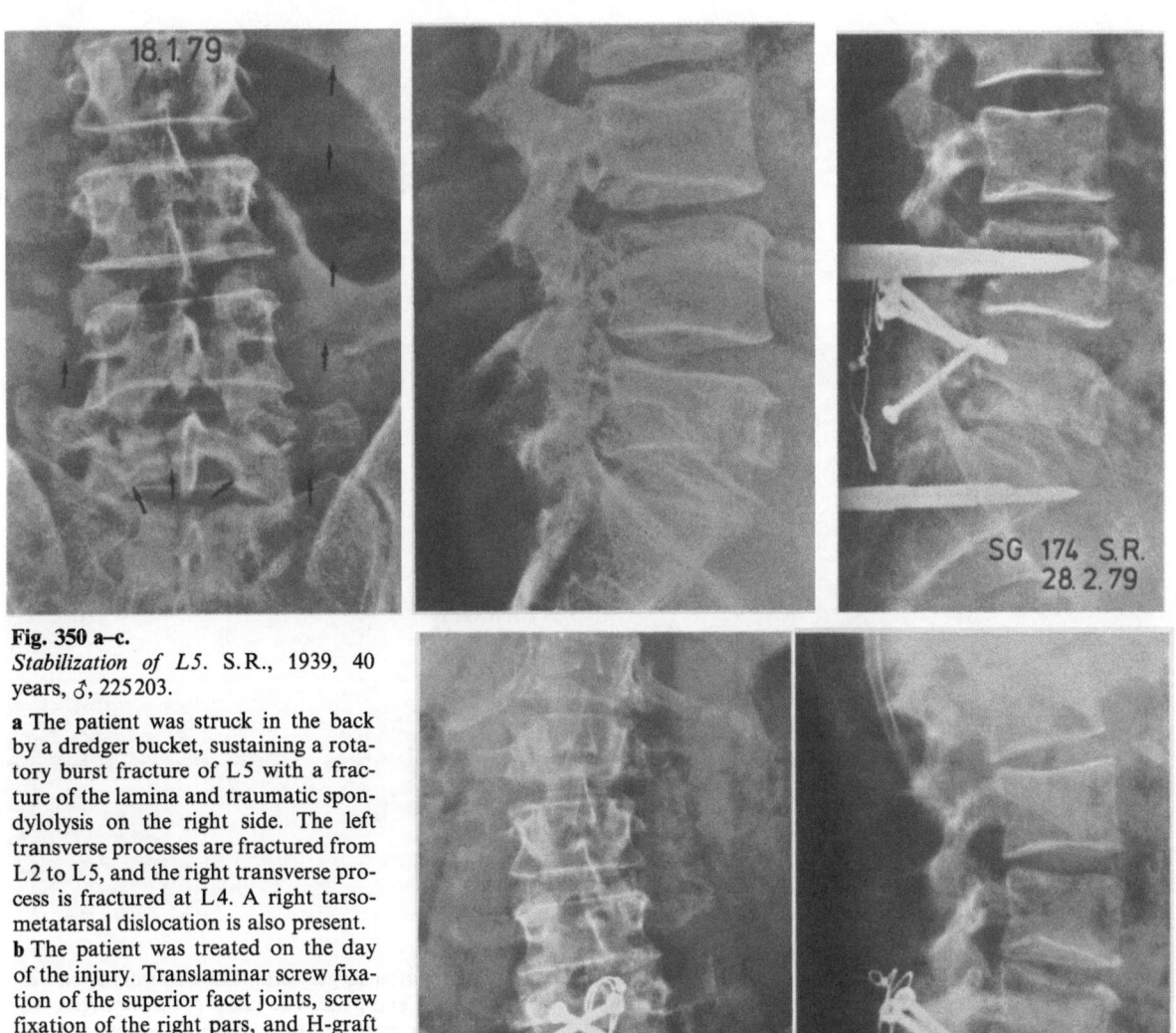

**Fig. 350 a–c.**
*Stabilization of L5.* S.R., 1939, 40 years, ♂, 225203.

**a** The patient was struck in the back by a dredger bucket, sustaining a rotatory burst fracture of L5 with a fracture of the lamina and traumatic spondylolysis on the right side. The left transverse processes are fractured from L2 to L5, and the right transverse process is fractured at L4. A right tarso-metatarsal dislocation is also present.
**b** The patient was treated on the day of the injury. Translaminar screw fixation of the superior facet joints, screw fixation of the right pars, and H-graft and wire fixation from L4 to S1. The caudal Schanz screws were anchored in the ilium. Ambulation was begun 5 days after surgery, and the ESSF device was removed at 13 weeks without further special treatment.
**c** At 51 months postinjury there is collapse of both discs. The patient has moderate lumbosacral complaints during strenuous work

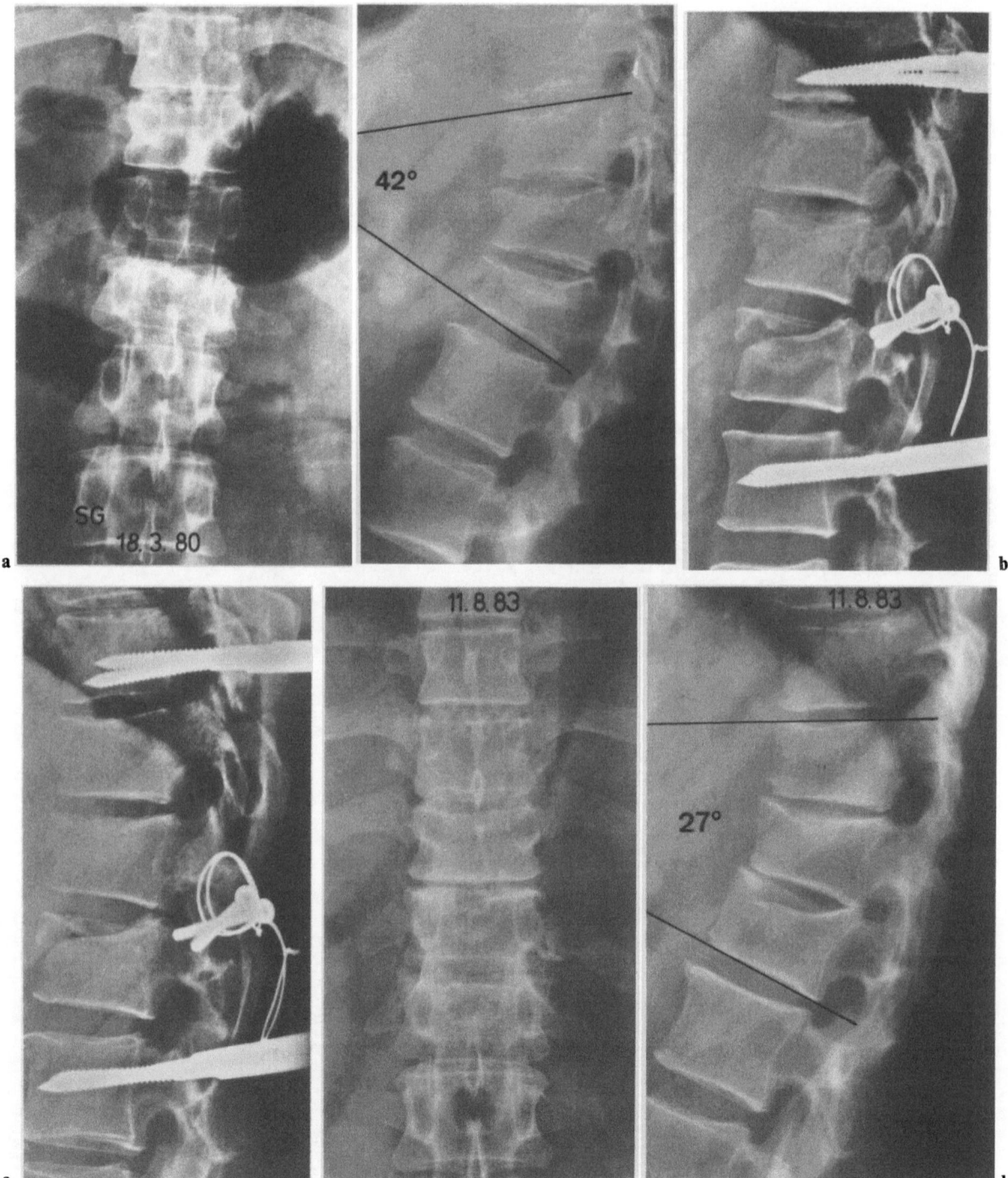

**Fig. 351 a–d.** Open-percutaneous stabilization with the simple ESSF device spanning four motion segments. S.M., 1942, 38 years, ♂, 237551.

**a** A traffic accident produced a wedge-compression fracture of T11 and incomplete burst fractures of T12 and L1. Total kyphotic deformity is 42°, and there is a root lesion of L1.
**b** At operation 8 days postinjury technique I was applied to T11–12, and a wire loop was secured around the T12 lamina and L1 spinous process. The ESSF device was applied percutaneously. The upper end plate of L1 remained compressed, and the vertebral body was not completely realigned. Ambulation was begun eight days postoperatively.

**c** At two months after surgery progressive consolidation was evident at the L1 end plate. The ESSF device was removed 13 weeks after surgery, and thus earlier than intended, because of psychogenic complaints. A hyperextension body cast was worn for seven weeks. The implants were removed due to pain over the site where the wire was twisted.
**d** At 29 months postfracture there is a 26° residual kyphosis due to incomplete realignment of the vertebral bodies and collapse of the discs. Even the wire loop could not prevent collapse of the disc at T12–L1. The patient has moderate complaints in the area of the L1 root lesion

### 11.1.5 Open or Open-Percutaneous Stabilization with the Simple ESSF Device Over More than Two Motion Segments (Fig. 351)

*Prerequisite:* Serial fracture of adjacent vertebrae. The posterior fusion may be limited to one or two motion segments.

*Principle:* Application of techniques I–III, open or open-percutaneous procedure. The ESSF device is prestressed in moderate distraction if not every motion segment bridged by the device is fused.

### 11.1.6 Stabilization of an Interbody Fusion with the ESSF Device (Figs. 352 and 353)

*Prerequisite:* Based on previous experience, interbody fusions are rarely indicated for injuries treated with the ESSF device. They should only be considered in the region of the lower thoracic spine. Lumbar spine injuries generally can be managed by the techniques of open or closed external fixation from a posterior approach.

*Principle:* An interbody fusion is performed from the posterior approach followed by open or percutaneous application of the ESSF device, or from the anterior approach with percutaneous application of the device. In both cases the device is prestressed in mild compression.

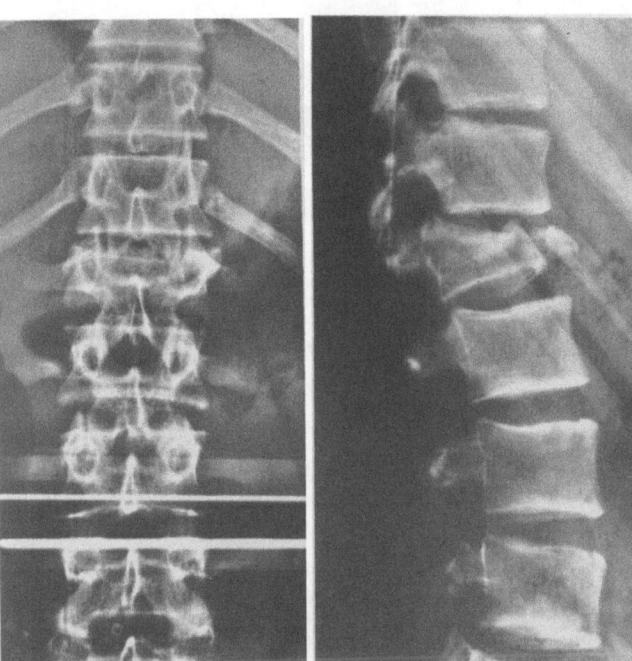

**Fig. 352 a–c.** Posterior interbody fusion and stabilization with the ESSF device. Z.U., 1962, 18 years, ♂, 235327.

**a** The patient was struck by a falling object, sustaining a rotatory crush-cleavage fracture of L1 with slight diastasis of the pedicles and displacement of an upper posterior wall fragment into the spinal canal, producing an incomplete conus syndrome.
**b** On the day of the injury the patient underwent a posterior interbody fusion of T12–L1 using a combination of techniques II and III. The patient ambulated 6 days after surgery, and the ESSF device was removed at 17 weeks; a hyperextension body cast was worn for an additional 6 weeks.
**c** At 15 months postinjury the fusions are consolidated, and there is collapse of the L1–2 disc. The patient has no complaints other than a mild disturbance of bladder function.
*Note:* Despite the good result we still question the cost-to-benefit ratio of posterior interbody fusions in spinal external fixation (cf. Sect. 8.1.11)

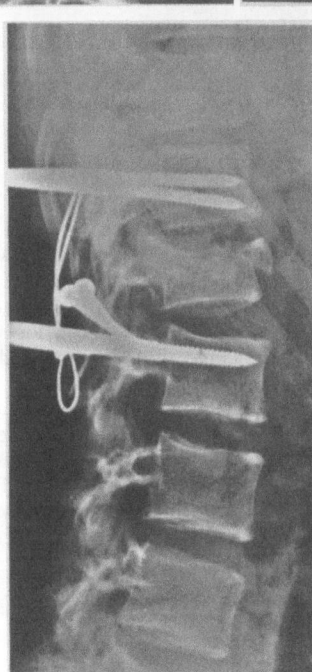
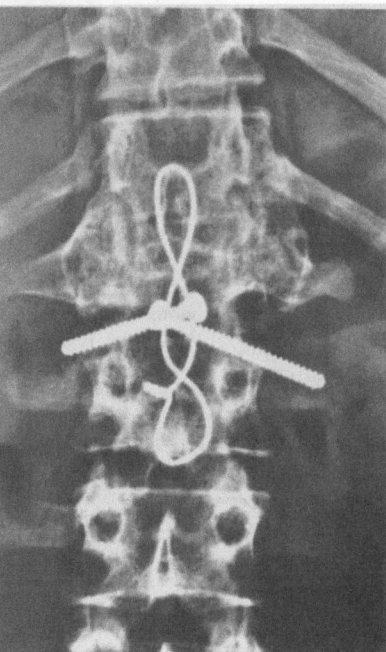
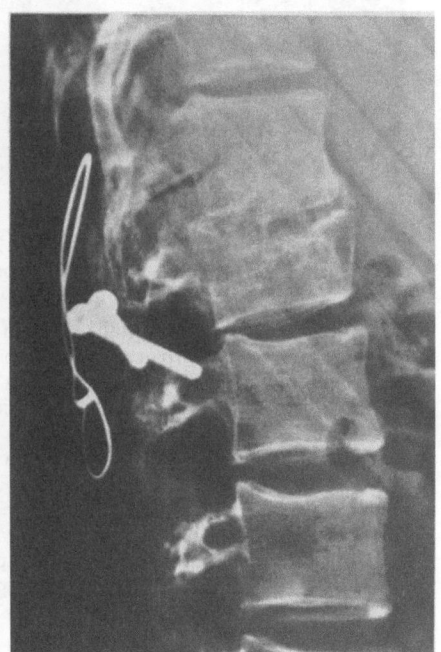

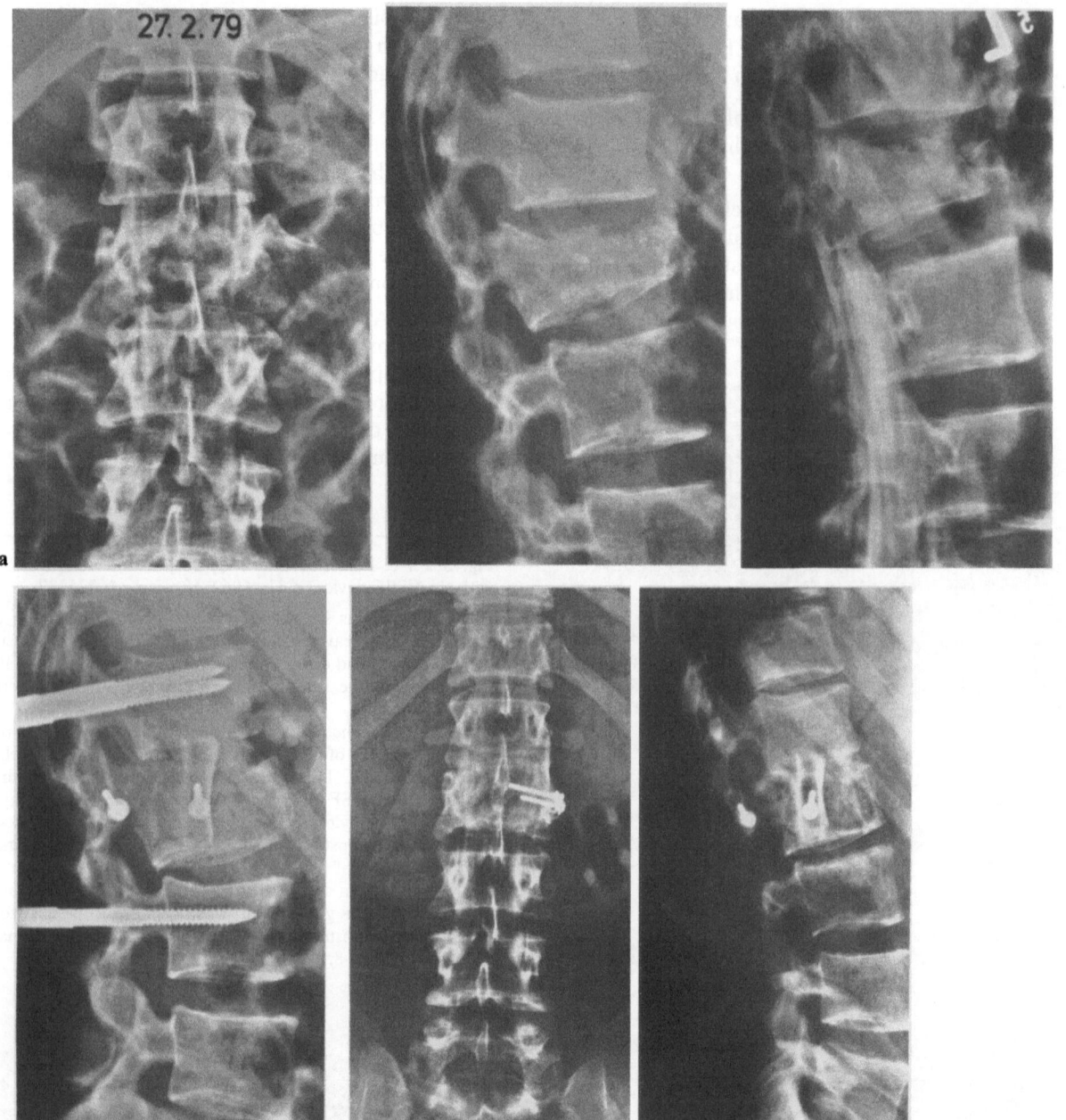

**Fig. 353 a–d.** Partial spondylectomy of L2, anterior interbody fusion and percutaneous stabilization with the ESSF device. S.G., 1958, 21 years, ♂, 157855.

**a** The patient fell from a scaffold to sustain a complete burst fracture of L1 with displacement of upper posterior wall fragments into the spinal canal, causing a partial cauda equina syndrome. The patient had associated fractures of the left metatarsals and ankle joint.
**b** Myelography demonstrated a fluid block at the level of L1.
**c** Two days postinjury an anterolateral decompression was carried out, a full-thickness bone graft from the iliac crest was inserted, and cancellous bone was applied anteriorly. A second corticocancellous graft was applied to restore

lateral bony coverage to the vertebral canal; this graft was attached with screws to the pedicle and fusion graft. In the same sitting the ESSF device was applied by the percutaneous method. Ambulation was begun 10 days postoperatively, the ESSF device was removed at 14 weeks, and a lumbar corset was worn for 6 weeks.
**d** At 25 months postinjury the fusion is undisplaced and consolidated, and the lower disc is collapsed. The patient has a residual sensory deficit at L3 on the left side and has moderate complaints during strenuous work. *Note:* Today we would still elect to do a posterior operation, and we would apply distraction primarily in an attempt to restore the lumen of the spinal canal

### 11.1.7 Percutaneous Application of the Simple ESSF Device or Coupled Assembly (Figs. 354 and 355)

*Prerequisite:* Injury to single or multiple vertebrae not requiring open reduction, open decompression or dural repair. Major surgery precluded by the patient's general condition (polytrauma).

*Principle:* Insertion of the Schanz screws under image intensification. Application of the simple ESSF device for trauma to one or more adjacent vertebrae, or the coupled assembly for trauma at multiple levels separated by undamaged vertebrae. The device is prestressed in moderate distraction or mild compression, depending on the type of injury.

**Fig. 354a–e.**
Legend see p. 348

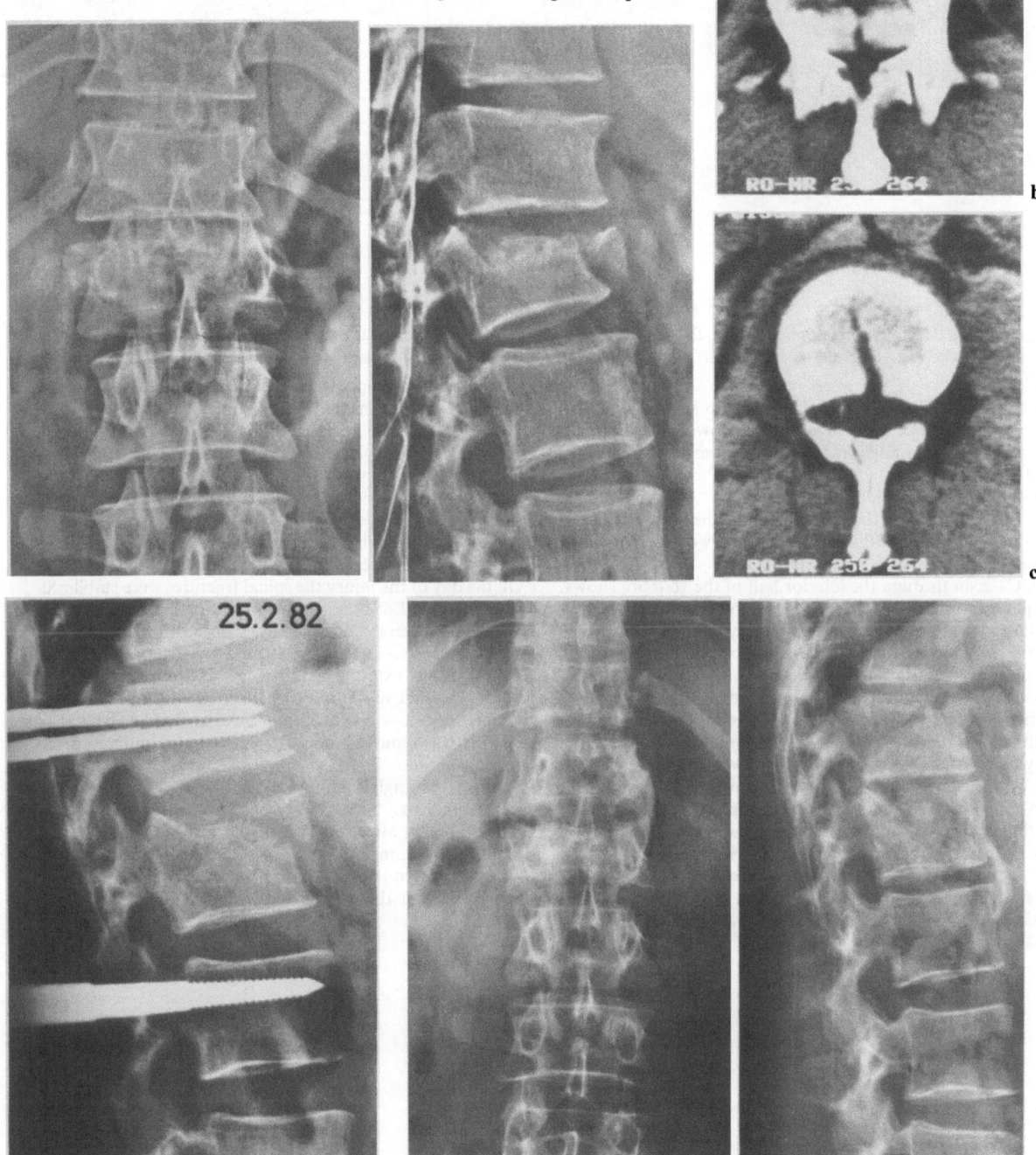

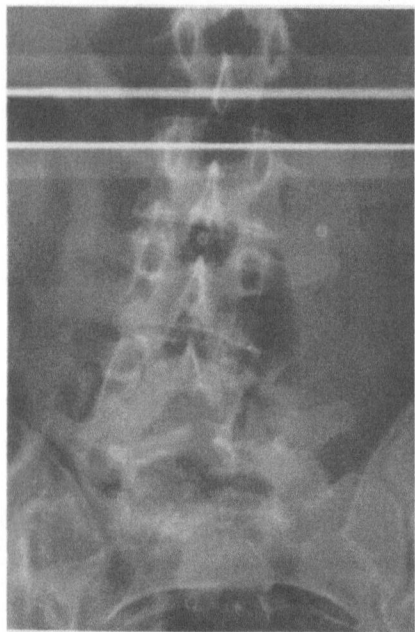

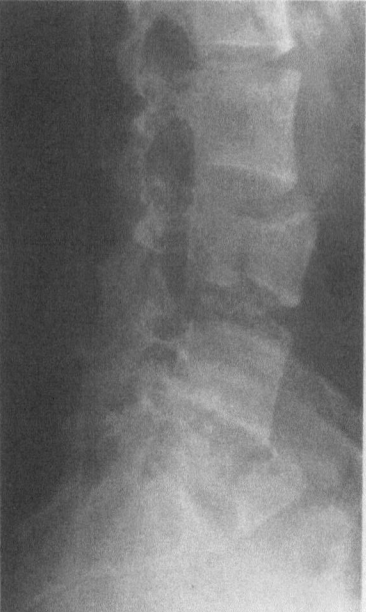

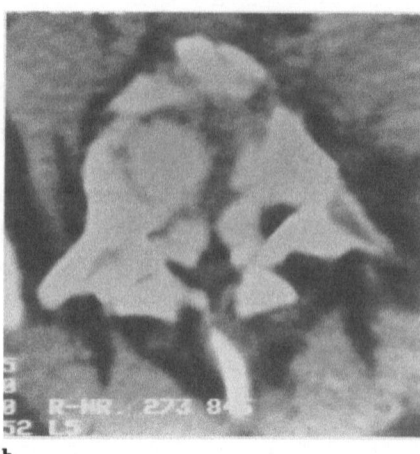

a

b

**Fig. 354 a–e.** Percutaneous application of the ESSF device for a crush-cleavage fracture of L1. N.M., 1939, 43 years, ♂, 250264.

**a** The patient fell from a height of 6 m to sustain a crush-cleavage fracture of L1 with marked narrowing of the spinal canal by posterior edge fragments, diastasis of the pedicles and a partial cauda equina syndrome. Psoriasis was also present in this individual.

**b** A CT scan through the superior half of the vertebra shows marked narrowing of the spinal canal by two posterior edge fragments.

**c** A CT scan through the inferior half of the vertebra shows a split fracture of the vertebral body and spinous process.

**d** Surgery was done two days postinjury. Due to severe psoriatic lesions over the injured area a closed reduction was carried out, and the ESSF device was applied percutaneously in moderate distraction. Good realignment of the vertebral body was obtained, and the edge fragments were reduced by the distraction. The patient was ambulated 2 days after surgery, and the ESSF device was removed at 26 weeks without further special treatment.

**e** At 16 months postinjury there is a slight residual kyphosis with collapse of both discs and spontaneous fusion across the left side of T2–L1 and the anterior side of L1–2. A screw track is visible in the right pedicle of T12. The patient has moderate back pain and ischialgia in addition to slight residual paralysis. The clinical result was rated as fair

**Fig. 355 a–e.** Percutaneous stabilization of L3 and L5 with a coupled ESSF assembly. E.E., 1959, 24 years, ♀, 273846.

**a** The patient attempted suicide by jumping from a fifth-floor window and sustained a complete burst fracture of L3 and a complete rotatory burst fracture (translational injury) of L5. She presented with partial paralysis in both legs, cerebral concussion, a skull fracture, serial rib fractures with a hematopneumothorax, and multiple fractures in three limbs, some very severe.

**b** A CT scan through L5 showed marked narrowing of the spinal canal by posterior wall fragments.

**c** On the day of the injury the spinal fractures were stabilized with a coupled ESSF assembly applied percutaneously; the lowermost Schanz screws were anchored in the ilia. The limb fractures were likewise treated by external fixation. A total of four external fixation devices were applied. The patient was first mobilized from bed to a wheelchair, and she was able to walk at about three months. The ESSF assembly was removed after 21 weeks and a lumbar corset applied.

**d** View of the angled fixation assembly in place on the recumbent patient.

**e** Status shortly after removal of the ESSF assembly: The fractures have consolidated in a satisfactory position, and the pareses have regressed. It is too early to make a final assessment, and the case is not included in the follow-up study.

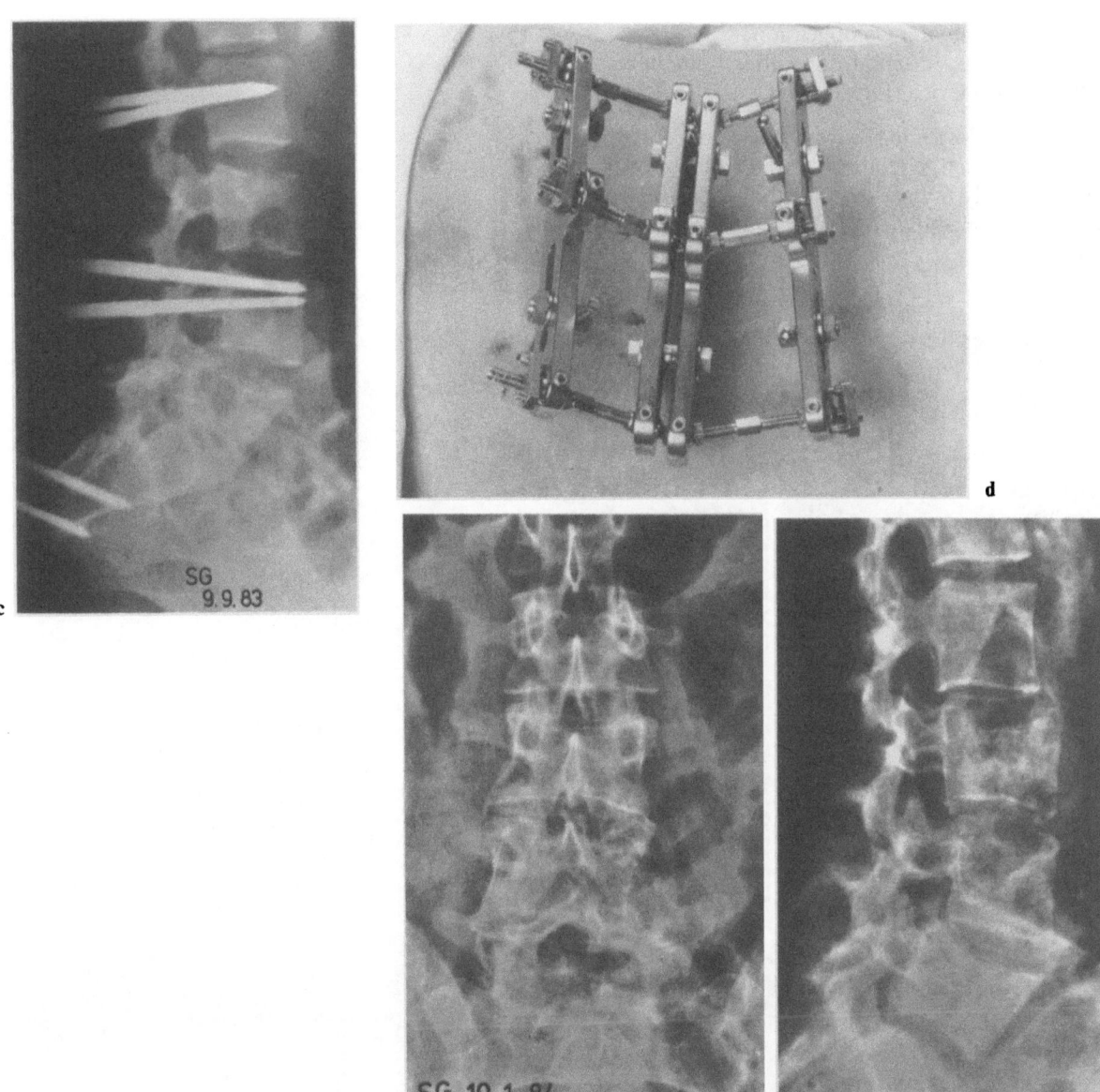

**Fig. 355 c–e**

## 11.1.8 Example of a Complication:
## Collapse of the Vertebral Body after Removal
## of the ESSF Device (Fig. 356)

If the ESSF device is removed before the fracture
has consolidated, a relatively rapid collapse of the
vertebral body many ensue. We have seen no case
in which a consolidated vertebra subsequently deformed.

Fig. 356a–d

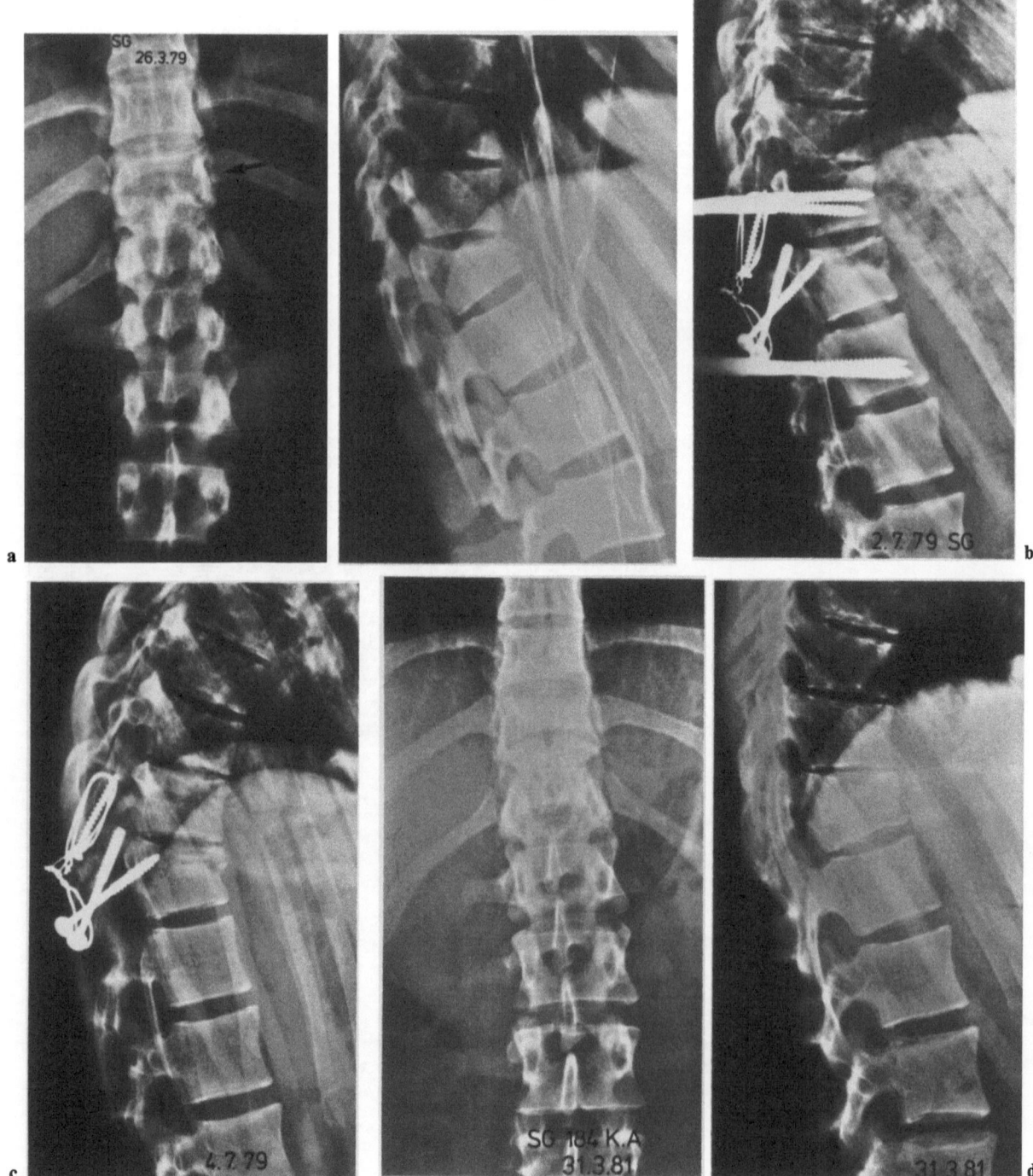

**Fig. 356 a–d.** Collapse of T11 following premature removal of the ESSF device. K.A., 1958, 21 years, ♀, 225873.

**a** A skiing accident resulted in a crush-cleavage fracture of T11 with fractures through both superior articular processes of T11, a facet dislocation at T10–11, a fracture of the T10 lamina, and mild compression fractures of T8–10. Operation on the day after injury. The T11 articular processes and T10 lamina were fixed with screws. Technique III was applied with stabilization from T10 to T12. Ambulation was begun five days later.
**b** Fourteen weeks after surgery an obvious defect was still present in the vertebral body; the ESSF device was removed.
**c** Two days later the vertebral body of T11 is collapsed, requiring an additional eight weeks' immobilization in a hypertextension body cast.
**d** At 24 months postinjury there is no further loss of correction. There is a residual kyphotic deformity, and both discs are collapsed. The patient is free of complaints and is able to engage in athletics

◀─────────────────────────────

## 11.2 Spondylitis

The antibiotic or tuberculostatic treatment is not described in the case reports. For this please refer to Sect. 9.

### 11.2.1 Two-Stage Procedure with Open Surgical Treatment (Figs. 357–360)

*Prerequisite:* Open surgical treatment necessitated by destruction, deformity, abscess or sequestrum.

*Principle:* Posterior fusion and stabilization with the ESSF device, debridement and installation of suction-irrigation drainage in the first sitting. Interbody fusion in the second sitting. Antibiotic therapy (cf. Sect. 9).

### 11.2.2 Exception: Single-Stage Procedure with Open Surgical Treatment (Fig. 361)

*Prerequisite:* This procedure is indicated only in cases of tubercular spondylitis which require supplementary posterior stabilization. With proper debridement and use of tuberculostatic drugs both before and after surgery, bone grafts implanted directly at the site of infection should heal without difficulty.

*Principle:* Debridement, interbody fusion, posterior fusion and stabilization with the ESSF device are performed in one sitting. Tuberculostatic agents are administered.

### 11.2.3 Indirect Treatment of Spondylitis with Percutaneous Application of the ESSF Device (Fig. 362)

*Prerequisite:* Spondylodiscitis with mild systemic symptoms, minimal osteolysis and no paravertebral abscessation. Causative organisms are sensitive to several antibiotics appropriate for long-term use.

*Principle:* Percutaneous stabilization of the spine. Long-term antibiotic therapy.

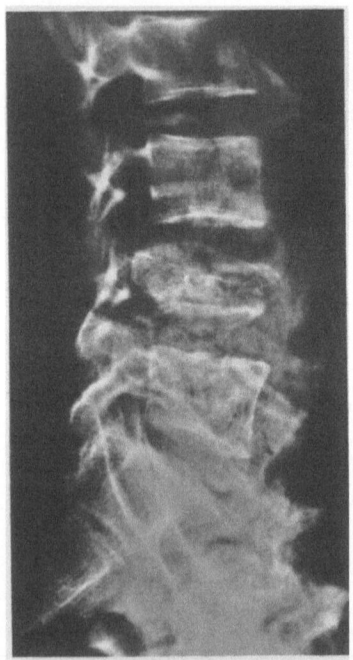

a

**Fig. 357 a–c.** Two-stage procedure for staphylococcal spondylitis of L4 without involvement of the disc. S.W., 1954, 23 years, ♂, 208 524.

**a** The patient was involved in a tractor accident, suffering a skull fracture and cerebral contusion, unilateral amaurosis, damage to the inner ear, and a renal contusion. He also sustained a complete burst fracture of L4. While in ICU the patient acquired a hematogenous spondylitis of L4 caused by *Staphylococcus aureus,* without adjacent disc involvement. The patient was septicemic and developed mild neurologic symptoms.

**b** In this first case of spondylitis treated with the ESSF device, we first managed the infection by surgical exposure, debridement, and interbody fusion with a full-thickness iliac block, followed by the placement of suction irrigation tubes. The iliac donor site was reconstructed with homologous bone and a Kirschner wire. Three weeks later a posterior bone graft was applied, and the ESSF device was applied from L3 to L5 in mild compression. The patient ambulated 7 days after the second operation, the ESSF device was removed at 12 weeks, and a body cast was worn for 4 weeks.

**c** At 45 months after surgery the fusion is consolidated, and the patient has no complaints referable to the spine

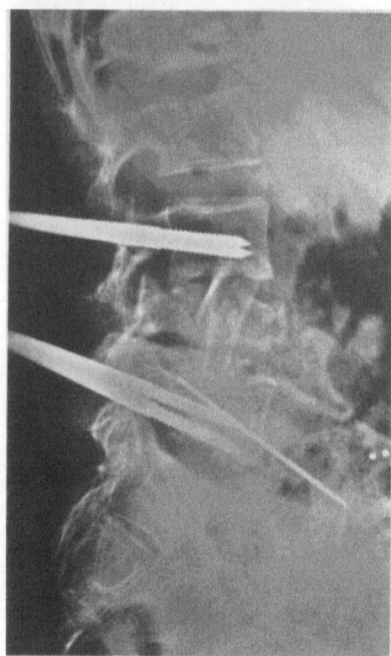

b

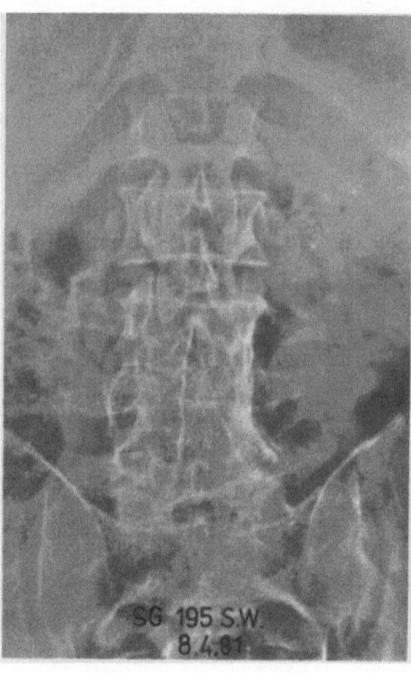

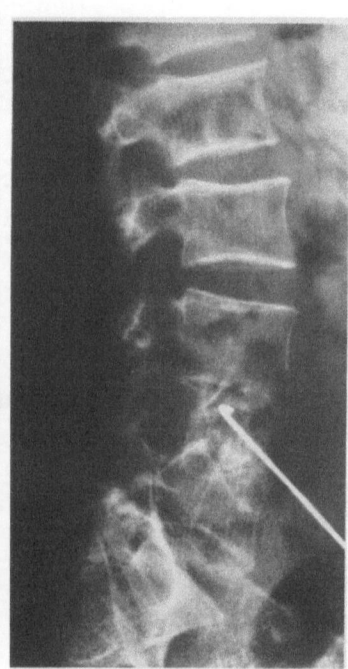

c

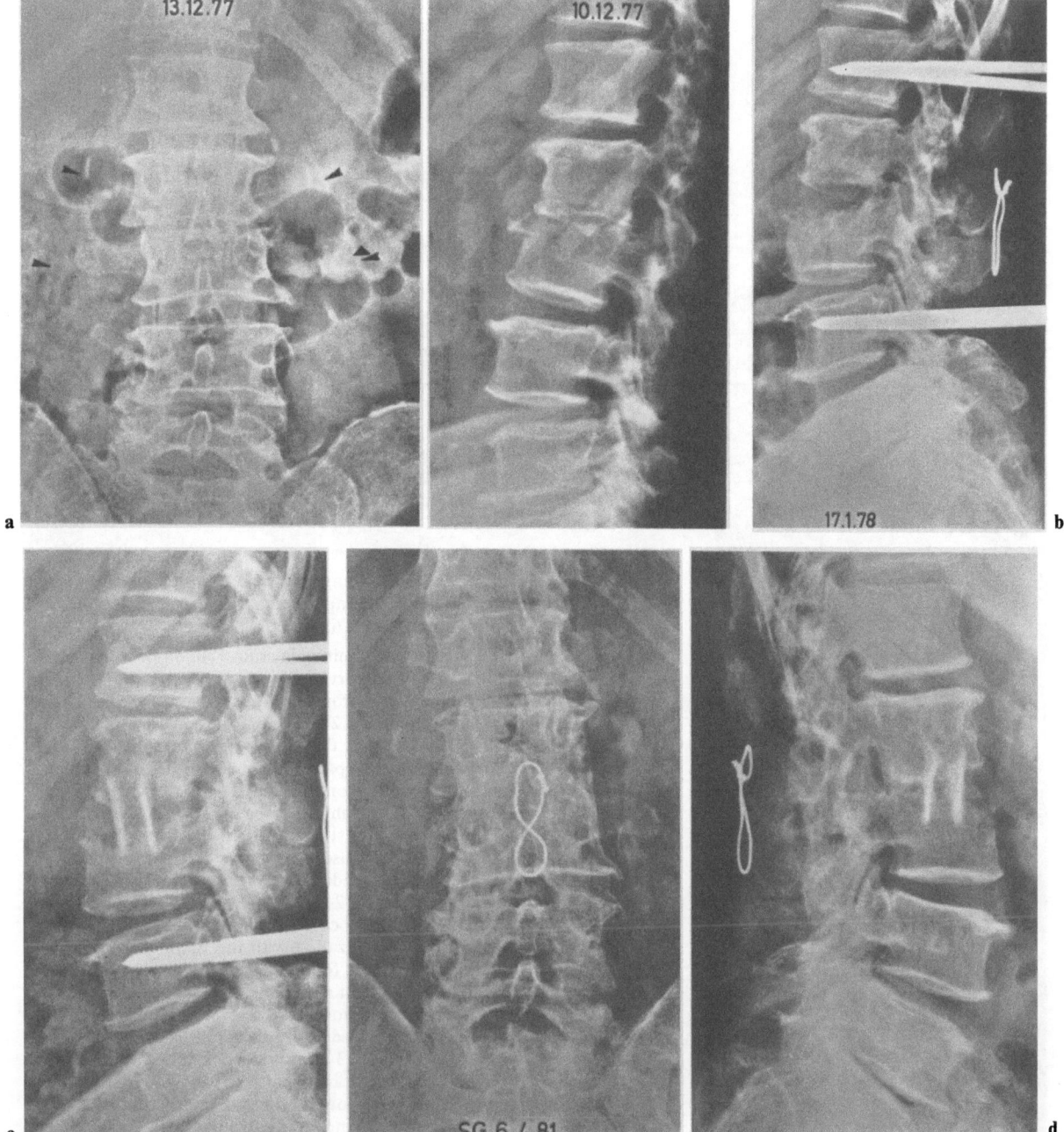

**Fig. 358 a–d.** Two-stage procedure for staphylococcal spondylitis involving the L2 disc space. G.J., 1909, 68 years, ♂, 214196.

**a** The patient had septicemia following conservative treatment abroad for spondylitis of L2–3 caused by *Staphylococcus aureus*. He had a large psoas abscess on the left side and mild neurologic symptoms.

**b** The first operation consisted of a posterior fusion of L2–3 and stabilization with the ESSF device from L1 to L4 in moderate distraction. The patient was repositioned, whereupon the abscess was evacuated and debrided, and suction irrigation was established. Ambulation was begun eight days after surgery.

**c** The second operation had to be delayed for eight weeks due to internal complications. The procedure consisted in an interbody fusion with a compression-resistant iliac bone graft. A wound smear obtained at that time was sterile. The patient ambulated six days after surgery, and the ESSF device was removed after 14 weeks, at which time a lumbar corset was prescribed.

**d** Forty months postoperatively the fusions are consolidated. The patient has no spine-associated complaints, and his activity level is normal for his age

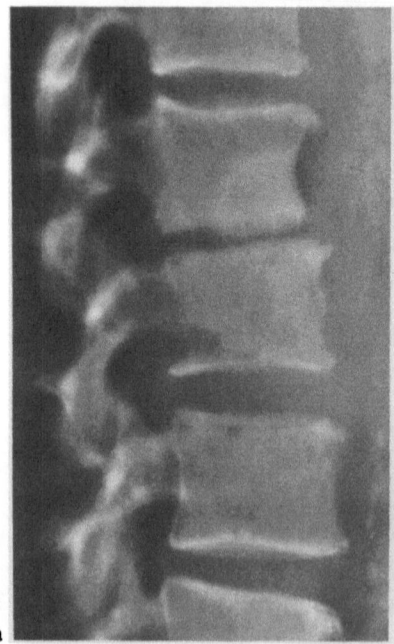
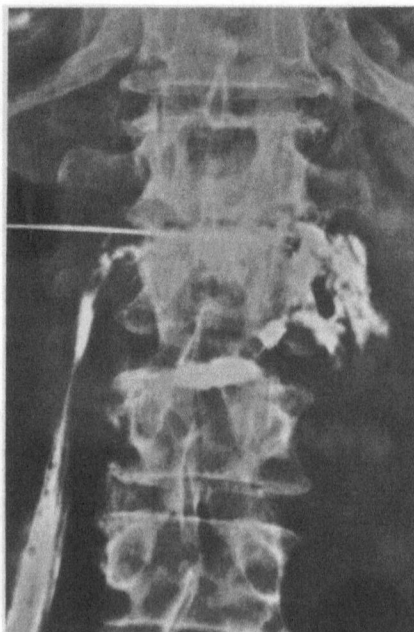
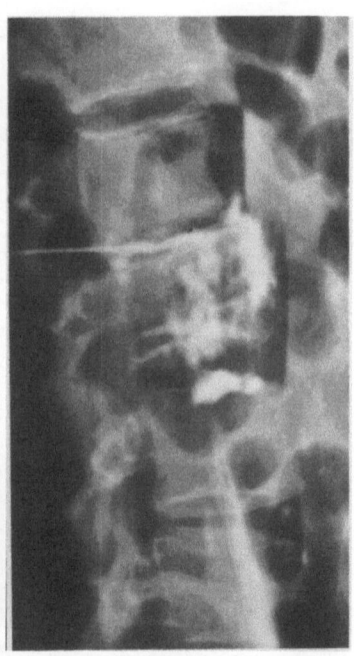

a

b

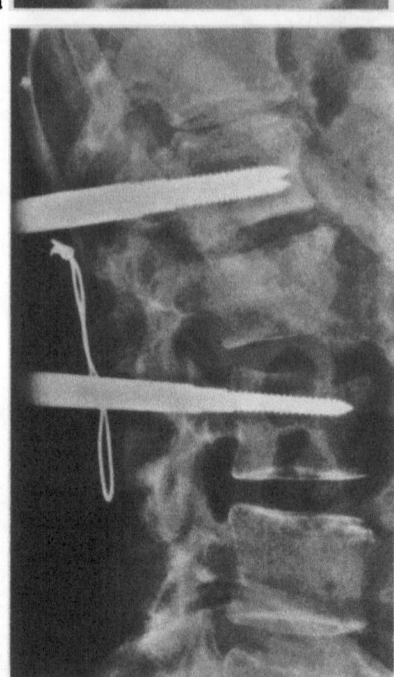

c

**Fig. 359 a–e.** Two-stage procedure with repositioning of the ESSF device during the treatment of *E. coli* spondylitis of L1–3. R.H., 1916, 65 years, ♂, 247749.

**a** The patient was admitted in critical condition, having been treated abroad conservatively for an *E. coli* spondylitis of L1–3. There was narrowing of the 1st disc space, and small foci were present in L2 and under the end plate of L3.

**b** During discography the contrast medium spreads through the 1st lumbar disc space, filling a left-sided paravertebral abscess of irregular contour and a small tubular paravertebral abscess on the right side. The spindle-shaped paravertebral depot of contrast material arising from that area is an artefact in the muscle. From the left paravertebral abscess the contrast medium flows through a channel in L2 to the center of the L2–3 disc.

**c** The first operation consisted in a posterior fusion from L1 to L3 and stabilization with the ESSF device over the same levels. This was followed by debridement and suction irrigation. The patient ambulated two days after surgery.

**d** The second operation was performed 19 days after the first. Because the need to resect additional bone from the upper part of the L3 vertebral body could not be ruled out, the caudal pair of Schanz screws was removed and reinserted one level lower. Then an interbody fusion from L1 to L3 was performed using two hydroxyl apatite blocks supplemented by cancellous bone in the upper segment and corticocancellous grafts in the lower segment. A wound smear showed no evidence of infection. Ambulation was started 2 days postoperatively, the ESSF device was removed at 22 weeks, and a 3-point brace and lumbar corset were worn a total of 12 weeks.

**e** At 29 months postoperatively the fusions are solid. The patient reports pain at the graft donor site but has no significant spine-associated complaints and is normally active for his age

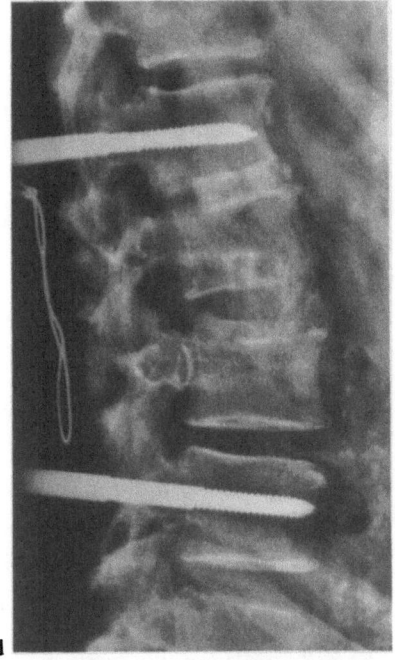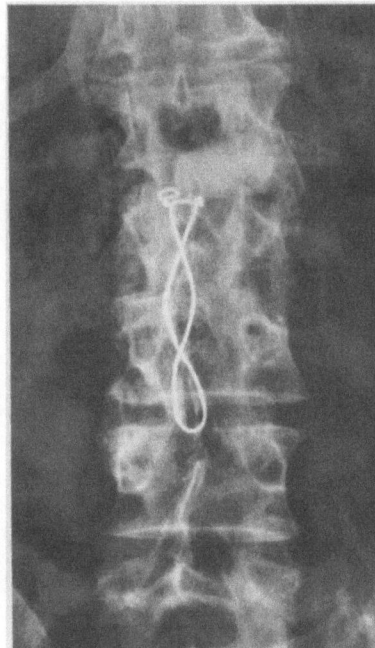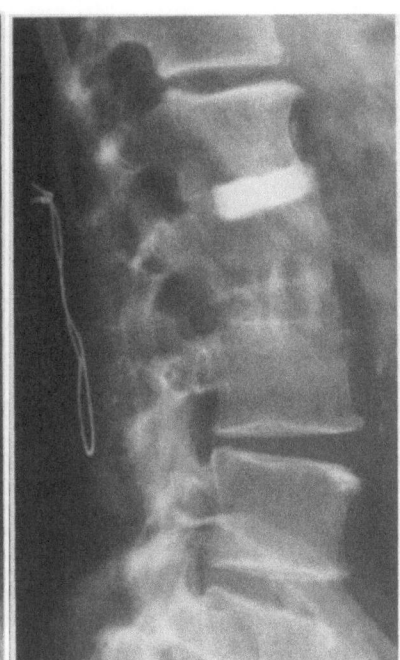

d

e

**Fig. 359 d, e**

→

**Fig. 360 a–e.** Two-stage procedure for tuberculous spondylitis of T11–12 with severe instability and paraplegia. K.L., 1910, 71 years, ♀, 246 527.

**a** The patient was admitted to another clinic for progressive sensory and motor deficits with urinary and fecal incontinence. She also had severe back pain with kyphotic deformity. Roentgenograms showed destruction of the T11 and T12 vertebral bodies.

**b** In myelography, a blockage of contrast medium was discovered at the T12 level. Tumor was suspected, and a broad decompressive laminectomy was performed, whereupon the neurologic deficits regressed. The deficits returned when the patient was ambulated.

**c** A myelogram obtained shortly before the patient was referred to our facility showed a marked narrowing of the dural sac at the T11–12 level with posterior displacement of T11.

**d** On admission the laminectomy wound was found to be contaminated, and aspiration of the spondylitic focus yielded pus. During the same anesthesia the spine was realigned, and the ESSF device was applied percutaneously from T10 to L1 in distraction. The neurologic deficits regressed quickly. The patient was able to ambulate 13 days after surgery. Two days later the focus was debrided and an interbody fusion was performed via the transthoracic route. The large defect was filled with methyl methacrylate and rib grafts. The cement plug was secured with a plate to prevent its posterior migration. The postoperative course was uneventful. The patient ambulated 3 days after surgery, the ESSF device was removed at 15 weeks, and a lumbar corset was applied.

**e** At 36 months the plate has become loose, but otherwise the area of the fusion is unchanged. The patient has moderate pain. Her walking distance is reduced but she is able to keep house without assistance. *Note:* Due to the size of the defect and the high degree of anterior and posterior instability, we saw at this time no other way of making the elderly woman ambulatory in the forseeable future.

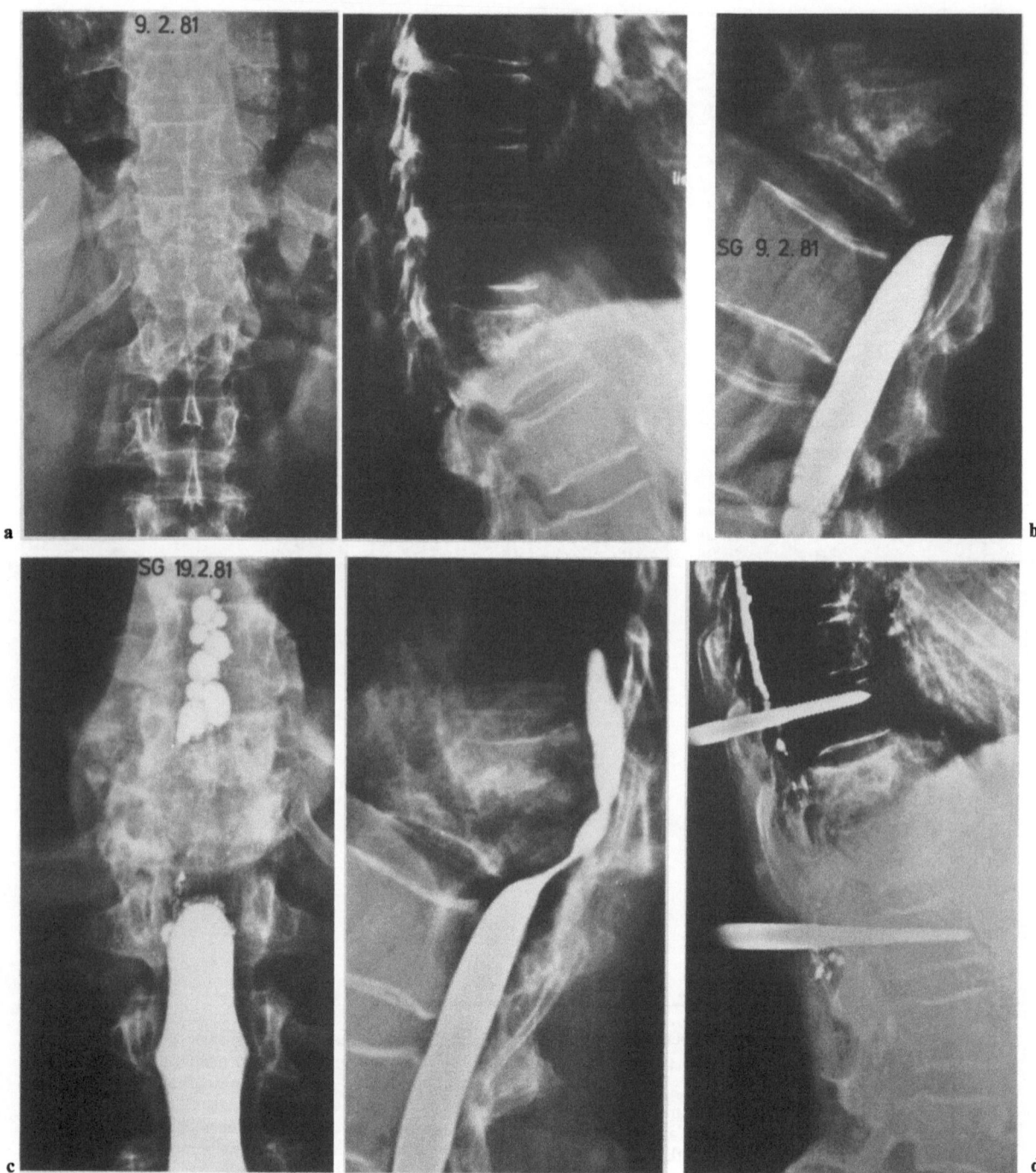

**Fig. 360a–d.** Legend see p. 355

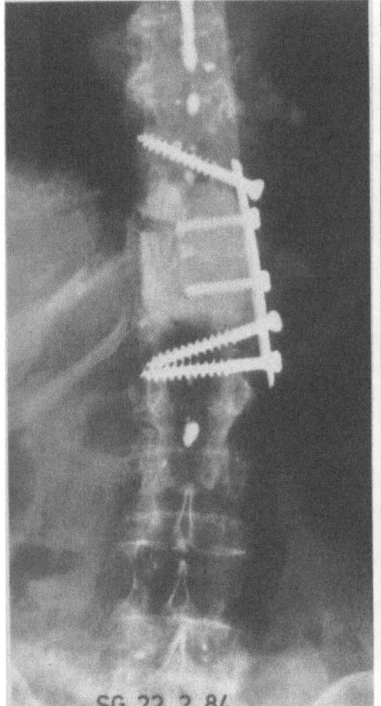

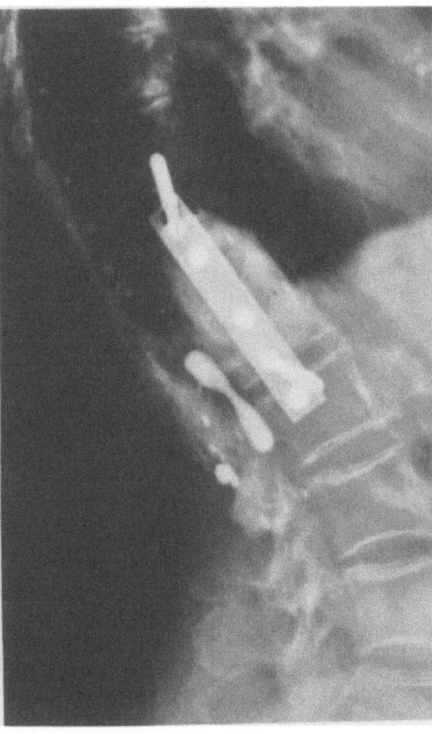

**Fig. 360e.** Legend see p. 355

**Fig. 361 a–d.** Single-stage procedure for tuberculous spondylitis of L3–4 with severe instability. P.M., 1906, 76 years, ♀, 259483.

**a** The patient presented with destructive changes about the L3–4 disc space, displacement of the L3 vertebra, kyphosis and scoliosis. She had mild but progressive neurologic deficits on the left side.

**b** Tomography, showing destruction at L3–4.

**c** In one sitting we performed a posterior fusion with cancellous bone grafting and stabilization with the ESSF device. The patient was then repositioned for debridement and an interbody fusion with cancellous bone and a full-thickness iliac block. An anterior plate was applied to secure the iliac graft. Severe osteoporosis precluded the use of a posterior tension band. This condition also greatly reduced the compression resistance of the interbody fusion; hence the ESSF device was applied in moderate distraction. The patient was permitted to walk 4 days after surgery, the ESSF device was removed at 17 weeks, and a lumbar corset was prescribed.

**d** Fifteen months postoperatively the fusion is consolidated, and residual scoliosis is present. The neurologic deficits have regressed completely. The patient is free of complaints and is normally active for her age

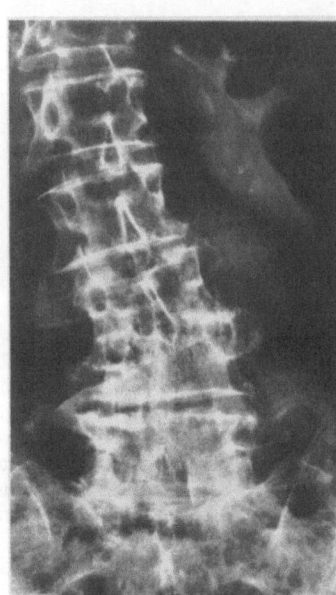

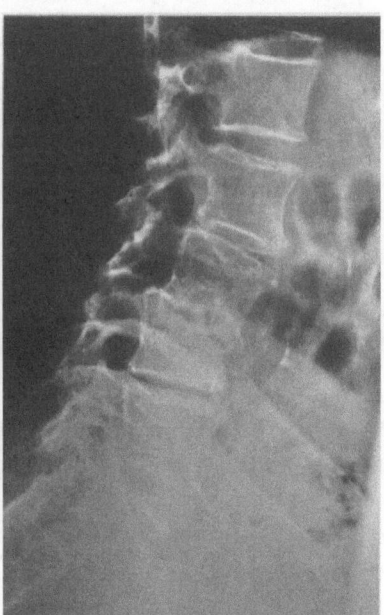

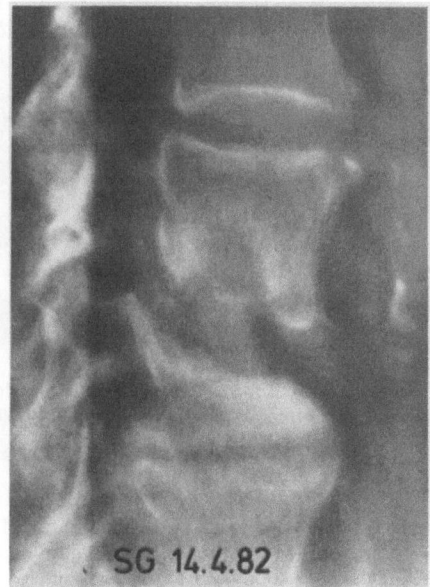

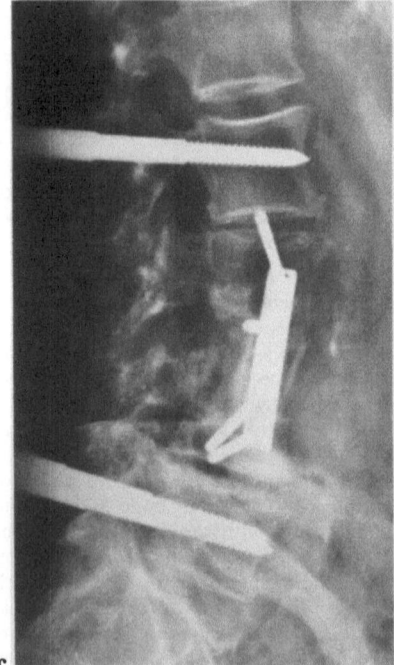
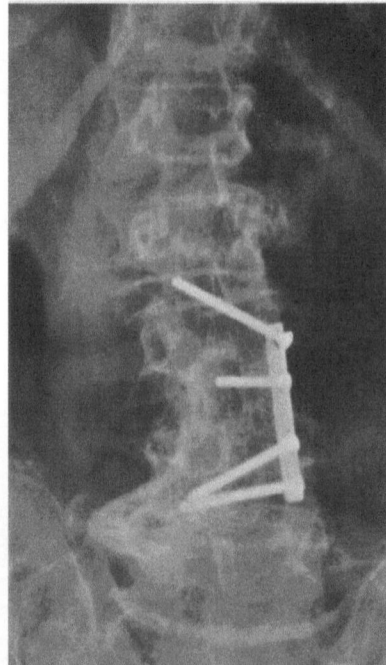
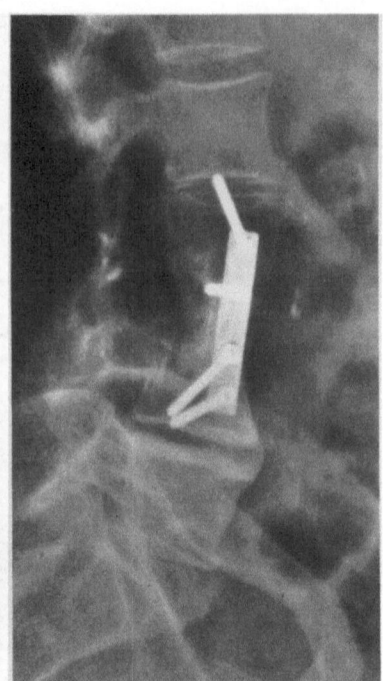

c                                                                      d

**Fig. 361 c, d.** Legend see p. 357

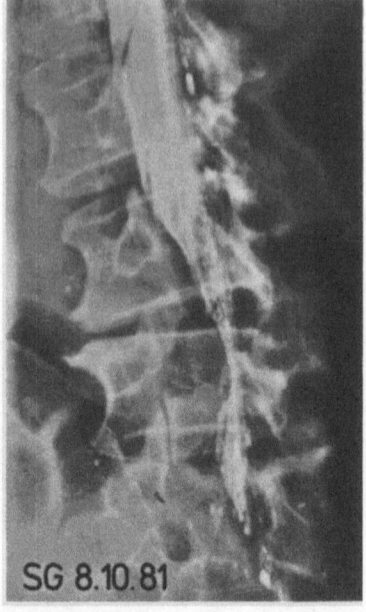
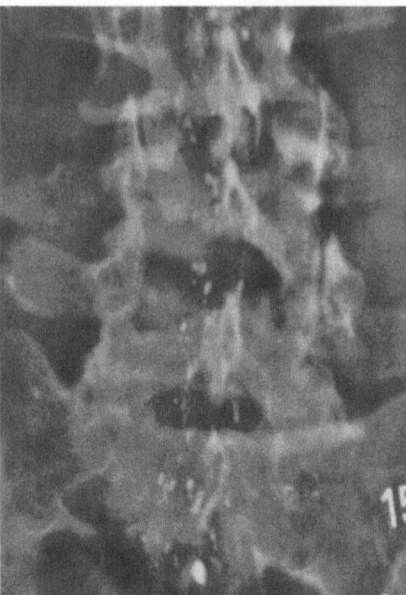
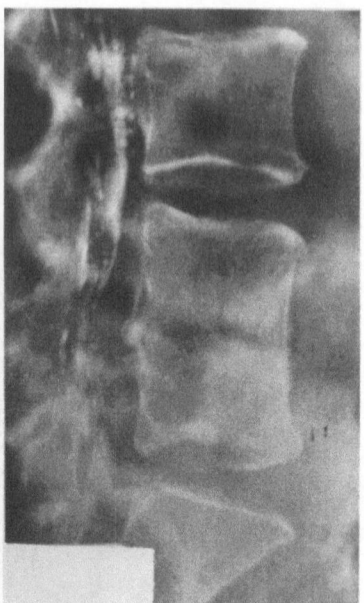

a    SG 8.10.81                                                        b

**Fig. 362 a–e.** Indirect treatment of staphylococcal spondylitis of L3–4. G.W., 1932, 48 years, ♀, 147203.

**a** Status three months prior to referral: discitis of L4–5 and an epidural abscess following surgery for a herniated disc. The epidural abscess was evacuated.

**b** On admission there was collapse of the L4 disc with rarefaction of the adjacent vertebral cancellous bone and a large cavity in the body of L5. The right inferior articular process of L4 was absent. The patient had a scoliotic deformity with back pain and ischialgia, and sensation in the right leg was impaired. Mild constitutional symptoms were present. CT disclosed a large abscess cavity in L5 and small foci in L4, with no evidence of an epidural abscess or disc herniation. Aspiration of the disc space revealed the presence of *Staphylococcus aureus*.

**c** The ESSF device was applied percutaneously in slight compression with the caudal Schanz screws anchored in the ilia. Ambulation was begun four days postoperatively.

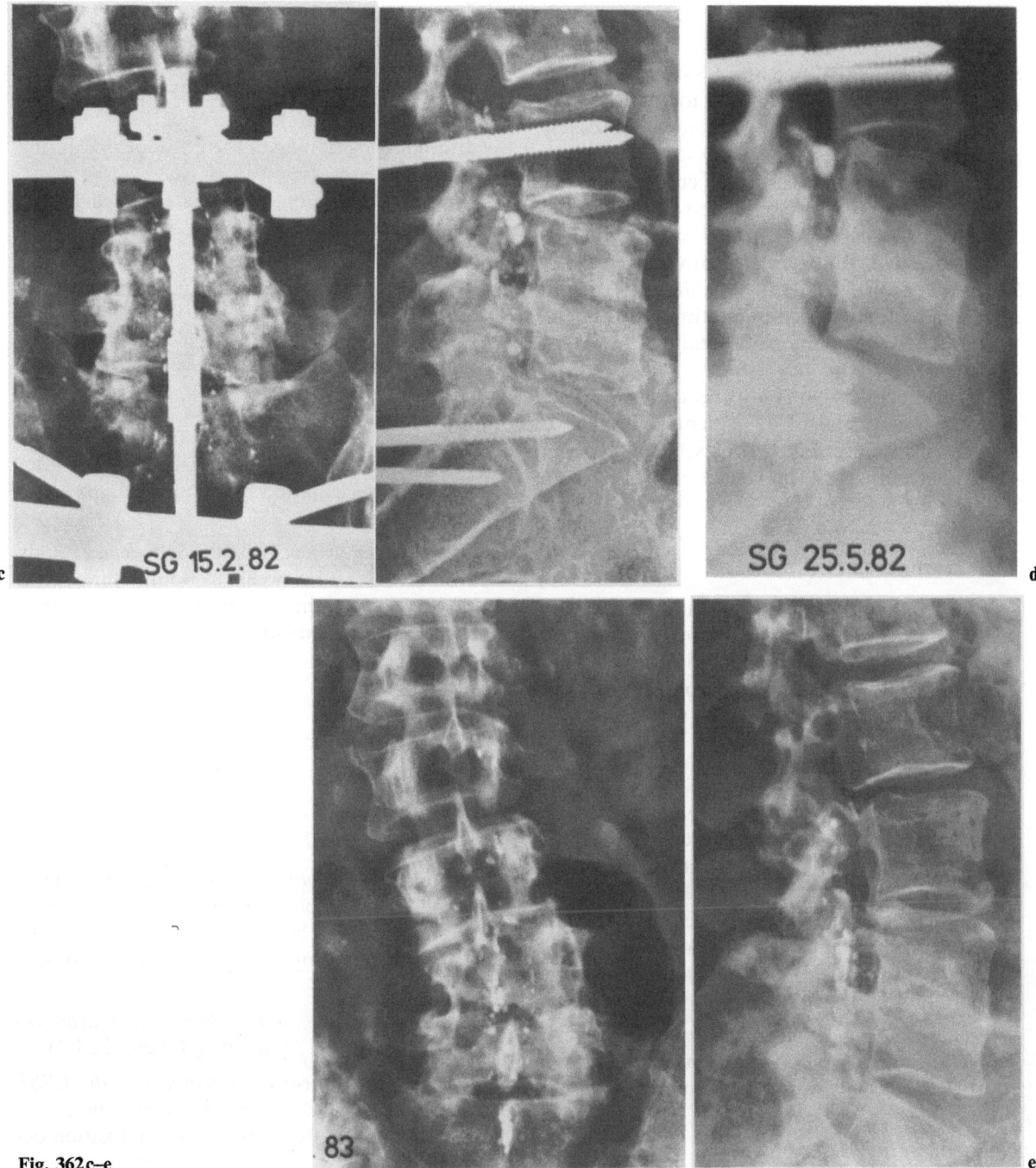

**Fig. 362c–e**

**d** At 18 weeks postoperatively there is spontaneous fusion of L4–5, and an abscess cavity is no longer visible. At this time, the ESSF device was removed, and subsequently a lumbar corset worn for four weeks.
**e** 19 months postoperatively, spontaneous anterior fusion is present. The degree of the scoliosis is the same as preoperatively. There are no signs of persisting infection. The patient has moderate complaints dependent upon physical activity. Ischialgia and sensory impairment as before disc surgery

## 12 Results of Treatment

Since 1977 we have used the ESSF device in 70 patients ranging in age from 15 to 76 years. The indications were as follows: fractures (59 cases), osteomyelitis (9 cases), instability secondary to extensive laminectomy (1 case), and chronic instability secondary to multiple operations (1 case).

The first 12 cases were treated with the conventional threaded rod external fixator of the ASIF. Three cases were stabilized with the ESSF device applied in a coupled configuration. All patients were followed regularly until treatment was concluded.

A recent follow-up study was done (MAGERL, in press) on a total of 52 patients (39 men, 13 women) who were followed closely for a period of at least one year. The results of the study are outlined below:

### 12.1 Fractures (T11–L5)

Forty-two fracture patients ranging in age from 15–56 years (average 33 years) were reviewed. Injuries were classified according to the system of MCAFEE et al. (1983), and neurologic complications according to FRANKEL et al. (1969).

#### 12.1.1 Injuries

*Types of injuries:* Three wedge-compression fractures, 3 incomplete burst fractures, 28 complete burst fractures, 6 flexion-distraction injuries, 2 translational injuries.

Two patients had two unstable injuries (L1–3, L3–5). Thirteen patients had 21 additional stable injuries of the cervical, thoracic and lumbar spine (19 vertebral body fractures).

*Neurologic complications:* Twenty patients had Grade D neurologic complications ranging from root lesions to an incomplete cauda equina syndrome.

*Concomitant injuries:* 16 patients.

#### 12.1.2 Treatment

*Time of operation:* 0–29 days, average of 7 days postinjury.

*Operative treatment:* ESSF device without fusion in 4 cases. ESSF device with posterior fusion in 36 cases (23 one-level fusions, 13 two-level fusions). ESSF device with posterior interbody fusion in 1 case. ESSF with spondylectomy and interbody fusion in 1 case.

Laminectomy: 3 cases.
Transpedicular vertebral-body cancellous bone graft: 3 cases.
Closed application of the ESSF device: 7 cases (5 after wound closure).
Closed repositioning of the ESSF device during treatment: 1 case.
Number of motion segments spanned by the ESSF device: 1 in 1 case, 2 in 38 cases, 4 in 3 cases (1 coupled assembly).

*Ambulation:* After 6 days on the average (2–41 days).

*Length of hospitalization:* Average of 26 days (13–49 days).

*Removal of ESSF device:* After 7–28 weeks. In the last 20 cases the device was removed after an average of 18.5 weeks. One early removal after 7 weeks was necessitated by a loose Schanz screw (cf. Sect. 12.1.4).

*Treatment after removal of the ESSF device:* Body cast in 11 cases (4–8 weeks), 3-point brace in 2 cases (6 weeks), lumbar corset in 15 cases (6–8 weeks). Fourteen patients did not require a brace or corset.

#### 12.1.3 Results of Treatment

*Length of follow-up:* 27 months (12–60 months).

*Nonunions:* None.

*Spontaneous anterior fusion:* 14 patients.

*Correction of traumatic kyphosis:* In 21 patients the kyphosis could be accurately assessed preoperatively and ranged betwen 20° and 42° (average 29°). The final postoperative kyphosis was 0°–20° (average 10°).

*Measurable collapse of vertebral bodies after removal of the device:* 3 patients (cf. Sect. 12.1.4).

*Collapse of disc spaces after removal of the ESSF device:* In most cases, damaged intervertebral discs collapsed shortly after removal of the fixation device. The resulting kyphotic angulation was approximately 4° per disc.

*Assessment of results:*
Excellent (no complaints or occasional moderate complaints during heavy physical labor): 22 patients.

Good (occasional moderate complaints without impairment of physical activity): 11 patients.

Fair (occasional moderate complaints during moderately heavy physical labor; unable to perform heavy labor): 7 patients.

Poor (constant complaints without invalidism; occasional analgesic therapy): 2 patients.

### 12.1.4 Complications

Nine complications occurred in nine patients:

- Partial collapse of a reduced vertebral body in three patients. Two were due to premature removal of the ESSF device. In one early case collapse was caused by a technical error during assembly of the ASIF threaded rod fixator. This patient also had severe osteoporosis secondary to lactose intolerance. Final kyphosis in these patients did not exceed 20°.
  Two of the patients required a subsequent interbody fusion because of pain. The clinical result was poor.
  The third patient required eight additional weeks of immobilization in a hyperextension body cast. Residual kyphosis was 15–18°. The clinical result was excellent.
- A superficial wound infection developed in one patient, and a seroma in another. These were treated by evacuation and aspiration, and an uneventful course ensued.
- Loosening of Schanz screws occurred in three patients. These screws had not been angled sufficiently at insertion and consequently broke through the lateral wall of the vertebral body. In one case severe pain and some febrile episodes necessitated removal of the device after seven weeks. This patient was then treated with a hyperextension body cast (seven weeks). In the remaining two patients the loosening was not recognized until the fixation device was removed. These patients were experiencing recurrent, radiating pain on motion (see Sect. 10.1) and a few episodes of intermittent fever.
- In one patient, painful skin tension around a Schanz screw had to be released with a second incision.

### 12.2 Spondylitis

Eight patients ranging from 23 to 76 years of age (average 54 years) were reviewed.

### 12.2.1 Causative Organisms, Localization, Findings

*Staphylococcus aureus* was causative in three cases (L2–3, L4, L4–5). Two cases had a hematogenous cause, and one was secondary to a laminectomy performed abroad. The patients with hematogenous spondylitis were in critical condition on admission following primary conservative treatment. One had a large psoas abscess. In the patient with postlaminectomy infection, an epidural abscess had been evacuated prior to referral. The spondylitis persisted. All three patients had mild neurologic symptoms.

*Escherichia coli* was causative in two patients (L1–2, L1–3), who were in critical condition following conservative therapy. One patient had a flat epidural abscess.

*Tuberculous spondylitis* was present in two cases (T11–12, L3). Both had massive destruction and instability. Mild neurologic symptoms were present in one case. The second patient, a woman, underwent a laminectomy abroad for incipient paraplegia. After ambulation was initiated, the paraplegia recurred due to gross instability. On admission the laminectomy wound was infected.

*Salmonella Emek* was causative in one patient (L2–3).

### 12.2.2 Treatment

*Operative treatment:*

*Two-stage procedure with direct focal treatment:* 6 cases. The average interval between the two procedures was 3 weeks.

*Single-stage procedure with direct focal treatment:* 1 case.

*Indirect treatment:* 1 case (postlaminectomy spondylitis caused by *Staphylococcus aureus*).

During direct focal treatment, corticocancellous blocks were inserted into the disc space in three patients, and hydroxyl apatite blocks impregnated with antibiotic (Nebacetin®) were implanted in three other patients (cf. Sect. 9.1). The seventh patient was a 71-year-old woman with tuberculous spondylitis of T11–12 and paraplegia. In view of the patient's age, we chose to use methyl methacrylate and rib grafts to fill the interbody defect.

*Ambulation:* All, but the first (Fig. 357) patients, began ambulation an average of 6 days (2–13 days) after surgery.

*Length of hospitalization:* Average of 54 days (24–105 days).

*Removal of the ESSF device:* After 17 weeks on the average (12–22 weeks).

*Further treatment:* Body cast in 1 case (6 weeks), 3-point extension brace in 4 cases (4–12 weeks), lumbar corset in 3 cases (4–6 weeks).

### 12.2.3 Results of Treatment

*Length of follow-up:* Average of 28 months (15–46 months).

*Nonunions:* None.

*Secondary deformity:* None.

*Recurrence of spondylitis:* None.

*Neurologic complications:* All regressed completely.

*Disability and complaints:* Two patients had no complaints and were able to return to their former occupations.

Four patients who already were retired were able to pursue their normal activities without significant complaints.

The patient with postlaminectomy *Staph. aureus* spondylitis had the same complaints as prior to the laminectomy.

The patient with tuberculous spondylitis and paraplegia complained of moderate pain. She wore a lumbar brace for long walks and still required two crutches at the conclusion of the study; subsequently she was able to walk without canes or crutches.

### 12.2.4 Complications

Three complications occurred in three patients:

- One hematoma at the donor site of the iliac graft, which was surgically evacuated.
- One case of skin tension at a Schanz screw, which was released by incision.
- One patient with staphylococcal sepsis had multiple internal complications which resolved with medical treatment.

### 12.3 Other Indications

This group included two patients 38 and 48 years of age.

The first patient underwent a posterior fusion of L3–4 due to instability and persistent pain secondary to previous laminectomies and fusions from L4 to S1. The ESSF device was applied from L3 to L4. The patient was ambulatory at 5 days and was discharged after 14 days. The ESSF device was removed after 12 weeks, and a lumbar corset was applied. The fusion united without complications. The result at 56 months was poor.

The second patient had to undergo an extensive laminectomy with removal of facet joints and neurolysis of the cauda equina due to progressive neurologic deficits one year after sustaining a complete burst fracture of L2. The site was stabilized by fusion and external fixation from L1 to L3. The patient was ambulatory at 5 days and was discharged after 63 days. The ESSF device was removed after 12 weeks, and a body cast was worn for 6 weeks. Consolidation of the fusion was obtained. After a transient exacerbation, the patient experienced a partial remission of neurologic symptoms. The result at 49 months was fair.

# 13 Discussion of the Method of Treatment

In the preceding chapters we have discussed indications and biomechanical principles, presented the results, and described the surgical technique in detail.

Now, we must raise several questions: What does the method accomplish? What are its risks, advantages and disadvantages? What developments may be expected in the future?

There is no question that external skeletal fixation of the spine is in every sense a demanding procedure. The question as to whether this method may be performed by other surgeons experienced in spinal surgery, may be answered positively. The results reported here represent the work of ten surgeons at our center.

Objections that have been raised against ESSF relate mainly to the transpedicular implantation of the Schanz screws and the risk of infection.

The principal danger of transpedicular screw implantation is the possibility of damage to neural structures. Another is the potential injury to the major blood vessels which lie anterior to the spine. Although the fact that no such injuries have yet occurred in our experience with this procedure does not refute these dangers, it does put them into perspective. Of course, a thorough knowledge of anatomy and a meticulous technique are absolute prerequisites for a safe operation.

The danger of deep infection by organisms introduced from the environment appears to be minimal if the Schanz screws are correctly introduced and anchored. In the cases treated to date we have observed no instance of deep infection, and only recently have we encountered a significant screw track infection. In this case gross loosening of the Schanz screw had developed as a result of faulty implantation. The ESSF device was removed at once and a plaster body jacket applied, whereupon the infection resolved completely.

R. WATKINS attempted in collaboration with A. BEKIER[1] to find evidence of smoldering infection in the tissues around former screw sites (not published). They did this by performing scintigraphic studies ($^{99m}$Tc-phosphate, $^{67}$Ga-citrate) on the first 23 patients, who were recalled to the center some time after their fractures had healed. No evidence of infection was found.

1 Director of the Nuclear Medicine Institute of the Kantonsspital St. Gallen

Another potential complication of spinal external fixation is the collapse of a vertebral body following removal of the device.

In 70 cases treated up to now there have been 5 instances of vertebral body collapse. Analysis of the cases showed conclusively that the vertebral bodies were not yet fully consolidated at the time the device was removed.

In 1972, TROJAN pointed out that a vertebral body, once healed, is no longer subject to collapse. However, later kyphotic angulation may occur at intervertebral spaces where discs have been damaged. This is entirely consistent with our own experience. Furthermore, our cases have shown that even a consolidated posterior fusion cannot prevent narrowing of the disc spaces. Evidently the bony mass of the posterior fusion undergoes plastic deformation when exposed to continuous bending loads. We have measured values of up to 6° kyphotic angulation per disc space (average 4°).

Misjudging the true nature of an injury, i.e. mistaking a distraction injury for a compression injury, may lead to the use of the ESSF device in an inappropriate mode. This risk arises mainly when the device is applied percutaneously. Two such cases occurred recently, and in both we were able to correct the error promptly. These cases underscore the importance of an accurate preoperative diagnosis. If doubt exists, open stabilization is preferred to the percutaneous technique, as this will restore tension resistance and permit the injury to be stabilized in distraction.

In analyzing the advantages and disadvantages of the ESSF device, one is struck first by the disadvantages that are inherent to external skeletal fixation. Above all, the ESSF entails a demanding postoperative course. It requires reliability and cooperation on the part of the patient and persons giving nursing care. The method is less comfortable and convenient than internal fixation techniques where no large brace or plaster body jacket is required postoperatively.

Despite the difficulties of postoperative care, the great majority of our patients readily accepted the spinal fixation device. There was only one case in which the device had to be removed prematurely because the patient was no longer able to tolerate it. It should be added that this patient also had difficulty tolerating a plaster jacket. The remaining patients considered freedom of movement to be more important than the inconveniences associated with the ESSF device.

The disadvantages are counterbalanced by a number of advantages:

- Owing to the adaptability of the fixation system, all types of lower thoracic and lumbar spine injuries may be managed in the biomechanically adequate fashion.
- The ability to apply the device percutaneously offers new possibilities of efficient and individualized stabilization in orthopedic and trauma surgery.
- In the open treatment of injuries, *all* necessary measures generally may be carried out through the less invasive posterior approach.
- Since bulky implants are not used, there is no problem with large "dead spaces" (decreased risk of infection!), there is less damage to the muscles, and more space is available for the application of bone graft.
- Compared to conventional systems, the device provides greater stability while immobilizing fewer vertebral segments. With monosegmental injuries the device must span at most one intact motion segment.
- The patient may be ambulated early without a body cast or large brace. Functional aftercare is possible. The length of hospitalization is reduced. There is little restriction of the patient's activity level, and some patients were able to perform light physical work in their profession.
- The ESSF device can be removed as an outpatient procedure without general anesthesia.
- Even extremely difficult stabilization problems can be managed with the ESSF device.
- The method has potential for further development.

Many fractures of the 12th thoracic vertebra and lumbar spine may be reduced by the conservative method of Boehler and stabilized in a hyperextension body cast. This raises the question of indications for the ESSF device in fracture management. In our view the ESSF device is indicated whenever safety and constancy of results are a prime concern. Operative treatment and application of the ESSF device provide a more complete reduction, a far more reliable retention, and aftercare without a cumbersome body cast.

In the past we considered severe osteoporosis to be a contraindication to the use of the ESSF, fearing that the Schanz screws could not gain solid purchase in the soft bone. To date, however, we have experienced no problems of bone purchase in elderly patients with both spondylitis and severe osteoporosis. Today we consider osteoporosis to be no more than a relative contraindication.

Until recently we did not anchor the ESSF device above the level of T9. In a recent case, however, we had to align and stabilize the upper thoracic spine percutaneously with the ESSF device in a woman with high thoracic spondylitis associated with rapidly progressive paralysis, sepsis and paralytic ileus. Abscess drainage and irrigation also were done percutaneously through the pedicles. The extremely critical condition of the patient precluded any other form of treatment. The patient has recovered well. Although treatment is not yet complete and we are dealing with only one patient, the case nevertheless offers evidence that the ESSF device is suitable in principle for stabilizations of the thoracic spine. However, until more experience is gained, we intend to restrict applications in the middle and upper thoracic spine to special cases.

The preceding discussions reflect the current state of development of the new system. What could future developments be?

There is no question that the prolonged fixation time, which also is characteristic for Boehler's conservative therapy, places a substantial burden on the patient, who is motivated to assume this burden only by the hope of recovery. As shown, the duration of the external fixation depends on the time required for the defects in the vertebral body to reossify. It is reasonable to assume that this process is hastened by the use of cancellous bone grafts. Hence, we shall resume packing defects with cancellous bone, as described in Sect. 8.1.11 whenever open treatment is used.

On the other hand, we feel that in the past we have relied too heavily on posterior fusions, and thus on open treatment, in an effort to forestall painful osteoarthritis and osteochondrosis. In fractures where spontaneous anterior fusion may be anticipated or in fractures with small vertebral body defects and without significant damage to the facet joints, we now advocate primary percutaneous stabilization. Should a post-traumatic pain syndrome develop, a posterior fusion of the involved motion segment is carried out secondarily.

Another possibility would be to remove the ESSF device following adequate consolidation of the posterior column (at about eight weeks) and to apply a hyperextension body cast. This would have the advantage of obviating further care of the device. Interestingly, the patients to whom we have presented this option have so far declined to have their fixators removed.

To date the ESSF device has been used in the treatment of fractures and spondylitis. It remains to be determined whether the principle of the ESSF would also be useful for the treatment of spinal deformities or for the reduction of spondylolytic vertebral displacements.

To date, virtually all problems of temporary stabilization of the thoracolumbar and lumbar spine may be solved using the ESSF. It is conceivable, that the application of the ESSF offers additional, new therapeutic options in orthopaedic surgery. For instance, deformations of the spine might be corrected gradually with a corresponding external fixator. This may, compared to the methods used presently, be both more efficient and more secure in respect to their inherent risks.

In order to complete the discussion of the method of treatment, we must point out a new fixation device not mentioned previously, since it was still in clinical trial at the time this paper was written. This is the so-called "fixateur interne" (DICK 1984; DICK et al., in press).

In the fixateur interne anchorage is also assured by modified Schanz screws, inserted through the pedicles into the vertebral body. The longitudinal connection is established by clamps and threaded rods. The direction of the Schanz screws may be chosen freely. Since the parts of the fixateur interne have no mobile connections, immobilization may also be restricted to the two vertebrae neighbouring the fractured one. Furthermore, as in the ESSF, the fixateur interne may be used in distraction, compression or in neutral mode.

These are the decisive advantages of this system compared to other methods of internal fixation. The fact that this is an internal fixation, makes it more advantageous for those cases, in which external fixation is unsought for, because of the necessary aftercare.

Primary stability is slightly, and long-term stability considerably less than in the ESSF (personal experience). Therefore, in the treatment of fractures using the fixateur interne, major defects in the vertebral bodies, *must* be filled with cancellous bone graft, since otherwise the Schanz screws could break in fatigue. Finally, it should be mentioned, that the fixateur interne is still fairly large.

The ESSF remains the most versatile, stable and secure of all fixation systems presently known. We will continue to apply it in appropriate cases, where the advantages outweight the involved technique and aftercare.

## 14 Remarks

The following figures (some modified) have been taken from previous publications.

Fig. 312, published in „Verletzungen der Brust- und Lendenwirbelsäule" by F. MAGERL (1980), Langenbecks Arch. Chir 352:427, with the kind permission of Springer-Verlag

Fig. 300, 301, 307, 317, 331, published in "External skeletal fixation of the lower thoracic and the lumbar spine", by F. MAGERL in "Current Concepts of External Fixation of Fractures" Ed. by H.K. UHTHOFF (1982), p. 353, with kind permission of Springer-Verlag.

Fig. 315, published in "Stabilization of the lower thoracic and lumbar spine: Comparative in vitro investigation of an external skeletal and various internal fixation devices" by F. SCHLÄPFER, O. WÖRSDÖRFER, F. MAGERL and S.M. PERREN in "Current Concepts of External Fixation of Fractures" Ed. by H.K. UHTHOFF (1982), p. 367, with kind permission of authors and Springer-Verlag.

Fig. 319, 324–333, 338, 347, 349, 358, published in "clinical application on the thoracolumbar junction and the lumbar spine" by F. MAGERL in "External Skeletal Fixation", Ed. by D.C. MEARS (1983), p. 553, with kind permission of Williams & Wilkins.

Fig. 305–307, 310, 331, 334, 340, published in "Stabilization of the lower thoracic and lumbar spine with external skeletal fixation" by F. MAGERL, in "Clinical Orthopaedics and Related Research" with kind permission of J.B. Lippincott Company.

# References

## The ASIF Threaded Rod External Fixator in General Orthopaedic and Trauma Surgery of the Extremities

B.G. WEBER

Ackroyd CE, O'Connor BT, De Bruyn PF (1983) The severely injured limb. Churchill Livingstone, Edinburgh London Melbourne New York

Adrey J (1970) Le fixateur externe d'Hoffmann couplé en cadre. Etude biomécanique dans les fractures de jambe. Thèse, Montpellier: Gead, Paris

Allen BL jr (1982) Book review of: Brunner CF, Weber BG: Special techniques in internal fixation. Springer, Berlin Heidelberg New York 1982. J Bone Jt Surg [Am] 64:797

Allen BL jr (1982) Reply to Schweizer G, Porsche P: Letter to the Editor ref. Book review of: Brunner CF, Weber BG: Special techniques in internal fixation: Springer, Berlin Heidelberg New York 1982. J Bone Jt Surg [Am] 64:1401

Anderson R (1937) New method of employing skeletal traction. Northwest Medicine, October, 1931. (Cited after Splints by Tower Co., Seattle, Washington/USA)

Anderson R: An automatic method of treatment for fractures of the tibia and the fibula. Surg Gynecol Obstet 58:639

Anderson R, O'Neill G (1944) Comminuted fractures of the end of the radius. Surg Gynecol Obstet 78:434

Behrens F (1982) Unilateral external fixation for severe lower extremity lesions: Experience with the ASIF (AO) tubular frame. In: Seligson D, Popo MH (eds) Concepts in external fixation. Grune & Stratton, New York

Behrens F, Searls K (1982) Unilateral external fixation experience with the ASIF "tubular" frame. In: Uhthoff HK (eds) (1982) Current concepts of external fixation of fractures. Springer, Berlin Heidelberg New York

Böhler L (1963) Die Technik der Knochenbruchbehandlung. Maudrich, Wien

Boltze W-H (1976) Der Fixateur externe (Rohrsystem). AO-Bulletin, Bern

Boltze W-H (1976) Le fixateur externe (système tubulaire). O-Bulletin, Bern

Boltze W-H, Fernandez DL, Schatzker J (1976) The external fixator (tubular system). AO-Bulletin, Bern

Boltze W-H, Chiquet C, Niederer PG (1978) Der Fixateur externe (Rohrsystem). Stabilitätsprüfung. AO-Bulletin, Bern

Brooker AF, Edwards CC (1979) External fixation. The current state of the art. Williams & Wilkins, Baltimore

Brunner C (1975) Arthrodesis of the ankle joint. In: Chapchal G (ed) The Arthrodesis. Thieme, Stuttgart

Brunner C, Weber BG (1981) Besondere Osteosynthesetechniken. Springer, Berlin Heidelberg New York

Brunner C, Weber BG (1982) Special techniques in internal fixation. Springer, Berlin Heidelberg New York

Burny F (1968) Etude par jauges de déformation de la consolidation des fractures en clinique. Acta Orthop Belg 34:917

Burny F (1976) Biomécanique de la consolidation des fractures. Mesure de la rigidité du cal in vivo. Etude théorique, expérimentale et clinique. Application à la théorie de l'ostéosynthèse. Thèse d'agrégation, U.L.S.

Burny F (1979) Strain gauges measurements of fracture healing. A study of 350 cases. In: Brooker AF, Edwards CC (eds) External fixation, the current state of the art. Williams & Wilkins, Baltimore

Burny FL (1979) Elastic external fixation of tibial fractures: study of 1421 cases. In: Brooker AF, Edwards CC (eds) External fixation. The current state of the art. Williams & Wilkins, Baltimore

Burny F (1982) Hoffmann external half frame fixation. In: Uhthoff HK (ed) Current concepts of external fixation of fractures. Springer, Berlin Heidelberg New York

Burny F, Donkerwolcke M, Saric O (1982) Elastic external fixation of tibial fractures: Influence of associated internal fixation. In: Uhthoff HK (ed) Current concepts of external fixation of fractures. Springer, Berlin Heidelberg New York

Charnley J (1953) Compression arthrodesis. Livingstone, Edinburgh London

Charnley J (pers. comm.) "Mechanical feeling".

Connes H (1973) Le fixateur externe d'Hoffman en double cadre. Techniques, indications et résultats. A propos de 160 observations. Gead, Paris

Connes H (1977) Hoffmann's external anchorage; techniques, indications and results. Gead, Paris

Cuendet S (1936) Procédé de réduction des fractures de la diaphyse des deux os de l'avant-bras à l'aide de l'appareil à broches jumelées. Livre jubilaire, Albin Lambotte, Vromant, Bruxelles

Debrunner AM (1970) Die operative Behandlung von Gonarthrosen. Ergebnisse und Indikationen. In: Nicod L (Hrsg) Die Gonarthrose, vol. 97. Huber, Bern Stuttgart Wien

Dehne E (1961) The natural history of the fractured tibia. Surg Clin North Am 41:1495

Dehne E (1974) Ambulatory treatment of the fractured tibia. Clin Orthop 105:192

Green SA (1981) Complications of external skeletal fixation. Causes, prevention and treatment. Thomas, Springfield/Ill.

Helal B (1975) Metatarsal osteotomy for metatarsalgia. J Bone Jt Surg 57-B:187

Hierholzer G (1975) Stabilisierung des Knochenbruchs beim Weichteilschaden mit Fixateur externe. Langenbecks Arch klin Chir 39:505

Hierholzer G, Chernowitz A (1982) External fixation, tubular ASIF set. In: Uhthoff HK (ed) Current concepts of external fixation of fractures. Springer, Berlin Heidelberg New York

Hoffmann R (1938) Rotules à os pour la réduction dirigée, non sanglante des fractures (ostéotaxis). Helv Med Acta 844

Hoffmann R (1942) Percutane Frakturbehandlung. Chirurg 14:101

Hoffmann R (1951) L'ostéotaxis, ostéosynthèse transcutanée par fiches et rotules. Gead, Paris

Ilizarov L, Soibelmann LM (1969) Some clinical and experimental data concerning bloodless lengthening of lower extremities. Experimentalnaja Kirurgija i Ortopedije 4:27

Ilizarov L (1976) Results of clinical tests an experience obtained from the clinical use of the set of Ilizarov compression-distration apparatus. Med Export, Moscow

Ilizarov L: Zit n. Cech O (1982) Stabilni osteosynteza v traumatologii a ortopedii. Avicenum, Praha

Jörg P (1984) Der Fixateur externe, Spindelsystem. Inaugural-Dissertation zur Erlangung der Doktorwürde der Med. Fakultät der Universität Bern

Judet R, Judet J, Lagrange L (1956) Traitement des pseudarthroses par la compression osseuse simple. Mém Acad Chir 82:402

Lambotte A (1907) L'intervention opératoire dans les fractures. Lamartin, Bruxelles

Lambotte A (1907) Le traitement des fractures. Masson, Paris

Lambotte A (1913) Chirurgie opératoire des fractures. Masson, Paris

Matheson JAL (1953) The force employed in compression arthrodesis of the knee. In: Charnley J (ed) Compression arthrodesis. Livingstone, Edinburgh London

McFarland B (1951) Pseudarthrosis of the tibia in childhood. J Bone Jt Surg [Br] 433:36

Mears DC, Fu F (1980) Modern concepts of external fixation. Clin Orthop 151:65

Mears DC (1983) External skeletal fixation. Williams & Wilkins, Baltimore London

Müller ME (1955) Die Kompressionsosteosynthese unter besonderer Berücksichtigung der Kniearthrodese. Helv Chir Acta 6:474

Müller ME (1957) Die hüftnahen Femurosteotomien. Thieme, Stuttgart

Müller ME, Allgöwer M (1958) Zur Behandlung der Pseudarthrosen. Helv Chir Acta 25:253

Müller ME, Allgöwer M, Willenegger H (1963) Technik der operativen Frakturenbehandlung. Springer, Berlin Göttingen Heidelberg

Müller ME (1966) Treatment of non-unions by compression. Clin Orthop 43:83

Müller ME (1967) Hip surgery. Twelve hip procedures. AO-Bulletin, Bern

Müller ME, Allgöwer M, Willenegger H (1969) Manual der Osteosynthese. Springer, Berlin Heidelberg New York

Müller ME, Allgöwer M, Willenegger H (1970) Manual of internal fixation of fractures. Springer, Berlin Heidelberg New York

Müller ME, Allgöwer M, Schneider R, Willenegger H (1977) Manual der Osteosynthese, 2nd ed. Springer, Berlin Heidelberg New York

Müller ME, Allgöwer M, Schneider R, Willenegger H (1979) Manual of internal fixation. Springer, Berlin Heidelberg New York

Nicholson OR (1957) Longitudinal osteotomy of the tibia (The "reed" osteotomy). J Bone Jt Surg [Br] 39:738

Pauwels F (1940) Grundriss einer Biomechanik der Frakturheilung. Verh Dtsch Orthop Ges 34

Pauwels F (1965) Grundriß einer Biomechanik der Frakturheilung. In: Pauwels F (Hrsg) Gesammelte Abhandlungen zur funktionellen Anatomie des Bewegungsapparates. Springer, Berlin Heidelberg New York

Pelet D, Berruex P (1976) Résultats après arthrodèse tibiotarsienne. Verh Soc Belge Chir Pied 101

Pelet D, Weber BG (1978) L'arthrodèse tibio-tarsienne pri-

maire dans les lésions traumatiques de l'astragale. Actual Méd Chir Pied 21:233

Perren SM, Hayes W (1971) Flexoral rigidity of compression plate fixation of fractures. Proc Second Nordic meeting on Medical and Biological Engineering, Oslo

Pohler O, Straumann F (1975) Charakteristik der AO-Implantate aus rostfreiem Stahl. AO-Bulletin, Bern

Pohler O, Straumann F (1975) Characteristics of the stainless steel ASIF/AO implants. AO-Bulletin, Bern

Sarmiento A (1970) A functional below-knee brace for tibial fractures. J Bone Jt Surg [Am] 52:295

Sarmiento A (1972) Functional bracing of tibial and femoral shaft fractures. Clin Orthop 105:202

Sarmiento A, Matta LL (1981) Closed functional treatment of fractures. Springer, Berlin Heidelberg New York

Schenk R, Willenegger H (1964) Zur Histologie der primären Knochenheilung. Langenbeck's Arch Klin Chir 308:440

Schenk R, Willenegger H (1967) Morphological findings in primary fracture healing. Symp Biol Hung 7:75

Schenk RK (1977) Histologie der Frakturheilung und der Pseudarthrosen. AO-Bulletin, Bern

Schenk RK (1978) Histology of fracture repair and nonunion. AO-Bulletin, Bern

Schenk RK (1979) Histologie de la consolidation des fractures et des pseudarthroses. AO-Bulletin, Bern

Schlössmann: cit. acc. Pauwels F (1965) Grundriß einer Biomechanik der Frakturheilung. In: Gesammelte Abhandlungen zur funktionellen Anatomie des Bewegungsapparates. Springer, Berlin Heidelberg New York

Schneider R (1982) Die Totalprothese der Hüfte. Huber, Bern Stuttgart Wien

Steinmann F (1919) Lehrbuch der funktionellen Behandlung der Knochenbrüche und Gelenkverletzungen. Enke, Stuttgart

Uhthoff HK (1982) Current concepts of external fixation of fractures. Springer, Berlin Heidelberg New York

Vidal J, Rabischong P, Adrey J, Bonnel F, Jamme M, Allieu Y (1969) Augmentation de l'efficacité de l'osteotaxis d'Hoffmann par l'utilisation de fixateurs couplés in cadre. 44e réunion de la SOFCOF, Paris

Vidal J, Rabischong P, Bonnel F, Adrey J (1970) Etude biomécanique du fixateur externe d'Hoffmann dans les fractures de jambe. Montpellier Chir 16:43

Vidal J, Buscayret C, Connes H, Paran M, Allieu Y (1976) Traitement des fractures ouvertes de jambe par le fixateur externe en double cadre. Rev Chir Orthop 62:433

Vidal J, Buscayret C, Connes H (1979) Treatment of articular fractures by "ligamentotaxis" with external fixation. In: Brooker AF, Edwards CC (eds) The current state of the art, vol 75. Williams & Wilkins, Baltimore

Vidal J, Melka J (1982) The double-frame external fixator. In: Uhthoff HK (eds) Current concepts of external fixation of fractures. Springer, Berlin Heidelberg New York

Wagner H (1972) Technik und Indikation der operativen Verkürzung und Verlängerung von Ober- und Unterschenkel. Orthopädie 1:59

Wagner H (1977) Surgical lengthening or shortening of the femur and tibia. In: Gschwend N et al. (eds) Progress in orthopaedic surgery, vol 1. Springer, Berlin Heidelberg New York, p 7

Watson-Jones R (1955) Fractures and joint injuries. Livingstone, Edinburgh

Weber BG (1961) Wie kommt der kindliche Einwärtsgang zustande, und was hat er zu bedeuten? Helv Paediat Acta 16:82

Weber BG (1961) Inwieweit sind isolierte extreme Torsionsvarianten der unteren Extremitäten als Deformitäten aufzufassen und welche klinische Bedeutung kommt ihnen zu? Z Orthop 94:287

Weber BG (1964) Grundlagen und Möglichkeiten der Zuggurtungsosteosynthese. Chirurg 35:81

Weber BG (1965) Kritisches zur Salter-Osteotomie. In: Chapchal G (Hrsg) Beckenosteotomie, Pfannendachplastik. Thieme, Stuttgart

Weber BG (1965) Die Behandlung der Sprunggelenks-Stauchungsbrüche nach biomechanischen Gesichtspunkten. Hefte Unfallheilkd 81:176

Weber BG (1967) Prophylaxe der Achsenfehlstellungen bei der Behandlung kindlicher Frakturen. In: Müller ME (Hrsg) Posttraumatische Achsenfehlstellungen an den unteren Extremitäten. Huber, Bern, S 95

Weber BG, Čech O (1973) Pseudarthrosen. Huber, Bern Stuttgart Wien

Weber BG (1974) Knöchel-Fußwurzel, Mittelfuß. In: Zenker R, Deucher F, Schink W (eds) Chirurgie der Gegenwart, Bd 4/1. Urban & Schwarzenberg, München Berlin Wien

Weber BG, Cech O (1976) Pseudarthrosis. Huber, Bern Stuttgart Wien

Weber BG (1981) Brüche von Knöchel und Talus. Bewährtes und Neues in Diagnostik und Therapie. Langenbecks Arch Chir 355:421

Weber BG, Brunner C (1981) The treatment of non-unions without electrical stimulation. Clin Orthop 161:24

Wolff J (1892) Das Gesetz der Transformation der Knochen. Hirschwald, Berlin

## The Threaded Rod External Fixator in Children and Adolescents

CH. BRUNNER

Bernbeck R (1947) Die pathologische Femurtorsion. Z Orthop 78:303

Müller ME (1955) Le traitement des subluxations résiduelles de la hanche par l'ostéotomie intertrochantérienne. Acta Orthop Belg 21:401

Müller ME (1966) Zwölf Hüfteingriffe. AO-Bulletin Beilageheft Nr. 1

Müller ME (1971) Die hüftnahen Femurosteotomien. Thieme, Stuttgart

Rippstein J (1955) Zur Bestimmung der Antetorsion des Schenkelhalses mittels zweier Röntgenaufnahmen. Z Orthop 86:345

## The Spinal External Fixation Device

F. MAGERL

Böhler L (1951) Die Technik der Knochenbruchbehandlung, 12th/13th edn, vol 1. Maudrich, Wien

Boucher HH (1959) A method of spinal fusion. J Bone Joint Surg [Br] 41:248

Bradford DS, Akbarnia BA, Winter RB, Seljeskog EL (1977) Surgical stabilization of fracture and fracture dislocations of the thoracic spine. Spine 2:185

Bryant CE, Sullivan JA (1983) Management of thoracic and lumbar spine fractures with Harrington distraction rods supplemented with segmental wiring. Spine 8:532

Convery FR, Minteer MA, Smith RW, Emerson SM (1978) Fracture-dislocation of the dorsal-lumbar spine. Acute operative stabilization by Harrington instrumentation. Spine 3:160

Daniaux H (1982) Technik und erste Ergebnisse der transpedikulären Spongiosaplastik bei Kompressionsbrüchen im Lendenwirbelsäulenbereich. Acta Chir Austr [Suppl] 43:79

Daniaux H (1983) Technik und Ergebnisse der transpedikulären Spongiosaplastik bei Brüchen im thorakolumbalen Übergangs- und Lendenwirbelsäulenbereich. Hefte Unfallheilkd 165:182

Denis F (1982) Updated classification of thoracolumbar fractures. Orthop Trans 6:8

Denis F (1983) The three column spine and its significance in the classification of acute thoracolumbar spinal injuries. Spine: 8:817

Dick W (1984) Innere Fixation von Brust- und Lendenwirbelfrakturen. Hans Huber, Bern Stuttgart Toronto

Dick W, Wörsdörfer O, Magerl F (in press) Mechanical properties of a new device for internal fixation of spine fractures, the fixateur interne. In: Schneider E and Perren SM (ed) Development in biomechanics, Vol II. Martinus Nijhoff, The Hague

Dickson JH, Harrington PR, Erwin WD (1978) Results of reduction and stabilization of the severely fractured thoracic and lumbar spine. J Bone Joint Surg [Am] 60:799

Ferguson RL, Allen BL Jr, Seay GB (1982) The evolution of segmental spinal instrumentation in the treatment of unstable thoracolumbar spine fractures. Orthop Trans 6:346

Flesch JR, Leider LL, Erickson DL, Chou SN, Bradford DS (1977) Harrington instrumentation and spine fusion for unstable fractures and fracture-dislocation of the thoracic and lumbar spine. J Bone Joint Surg [Am] 59:143

Frankel HL, Hancock DO, Hyslop G et al. (1969) The value of postural reduction in the initial management of closed injuries of the spine with paraplegia and tetraplegia, part I. Paraplegia 7:179

Gertzbein SD, MacMichael D, Tile M (1982) Harrington instrumentation as a method of fixation in fractures of the spine. J Bone Joint Surg [Br] 64:526

Gumley G, Taylor TKF, Ryan MD (1982) Distraction fractures of the lumbar spine. J Bone Joint Surg [Br] 64:520

Holdsworth FW (1963) Fractures, dislocations and fracture-dislocations of the spine. J Bone Joint Surg [Br] 45:6

Holdsworth FW (1970) Fractures, dislocations and fracture-dislocations of the spine. J Bone Joint Surg [Am] 52:1534

Jacobs RR, Schläpfer F, Mathys R Jr, Perren SM (1980) A new spinal instrumentation system for dorsal-lumbar spinal fractures. J Biomech 13:801

Kägi F, Magerl F, Jeanneret B (1983) Diagnostische Wirbelsäulenpunktion. Münch Med Wochenschr 125:901

Kaufer H (1975) The thoracolumbar spine. In: Rockwood CA, Green DP (eds) Fractures, vol 2. Lippincott, Philadelphia Toronto, p 861

Kaufer H, Hayes JT (1966) Lumbar fracture dislocation. J Bone Joint Surg [Am] 48:712

King D (1944) Internal fixation for lumbosacral fusion. Am J Surg 66:357

King D (1948) Internal fixation for lumbosacral fusion. J Bone Joint Surg [Am] 30:560

Kostuik JP (1983) Anterior spinal cord decompression for lesions of the thoracic and lumbar spine, techniques, new methods of internal fixation results. Spine 8:512

Lesoin F, Bouasakao N, Cama A, Lozes G, Combelles G, Jomin M (1982) Posttraumatic fixation of the thoraco-lumbar spine using Roy-Camille plates. Surg Neurol 18:167

Lindahl S, Willén J, Nordwall A, Irstam L (1983) The crush-cleavage fracture, a "new" thoracolumbar unstable fracture. Spine 8:559

Louis R (1977) Les théories de l'instabilité. Rev Chir Orthop 63:423

Luque ER (1982) Segmental spinal instrumentation in the treatment of fractures of the spine. Orthop Trans 6:22

Magerl F (1979) Die Behandlung von Wirbelsäulenverletzungen. Kongressbericht 19. Tagung der Oesterreichischen Gesellschaft für Chirurgie und der angeschlossenen Fachgesellschaften 1978 in Kremsmünster, Bd II. Egermann, Wien, S 859

Magerl F (1980) Verletzungen der Brust- und Lendenwirbelsäule. Kongressbericht. Langenbecks Arch Chir 352:427

Magerl F (1982) External skeletal fixation of the lower thoracic and the lumbar spine. In: Uhthoff HK (ed) Current concepts of external fixation of fractures. Springer, Berlin Heidelberg New York, p 353

Magerl F (1983a) External skeletal fixation of the lower thoracic spine. In: Vécsei V (ed) Traumatology of the spinal column. Proceedings of the 1. Viennese Workshop, International College of Surgeons, Austrian Section, part II. Informatica, Vienna, p 275

Magerl F (1983b) Clinical application on the thoracolumbar junction and the lumbar spine. In: Mears DC (ed) Exernal skeletal fixation. Williams & Wilkins, Baltimore London, p 553

Magerl F (1984, to be published) Stabilization of the lower thoracic and lumbar spine with external skeletal fixation. Clin Orthop 189

Magerl F, Schenk R, Müller W (im Druck) Klinische Erfahrungen mit geformten porösen Hydroxylapatitblöcken. Vortrag gehalten am 21. Kongress der Deutschen Gesellschaft für Plastische- und Wiederherstellungschirurgie, 1983, Giessen

McAfee PC, Yuan HA, Frederickson BE, Lubicky JP (1983) The value of computed tomography in thoracolumbar fractures. J Bone Joint Surg [Am] 65:461

Ottolenghi CE (1954) Diagnosis of orthopaedic lesions by aspiration biopsy, results of 1061 punctures. J Bone Joint Surg [Am] 37:443

Ottolenghi CE (1969) Aspiration biopsy of the spine. Technique for the thoracic spine and results of twenty-eight biopsies in this region and over-all results of 1050 biopsies of other spinal segments. J Bone Joint Surg [Am] 51:1531

Roy-Camille R, Saillant G, Berteaux D, Salgado V (1976) Osteosynthesis of thoraco-lumbar spine fractures with metal plates screwed through the vertebral pedicles. Reconstr Surg Traumatol 15:2

Roy-Camille R, Berteaux D, Saillant G, Judet H, Salgado V (1977) Ostéosynthèse des fractures du rachis dorso-lombaire avec plaques vissées dans les pédicules vertébraux. Résultats mécaniques dans 66 observations. Int Orthop 1:121

Roy-Camille R, Saillant G, Marie-Anne S, Mamoudy P (1980) Behandlung von Wirbelfrakturen und -luxationen am thorako-lumbalen Übergang. Orthopäde 9:63

Ruge D (1977) Spinal cord injuries. In: Ruge D, Wiltse LL (eds) Spinal disorders, diagnosis and treatment. Lea & Febiger, Philadelphia

Saillant G (1976) Etude anatomique des pédicules vertébraux, application chirurgicale. Rev Chir Orthop 62:151

Schläpfer F, Magerl F, Jacobs R, Perren SM, Weber BG (1980) In vivo measurements of loads on an external fixation device for human lumbar spine fractures. In: Conference on engineering aspects of the spine., C 131/80. Institution of Mechanical Engineers, London, p 59

Schläpfer F, Wörsdörfer O, Magerl F, Perren SM (1982) Stabilization of the lower thoracic and lumbar spine: Comparative in vitro investigation of an external skeletal and various internal fixation devices. In: Uhthoff HK (ed) Current concepts of external fixation of fractures. Springer, Berlin Heidelberg New York, p 367

Schläpfer F, Magerl F, Perren SM, Nigg B (to be published) Estimation of the in vivo load in the lower spine based on a semidirect approach. Paper presented at the 9th International Congress of Biomechanics, August 1983, Waterloo, Canada

Tarlov IM (1972) Acute spinal cord compression paralysis. J Neurosurg 36:10

Trojan E (1972) Langfristige Ergebnisse von 200 Wirbelbrüchen der Brust-Lendenwirbelsäule ohne Lähmung. Z Unfallmed Berufskr 65:122

Weiss M (1975) Dynamic spine alloplasty (spring-loading corrective devices) after fracture and spinal cord injury. Clin Orthop 112:150

White JR (1975) Pathology of spinal cord injury in experimental lesions. Clin Orthop 112:16

Whitesides TE Jr (1977) Traumatic kyphosis of the thoracolumbar spine. Clin Orthop 128:78

Whitesides TE, Ghazanfar Ali Shah S (1976) On the management of unstable fractures of the thoracolumbar spine. Rationale for use of anterior decompression and fusion and posterior stabilization. Spine 1:99

Wörsdörfer O (1981) Operative Stabilisierung der thorakolumbalen und lumbalen Wirbelsäule: Vergleichende biomechanische Untersuchungen zur Stabilität und Steifigkeit verschiedener dorsaler Fixations-Systeme. Habilitationsschrift, Universität Ulm

Yosipovitch Z, Robin GC, Makin M (1977) Open reduction of unstable thoracolumbar spinal injuries and fixation with Harrington rods. J Bone Joint Surg [Am] 59:1003

# Subject Index

C. F. Brunner, B. G. Weber

# Special Techniques in Internal Fixation

Translated from the German by T. C. Telger

1982. 91 figures. X, 198 pages. ISBN 3-540-11056-9

**Contents:** Lag Screws. – Wire Loop. – Combination of Wire Loop and Screw. – Kirschner Wire. – Combination of Kirschner Wire and Wire Loop. – Anti-glide Plate. – Plating of the Vertebral Column. – Internal Fixation Plates with a Specialized Form or Function. – Medullary Nail. – External Fixator. – Concluding Remarks. – References. – Subject Index.

"The textboook on internal fixation by Brunner and Weber is a very well-organized, copiously illustrated book that demonstrates unusual and occasionally elegant applications to fracture and bone-fixation problems of the internal-fixation devices and techniques devised by the Swiss AO group. It is not a textbook for inexperienced bone surgeons, as many of the techniques it presents are controversial in their application, and clinical series proving their efficacy are not presented. As is typical of most European textbooks in the field, this is a series of very well-illustrated and well-documented anecdotal cases. For the bone surgeon seeking a new way to solve a difficult or unusual problem or seeking a way to solve a common problem in a more elegant manner the text is extremely useful and reflects the extensive experience of the Swiss AO Group.

For the most part this book is aimed at a highly specialized reader: the fracture surgeon experienced in Swiss fracture-fixation techniques. The casual reader in the field of fracture treatment will find it a very entertaining, well-illustrated, and interesting textbook to peruse." *The New England Journal of Medicine*

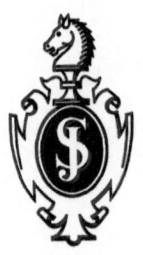

Springer-Verlag
Berlin
Heidelberg
New York
Tokyo

# Treatment of Fractures in Children and Adolescents

Editors: **B. G. Weber, C. Brunner, F. Freuler**

In collaboration with numerous experts

Translated from the German by P. A. Casey

1980. 462 figures, 31 tables. XII, 408 pages. ISBN 3-540-09313-3

**Contents:** Basic Histomorphology and Physiology of Skeletal Growth. – Fracture Healing in the Growing Bone and in the Mature Skeleton. – Treatment of Fractures in Children. – Birth Injur. Thoracic, Abdominal, and Multiple Injuries. The Battered Child. – Fractures of the Clavicle and Scapula. – Fractures of the Proximal Humerus. – Fractures of the Shaft of the Humerus. – Fractures of the Medical Epicondyle. – Supracondylar Fractures of the Humerus. – Fractures of the Elbow. – Shaft Fractures in the Forearm. – Fractures of the Distal Forearm. – Fractures of the Hand. – Fractures and Dislocations of the Vertebral Column. – Fractures of the Pelvis and Acetabulum. – Fractures of the Proximal Femur. – Fractures of the Shaft of the Femur. – Fractures In and Around the Knee Joint. – Fractures of the Proximal Tibial Metaphysis. – Fractures of the Lower Leg. – Malleolar Fractures. – Fractures of the Talus and Calcaneus. – Fractures of the Tarsal Bones, Metatarsals, and Toes. – Amputations in Children. – Summary. – Subject Index.

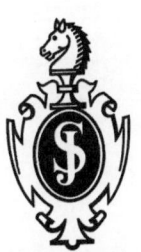

Springer-Verlag
Berlin
Heidelberg
New York
Tokyo

"It is not often that a medical book is published and remains a standard work of reference for a long period of time. Undoubtedly *Treatment of Fractures in Children and Adolescents* falls into this category, as there are very few books that deal with these fractures in such depth and detail ...

As is stated in the preface of this book, treatment of fractures relies on knowledge, logic and ability, and all these concepts run through the pattern of this book. The book itself is large but is not meant to be used as an encyclopaedia of fractures in children but rather as a standard work written by authors who draw on their own personal experience in this very difficult field of orthopaedics. The book, with its excellent bibliography, is intended for orthopaedic surgeons at all levels of training and it should be bought by every medical library."

*Injury*